Handbook of

INSTITUTIONAL PHARMACY PRACTICE

Third Edition

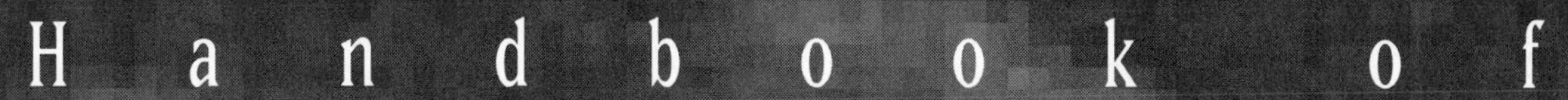

Handbook of

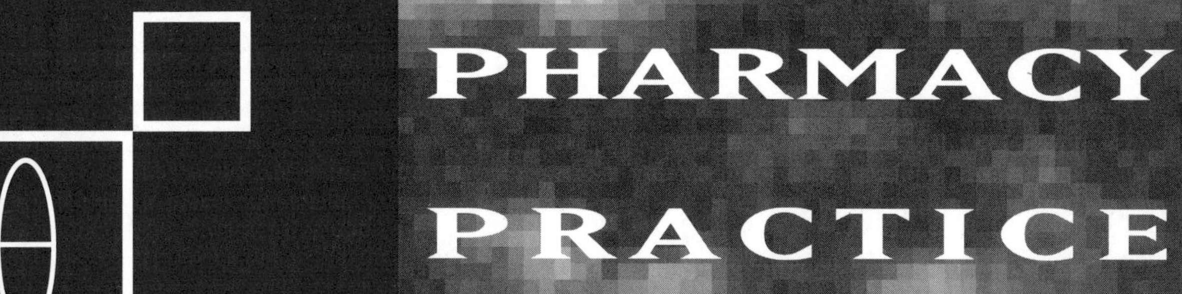

INSTITUTIONAL PHARMACY PRACTICE

Third Edition

Thomas R. Brown,
Editor

M.S., Pharm.D., FASHP
Professor and Chair,
Department of Pharmacy
Administration
School of Pharmacy
University of Mississippi

ASHP

Correspondence should be sent in care of the publisher, American Society of Hospital Pharmacists, 4630 Montgomery Avenue, Bethesda, MD 20814.

The information presented herein reflects the opinions of the authors and reviewers. It should not be interpreted as official policy of ASHP or as an endorsement of any product(s).

Produced by the American Society of Hospital Pharmacists' Special Projects Division.

ISBN: 1-879907-03-8

DEDICATION

To

Mickey and Mary Smith

Foreword

The American Society of Hospital Pharmacists (ASHP) is pleased to publish the third edition of the *Handbook of Institutional Pharmacy Practice*. The book's crowning feature is that there is something in it for everyone—from first-year pharmacy students to seasoned practitioners. Although each chapter can stand alone as a sound overview of a specific practice area or topic, the *Handbook* as a whole serves as a comprehensive guide to institutional practice.

It would be fair to say that the scope of pharmacy practice has changed a great deal since the first edition of the *Handbook* was published in 1979—more than a decade ago. The first edition had a chapter entitled "The Future of Institutional Pharmacy." The future is now. Just as pharmacists and the practice of pharmacy have changed with the times to reflect the evolution of health care, so has the *Handbook*.

The editor of this edition, Dr. Thomas R. Brown, has done a superb job of bringing together experts in their respective areas of pharmacy to write about the subjects they know best. Producing a text that encompasses so many aspects of institutional pharmacy practice is no easy task. The efforts of Dr. Brown and the 60 authors are to be commended.

A chief part of ASHP's mission is to ensure that our members have the products and services they need to provide high-quality pharmaceutical services. The *Handbook*, which is an excellent orientation to the contemporary world of institutional pharmacy practice, is a welcome addition to our array of publications. It is our hope that, in its pages, readers will find ways to foster the efficacy, safety, and cost-effectiveness of drug use in their practice settings for the benefit of our profession and, above all, our patients.

ASHP is proud to be associated with this fundamental tool for practitioners and students who want to know more about practice in organized health care.

Joseph A. Oddis, Sc.D.
Executive Vice President
ASHP

Preface

The third edition of the *Handbook of Institutional Pharmacy Practice* is published by the American Society of Hospital Pharmacists. Dr. Mickey C. Smith and I had hoped more than 10 years ago that this book would be an ASHP product. For a variety of reasons, none of which seem important now, it was not, but at long last the book is being published and marketed by ASHP and I am very pleased.

The focus of the book has changed very little, although it is not as encompassing as the previous editions. The diverse and often complex specialty areas of practice make it unlikely that a single reference can adequately do justice to every topic required in a text of this magnitude; therefore, it is prudent for specialized areas of practice to be presented in more detail in other texts.

This book is intended for both student and practitioner. It is hoped that it will provide practical information for the student with little or no experience in institutional pharmacy and serve as a ready reference for practitioners who seek answers to problems in practice. The intent was to ensure that the practical orientation be adequately conceived through relevant theory such that the reader could explore the subject in as much depth (even beyond the chapter) as he or she wishes.

It would be extraordinarily difficult for one person to author a text of this magnitude. Accordingly, the most acceptable alternative has been to seek the best people available, with due consideration for both their knowledge of subject matter and their writing skills. Advice and counsel from ASHP have been exceedingly helpful in identifying skilled individuals as contributors, and insofar as possible, practitioners have been sought as authors.

The editor is well aware that entire books could be written on subjects for which a single chapter is provided in this text. It is hoped that the authors have provided the reader with:

1. An appreciation for the nature and scope of the subject;
2. Examples, when appropriate, of practical applications; and
3. Sufficient discussion and additional resources to allow for and encourage independent study.

The reader is strongly encouraged to purchase a copy of *Practice Standards of the ASHP* as a companion to this book and his or her practice in pharmacy. It is an invaluable collection of statements, guidelines, technical assistance bulletins, and therapeutic guidelines that "provide a point of reference for pharmacists' use in evaluating institutional programs and services." In the opinion of this editor, every pharmacy practitioner should be required to read these standards.

This book is not intended to be all things to all institutional practitioners. Read it, study it, and by all means go beyond it.

Thomas R. Brown

Acknowledgments

More than 10 years ago, Dr. Mickey Smith and I began work on the first edition of the *Handbook.* We locked ourselves away for a couple of days and began the development of a list of topics which, after several revisions, became the table of contents for the first edition. The topic areas were derived from the *ASHP Guidelines on the Competencies Required in Institutional Pharmacy Practice.* These guidelines provided for us, as editors, clear evidence of the oft-espoused hypothesis that ASHP established, through its membership and leadership, and published the reference standards for hospital pharmacy practice. In our minds as editors, hypothesis became axiom with the first and second editions.

I am grateful to ASHP for its contributions to the publication of this edition. Special appreciation goes to Jim Caro, Susan Dombrowski, Daria Delfino, and Marie Smith. It has been my pleasure to work with these individuals.

This work would not be possible without the collective efforts of a number of talented contributors. Their knowledge and writing skills are important to this work as well as to the profession; they are very much appreciated. To those contributors who met their deadlines, I owe a special debt of gratitude. Should a manual be written on how to edit or write a book of this magnitude, the premier chapter should be titled, "Authoring, Timeliness, and Editing: A Pathologic Dilemma." At the University of Mississippi, special recognition is given to Debbie Prestage, who managed the word processing, mailings, file management, much of the telephoning, and this editor, to the extent possible. Without her skills and patience, I could not have maintained what sanity I have.

Mickey Smith and I have been special friends and colleagues for many years, and a debt of gratitude is owed to him for his example over many years.

Finally, my family has endured my pleasure in working on this book, and I have benefited from their support. Thanks are due my wife, Bonnie, who underwent two surgical procedures during the time this book was being completed; Dennis, whose military time was spent, in part, in a certain desert during this work; and Jeffrey, who provided laughter as my best medicine. I am likewise grateful to my parents, who always wanted to know, as did I, "When will you finish?"

Contributors

Paul W. Abramowitz, Pharm.D.
Director of Pharmaceutical Services, The University of Minnesota Hospital and Clinic, Associate Professor, College of Pharmacy, The University of Minnesota, Minneapolis, Minnesota

David S. Adler, Pharm.D.
Professor and Vice Chairman of Clinical Pharmacy, Division of Clinical Pharmacy, University of California, School of Pharmacy, San Francisco, California

Vance L. Alexander, M.S., J.D.
Associate Director and Associate Professor, The University of Alabama Hospital, Birmingham, Alabama

Elizabeth L. Allan, M.S., R.Ph.
Research Associate, Department of Pharmacy Care Systems, Auburn University, Auburn, Alabama

Stephen J. Allen, M.S.
Director of Pharmacy Services and Central Supply, Children's Hospital National Medical Center, Washington, D.C.

Ann B. Amerson, Pharm.D.
Professor, College of Pharmacy, Director, Drug Information Center, University of Kentucky, Chandler Medical Center, Lexington, Kentucky

Kenneth N. Barker, Ph.D.
Professor of Pharmacy Administration, School of Pharmacy, Auburn University, Auburn, Alabama

Harold J. Black, M.S.
Director of Pharmacy, Assistant Professor of Pharmacy, Special Assistant to The University of Iowa Hospitals and Clinics Director, Pharmacy Department, College of Pharmacy, The University of Iowa, The University of Iowa Hospitals and Clinics, Iowa City, Iowa

Larry E. Boh, M.S.
Associate Professor, University of Wisconsin, Center for Health Sciences, School of Pharmacy, Madison, Wisconsin

Thomas R. Brown, M.S., Pharm.D., FASHP
Professor and Chair, Department of Pharmacy Administration, School of Pharmacy, University of Mississippi, University, Mississippi

Clyde Buchanan, M.S.
Director, Emory University Hospital, Department of Pharmaceutical Services, Atlanta, Georgia

Barry L. Carter, Pharm.D., F.C.C.P.
Associate Professor and Assistant Head for Ambulatory Care, Department of Pharmacy Practice, College of Pharmacy, University of Illinois at Chicago, Chicago, Illinois

Rudolph Choich, Jr., M.Sc., M.B.A.
Director, Department of Pharmacy Services, University Hospitals of Cleveland, Cleveland, Ohio

Wayne F. Conrad, Pharm.D.
Professor of Pharmacy Practice, College of Pharmacy, University of Cincinnati, Cincinnati, Ohio

James W. Cooper, Jr., Pharm. Ph.D., F.C.P., F.A.S.C.P.
Professor and Head, Department of Pharmacy Practice, Director of Pharmacy, College of Pharmacy, University of Georgia, Athens, Georgia

Frederic R. Curtiss, Ph.D, R.Ph.
Certified Employee Benefits Specialist and President, The Reimbursement Update, Lewisville, Texas

Clarence L. Fortner
Scientific and Medical Affairs Executive, Adria Laboratories, Joppa, Maryland

Malcolm T. Foster, Jr., M.D.
Professor and Associate Chairman, Chief, Division of Infectious Diseases, Department of Internal Medicine, University of Florida Health Science Center, Jacksonville, Florida

Christine Gabos, Pharm.D.
Assistant Director of Pharmacy, Suburban General Hospital, Norristown, Pennsylvania

Aileen M. Grimm, Pharm.D.
Drug Information Specialist, Department of Pharmacy, Thomas Jefferson University Hospital, Philadelphia, Pennsylvania

James M. Hethcox
Associate Director of Pharmacy, Rush-Presbyterian-St. Luke's Medical Center, Chicago, Illinois

Robert J. Holt, M.A.
Director, Continuing Education Department, Assistant Professor of Pharmacy Practice, College of Pharmacy, University of Oklahoma, Oklahoma City, Oklahoma

Leigh E. Hopkins, Pharm.D.
Assistant Director, Drug Information and Research, Department of Pharmacy, Thomas Jefferson University Hospital, Philadelphia, Pennsylvania

Joseph D. Jackson, Ph.D.
Director, Health Economics, Worldwide Pharmaceutical Operations, The Du Pont Merck Pharmaceutical Company, Wilmington, Delaware

Philip E. Johnston, Pharm.D.
Assistant Director for Clinical Services, Department of Pharmacy, Vanderbilt University Medical Center, Nashville, Tennessee

Thomas D. Keith, M.S., Pharm.D.
Director, Department of Pharmacy, University Medical Center, Clinical Associate Professor and Assistant Dean for Jacksonville Programs, Jacksonville, Florida

William N. Kelly, Pharm.D.
Assistant Vice President and Director, Pharmacy and Drug Information Service, Hamot Medical Center, Erie, Pennsylvania

Michael L. Kleinberg, M.S., FASHP
Director, Professional Services, IMMUNEX Corporation, Associate Clinical Professor, University of California-San Francisco, Seattle, Washington

James R. Knight, D.Ph., M.S.
Director, Department of Pharmaceutical Services, Vanderbilt University Medical Center, Nashville, Tennessee

Karen E. Koch, Pharm.D.
Assistant Professor of Clinical Pharmacy Practice, University of Mississippi, Assistant Director for Clinical Services, Clinical Pharmacist, North Mississippi Medical Center, Tupelo, Mississippi

Herman L. Lazarus, M.S., R.Ph.
Director of Pharmacy Services, The University of Alabama, Birmingham, Alabama

Donald E. Letendre, Pharm.D.
Director, Accreditations Service Division, American Society of Hospital Pharmacists, Bethesda, Maryland

Alex C. Lin, Ph.D.
Assistant Professor, Division of Pharmacy Practice and Administration, College of Pharmacy, University of Cincinnati Medical Center, Cincinnati, Ohio

Arthur G. Lipman, Pharm.D.
Professor of Clinical Pharmacy, Department of Pharmacy Practice, College of Pharmacy, University of Utah, Salt Lake City, Utah

Dennis W. Mackewicz, Pharm.D.
Senior Associate Director, Pharmacy Services, Memorial Medical Center, Long Beach, California

Lee A. Mork, M.S.
Professional Services Associate, Upsher Smith Laboratories, Inc., Minneapolis, Minnesota

Jeanine Mount, Ph.D., R.Ph.
Assistant Professor, Social and Behavioral Pharmacy, School of Pharmacy, University of Wisconsin, Madison, Wisconsin

John Murray, B.S., R.Ph.
Clinical Pharmacist, Nutrition Support, Duke University Medical Center, Durham, North Carolina

Steven P. Nelson, M.S.
Senior Assistant Director, Inpatient Care, The University of Iowa Hospitals and Clinics, Iowa City, Iowa

Michael R. Norwood, Pharm.D.
Director, Home Infusion Services, St. Joseph Hospital and Medical Center, Tacoma, Washington

Gary M. Oderda, Pharm.D., M.P.H.
Professor and Chairman, Department of Pharmacy Practice, College of Pharmacy, University of Utah, Salt Lake City, Utah

Robert E. Pearson, M.S.
Associate Professor, School of Pharmacy, Auburn University, Auburn, Alabama

Larry Pelham, M.S., R.Ph.
Administrator, Home Health Care Services, St. Joseph Hospital and Medical Center, Tacoma, Washington

Lawrence J. Pesko, M.S.
Associate Director of Pharmacy Services, Assistant Professor of Pharmacy, Medical College of Virginia Hospitals, Virginia Commonwealth University, Richmond, Virginia

Pamela A. Ploetz, B.S.
Associate Professor, Clinical Pharmacy Services, Clinical Associate Professor, University of Wisconsin School of Pharmacy, University of Wisconsin Hospital and Clinics, Madison, Wisconsin

Hazel H. Seaba, M.S.
Drug Information Specialist, Department of Pharmacy Services, Meriter Hospital, Inc., Madison, Wisconsin

Marie A. Smith, Pharm.D.
Director, Special Projects Division, American Society of Hospital Pharmacists, Bethesda, Maryland

Mickey C. Smith, Ph.D.
Frederick A.P. Barnard Distinguished Professor of Pharmacy Administration, School of Pharmacy, University of Mississippi, University, Mississippi

William E. Smith, Pharm.D., M.P.H.
Research Associate, Department of Pharmacy Care Systems, Auburn University, Auburn, Alabama

Harlan C. Stai, R.Ph.
Executive Vice President, Owen Healthcare, Inc., Houston, Texas

Bonnie L. Svarstad, Ph.D.
Professor of Social and Behavioral Pharmacy, School of Pharmacy, University of Wisconsin, Madison, Wisconsin

Albert J. Szkutnik, R.Ph.
Pharmacy Support Services, Walter Reed Army Medical Center, Washington, D.C.

Mark W. Todd, Pharm.D.
Associate Director, Department of Pharmacy, University Medical Center, Clinical Associate Professor, College of Pharmacy, University of Florida, University Medical Center, Jacksonville, Florida

Mary Monk Tutor, M.S.
Graduate Assistant, University of Mississippi, School of Pharmacy, University, Mississippi

Katherine Trexler, B.S., R.Ph.
Clinical Pharmacist, Nutrition Support, Duke University Medical Center, Durham, North Carolina

Allen J. Vaida, Pharm.D.
Assistant Vice President and Director of Pharmacy Services, Suburban General Hospital, Norristown, Pennsylvania

Albert I. Wertheimer, Ph.D.
Dean, School of Pharmacy, Philadelphia College of Pharmacy and Science, Philadelphia, Pennsylvania

Sara J. White, M.S.
Professor and Associate Director of Pharmacy, University of Kansas Medical Center, Kansas City, Kansas

Andrew L. Wilson, Pharm.D.
Department of Pharmacy Services, St. Louis University Hospital, St. Louis, Missouri

Thomas W. Woller, M.S.
Assistant Director, Department of Pharmaceutical Services, The University of Minnesota Hospital and Clinic, Assistant Professor, Department of Pharmacy Practice, University of Minnesota College of Pharmacy, Minneapolis, Minnesota

David C. Wordell
Pharmacy Systems Supervisor, Pharmacy and Drug Information, Hospital of the University of Pennsylvania, Philadelphia, Pennsylvania

William A. Zellmer
Editor, *American Journal of Hospital Pharmacy* and *Clinical Pharmacy*, Vice President of Professional and Government Affairs, American Society of Hospital Pharmacists, Bethesda, Maryland

Reviewers

The editor and ASHP gratefully acknowledge the following individuals who donated their expertise in reviewing the chapters for this book:

Jon T. Albrecht
Robert S. Beardsley
Caryn M. Bing
Beverly L. Black
Jeffrey A. Bourret
Carla J. Brink
David B. Brushwood
Susan A. Cantrell
James P. Caro
Renato Cataldo Jr.
Toby Clark
Charles P. Coe
Susan Cook
Linda M. Cortese
Stephanie Y. Crawford
Fredric R. Curtiss
Michael P. Davis
Neil M. Davis
SR. Mary L. Degenhart
Susan R. Dombrowski
Rena Eatherton
Patricia A. Ensor
Kenneth G. Jozefczyk
Samuel H. Kalman
Jacqueline Z. Kessler
Catherine Nichols Klein
Stan F. Lowe, Jr.
Ray R. Maddox
Jeannell M. Mansur
Alicia S. Miller
Kristen W. Mosdell
Charles E. Myers
L. Michael Posey
Paul J. Ranelli
Bruce E. Scott
Marie A. Smith
Gene L. Stauffer
Marc R. Summerfield
Brian G. Swift
C. Richard Talley
Roberta M. Tankanow
James A. Visconti
Lee A. Wanke
Gordon S. Willcox
William A. Zellmer

Table of Contents

CHAPTER 1

Health Care Institutions and the Health Care System: A Historical Perspective

ALBERT I. WERTHEIMER and FREDERIC R. CURTISS

"If you are not part of the solution, then you must be part of the problem." — **Eldridge Cleaver, *Soul on Ice***[1]

It is essential for the pharmacist as well as any helping professional to understand the environment or universe in which we function. The health care delivery system is the second largest industry in the United States, and it is important for us to know who does what and the means for reaching them. Moreover, by understanding the area of activity and the capabilities and limitations for each of the nearly 400 professions and subprofessional groups identified within that system, we are better able to make informed decisions. The conscientious pharmacist will know where patients may be served and how they may be referred, the differences in costs and prices for various types of care, and the legal, organizational, political, and, most important, economic considerations involved in the delivery of health care services. We owe patients no less than this.

Pharmacists in patient care settings will be called upon to answer questions and provide explanations to patients and to their families and friends. Taking time to explain the details of a particular diagnostic test or to discuss the advantages and safeguards of transferring a patient to a given facility may be more valuable, and surely less harmful, than simply dispensing drugs intended to deal with problems such as anxiety arising from the uncertainty surrounding these events.

The first step to take in becoming a problem solver for patients is to gain a perspective on the U.S. health care delivery system. This perspective then should help us to serve patients seeking referral and information, as well as to be a reliable and trusted source of drugs and related products.

PERSPECTIVE ON THE HEALTH CARE SYSTEM

Health has to do with well-being and the ability to engage in the activities that we want to be able to do. As such, "health" is a personal and emotional matter. Small wonder, then, that the availability, quality, and cost of health care services are important social and political issues. This prominence in the social and political arenas guarantees political debate and legislation intended to improve the quality of the health care system or access to it, or to moderate its cost. In the 1980's and beyond, the focus is on the cost of health care services and ways to moderate these costs. This focus on *costs* contrasts with the greater attention paid to *access* to health care services during the 1950's and 1960's and to the *quality* of health care in the 1970's.

Concern regarding the cost of health care has led to significant legislative changes by Federal and State legislators and regulatory changes by Federal and State agencies. These changes are affecting the financing of health care services. As the method of payment for services and the financial incentives change, significant effects are being seen in the organizational structure of the health care system. Proprietary companies, once insignificant in the health care delivery system, are now becoming increasingly important determinants of the shape of this system. Financial incentives are causing a change in focus away from the acute care hospital as the center of the health care system to alternative care delivery sites, including emergency and surgical care centers and home health care. Although the direction of future changes may be difficult to predict, what is not speculative is that change in the structure of the health care delivery systems will be commonplace throughout the 1990's and probably into the 21st century. The pharmacist will be better prepared to serve patients in this changing environment by understanding the current health care delivery system, including its shortcomings, and how this system evolved.

In our study of the health care delivery system, the first thing that strikes us is that it is not really a "system" at all, but rather a quasisystem of health care delivery that often lacks organization and a rational distribution of services. Gaps and overlaps, undercare and overcare result in many patients not receiving the care they need and others receiving perhaps too much care.[2] Moreover, virtually all care commands high prices. Throughout this and any examination of the health care delivery system, it is particularly helpful to think of the major issues, problems, and solutions in terms of three evaluative parameters: *cost*, *quality*, and *access*.

In our analysis of the health care system, it will become clear that the problems associated with the delivery of health care have not gone unanswered. Indeed, the number of proposed solutions probably exceeds the number of problems. Remember that the generation and choice of solutions are probably directed as much by politics and emotion as by rationality. Appropriate balance often is not achieved among the parameters of access, quality, and cost. Our analysis here will involve a review of the major shortcomings in current "systems" of health care delivery in the hope of obtaining insight to help us in our task of providing efficient, optimal care.

Maldistribution of Personnel

The U.S. health care delivery system probably has sufficient resources to meet all patient needs, but proper distribution of these resources is still problematic. Geographic distribution of manpower, particularly physicians, is a major concern of experts and planners in health care. Some states have a ratio of more than 1,000 persons for each practicing physician, while others have just over 400.[3] Many communities are completely without physician services, while some urban and suburban areas of the country report physician-to-population ratios two and three times that of rural and economically depressed urban areas.[4,5] Furthermore, the percentage of physicians reporting patient care as their major activity has declined to about 85 percent.[6]

Efforts intended to encourage physicians to establish practice in "physician shortage areas" have been attempted by Federal, State, and local governments and by many private institutions.[7] And despite significant spending in these programs, population size continues to influence practice location for many categories of physicians; the best predictors of distribution of physicians are median area income[8] and factors unrelated to the health care needs of the population.[9]

Maldistribution of the total number of practicing physicians also is coupled with an inadequate distribution by type of practice. The "specialty" of general practice has a particularly acute physician shortage. The proportion of physicians in general practice has declined steadily over the years to less than 15 percent in 1981, and this figure includes more than 7,000 physicians in family practice.[6] The specialties, particularly surgery, continue to attract an increasing proportion of physicians, and American specialty boards now number 23. The fastest growing physician specialties over the 10-year period from 1971 to 1981 were radiology, neurology, and gastroenterology.

Adequate distribution of physicians is a concern extending even beyond maldistribution by geography and type of practice. As we have seen, the proportion of physicians engaged in direct patient care has decreased to the point where only four out of five physicians are treating patients directly.[10] Furthermore, specialization has decreased patient access to general practitioners. Access to the health care delivery system for the poor and for minorities is even poorer than it is for whites, with the portal of entry being the hospital emergency room or outpatient department or the community clinic rather than private practitioners.[11] In addition, in 1982 women physicians accounted for less than 10 percent of the total number of physicians, but that figure rose to 15.3 percent in 1986.[12]

Although other providers such as dentists, pharmacists, and nurses may not be quite as maldistributed as physicians, their distribution usually parallels that of physicians, contributing to the problem of difficult access to care for many persons.

Maldistribution of Facilities

Hospitals and other health care institutions may be defined by several characteristics, such as ownership, types of service rendered, size, average length of patient stay, etc. General acute care hospitals have become the center for the delivery of health care services in the United States over the last 50 years. The average length of patient stay in these short-term hospitals is less than 30 days. These are the most numerous of health care facilities, with approximately 4.4 beds per 1,000 population throughout the United States.[13] In contrast to health care systems in other developed countries, the majority of hospitals in the United States are nongovernmental facilities. Acute care hospitals also are classified as to whether they are teaching institutions and, often, according to specialization and intensity of care. For example, some categories of specialty hospitals are those for children, mental diseases, women, cancer, alcohol rehabilitation, and drug rehabilitation. Some hospitals, particularly small rural hospitals, are equipped to handle only primary care patients and refer patients requiring more intensive or sophisticated services to other hospitals that possess intensive care units (ICU's), coronary care units (CCU's), burn units, etc. Hospitals providing sophisticated services, usually teaching hospitals, often are referred to as "tertiary care facilities" and are equipped to handle the most severely ill patients and those with rare diseases or other special needs.

Hospitals with the average length of stay of 30 days or more are referred to as "long-term hospitals." Examples include hospitals focusing their care on mental illness, tuberculosis, rehabilitation, and some cancers. Long-term care services of a less acute nature are also provided by long-term care (LTC) facilities, generally referred to as "nursing homes." Although there was an average of 4.4 short-term hospital beds per 1,000 population throughout the United States in 1982, there was not an even distribution of hospitals and other health care facilities according to geographic area and urban versus rural setting.[14] Because of this maldistribution of health care facilities and services, care is not accessible to many population groups. National studies of medical care utilization indicate that persons who need health care are not necessarily those most likely to receive it.[15] In particular, nonwhites, rural farm people, the poor, the uninsured, and those who do not have a regular source of care have been found to have less access than they "should," based on medical evaluation of severity of reported symptoms.

Various health plans have advocated a 30-minute travel time to general hospitals as a criterion of accessibility. According to this standard, 10 percent of the entire population (extrapolated from one State under study) and nearly 20 percent of rural residents live in areas of inaccessibility to health care services.[16]

Accessibility to care is a function of more than the availability of services, however. Utilization of services is also affected by economic and cultural barriers. Perceived symptoms and ability to pay are the major predictors of utilization of health services, and cultural barriers (e.g., cultural differences, expectations, and differential ordering of values) still exist when economics is no longer a barrier.[17] Furthermore, organizational barriers to entry, such as long queues to obtain services and long travel time to care in some areas, still exist.[18] These organizational barriers contribute to problems of differential access, and perpetuation of two levels of health care in this country, i.e., a level of care for the poor and a separate level of care for the nonpoor.[19-21] Furthermore, while distribution statistics directly address the issues of patient access and efficiency in the delivery of services, variations in individual community requirements for health care are disregarded. Patterns of utilization of services (demand), as well as local health care needs, also should be considered. The supply of care, in terms of both health manpower and health facilities, is of principal interest as it relates availability of care to the needs of the local population.

REGIONALIZATION

The concept of regionalization of health care providers represents one approach to combating the maldistribution of personnel and facilities. The concept is based on tiered levels of care and adequate referral relationships. Primary ambulatory care is provided in small towns and rural areas. Secondary level care is provided by community hospitals in larger towns, such as the county seat. These community hospitals are linked to medical centers that provide tertiary care. Very specialized procedures may be performed by experts located in university teaching facilities. This tiered system of regionalized care requires local responsibility for medical care for specific population groups and formal and informal referral mechanisms to allow access to the proper level of care for all persons.

ORGANIZATIONAL CHANGES IN DELIVERY OF CARE

The social goal of making necessary and proper health care readily available to everybody has spawned major changes in the organization of health care services in the United States. Not many years ago, medical care was delivered from black bags toted by "family docs" who traveled from house to house, generally treating patients in their homes. Most of these practitioners worked alone, out of their own houses or possibly out of small, rented offices. Indeed, all of health care was organized as a "cottage industry," each individual practitioner working independently of other practitioners and facilities.

Today, physician solo practices are much less common. Solo physicians are more likely to practice in urban locations and in counties where per capita incomes are relatively high.[22] Solo physicians are more highly concentrated in the older portions of the United States, such as New England and the mid-Atlantic areas, whereas the number of physicians in organized group practice is significantly greater in the Pacific Coast States. The Council on Medical Services of the American Medical Association (AMA) defines medical group practice as the delivery of medical services "by three or more physicians formally organized to provide medical care, consultation, diagnosis and/or treatment through the joint use of equipment and personnel, and with income from medical practice distributed in accordance with methods previously determined by members of the group."

Group practice has become increasingly popular as an organizational form and may be defined by the following three categories: single-specialty groups, composed of physicians who restrict their practice to one specialty; general practice groups, composed of general practitioners only (or family medicine practitioners); and multispecialty groups, consisting of physicians in at least two major specialties. General practice groups possess characteristics that overlap with the other two groups, composed only of general practitioners (or family medicine practitioners), and multispecialty groups, consisting of physicians in at least two major specialties. General practice groups possess characteristics that overlap with the other two groups, resembling single-specialty groups in the provision of more diversified medical care services.

Pharmacy, like medicine, shows less resemblance to a cottage industry today. More and more health care is being delivered through institutions. Hospitals and chain pharmacies* have recorded steady, substantial increases in prescription dispensing. In the early 1900's, independent community pharmacies dispensed virtually all prescriptions filled in this country. Today, hospitals dispense prescriptions to outpatients as well as deliver drugs and intravenous solutions to inpatients, and chain pharmacies now dispense 27 percent of all retail prescriptions in the United States.[23] Many medical clinics also have incorporated pharmacy services in their delivery of care. This trend toward institutional pharmacy practice is in sharp contrast to the one-man drugstores and apothecaries that were so characteristic at the turn of the century. Small pharmacies continue to be replaced by large pharmacies having several millions of dollars of sales each year. In 1990, outpatient prescriptions came from the following sources: chain pharmacies, 39 percent; independent pharmacies, 45 percent; grocery and supermarket pharmacies, 10 percent; mail order pharmacies, 4 percent; and physician dispensers, 2 percent.[24]

In general, the changes in the organization of health care services might be described as centralization and institutionalization. A related, but perhaps parallel, shift in the organizational structure has been coined "corporatization," referring to corporate-oriented health care delivery.[25] Many of these corporate-oriented delivery systems involve proprietary providers such as investor-owned chains of hospitals, nursing homes, home health agencies, medical equipment suppliers, and dialysis centers that sell patient services for a profit. For example, for-profit companies owned 1,118 hospitals with 131,109 beds in 1983 and managed another 282 hospitals with 35,499 beds, and in 1986 the number of proprietary hospitals rose to 834 with 106,716 beds.[26]

---

* A chain pharmacy is defined by the National Association of Chain Drugstores (NACDS) as common ownership of four or more retail pharmacies.

Hospitals also are investigating shared services and other forms of horizontal integration, such as multihospital systems, in order to optimize management efficiencies and increase access to capital.

ALTERNATE DELIVERY MODES

At the same time that corporatization is taking place in the delivery of health care services in the United States, there is a seemingly dichotomous trend developing in which the hospital is no longer the principal and central source of care. "Alternate care" services are now being touted as substitutes for more expensive hospital care. Although some of these alternate care modes involve centralized delivery structures, such as health maintenance organizations (HMO's), restructured hospital outpatient departments (OPD's), neighborhood health centers, and prepaid group practices (PGP's), often these alternate care services are provided in freestanding centers. Particularly popular in the 1980's were the freestanding primary care clinics, freestanding emergency care units (referred to as "emergicenters"), ambulatory "surgicenters," birthing centers, retail dentistry outlets, and freestanding urgent care units (referred to as "urgicenters").[27] These alternate care services tend to be more consumer oriented in that patients can stop in without appointments and receive care after only a short time. Most alternate care facilities feature longer hours than physicians' offices, typically ranging from 16 to 24 hours a day.

The number of alternate care service sites is expected to increase greatly, particularly since the predicted surplus of physicians in the United States has materialized during the late 1990's. The growth of alternate care facilities increases access to primary health care services for much of the population. However, many alternate care centers will handle only certain patient cases, often based on an ability to pay, and these centers may not be integral parts of referral networks that provide continuity of care.

The HMO is an alternate care organizational structure that has become an important part of the U.S. health care delivery system. HMO's provide comprehensive health care services in exchange for a fixed monthly premium amount, negotiated and paid in advance. The number of HMO's in the United States grew from 72 in 1973 to an estimated 614 in 1983, serving 32.6 million people nationwide, approximately 14 percent of the entire population.[28] Accelerated growth for HMO's is expected as the capitation payment method becomes increasingly popular among insurance companies, employers, and Federal and State governments. However, HMO's have shown disappointingly slow growth in low-income communities and, because of the large amount of capital required, may not be feasible for serving nonurban populations.[29] Also, despite evidence that properly structured ambulatory care service can reduce higher-cost hospitalization,[30] HMO's and PGP's have been criticized for achieving savings by making it more difficult for patients to obtain appointments and requiring long waiting times for care.[31] What *is* clear is that HMO's have significantly lower hospitalization rates than traditional health insurance programs.[32]

The competitive struggle for patients has spawned another alternate care delivery structure, referred to as a preferred provider organization (PPO). PPO's generally offer comprehensive health care services to insurance companies, employers, and other payers at a discounted rate in exchange for being designated as the "preferred provider" for the given population of patients.[33] Many of the PPO's have been formed by hospitals in an effort to compete with HMO's and other hospitals.[34]

Home health care is expected to show perhaps the most dramatic growth in the next 10 years. Home care can be a less expensive substitute for institutional care, and many fairly acute and intensive services are now being provided in the home environment.[35] Also, many patients have been shown to prefer the comfort and familiarity of the home as the site of care.[36] Yet the growth of home health care services will depend on both the generation of evidence that these are indeed substitutes for institutional care rather than additions to it and the development of payment mechanisms that recognize home care products and services as covered benefits.

MANAGED CARE

Perhaps the most significant event of the late 1980's was the advent of a concept generally referred to as "managed care," which aptly describes the concept. HMO's, in their continuing efforts to contain costs, had already effected great savings through the use of outpatient surgery and other procedures by obtaining favorable contract prices with selected hospitals and PPO's. Now, the latest endeavor is to determine the extent of care to be provided to each patient and to manage the care. Needless to say, physicians have not greeted this concept with enthusiasm; however, acceptance by physicians is growing.

For example, when a physician or surgeon wants to hospitalize a patient to conduct a specific diagnostic study, he or she will have to obtain prior authorization from a case manager at the HMO offices. Authorization is usually obtained from a nurse, although physicians are also used. The patient's doctor describes the rationale for the proposed hospital admission and diagnostic work. The case manager may seek to determine if preliminary tests have been conducted, and then may approve or deny the request. If it is refused, an alternative is proposed. If the request is approved, it may be for a specified hospital or clinic, and the approval may be for a maximum length of stay or have limits on what may be done without further approval. Case management may determine what specialist or PPO the patient will be referred to, much of this based upon a goal of containing costs without reducing the quality of care and services.

This involvement by persons on the administrative and business side in the medical care decision-making process is the latest step in a growing trend that has continued since the coverage for second opinions was added to health insurance policies in the 1970's.

THE PRICE OF HEALTH CARE

Health care spending has become one of the major social and political issues of the 1980's. An estimated $458 billion was spent for health care in the United States in 1986, or approximately $1,837 per person. This amount was equal to 11.5 percent of the total output of all goods and services and grew 12.5 percent over the previous year, during a time when the economy as a whole was in recession. As a country, we spend more of our gross national product on health care services than any other country in the world, and in just 20 years we have doubled the percentage of the gross national product that is spent on health care.[37] Part of this tremendous spending of course is due to greater access to care, resulting in higher utilization of services. However, a larger part of this increase in health care spending is due to higher prices and inflationary increases in those prices. Politicians are increasingly inclined to claim that too much is being spent on government-financed health programs. Economists and others suggest that we would be just as healthy a population if we spent half of what we do today on health care services and addressed ourselves more to those factors that have a significant effect on health status: smoking, drinking, overeating, stress, and insufficient exercise.

Medicare and Medicaid and Health Insurance

Economists attribute much of health care spending and the spiraling costs to the Medicare and Medicaid entitlement programs and to private health insurance. Because health care services are financed through these programs, the users (patients) are effectively insulated from the price of these services. Most of the reforms being proposed today for the financing of health care services include features that reintroduce the factor of price to the patient at the point at which health care services are purchased.

The greatest impact on the U.S. health care system in the last two decades has perhaps been the enactment of Medicare and Medicaid legislation. When Medicaid was initiated on July 30, 1965, under Public Law (P.L.) 89-97, the predominant view was that an infusion of money into the system would correct many of its deficiencies.[38] Now it seems difficult to understand how Congress could have been persuaded to appropriate funds for health care without attention to the organization of services. Medicare and Medicaid enactment fueled rising health care expenditures by paying hospitals their actual costs. This caused hospitals to be largely unconcerned about their operating costs. Reimbursing physicians at prices set by physicians also contributed to spiraling health care prices and spending. With Medicaid patients being totally insulated from the price of health care services and Medicare patients having only a small degree of price sensitivity, and with no effective means to control utilization, health care spending in these government programs grew from less than $2 billion in 1966[39] to over $80 billion in 1984.[40]

Proposals for reform of Medicare and Medicaid include restrictions on eligibility, greater cost sharing by Medicare beneficiaries and Medicaid recipients, and new reimbursement systems with altered financial incentives for hospitals, physicians, and other providers. These reforms directly affect the delivery of health care services to approximately 20 percent of the U.S. population, i.e., the elderly, the disabled, and those with severe kidney disease, through the Medicare program and the poor through the Medicaid program. However, changes in Medicare and Medicaid reimbursement methods also tend to have a major influence on the structure and delivery of health care services to the entire population. After 15 years of relatively little change in government reimbursement methods and with the government share of total health care spending increasing from 20 percent to more than 40 percent, the first major reform occurred with Public Law 97-35, the Omnibus Budget Reconciliation Act of 1981. This legislation significantly affected Medicaid programs in several ways, primarily by allowing State Medicaid agencies greater flexibility in setting eligibility criteria for recipients, requiring copayments of patients at the time when they use services, and establishing limits and fixed rates of payments to hospitals and physicians.[41] Even more dramatic changes were prescribed by Congress the following year when a prospective pricing system was adopted for Medicare payments to hospitals.[42] The new payment method established fixed prices for specific patient cases, categorized according to the admission diagnosis of the patient in 1 of 470 diagnosis-related groups (DRG's).

As revolutionary as these changes were, they still were not perceived as sufficient to bring government spending for health care services under control. As the solvency of the Medicare Hospital Insurance Trust Fund was called into question in the early 1980's, a 13-member Advisory Council on Social Security was commissioned. Its recommendations included new sources of revenue, such as increased taxes on alcohol and tobacco, and new limits on eligibility and coverage, as well as ways to reduce the use of health care services and payments to health care providers.[43] A parallel but separate report on the Medicaid program was released by the Center for the Study of Social Policy in early 1984. The study recommended the use of prepaid capitated financing by the Federal Government and called for reform of long-term care for the elderly and mentally retarded,[44] which accounted for approximately 50 percent of the entire Medicaid budget in most states.

Private health insurance, including Blue Cross and Blue Shield and commercial companies such as Aetna, Metropolitan, and Prudential, account for approximately 30 percent of health care financing. The role of private health insurance in financing of services grew most dramatically after World War II, when the U.S. Supreme Court ruled that fringe benefits, including health insurance, were a legitimate part of the bargaining process in labor contract negotiations with management. Since that time the number of persons insured has increased greatly, and health insurance coverages have broadened significantly. In a chicken versus egg manner, health insurance became necessary to protect people from personal bankruptcy resulting from the use of costly medical care services, and simultaneously fueled inflationary increases in health care spending by insulating users for these services from their cost.

Blue Cross and Blue Shield plans are tax-exempt organizations, tied by membership to the national Blue Cross/Blue Shield Association (BCA), but otherwise are independent corporations. The "Blues" and the commercial insurers historically have had less influence than Medicare and Medicaid on the structure of the U.S. health care delivery system. However, these companies are making increased efforts to control health care prices and spending, as they have watched their payments to providers balloon and subsequently have had to increase their premiums to employers and individual subscribers.

Prepaid capitated financing of health care in the United States would help control health care prices and the use of services, as well as promote further centralization and institutionalization in the structure of the health care delivery system. If prepaid capitation financing does not bring health care spending under control, the obvious alternative is a nationalized health care system in which the government is the provider as well as the payer for health care services to the entire population.

QUALITY OF CARE

There is more than price at issue, and the impact of Medicare and Medicaid legislation has been felt in more than economic terms. Federal legislation has influenced the quality of health services provided to beneficiaries, and to the entire U.S. population, by tying Medicare payments to accreditation standards for facilities, licensure, and other certification requirements for personnel and by mandating the establishment of watchdogs, such as pharmacy and therapeutics (P&T) committees in hospitals and utilization review mechanisms for hospitals and ambulatory care facilities. The utilization of services, quality of program administration, and relationships between providers of health services and fiscal intermediaries all have come under scrutiny as government has increased its role in health care delivery.[45]

Superior quality of health care services in the United States often is cited as the reason for the high cost of these services. Certainly, there is some direct and proportional relationship between quality and cost. Yet we still are unable to measure quality precisely and therefore also are unable to determine the "price" of quality. Quality assurance (QA) has become commonplace in hospitals, and QA programs are mandated by the conditions of participation for the Medicare program. Most QA programs attempt to define standards and measure performance according to the parameters of structure, process, and outcome of hospital services. Proposed changes in the Medicare conditions of participation would give hospitals greater flexibility in designing these QA programs and monitoring the quality of hospital services.[46] These newer Medicare conditions signal clearly that the issue of quality of health care services will take a back seat to concerns regarding the costs of these services during the 1990's.

The quality of health care services in the United States is protected by more than accreditation of health care facilities, educational institutions and teaching programs, and the licensure of personnel. Peer review also is performed in an attempt to protect quality. Peer review is both formal and informal and may be retrospective, current, or prospective in nature. Retrospective peer review involves examination of patient chart information in a case-by-case medical audit or employs a computerized review of this information, sometimes referred to as patient care monitor (PCM).[47] Hospital charts usually are the basis for evaluation, but physician office records also may be used in the retrospective peer review process.[48]

Concurrent review is becoming a more common means of health care evaluation, and may be more effective because it involves evaluation of care as it is rendered. Major aspects of concurrent review are hospital admission certification, continued stay review, and discharge planning. Admission certification is concerned with appropriateness of institutionalization. Continued stay review monitors the length of stay of patients according to their diagnosis, severity of illness, and major complications. Discharge planning involves weighing alternative courses of action regarding discharge, such as extended care versus hospitalization, home care versus extended care, and the need for specific health care services after discharge. Prospective review involves the establishment of standards of care and the design and implementation of provider education programs to meet these standards.

Efforts to protect the quality of health care services also include some indirect methods, such as voluntary and compulsory continuing education for practitioners and relicensure of personnel via reexamination. These methods will probably become more important in the future, particularly as health care technology and the amount of health care information continue to grow. Continuing education and reexamination for licensure are only indirect methods of quality protection, however, since they tell us what the practitioner has learned or should be doing, not what is actually being done or the consequent health care outcome.

Utilization review (UR) is a more direct, but not necessarily more effective, means of protecting the quality of health care services. UR first was formalized in 1972 with the establishment of professional standard review organizations (PSRO's) by the 1972 Amendment to the Social Security Act (P.L. 92-603). The purpose of the PSRO program was to ensure that health care services and items for which payment was made by the government through Medicare, Medicaid, and other programs are medically necessary, conform to certain professional standards, and are delivered effectively and efficiently. Overall, PSRO's had only limited success in achieving these goals, largely as a result of the obstacles that plague all UR activities, i.e., the use of incomplete and inaccurate medical record information as the basis for monitoring and evaluating health care services and outcomes, and a reluctance on the part of organized medicine to control those practitioners who deviate from ethical and professional norms.[49] PSRO's were replaced by peer review organizations (PRO's) in 1984 in an attempt to improve control of hospital utilization under the Medicare Prospective Payment System by examining the medical necessity and appropriateness of hospital admissions and hospital services to Medicare patients.[50] We will be better able to measure the performance of PRO's as opposed to other quality protection efforts because PRO's will focus primarily on the costs associated with medically unnecessary or inappropriate services.

LONG-TERM SERVICES

Long-term care is the fastest-growing segment of the U.S. health care industry. In terms of revenues and spending, nursing homes dominate the long-term care sector.[51] The other institutional components of long-term care include chronic disease hospitals, domiciliary care facilities, and retirement homes, sometimes referred to as "lifecare" centers. Many personal and supportive care services are also provided in the home and in noninstitutional environments to the elderly, chronically infirm, and mentally retarded; therefore, counting the long-term care population is difficult. Moreover, many long-term care services, particularly supportive and personal care, are delivered by friends and relatives.

Nursing homes are so designated on the basis of scope and organization of services and the level of care required by the patient. Chronic disease facilities include institutions for mental retardation, tuberculosis, and the mentally ill, among others. Domiciliary care institutions essentially are living accommodations without health-related services. Personal care institutions, which provide services related to activities of daily living, such as dressing, eating, walking, etc., and sheltered care institutions, which provide a protective environment and occasional personal service, complete this category of health care-related institutions.

Long-term care institutions, particularly nursing homes, have been found to suffer from major deficiencies such as unsatisfactory compliance with various codes and regulations and inappropriate patient placements.[52,53] Nursing homes seem chronically prone to fail to meet Federal requirements for Medicaid and Medicare programs.[54] Required medical and nursing attention was not being rendered to patients in these facilities, and noncompliance with prevailing safety codes was widespread. A comprehensive report by the U.S. General Accounting Office (GAO) in 1983 highlighted several problems and challenges for the nursing home industry: (1) the availability of nursing home services varies widely from State to State; (2) some elderly persons are unable to gain access to nursing homes; (3) unavailability of nursing home beds may be due in part to unnecessary use of nursing homes by some persons; (4) the new Medicare Prospective Payment System for hospital reimbursement may unintentionally increase the demand for nursing home beds and thereby further reduce the availability of nursing home services to some persons; and (5) efforts by States to keep their Medicaid costs down by limiting reimbursement, the supply of beds, or both, are expected to continue to restrict the availability of beds for the elderly at a time when the demand for these beds is growing significantly.[55]

Remedial efforts in the provision of long-term care services are hampered by inadequate participation by consumers, community advisory groups, and even physicians. Physician services are in short supply in long-term care because such care is a neglected aspect of the medical student's socialization process; when combined with the very nature of long-term care (i.e., little hope for real improvement in patients' health status), this often results in provider apathy and apparent indifference. Some claim that too few physicians are involved in nursing home care in the community, and of those involved, even fewer devote much attention to such patients on a regular basis.[56]

Major reform in long-term care services appears unavoidable. The increasing proportion of elderly persons in the population will come into direct conflict with further legislative efforts to cut spending at the Federal and State levels. One alternative in the financing of long-term care may involve a greater role for the private health insurance industry.[57]

PATIENT MANAGEMENT

Patient misplacement is a major problem in health care delivery, with many thousands of patients placed in facilities inappropriate to their needs.[58] Misplacement contributes to great inefficiencies in economic terms, as well as to inappropriate personal care of the patient. The factors contributing to misplacement of patients are many, including the lack of suitable alternatives to institutionalization, reimbursement based on factors other than patient needs, and the insensitivity of utilization review to detect much care that is inappropriate or unnecessary.

In order to place patients where they could receive all of the services they need, the concept of progressive patient care was developed and promoted by the U.S. Public Health Service in the early 1960's. Six levels of care were delineated, and judgments could be made to transfer patients so that a person would not occupy a bed associated with unnecessary services and concomitant costs. The six levels are:

1. *Intensive care*. For critically and seriously ill patients. All necessary lifesaving emergency equipment, drugs, and supplies are immediately available.
2. *Intermediate care*. For patients requiring a moderate amount of nursing care. Emergency care and frequent observation rarely are needed.
3. *Self-care*. For ambulatory and physically self-sufficient patients requiring tests or convalescence.
4. *Long-term care*. For patients requiring skilled, prolonged medical and nursing care.
5. *Home care*. For patients who can be cared for adequately in the home with the addition of specific services delivered to them by visiting nurses or others.
6. *Outpatient care*. For ambulatory patients requiring specific diagnostic or treatment services on a scheduled basis, primarily through clinics.

A general preference for analyzing structure and process components of health care rather than health outcomes inhibits improvements in the patient misplacement problem.

COORDINATION OF SERVICES AND CONTINUITY OF CARE

Specialization of medical practice and the independence of providers at various levels in delivery of health care services contribute to a lack of continuity of care; better coordination of care is needed and may be achieved through more comprehensive and sophisticated information systems and more communication among practitioners. The practice of medicine and the delivery of health care services demand oral and written communications among other providers as well as patients. However, the quality and quantity of communication are concerns voiced by experts, planners, and providers. Interprofessional communication often is strained, causing inadequate coordination of services and threatening the quality of care.[59-62]

Referral networks are illustrative of interpersonal relationships among providers, both intraprofessionally and interprofessionally. The failure of physicians to use the referral process adequately and to effectively use the information available to primary care physicians leads to inefficiencies in the provision of health care services.[63,64] The referral process also may be viewed as a means for the medical profession to exert control over the health care delivery system and its own members.[65]

Provider-patient interaction also is plagued by an inadequate exchange of information. Social distance and status differentials impair physician-patient communication,[66,67] and pharmacist-patient communication is compromised because of physical barriers such as the prescription counter and a time commitment to the technical tasks involved in dispensing prescriptions. Furthermore, evidence suggests that even when support personnel are used in pharmacies, presumably to free pharmacist time for greater patient interaction, patient contact actually may decrease rather than increase.[68]

EXPANSION OF PROVIDER ROLES

Physicians are the captains in the health care delivery system. Physicians admit and discharge patients from hospitals, write prescriptions for drugs and diagnostic tests, refer patients to other providers, etc. These functions are restricted to physicians through State medical practice act and physician licensure requirements. However, many nonphysician providers are assuming expanded roles in specialty areas as a means to increase productivity in the health care system. Productivity can be increased through the use of paramedical or support personnel.[69-72] Most studies have shown that nonphysician practitioners in these expanded roles deliver primary care of quality comparable to that delivered by physicians.[73-77] Yet despite this evidence and the need for greater productivity, several factors augur limited expansion of nonphysician roles. Patient acceptance of support personnel in surrogate physician roles is an important factor.[78-80] Physician resistance to expanded roles for nonphysician providers is a significant limiting factor.[81]

Greater interprofessional cooperation and a more appropriate division of labor in health care would lead to a more efficient delivery system. However, State legislation will be necessary to bring about change in statute and regulation to permit overlap in responsibility and authority in patient care among health professionals.

Consumer Participation

Delivery of health care services in the United States involves more than a simple provider-patient relationship. Many third parties are important in the delivery of care. As we have seen, government is playing a greater role in all aspects of health care; employers are having greater influence in the delivery of health care services through business coalitions.[82] Consumer participation in planning and management of health care programs was mandated by Federal legislation in 1972 (P.L. 92-603) and in 1974 (P.L. 93-641) and has continued to be included in all subsequent health care legislation.[83]

At the same time, several forces have been at work to limit greater consumer participation in planning and regulation of the health care industry. The role of the consumer sometimes is unclear in Federal legislation. Health practitioners may be reluctant to consider their work in terms of a service industry responsive to consumer input,[84] and providers dominate the accreditation process, licensure boards, and total health care management.[85]

MALPRACTICE

Medical malpractice suits by patients precipitated a near crisis in the middle 1970's.[86] Malpractice insurance premiums had increased to the point where some U.S. physicians were paying as much for malpractice insurance as the physicians in other countries earned in an entire year.[87] Nearly every State responded by approving legislation oriented toward arbitration and other quasilegal approaches to resolving medical disputes, setting limits on malpractice awards, or establishing malpractice insurance pools.[88] Nevertheless, medical malpractice problems persist, and medical malpractice insurance rates increased an average of 20-30 percent in 1983.[89] For example, a neurosurgeon in Long Island, New York, may pay $66,500 a year in premiums or as much as $199,400 with a poor loss experience record. Some physicians have gone "bare," dropping medical malpractice insurance altogether, as a result of these high insurance premiums.

The sources of the malpractice problem, apparently unique to the U.S. health care system, are unclear. The U.S. health care system may be partly responsible because of its commercial nature, creating a demanding patient who is inclined to rush off to the courts if things go wrong; an impersonal provider-patient relationship in the delivery of health care also has been cited.[90] Medical incompetence appears to be a factor in many of the malpractice cases.[91] The growth of medical malpractice law as a specialty predicts further increases in the number of malpractice suits and concomitant expense in the health care delivery system.[92]

SUMMARY

The U.S. health care delivery system is a complex mix of facilities and practitioners, financed via myriad increasingly centralized payment mechanisms. Increasing centralization and institutionalization may bring providers together but not necessarily result in better coordination of care and patient management. The delivery of health care in the United States will continue to be the subject of much sociopolitical debate until health care spending is contained. Inevitably, society will be faced with making increasingly difficult decisions regarding the structure and financing of the health care delivery system. "Access" may have to be more restricted and perhaps "quality" compromised in some manner in order to contain "cost."

REFERENCES

1. Cleaver E: *Soul on Ice*, New York, Laurel/Dell, 1992.
2. McLaughlin CP, Sheldon A: *The Future and Medical Care*. Cambridge, MA, Ballinger, 1974.
3. U.S. Department of Health, Education, and Welfare: Press release. January 8, 1976.
4. Fahs I, Peterson O: Towns without physicians and towns with only one: A study of four states in the Upper Midwest. *Am J Public Health* 58:1200, 1968.
5. Elesh D, Shollaert PT: Race and urban medicine: Factors affecting the distribution of physicians in Chicago. *J Health Soc Behav* 13:236-250, 1972.
6. Bidese CM, Danais DG: *Physician Characteristics and Distribution in the U.S.* Chicago, American Medical Association, 1982.
7. Eisenberg BS, Cantwell JR: Policies to influence the spatial distribution of physicians: A conceptual review of selected programs and empirical evidence. *Med Care* 14:455-468, 1976.
8. Guzick DS, Jahiel RI: Distribution of private practice offices of physicians with specified characteristics among urban neighborhoods. *Med Care* 14:469-488, 1976.
9. Fuchs VR, Kramer MJ: *Determinants of Expenditures for Physicians' Services in the United States, 1948-1968*. National Bureau of Economic Research, Paper No. 17, DHEW Publication No. (HSM) 733013. Washington, DC, U.S. Government Printing Office, December 1972.
10. Anon: *Health—United States 1988*. DHHS Publication No. (PHS) 831232. Hyattsville, MD, U.S. Department of Health and Human Services, December 1988.

11. Ginzberg E: A new physician supply policy is needed. *JAMA* 250:2621-2622, 1983.
12. Anon: *Physician Characteristics and Distribution in the U.S., 1988*. Chicago, American Medical Association, 1989.
13. Roemer MI: *An Introduction to the U.S. Health Care System*. New York, Springer, 1982.
14. U.S. National Center for Health Statistics: *Vital and Health Statistics*. Series 10, Nos. 9( ), 64(1968), 74( ), 75(1969), 87(1971); Series 3, No. 7( ); Series 11, No. 125( ).
15. Taylor DG, Aday LA, Anderson R: A social indicator of access to medical care. *J Health Soc Behav* 16:39-49, 1975.
16. Bosanac EM, Parkinson RC, Hall DS: Geographical access to hospital care: A 30-minute travel time standard. *Med Care* 14:616-624, 1976.
17. Berkanovic E, Reeder LG: Can money buy the appropriate use of services? Some notes on the meaning of utilization data. *J Health Soc Behav* 15:93-99, 1974.
18. Aday LA: Economic and noneconomic barriers to the use of needed medical services. *Med Care* 13:447-456, 1975.
19. U.S. National Center for Health Statistics: *Health Characteristics of Low Income Persons*. Public Health Service Publication No. 73-500, Series 10, No. 74, 1972.
20. Leo PA, Rosen G: A bookshelf on poverty and health. *Am J Public Health* 59:591, 1969.
21. Smith DB, Kaluzny AD: Inequality in health care programs: A note on some structural factors affecting health care behavior. *Med Care* 12:860-870, 1974.
22. Lorant JH: *Characteristics of Group and Solo Physicians, Practices, and Populations Served. Profile of Medical Practice*. Chicago, Center for Health Services, Research and Development, American Medical Association, 1974.
23. Anon: American Druggist annual pharmacy survey. *Am Druggist* 187(5):12, 16, 1983.
24. Smith MI: Pharmaceutical Data Services, Inc. Personal communication, January 19, 1990.
25. Anon: Perspectives. The corporatization of American health care. *Wash Rep Med Health* 37(45):Suppl 4p, 1983.
26. Anon: Management companies' progress enables industry to maintain growth pattern. In *1988 Directory of Investor-Owned Hospitals and Hospital Management Companies*, Little Rock, Federation of American Hospitals, 1989.
27. Anon: Perspectives. Doctor surplus breeds new practice forms. *Wash Rep Med Health* 37(17):Suppl 4p, 1983.
28. U.S. Public Health Service: *National Directory of HMOs*. Department of Health and Human Services, Washington, DC, 1989.
29. Blendon RJ: The reform of ambulatory care: A financial paradox. *Med Care* 14:526-534, 1976.
30. Bellin SS, Geiger HJ, Gibson CD: The impact of ambulatory health care services on the demand for hospital beds. *N Engl J Med* 280:808, 1969.
31. Tessler R, Mechanic D: Consumer satisfaction with PGP: A comparative study. *J Health Soc Behav* 16:95-113, 1975.
32. Greenlick MR, Lamb SJ, Carpenter TM, et al: Kaiser-Permanente's Medicare plus project: A successful Medicare prospective payment demonstration. *Health Care Fin Rep* 13(4):85-97, 1983.
33. Lundy RW, Blacker RA: Preferred provider organizations: The latest response to healthcare competition. *Healthcare Fin Mgt* 13(7):14-18, 1983.
34. Kuntz EF: Hospitals forming PPO's to fend off HMO rivals. *Mod Healthcare* 13(2):22-24, 1983.
35. Curtiss FR: Third party reimbursement for home parenteral nutrition and IV therapy. *NITA J* 6:193-197, May/June, 1983.
36. Anon: *The Elderly Should Benefit from Expanded Home Health Care but Increasing These Services Will Not Insure Cost Reductions*. Report No. IPE-83-1, Gaithersburg, MD, U.S. General Accounting Office, December 7, 1982.
37. Gibson RM, Waldo DR, Levit KR: National health expenditures. *Health Care Fin Rev* 5(l):1-31, 1983.
38. Breslow L: The organization of personal health services. *Millbank Mem Fund* 50(4):365, 1972.
39. Muse DN, Sawyer D: *The Medicare and Medicaid Data Book, 1981*. Office of Research and Demonstrations, Healthcare Financing Administration, Baltimore, MD, April 1982.
40. Anon: Reagan budget: What's new? *Wash Rep Med Health* 38(6):Suppl 6p, 1984.
41. Anon: Medicaid program; miscellaneous Medicaid provisions-increased state flexibility. *Fed Reg* 46(190):48524-48561, 1981.
42. Anon: Medicare program: Prospective payment for Medicare inpatient hospital services; final rule. *Fed Reg* 49(FR):233-340, 1984.
43. Anon: Advisory Council on Social Security recommends major Medicare reforms. *Hotline* November 15, 1983.
44. Anon: Report recommends drastic Medicaid program reform. *Hosp Week* 20(6):1, 1984.
45. Costanzo CA, Vertinsky L: Measuring the quality of health care: A decision oriented typology. *Med Care* 13:417-431, 1975.
46. Anon: Medicare and Medicaid programs; conditions of participation for hospitals: Proposed rule. *Fed Reg* 48(2):299-315, 1983.
47. Novick LF, Dickinson K, Asnes R, et al: Assessment of ambulatory care: Application of the tracer methodology. *Med Care* 14:1-12, 1976.
48. Wirtschafer DD, Mesel E: A strategy for redesigning the medical record for quality assurance. *Med Care* 14:68-76, 1976.
49. Bellin LE: PSRO-quality control? Or gimmickry? *Med Care* 12:1012-1018, 1974.
50. Anon: Medicare: Utilization and quality control peer review organization (PRO) area designations and definitions of eligible organizations; final rule and notice. *Fed Reg* 49(39):7201-7210, 1984.
51. Scanlon WJ, Feder J: The long-term care marketplace: An overview. *Healthcare Fin Mgt* 14(1):18, 19, 24-26, 28, 30, 34, 36, 1984.
52. Comptroller General of the United States: *Problems in Providing Proper Care to Medicaid and Medicare Patients in Skilled Nursing Homes*. Report B-16403 (13), Washington, DC, U.S. Government Printing Office, 1970.
53. Zimmer JG: Characteristics of patients and care provided in health related and skilled nursing facilities. *Med Care* 13:992-1010, 1975.
54. Ruchlin HS, Levey S, Miller C: The long-term care marketplace: An analysis of deficiencies and potential reform by means of incentive reimbursement. *Med Care* 13:979-991, 1975.
55. Anon: *Medicaid and Nursing Home Care: Cost Increases and the Need for Services Are Creating Problems for the States and the Elderly*. Publication No. GAO-IPE-84-1, Washington, DC, U.S. Government Accounting Office, October 21, 1983.
56. Solon JA, Greenwalt LF: Physicians' participation in nursing homes. *Med Care* 12:486, 1974.
57. Lifson A: Financing long-term care: HIAA's evaluation. *Healthcare Fin Mgt* 14(3):64-65, 1984.
58. Fincham JE, Wertheimer A: *Pharmacy and the U.S. Health Care System*. New York, Pharmaceutical Products Press, 1991.
59. Starfeld DH, Simborg DW, Horn SD, et al: Continuity and coordination in primary care: Their achievement and utility. *Med Care* 14:626-636, 1976.
60. Banta HD: Role strains of a health care team in a poverty community. *Soc Sci Med* 6:697-722, 1972.
61. Nathansan CA, Becker NH: Physicians, nurses and clinical records. *Med Care* 11:213-233, 1973.
62. Brown CA: The division of laborers: Allied health professions. *Int J Health Serv* 3:435-444, 1973.
63. Clute KF: *The General Practitioner: A Study of Medical Education and Practice in Ontario and Nova Scotia*. Toronto, University of Toronto Press, 1963.
64. Clark DA, Kroeger HH, Altman I, et al: The office practice of internists: III. Characteristics of patients. *JAMA* 193:916-923, 1965.
65. Shortell SN: *A Model of Physician Referral Behavior: A Test of Exchange Theory in Medical Practice*. Chicago, University of Chicago, Center for Health Administration Studies, Reserve Series, 1972.
66. Freidson E: *Professional Dominance*. Chicago, Atherton, 1970.

67. McKinley JB: Who is really ignorant—physician or patient? *J Health Soc Behav* 16:3-11, 1975.
68. Dickson WM, Rodowskas CA: Verbal communication of community pharmacists. *Med Care* 13:486-498, 1975.
69. Lees REM: Physician time-saving by employment of expanded-role nurses in family practice. *Can Med Assoc J* 108:871-875, 1973.
70. Rafferty J: *Health Manpower and Productivity*. Lexington, MA, Lexington Books, 1974.
71. Hepler CD: A primer on productivity. *Top Hosp Pharm Mgt* 1:55, 1981.
72. McGhan WF, Smith WE, Adams DW: A randomized trial comparing pharmacists and technicians as dispensers of prescriptions for ambulatory patients. *Med Care* 21:445-453, 1983.
73. Lewis CG, Resnick BA: Nurse clinics and progressive ambulatory patient care. *N Engl J Med* 277:1236-1245, 1967.
74. Charney E, Kitzman H: The child-health nurse (pediatric nurse practitioner) in private practice: A controlled trial. *N Engl J Med* 285:1353-1358, 1971.
75. Sackett DL, Spitzer WO, Gent M, et al: The Burlington Randomized Trial of the nurse practitioner: Health outcomes of patients. *Ann Intern Med* 80:137-145, 1974.
76. Levine DM, Morlock LL, Mushlin AI, et al: The role of new health practitioners in a prepaid group practice: Provider differences in process and outcomes of medical care. *Med Care* 14:326-347, 1976.
77. McCloud BC: Clinical pharmacy: The past, present and future. *Am J Hosp Pharm* 33:29-38, 1976.
78. Litman T: Public perception of the physician's assistant—a survey of attitudes and opinions of rural Iowa and Minnesota residents. *Am J Public Health* 62:343-346, 1972.
79. Weinstein P, Demers JL: Rural nurse practitioner clinic: The public's response. *Am J Nurs* 74:2022-2026, 1974.
80. Lawrence LS: Patient acceptance of the family nurse practitioner. *Med Care* 14:356-364, 1976.
81. Wriston S: Nurse practitioner reimbursement. *J Health Politics Policy Law* 6:444-462, 1981.
82. Anon: *Managing Health Costs: Strategies for Coalitions and Business*. Washington, DC, Clearinghouse on Business Coalitions for Health Action, Chamber of Commerce of the United States, 1982.
83. Metsch JM, Veney JG: Consumer participation and social accountability. *Med Care* 14:283-293, 1976.
84. Wingate MB, Silver T, McMillen M, et al: Obstetric care in a family health oriented university associated neighborhood health center. *Med Care* 14:315-325, 1976.
85. Stein OH: The use of a nurse practitioner in the management of patients with diabetes mellitus. *Med Care* 12:885-890, 1974.
86. Anon: Survey shows liability law gains in '75. *Am Med News* 19:1, 1976.
87. Klein R: Few suits in British medicine. *Washington Post* May 23, 1976.
88. Congressional Record Proceedings: Medical Malpractice Reinsurance Program. *Congr Rec* 121:5302, 1975.
89. Taravella S: Physicians faced with ballooning malpractice rates. *Lauer Rep* 1(5):2-3, 1983.
90. Mechanic D: *Public Expectations and Health Care*. New York, Wiley-Interscience, 1972.
91. Klaw S: Bad medicine: When practice makes imperfect. *Washington Post* December 21, 1975.
92. Holder AR: *Medical Malpractice Law*. New York, John Wiley & Sons, 1975.

CHAPTER 2

The Social Systems Perspective on Patient Care

BONNIE L. SVARSTAD and JEANINE K. MOUNT

Better understanding of patients' feelings, beliefs, and behavior is important for several reasons. First, studies have shown repeatedly that patient noncompliance with prescribed regimens continues to be a major public health problem that cannot be reduced without more effective communication between patients and practitioners.[1,2] Second, improved understanding of and communication with patients also can substantially influence patients' ability to cooperate during painful or noxious procedures;[3] frequency of postoperative complications and length of stay;[4-6] need for sedative-hypnotics and analgesics;[4-6] satisfaction with services;[7] and sense of control and well-being.[8,9] Practitioners also require good understanding of patients to assess better patients' needs and provide more humane care.[10] For example, it is difficult to obtain complete and accurate information from patients if we ignore the social and psychological factors that can influence patients' willingness to fully report their pain and discomfort, the medications they are taking, and side effects they have experienced.

How can we better understand patients and drug use in the institutional setting? In the first section of this chapter, we provide a brief overview of two alternative perspectives on patients and drug use in this setting: the physiologic or biomedical perspective and the social systems perspective. We argue that the biomedical view is too narrow because it fails to consider patients' social and psychological needs, caregiving relationships, the treatment environment, and the larger sociocultural context. The social systems perspective is more suitable because it provides a holistic orientation. It recognizes the interdependence of natural systems, the stresses and demands of illness and caregiving, and the different ways in which patients and providers adapt to their situation.

In the second section, we discuss several ways in which a social systems perspective has been used to examine the nature and outcome of care in hospitals and nursing homes. Even if it were possible to present a detailed review of the social research in this area, such a review is beyond our purposes. Instead, we provide selected examples of the ways in which social factors can influence patients' responses to asthma, recovery from surgery, pain reporting, sense of well-being, and use of psychoactive medications in the institutional setting.

PERSPECTIVES ON THE PATIENT AND DRUG USE IN INSTITUTIONS

The Biomedical Perspective

Although health care professionals are becoming increasingly aware of the social and psychological dimensions of illness and patient care, many still rely on a physiologic or biomedical approach when assessing their patients' needs and responses.[10,11] This approach is based in the biological sciences and does not explicitly consider social, cultural, or psychological factors that can have direct or indirect effects on symptom reporting, patterns of drug use, or outcomes of treatment in institutional settings. It assumes that diseases result primarily from physical causes and that variations in the patient's symptoms and behavior during illness reflect the severity or stage of disease. It further assumes that drugs will be prescribed and consumed according to the patient's physical needs and the health care provider's scientific knowledge and criteria, as depicted in figure 2-1. A final assumption is that treatment outcomes are determined largely by physiologic or biologic processes.

This type of approach has several weaknesses. First, the patient's feelings, beliefs, and behavioral reactions to illness and treatment are neglected because the patient is viewed simply as a passive organism whose rehabilitation or recovery depends solely on the availability and appropriate use of medical technology, such as drugs, devices, and surgery. Second, it assumes that inappropriate drug prescribing and administration are caused by a lack of scientific knowledge. Efforts to improve drug use in institutional settings that have relied on the biomedical perspective have not always achieved desired results.[2] This may be because such efforts overemphasize the importance of scientific information and underemphasize the importance of nonmedical factors, such as patient demand, economic pressures, staffing patterns, and the provider's personal beliefs and norms.[2,12]

The Social Systems Perspective

The social systems perspective encourages us to consider a more holistic orientation to understanding institutionalized patients and the drug-use process in institutional settings. Mount[11] has described a broader application of this approach to analyzing events in pharmacy and health care. The three main assumptions underlying this approach are as follows:

1. The interdependence of natural systems,
2. The stresses and demands of illness and caregiving, and
3. Variations in illness and caregiving behavior.

Let us begin by looking at the first assumption. Proponents of the social systems perspective[10] suggest that we cannot fully understand patient symptoms and response to treatment unless we consider the full range of naturally occurring systems, including: molecules, cells, tissues, organs, and organ systems; the patient-provider relationship and other two-person systems; the family and other social groups; the treatment environment; and the larger social, cultural, political, and economic contexts. Each of these "systems" has distinctive properties that can and should be studied with scientific methods, and each system can be influenced by the larger system(s) of which it is a part. To understand these links, we must integrate concepts and principles from diverse disciplines, including the physical and biological sciences and the different social and behavioral sciences. No single discipline or theoretical perspective is likely to provide a complete understanding of institutionalized patients, their needs, and their behavior.

This implies that we cannot understand patients and their needs without considering different levels of phenomena and their interrelationships, as depicted in figure 2-2. According to this model, patients are more than passive organisms.

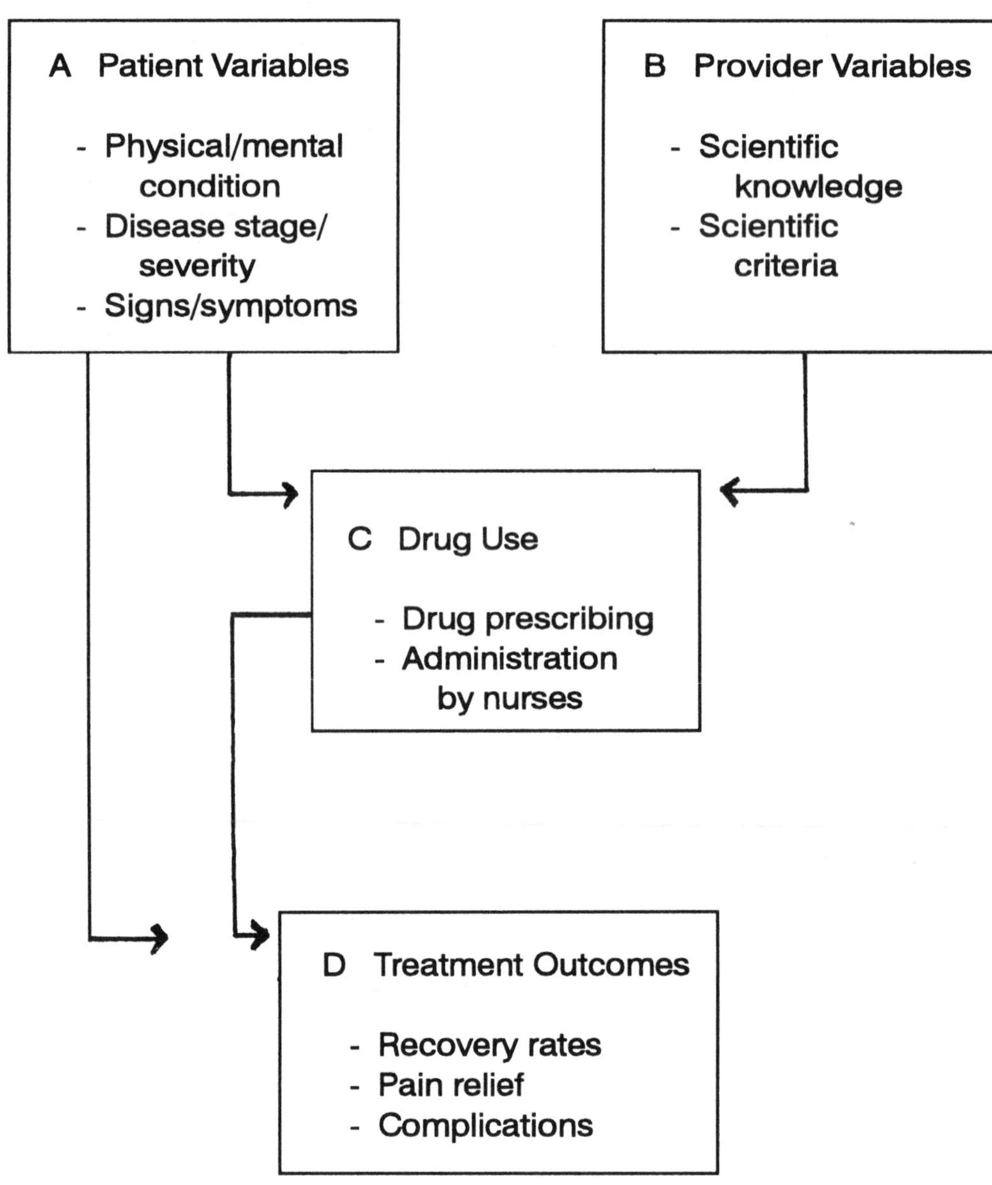

Figure 2-1. Biomedical model of patient care and drug use

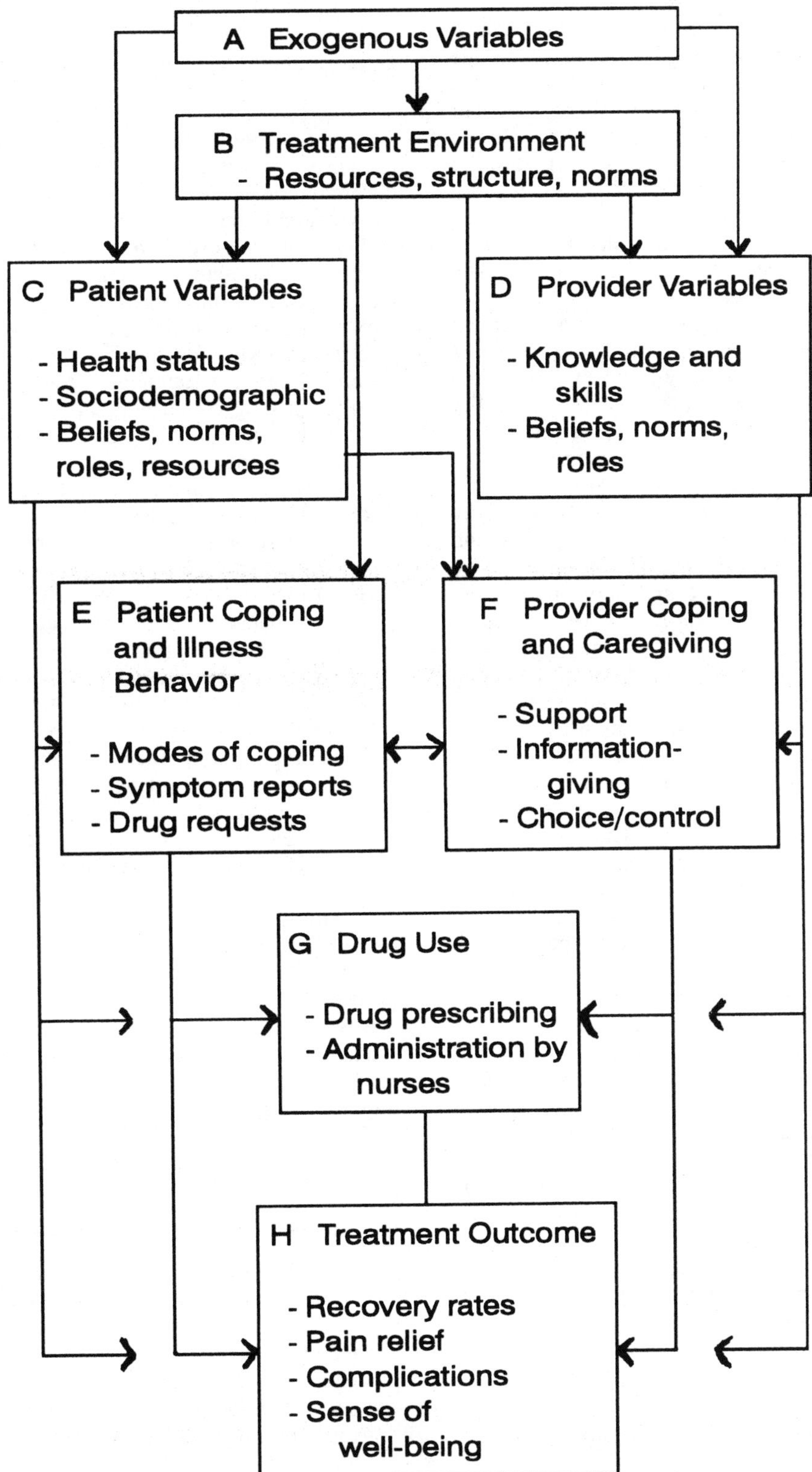

Figure 2-2. Social systems model of patient care and drug use

They are thinking, feeling human beings with diverse physical conditions, personal beliefs, and modes of coping with illness and medical treatment (see boxes C and E, figure 2-2). Providers are more than applied scientists. They, too, are thinking, feeling human beings whose decisions and behaviors are shaped by professional education and socialization. Providers are influenced by the larger sociocultural and economic context (box A), the institution or environment in which they work (box B), their personal beliefs and norms about caregiving (box D), and their patients' expectations or demands (box E). Similar models have been proposed for the study of nursing practices and the care of nursing home residents.[13,14]

The second assumption of the social systems perspective is that both patients and providers are confronted with a wide variety of potentially stressful, threatening, or challenging events. For patients, there are many threats associated with the physical, psychological, or social consequences of illness or disability, as well as threats associated with the treatment environment and staff-patient relationships. For example, patients who are hospitalized for a myocardial infarction experience the threat to life, as well as threats to self-esteem and identity, their social roles and relationships, and their emotional well-being.[15-17] In today's highly technological hospitals, patients also face a confusing and frightening array of drugs and devices, machines, specialists, specialty care units, and support and servicing departments.[18] Those who require long-term care in nursing homes or other highly restrictive institutional settings face potential threats to their sense of well-being, including increased dependence on others, loss of autonomy or control over day-to-day activities, and social isolation.[8,9]

Of course, institutional caregivers and staff also are confronted with a variety of situations that are stressful or difficult to manage.[19] Scientific knowledge, time, and administrative support often are limited. Third-party payers frequently place constraints on the services that can be provided. Equipment requires careful monitoring and does not always function as it should. Effective communication and coordination with specialists and support departments is difficult to accomplish. Another source of stress is the patient or family who can be very demanding and unappreciative, noisy, combative, or totally dependent on staff.

Another major assumption is that patients have very different ways of perceiving, evaluating, and responding to a given illness and medical treatment. Thus, it is important to distinguish between patients' illness and their "illness behavior."[19] We also must recognize that providers differ in the way they perceive, evaluate, and try to cope with the situational demands and conditions with which they are confronted. We must distinguish between providers' technical knowledge, skills, and strategies and their personal beliefs, norms, roles, and caregiving strategies.[13] Whether they provide patients with an adequate level of psychosocial support, information, and choice over life decisions becomes as important as provision of adequate technical care.

SOCIAL RESEARCH ON THE PATIENT AND DRUG USE IN INSTITUTIONS

In recent years, researchers have shown increased interest in the social factors that can influence the nature and outcome of patient care in hospitals and nursing home settings. Some areas have been studied extensively, whereas other important issues have not yet received the attention they deserve. The following examples illustrate several areas of current research interest.

Patients' Modes of Coping

There is considerable debate about the origins and impact of different strategies for coping with illness and disability.[15-17] It is clear, though, that patients employ different modes of coping with the same condition and that individual differences can play an important role in patients' ability to prevent excessive fear or "panic" when faced with a potentially stressful situation or event. For example, there are considerable differences in the extent to which patients seek or avoid information, turn to or withdraw from others, take responsibility for their own care or "give up," and use different cognitive techniques (e.g., denial, intellectualization) for dealing with acute pain and distress.

If clinicians do not explicitly consider these coping patterns, they may inaccurately estimate the severity of the patient's medical condition, medication needs, and need for discharge counseling. For example, researchers[20-22] have shown that some patients with asthma are more likely to report feeling scared and afraid of dying or being left alone during an asthma attack and that there is a weak correlation between patients' level of fear and their objectively measured pulmonary function levels. This suggests that patients' reactions are a function of personality or behavioral factors in addition to their actual medical condition. Research[22] also shows a close relationship between the patients' coping style, their request for pro re nata (PRN) medication, and physicians' prescribing of oral corticosteroids. Compared with other patients, "panicky" patients requested and used more medication both while hospitalized and when discharged, thus being exposed to increased risks of side effects and overuse. How these patients influence their physicians' prescribing decisions is not clear. It is believed, though, that they receive more intensive drug regimens because their subjective reports make them appear to have a worse condition. In contrast, other patients may present a "serene picture of well-being" and result in earlier discharge, less intensive drug regimens, and possibly less discharge counseling. These patients may continue to minimize or disregard their asthmatic distress and not follow scheduled drug regimens. This would expose them to a different set of potentially serious consequences.[22]

Psychosocial Support and Recovery From Surgery

Since the 1970's, there has been a dramatic increase in research examining the availability of psychosocial support and various kinds of information on the patient's adaptation and recovery from different physical conditions and medical procedures.[4,5] Mumford et al.[4] reviewed 34 experimental studies testing the effects of various psychosocial interventions on recovery from surgery and heart attacks. In general, the evidence is quite strong: patients given higher amounts of psychosocial support and information by their providers have significantly shorter hospital stays, fewer physical complications, and lower use of narcotic analgesics, tranquilizers, and sleep medications. An early study involved 97 patients receiving elective intra-abdominal operations.[23] Those who were assigned to the experimental group received detailed instruction and encouragement from an anesthetist the night before surgery. They were told the nature of the pain to be experienced, what would be done at various times, how to relax, how to turn, and how to use the trapeze. To prevent bias, the prescribers and nurses were unaware of which patients were assigned to the experimental and control groups. As predicted, the patients in the experimental group required about one-half the narcotic analgesics required by the other patients and were able to leave the hospital on an average of 2.7 days earlier.

Other investigators have examined the effects of special instruction on the patients' reactions to a painful or noxious diagnostic procedure. A good example is a study that examined 48 patients receiving an endoscopic examination.[3] The study's purpose was to test several hypotheses derived from social psychological theory about the ways in which people generally react to threatening events. As predicted, patients were less likely to experience negative affective or emotional reactions if they received "sensory information" that enabled them to anticipate accurately what they would feel during the endoscopic examination (e.g., how the drug would affect them, how it would feel to have air pumped into the stomach). Second, patients were better able to perform painful or noxious tasks if they received detailed instruction about how to perform the given tasks (e.g., how to control their breathing and tube swallowing). Although the findings varied somewhat by the type of instruction provided, the patients receiving special instruction generally showed more stable heart rates, had a lower frequency of gagging, achieved better control over tube swallowing, and required less diazepam than did the patients not receiving special instruction.

Despite strong evidence that psychosocial interventions have beneficial effects on patients' well-being and length of hospital stay, Devine and colleagues[6] have questioned whether these benefits can be obtained in the current environment when such interventions are implemented by existing hospital staff (rather than academic researchers). To answer these questions, they conducted a three-hour, two-stage, in-service workshop for hospital staff nurses. The experimental program included a presentation of past research on the effects of psychosocial support and patient education, feedback based on preworkshop data collection, and strategies for increasing the level of "psychoeducational care" provided. The strategies for increasing psychoeducational care included individual consultation with staff nurses and meetings with the head nurses to enhance administrative support. The workshop was evaluated in terms of its effects on 148 patients who had a cholecystectomy or other abdominal surgery after the in-service workshop. After the workshop, the patients used fewer antiemetics and sedative-hypnotics and had shorter hospital stays than did patients having surgery before the workshop.

Family and Social Group Influences on Pain Reporting

Although health professionals long have noted that pain is a subjective experience, it was not until the 1950's that researchers began to examine systematically the social and cultural factors that can increase or decrease the patient's perception of pain, the degree of discomfort reported, and the amount of medication requested. In a classic sociological study, Zborowski[24] demonstrated that patients from different ethnic backgrounds had very different reactions to pain, even though they were suffering from similar physical problems (i.e., herniated discs and spinal lesions). For example, Jewish and Italian patients tended to have a more emotional response to pain; they felt freer to discuss their pain, complain about it, groan and cry, and ask for relief. In contrast, patients from other backgrounds tried to deny their pain and appear more stoic. Based on observational and interview data, Zborowski concluded that the patients had learned different ways of reacting to pain and that they simply were behaving in a manner that was "expected, accepted, and approved" by their families and others in their community.

Over the past 30 years, there have been many experimental and nonexperimental studies confirming and extending Zborowski's basic hypothesis about the important influence of social factors on pain reporting and the use of pain relievers.[25,26] One of the more consistent findings is that males report fewer physical symptoms than females and typically have a lower level of analgesic use.[27-29] Although physical differences partially explain these gender differences in symptom reporting and drug use, they do not fully account for the observed differences. Thus, social researchers have explored other explanations. For example, studies of children's illness behavior suggest that boys and girls acquire different beliefs and ways of coping with pain through the process of socialization into traditional male and female roles: girls are encouraged to express their pain, whereas boys are encouraged to deny their pain and avoid "feminine" or "sissy-like" behaviors.[29] Consequently, men may be less likely to complain about and seek relief from pain unless they are encouraged to do so by their caregivers.

Others have observed that older patients consistently report less pain than might be anticipated on the basis of physical findings or known patterns of morbidity[30] and that elderly patients on medical and surgical units are prescribed and consume fewer analgesics, particularly narcotic analgesics.[31,32] There are several possible explanations. According to the biomedical perspective, physicians' and patients' behaviors can be explained in biomedical and pharmaceutical terms:

> . . .This may be partly explained by a lower incidence of pain in the elderly, which has been suggested by their increased threshold and tolerance to experimental pain induced by radiant heat. Alternatively, this population may have enhanced responsiveness to analgesic medications. Pain relief after morphine injection is greater in the elderly, perhaps due to prolonged plasma half-life, and other analgesics may have greater action because of decreased metabolism and elimination. Finally, it is possible that concern about the increased risk of side effects in older patients leads to undertreatment of their pain. . . .It is apparent that further efforts need to be made to educate physicians about the use of these agents in the treatment of pain (p. 441).[32]

An alternative explanation—and the one that we support—is based on the social systems perspective. It suggests that observed age differences in pain reporting and analgesic use reflect broader social and cultural processes.

These include the subtle effects of "ageism" or negative stereotypes held by society, health professionals, and the elderly themselves.[33-36] Thus, older patients may have similar or greater levels of discomfort than younger patients but report less pain and request less medication because they expect or accept greater pain with advancing age,[30,37,38] because they are more deferential when interacting with physicians,[36] or because they fear inconveniencing nurses and others with their complaints.[39] Similarly, physicians may direct less energy toward the assessment and treatment of pain in older patients because they have learned to view older people as less competent, less interesting, or less worthy.[40] This explanation is consistent with data showing that physicians generally spend less time with older patients,[41] are less likely to perform routine cancer screenings on older women,[42] and provide less curative treatment for older patients with cancer.[43,44]

Environmental Influences on Nursing Home Residents' Well-Being

Another interesting set of studies suggests that social and environmental restrictions in choice and control over daily activities can have negative effects on the physical health, memory, morale, and general sense of well-being of residents in nursing homes.[8,9,45] Although there has not been a great deal of work in this area, experimental studies are consistent: patients who are given more autonomy or opportunities for self-determination tend to have higher morale, become more alert, and show greater improvement in their health status.[8] Whether increased control over drug-related decisions can have similar beneficial effects is a question that deserves careful study by pharmacists in health care institutions.

Effects of Staff Attitudes on PRN Drug Administration

Staff attitudes toward the patient often are cited as an essential factor contributing to the quality of patient care in general and the quality of staff-patient interaction in particular.[13] Surprisingly, only a few studies specifically examine whether and how staff perceptions influence medication use among institutionalized patients. Existing data suggest that nurses have variable drug philosophies and preferences and that these perceptions can play an important role in the patient's use of PRN medications, including medications for pain, sleep, and anxiety.[46-48] For example, Parker[46] found considerable variation in the degree to which medical patients were involved in the nurse's decision to administer a PRN hypnotic medication. One-half of the doses were requested initially by the patient, 30 percent were given after the nurse offered the medication, and 20 percent were administered without any discussion. Of the last group, one-half of the patients were unaware that they had received a sleep medication and did not think they needed it. Interestingly, the majority of these "routine" PRN doses were administered by the same nurse.

In their study of pain management, Fagerhaugh and Strauss[47] found wide variation in nurse beliefs about who should give drug information, how much information should be given, how much pain the patient should endure before calling a nurse, the amount of control that patients should have, when the nurse should consult the physician for changes in the order, and other drug-related issues. They also observed that physicians varied in the amount of discretion they allowed nurses and that nurses varied in their interpretation of physicians' orders. Some nurses consistently gave the lowest amount permitted, whereas others consistently gave the highest amount permitted. Given these opposing views and practices, the researchers were not surprised to find considerable patient confusion, dissatisfaction, and mistrust, along with a high level of conflict in patient-nurse and nurse-nurse interactions.

How and why do these different medication philosophies develop? How do these staff perceptions ultimately influence the quality of pain relief and other treatment outcomes? What should be the role of the institutional pharmacist under these circumstances? Despite increased concern about the undertreatment of pain in hospitals and nursing homes, these questions remain unexplored.

Organizational Factors Affecting Psychotropic Drug Use

In recent years there has been increased interest in organizational variables and their effect on the quality of patient care in hospitals and nursing homes. Organizational factors that have proven to be important include type of ownership and control, size, staffing patterns, and presence of a "custodial" versus a "rehabilitative" treatment orientation.[14,49]

Whether these factors also influence the quantity or quality of drug prescribing and administration is a question that has been examined in only a few studies, all dealing with antipsychotic drug use.[50-54] Two conclusions can be drawn. First, there is extraordinary variation in the rate of antipsychotic prescribing from one nursing home to another. Ray and colleagues[50] were the first to draw attention to this pattern, noting that the percentage of residents who received antipsychotics on a chronic basis varied from 0 percent to 46 percent in their sample of 173 Tennessee facilities. Researchers in Washington State[54] also reported wide variation in the routine use of these medications, ranging from 5.9 percent to 52.3 percent in their sample of 38 nursing homes. Second, the reasons for this variation are not well understood. Illinois researchers using a Medicaid data base found a weak correlation between selected nursing home characteristics and antipsychotic drug use, leading them to speculate that facility characteristics are unimportant.[51] On the other hand, Wisconsin researchers included both Medicaid and privately funded nursing home residents and found that the quality of psychotropic prescribing was correlated significantly with the level of registered nurse staffing: quality of drug use was higher in facilities with higher levels of registered nurse staffing.[52,53] Data showing a positive correlation between nurse staffing and the appropriate use of antipsychotics confirm what many practitioners, researchers, and lay persons have suspected for a long time. However, many questions must be answered before we can draw any firm conclusions. First, we need to understand the inconsistent results from one study to another. Are they because of differences in sampling, sources of data, and measurement, or are they because of differences in nursing home policies or practices? Second, we need to establish the causal order and explanation for the positive correlation between nurse staffing and the quality of antipsychotic drug prescribing. Does a high level of registered nurse staffing lead to better-quality drug use, or is it the other way around? Perhaps facilities with better medical, social, and pharmacy services are more successful in recruiting registered nurses. If prospective studies establish that better staffing leads to better-quality drug use, then we still need to understand how and why a higher level of nurse staffing leads to higher-quality drug use. In any case, we need a much better understanding of the environmental barriers to quality drug use in institutional settings.

CONCLUSION

Being attentive to the patient's psychosocial needs is no easy task. It requires new ways of thinking about patients and recognizing the potential importance of staff-patient relationships for the patient's recovery and well-being. In this chapter we have just scratched the surface in discussing current knowledge about patients in hospitals and nursing homes. Likewise, researchers have just scratched the surface in documenting the link between patients' psychosocial needs and the quality and cost of health care. We advise the reader to consider the relevance of this link when reading the chapters that follow.

REFERENCES

1. Svarstad B: Patient-practitioner relationships and compliance with prescribed medical regimens. In Aiken L, Mechanic D (eds): *Applications of Social Science to Clinical Medicine and Health Policy*. New Brunswick, Rutgers University Press, 1986, pp 438-459.
2. Svarstad B: Sociology of drugs in health care. In Wertheimer A, Smith M (eds): *Pharmacy Practice: Social and Behavioral Aspects*. Baltimore, Williams & Wilkins, 1989, pp 197-211.
3. Johnson JE, Leventhal H: Effects of accurate expectations and behavioral instructions on reactions during a noxious medical examination. *J Soc Psychol* 29:710-718, 1974.
4. Mumford E, Schlesinger H, Glass G: The effects of psychological intervention on recovery from surgery and heart attacks: An analysis of the literature. *Am J Public Health* 72:141-151, 1982.
5. Devine E, Cook T: Clinical and cost-relevant effects of psychoeducational interventions with surgical patients: A meta-analysis. *Res Nurs Health* 9:89-105, 1986.
6. Devine E, O'Connor F, Cook T, et al: Clinical and financial effects of psychoeducational care provided by staff nurses to adult surgical patients in the post-DRG environment. *Am J Public Health* 78:1293-1297, 1988.
7. Ley P, Bradshaw PW, Kincey JA, et al: Increasing patients' satisfaction with communications. *Br J Soc Clin Psychol* 15:403-413, 1976.
8. Rodin J: Aging and health: Effects of the sense of control. *Science* 233:1271-1276, 1986.
9. Rodin J: The application of social psychology. In Lindzey G, Aronson E (eds): *Handbook of Social Psychology* (3rd ed). New York, Random House, 1985, pp 805-881.
10. Engel GL: The clinical application of the biopsychosocial model. *Am J Psychiatry* 137:534-544, 1980.
11. Mount J: Contributions of the social sciences. In Wertheimer A, Smith M (eds): *Pharmacy Practice: Social and Behavioral Aspects*. Baltimore, Williams & Wilkins, 1989, pp 1-15.
12. Schwartz R, Soumerai S, Avorn J: Physician motivations for nonscientific drug prescribing. *Soc Sci Med* 28:577-582, 1989.
13. Wright L: A reconceptualization of the "negative staff attitudes and poor care in nursing homes" assumption. *Gerontologist* 28:813-820, 1988.
14. Pillemer K: Maltreatment of patients in nursing homes: Overview and research agenda. *J Health Soc Behav* 29:227-238, 1988.
15. Cohen F, Lazarus RS: Coping with the stresses of illness. In Stone GC, Chen F, Adler NE, et al (eds): *Health Psychology - A Handbook*. San Francisco, Jossey-Bass, 1979, pp 217-254.
16. Cohen F, Lazarus RS: Coping and adaptation in health and illness. In Mechanic D (ed): *Handbook of Health, Health Care, and the Health Professions*. New York, Free Press, 1983, pp 608-635.
17. Wortman C, Conway T: The role of social support in adaptation and recovery from physical illness. In Cohen S, Syme SL: *Social Support and Health*. Orlando, Academic Press, 1985, pp 281-302.
18. Strauss A, Fagerhaugh S, Suczek B, et al: *Social Organization of Medical Work*. Chicago, University of Chicago Press, 1985.
19. Mechanic D: *Medical Sociology* (2nd ed). New York, Free Press, 1978.
20. Konsman, RA, Dahlem NW, Spector S, et al: Observations on subjective symptomatology, coping behavior, and medical decisions in asthma. *Psychosom Med* 39:102-119, 1977.
21. Dirks JF, Jones NF, Kinsman RA: Panic-fear: A personality dimension related to intractability in asthma. *Psychosom Med* 39:120-126, 1977.
22. Dahlem NW, Kinsman RA, Horton DJ: Panic-fear in asthma: Requests for as-needed medications in relation to pulmonary function measurements. *J Allergy Clin Immunol* 60:295-300, 1977.
23. Egbert LD, Battit GE, Welch CE, et al: Reduction of postoperative pain by encouragement and instruction of patients. *N Engl J Med* 270:825-827, 1964.
24. Zborowski M: Cultural components in response to pain. *J Soc Issues* 8:16-30, 1952.
25. Kotarba JA: *Chronic Pain: Its Social Dimensions*. Beverly Hills, Sage Publications, 1983.
26. Osterweis M, Kleinman A, Mechanic D (eds): *Pain and Disability: Clinical, Behavioral and Policy Perspectives*. Committee on Pain, Disability, and Illness Behavior, Institute of Medicine, Washington, DC, National Academy Press, 1987.
27. Nathanson CA: Sex, illness, and medical care: A review of data, theory, and method. *Soc Sci Med* 11:13-25, 1977.
28. Verbrugge LM: Sex differences in legal drug use. *J Soc Issues* 38:59-76, 1982.
29. Lewis CE, Lewis MA: The potential impact of sexual inequality on health. *N Engl J Med* 297:863-869, 1977.
30. Mechanic E, Angel R: Some factors associated with the report and evaluation of back pain. *J Health Soc Behav* 28:131-139, 1987.
31. Goldberg R, Mor V, Wiemann M, et al: Analgesic use in terminal cancer patients: Report from the National Hospice Study. *J Chronic Dis* 39:37-45, 1986.
32. Portenoy R, Kanner R: Patterns of analgesic prescription and consumption in a university-affiliated community hospital. *Arch Intern Med* 145:439-441, 1985.
33. Butler R: *Why Survive? Being Old in America*. New York, Harper and Row, 1975.
34. Cohen E: The elderly mystique: Constraints on the autonomy of the elderly with disabilities. *Gerontologist* 28:24-31, 1988.
35. Radecki S, Kane R, Solomon D, et al: Are physicians sensitive to the special problems of older patients? *J Am Geriatr Soc* 36:719-725, 1988.
36. Lipton H, Lee P: *Drugs and the Elderly: Clinical, Social, and Policy Perspectives*. Stanford, Stanford University Press, 1988.
37. Tornstram L: Health and self-perception: A systems theoretical approach. *Gerontologist* 27:264-270, 1975.
38. Ferrell BA, Ferrell BR: Assessment of pain in the elderly. *Geriatr Med Today* 8:123-134, 1989.
39. Ferrell BA, Ferrell BR, Osterweil D: Pain in the nursing home. *J Am Geriatr Soc* 38:409-414, 1990.

40. Miller D, Lowenstein R, Winston R: Physicians' attitudes toward the ill aged and nursing homes. *J Am Geriatr Soc* 24:498-505, 1976.
41. Keeler E, Solomon D, Beck J, et al: Effect of patient age on duration of medical encounters with physicians. *Med Care* 20:1101-1108, 1982.
42. Radecki S, Kane R, Solomon D, et al: Are physicians sensitive to the special problems of older patients? *J Am Geriatr Soc* 36:719-725, 1988.
43. Samet I, Hunt W, Key C, et al: Choice of cancer therapy varies with age of patient. *JAMA* 255:3380-3385, 1986.
44. Greenfield S, Blanco D, Elashoff R, et al: Patterns of care related to age of breast cancer patients. *JAMA* 257:2766-2770, 1987.
45. Ryden M: Morale and perceived control in institutionalized elderly. *Nurs Res* 33:130-136, 1984.
46. Parker WA: Effect of hospitalization on patient use of hypnotics. *Am J Hosp Pharm* 40:446-447, 1983.
47. Fagerhaugh SY, Strauss A: *Politics of Pain Management: Staff-Patient Interaction.* Menlo Park, CA, Addison-Wesley, 1977.
48. Lund M: The social organization of drug management in two nursing homes. Unpublished Ph.D. dissertation, Graduate College of the University of Illinois at the Medical Center, Chicago, 1979.
49. Hawes C, Phillips CD: The changing structure of the nursing home industry and the impact of ownership on quality, cost, and access. In Gray BS (ed): *For-Profit Enterprise in Health Care.* Washington, DC, National Academy Press, 1986, p. 492.
50. Ray WA, Federspiel CF, Schaffner W: A study of antipsychotic drug use in nursing homes: Epidemiologic evidence suggesting misuse. *Am J Public Health* 70:485-491, 1980.
51. Buck JA: Psychotropic drug practices in nursing homes. *J Am Geriatr Soc* 36:409-418, 1988.
52. Mount J: Facility predictors of quantity and quality of antipsychotic drug use among nursing home residents: Anticipating OBRA 87. Poster presented at the annual meeting of the Association for Health Services Research, Arlington, VA, June 17, 1990.
53. Svarstad B, Mount J: Nursing home resources and tranquilizer use among the institutionalized elderly. *J Am Geriatr Soc* 39:869-875, 1991.
54. Doane KW, Schrempp CO, Bell RA, et al: Prevalence of neuroleptic use in nursing homes. *Consult Pharm* 44:367-370, 1989.

CHAPTER 3

The Hospital and the Department of Pharmaceutical Services

PAUL W. ABRAMOWITZ and LEE A. MORK

INTRODUCTION

Institutional pharmaceutical services have developed and evolved tremendously over the past 20-30 years. Hospital pharmacy practice has changed from a profession concerned chiefly with the bulk preparation and distribution of drug products to one centered on ensuring optimal drug therapy in patients.[1-3] Whereas hospital pharmacists were charged with maintaining large drug stocks on nursing units, many now provide individualized patient therapies. The predominant activity of hospital pharmacists used to be ensuring that drug preparations were chemically and pharmaceutically correct; now they are as concerned that the patients' drug therapy is the most appropriate to treat their disease and is initiated, monitored, and changed correctly. The practice of hospital pharmacy has therefore become one encompassing all aspects of drug therapy, from the procurement of drugs and drug delivery devices, to their preparation and distribution, and to their most appropriate selection and use in each patient.

There are approximately 6,780[4] hospitals in the United States, the majority of which provide acute care. Recent trends in health care directed toward the expansion of ambulatory care have caused the acuity of hospitalized patients to rise. This has been due to the growth of ambulatory surgery, home intravenous therapy, preadmission diagnostic testing, and other methods of treating patients who were formerly hospitalized in the ambulatory clinic or in the home.[5] In part it has been prompted by financial constraints in the health care industry. Some have predicted that by the year 2000, the hospital will become a large intensive care unit.[6]

Hospital-affiliated ambulatory clinics have grown tremendously, along with emergency care centers and other ambulatory care sites either owned by or affiliated with hospitals. In addition, the rapid growth of health maintenance organizations (HMO's), preferred provider organizations (PPO's), and multihospital systems has caused hospital organizational structures to be modified or changed and has also increased competitiveness. These factors have further influenced the scope of pharmaceutical services delivered in institutional settings.

The objective of this chapter is to provide the reader with an overall understanding of the practice of institutional pharmacy. To accomplish this, a knowledge of the Department of Pharmaceutical Services in a hospital, and also the hospital in general, is required.

HOSPITAL CLASSIFICATION

Hospitals can be classified in the following ways: (1) by ownership (e.g., for profit or nonprofit), (2) by type of care provided (e.g., tertiary), and (3) by teaching affiliation (e.g., university affiliated).[7-9] Often, each of the three classifications is used to categorize an institution. For example, a hospital can be classified as a State-owned, tertiary-care teaching facility. In contrast, a hospital might be considered a private, primary care, community hospital or a private, for-profit, teaching-affiliated, specialty hospital.

Classification by Ownership

Hospital ownership can be described as either governmental or private. Government-owned hospitals include those owned by Federal, State, county, or municipal governments. Government-owned hospitals generally receive at least some funding from a branch of the government and are responsible to it, meaning that the hospital is ultimately responsible to Congress, a State legislature, or a county board. Examples of federally owned hospitals include the armed services (e.g., Walter Reed Hospital in Washington, DC) and Veterans Administration facilities. Many State-owned hospitals are affiliated with State university systems. Other State institutions include the smaller State psychiatric and rehabilitation facilities. County or municipal hospitals include but are not limited to general-care facilities. County facilities often provide care to patients who are unable to pay for services. Los Angeles County Hospital and Cook County Hospital in Chicago are examples of this type.

Privately owned hospitals are responsible for their own funding; that is, they generally do not receive tax dollars for their operation. Private hospitals are typically owned and operated by religious organizations, nonsectarian organizations, or other corporations. Many community hospitals, including St. Joseph Hospital in Pontiac, MI, (operated by the Sisters of Mercy) and Lutheran General Hospital in Chicago (operated by Lutheran General Care Systems), are privately owned. Some privately owned hospitals are associated with universities, such as the University of Chicago Hospital and the Hospital of the University of Pennsylvania. Hospitals such as St. Mary's Hospital in Rochester, MN, owned by the Mayo Clinic, and Cedar-Sinai in Los Angeles are also private hospitals. The Humana Hospital Sunrise, in Las Vegas, owned by Humana, Inc., and the West Florida Regional Medical Center, in Pensacola, FL, owned by the Hospital Corporation of America, are also examples of private hospitals.

Government-owned hospitals are always classified as not-for-profit (i.e., they do not pay profits or dividends to owners or shareholders), but private hospitals may be classified as either not-for-profit or for-profit. The vast majority of private hospitals in the United States are not-for-profit; however, the number of for-profit hospitals is growing. Humana Inc., Hospital Corporation of America, Healthtrust, Inc.-The Hospital Company, and Charter Medical Corporation are examples of corporations operating for-profit hospitals in this country. Together they own approximately 542 hospitals.[10]

Classification by Care Provided

Hospitals are also classified according to the type of care that they provide. In general, hospitals may be classified as providing either acute or chronic care. Acute care hospitals admit patients who have either temporary or chronic illnesses that can be treated in relatively short periods of time. Chronic care or long-term care hospitals provide for patients requiring either permanent or prolonged hospitalization for rehabilitation or inability to be managed in the ambulatory setting. Many psychiatric hospitals, rehabilitation hospitals, and select Veterans Administration hospitals can be characterized as chronic care hospitals, whereas most of the Nation's hospitals are acute care.

Care provided at acute care hospitals can be classified as being primary, secondary, or tertiary. Primary care is the starting point for entry into the health system. Primary care patients are typically admitted by a family practitioner, internist, pediatrician, or general surgeon. An example of a primary care patient would be one admitted for an emergency appendectomy. Secondary care is defined as referral services that are intermediate in intensity, for example, referral to a specialist. A patient who receives a referral from his or her general practitioner to a cardiologist that results in a hospital admission for evaluation and treatment of coronary artery disease is an example. Tertiary care refers to a setting where patients are referred for very intensive subspecialty care. Tertiary care requires the services of a physician and a hospital equipped to treat extremely complex problems less frequently seen or managed in a community hospital setting. Examples might include the treatment of cystic fibrosis, organ transplantation, or the management of neoplastic disease. Although many community hospitals provide primary care, patients are often referred to nearby university hospitals to receive tertiary care. Although university hospitals generally provide tertiary care, they also often treat a combination of primary, secondary, and tertiary care patients. Hospitals may further distinguish themselves by treating either a wide variety of disease states (general hospitals) or by treating patients with only selected diseases (specialty hospitals). For example, the University of Wisconsin Hospital and Clinic in Madison treats patients with many different disease states and would be classified as a general, tertiary care facility. On the other hand, the University of Texas M.D. Anderson Cancer Center in Houston primarily treats patients with cancer and would be considered a specialty tertiary care hospital.

Classification by Teaching Affiliation

Finally, hospitals may be classified as teaching, teaching-affiliated, or nonteaching institutions. Teaching hospitals are defined as those that operate residency training programs in medicine, surgery, pediatrics, and other specialty areas. In such institutions, residents provide patient care under the supervision of the hospital's medical staff. Teaching hospitals may be the primary teaching site for a college of medicine. In this case, they are usually referred to as "primary teaching hospitals" and serve as a training site for medical students, residents, and fellows. Hospitals that do not operate their own residency training programs but serve as a training site for residents or students from a nearby university hospital are often referred to as "teaching-affiliated hospitals." Hospitals having no residency training programs and no university hospital affiliation would be termed "nonteaching."

THE HOSPITAL'S GOVERNANCE AND ORGANIZATIONAL STRUCTURE

Governance

Hospitals have a governing body that is given the ultimate authority over the actions of the institution. This usually takes the form of a board of directors, a board of governors, or a board of trustees. In for-profit hospitals, the governing body is either the corporation's board of directors or a separate hospital board. In university hospitals, the hospital may have its own board of directors, or it may be governed by the university's board of trustees. In most cases, hospitals (government or private, for profit or non-profit) have their own governing board, because of the special nature of the hospital's business and the societal needs it serves. The hospital's board is often, however, responsible to the board of the parent body, such as the university, the corporation, or the State legislature.

The hospital's governing body has the responsibility to provide the overall mission and goals to the hospital, to evaluate its progress toward achieving the mission and goals, and thus to ensure that the hospital serves its community. The hospital's governing body also has fiduciary responsibility for the organization, to ensure financial appropriateness. The governing body of the hospital, in consultation with the hospital staff, the community the hospital serves, and the larger organization that the hospital may be a part of, selects the hospital director.

Hospitals are also responsible to various accrediting and licensing bodies. The Joint Commission on Accreditation of Healthcare Organizations (JCAHO) grants accreditation to hospitals and reviews their activities at least every 3 years.[11]

The accreditation process consists of evaluating the care and services provided by a hospital against a published list of standards. Loss of accreditation by JCAHO may make it difficult for a hospital to obtain some types of reimbursement for its services, or may discourage patients and physicians from using the hospital. State and local boards of health, medicine, pharmacy, and nursing may also have authority for the provision of certain types of services. For example, a State board of pharmacy may require a hospital to change its procedure for the labeling of intravenous admixtures, and a State board of nursing may require changes in drug administration practices.

Organizational Structure of the Hospital

The organizational structure of a hospital generally consists of several levels of management. The hospital director represents the uppermost level of hospital management. Depending on the institution, the hospital director may be called a hospital president or chief executive officer (CEO). The hospital director is responsible for carrying out the directives of the hospital's board. The director manages hospital operations, finances, and personnel. In addition, the director is responsible for maintaining effective medical staff relations. The director will periodically report the hospital's progress in achieving its mission and goals to the hospital's board. In a university hospital, the hospital director often reports to both the hospital's board of directors and a university official, such as a vice president for health sciences.

Assisting the CEO or hospital director in the management of the hospital is a second level of managers, which usually includes a chief operating officer (COO), a chief financial officer (CFO), and a director of nursing. This model is the most common seen in hospitals. These "level 2" administrators may have the titles of hospital associate directors, senior vice presidents, etc., depending on the organization.

The COO is responsible for managing the day-to-day operations of the hospital. The responsibilities of the COO usually include all departments contributing to hospital operations, with the exception of the departments of nursing and the departments concerned with financial management. Most clinical and nonclinical departments of the hospital are the responsibility of the COO. This would include departments such as pharmacy, laboratories, radiology, medical records, physical therapy, materials management, environmental services, facilities, security, and dietary services.

The CFO is responsible for the hospital's fiscal management, including the management of all revenues and expenses the hospital incurs. This usually includes departments responsible for financial accounting, patient accounting, and reimbursement management. In some cases, the CFO is also responsible for the hospital's information systems departments.

The director of nursing is responsible for the hospital's largest labor pool, its nurses. Nurses often represent as much as one-third of all hospital personnel. Nurses provide by far the greatest amount of direct patient care in a hospital. There are usually multiple nursing departments reporting to a director of nursing. These departments are frequently arranged by patient type. For example, a hospital may have medical, surgical, pediatric, critical care, and ambulatory nursing departments, each with a departmental director. Nurse managers report to the nursing directors, and each has responsibility for a particular patient care area.

In medium- to large-sized hospitals, that is, hospitals with more than 250 beds, a third level of hospital administrators may also be present to assist the COO and CFO in management. These "level 3" administrators may be called hospital assistant directors or vice presidents. They will each have administrative responsibility for several departments. Figure 3-1 illustrates a hospital organizational structure with three administrative levels. "Level 3" hospital administrators have hospital department heads reporting to them and serve as facilitators to ensure that the hospital's multiple departments are moving in a unified direction.

Department heads or department directors are the next level of management in a hospital. Since each nursing department may have a department director, as do financial departments, so do the other clinical and support departments of the hospital. These clinical and support department directors usually report to an assistant hospital director or to the COO. They have responsibility for managing and directing all aspects of a particular hospital service, such as a pharmacy service. Department directors have fiscal, operational, and patient care responsibilities for their individual services. The director of pharmaceutical services usually is a department director reporting to either a "level 2" or "level 3" administrator.

Although the hospital organizational structure described above and depicted in figure 3-1 may be commonly seen, others do exist. Hospitals organized along "product lines" are becoming more common. In this type of organizational structure, administrators exist for various groupings of patient types that the hospital treats. For example, there may be an administrator for pediatrics, for cardiovascular care, for oncology, etc. These administrators, in turn, will have responsibility for all services required to treat and manage these patient types. In this organizational structure, a director of pharmacy may report to multiple hospital administrators.

Finally, it should be noted that in several hospitals, the director of pharmacy position has been elevated to a hospital assistant director or vice president level. This is generally in recognition that the pharmacy is a very important and extensive clinical service. A unique reporting situation exists at the University of Texas M.D. Anderson Cancer Center in Houston. Here the pharmacy department is a clinical division within the Health Sciences Center, and the director of pharmacy reports directly to the vice president for health sciences rather than to a hospital administrator.[12] In this regard, it is recognized as similar to the medical clinical departments of the Health Sciences Center.

THE MEDICAL STAFF

The medical staff, and thus the medical clinical departments of a hospital, have a unique relationship with the hospital in that they generally are not considered hospital departments. This is because members of the medical staff of a hospital are usually not hospital employees as are nurses, pharmacists, and others. Usually the medical staff members are in private practice, and are thus self-employed. They may also be faculty members employed by a school of medicine. Physicians may also be employed by an HMO

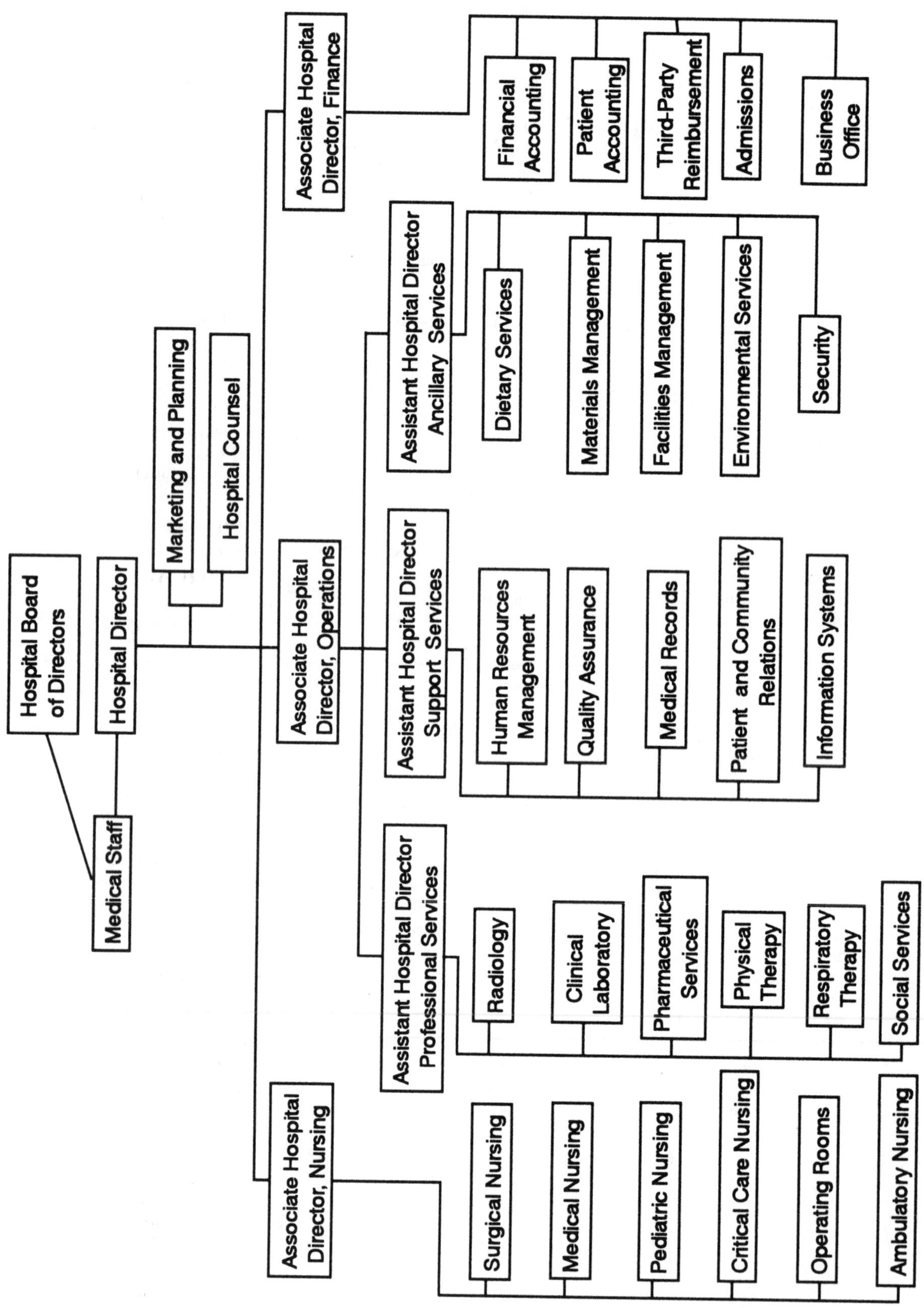

Figure 3-1. Example of a hospital organizational chart

that contracts with the hospital. In these circumstances, physicians are granted privileges to use the hospital to treat their patients. Medical departments, such as a department of medicine or pediatrics, are usually not hospital departments but rather departments of a medical school or departments of the medical staff itself.

In some cases, physicians may be employees of the hospital. Examples include hospitals that directly employ medical residents. Other medical staff might be hired and paid directly by a hospital, such as a physician who is the hospital's infection control officer.

Although not directly employed by the hospital, the medical staff has its own organizational structure linking it to the hospital's organization. The medical staff of the hospital usually elects a chief of staff, who will serve as its liaison to the hospital director. The chief of staff and the hospital director work together to resolve issues and to keep the hospital staff and medical staff working together to achieve mutual goals of providing quality patient care.

The medical staff itself is governed by an executive committee of the medical staff. This committee is responsible to the governing body of the hospital and comprises elected members of each major section of the medical staff. The hospital director is a member of this committee. The executive committee of the medical staff serves to oversee the activities of the medical staff in the hospital and is responsible for recommending the granting of clinical privileges to physicians. It is also responsible for conducting various quality assurance programs that ensure medical care is appropriate.

The executive committee of the medical staff usually delegates its responsibilities to several committees that report to it. These often include a pharmacy and therapeutics committee, a quality assurance committee, a credentialing committee, and others. These committees gather and analyze information and make recommendations to the executive committee.

THE MISSION AND PURPOSE OF THE DEPARTMENT OF PHARMACEUTICAL SERVICES

Departments of pharmaceutical services in hospitals today are responsible for providing and managing all aspects of drug use. This translates into the provision of comprehensive product and clinical pharmaceutical services or pharmaceutical care. A breakdown of the types of services provided will be discussed later in this chapter. The mission of a department of pharmaceutical services in a hospital is, therefore, to provide optimal drug therapy for all patients and to ensure the highest quality and most cost-effective care.[13] In addition, the mission of many departments of pharmaceutical services include teaching and generating new knowledge through research.

The department of pharmaceutical services is responsible to the hospital organization and to its patients. It works in conjunction with the medical and nursing staff of the hospital and the other hospital departments in providing service. A sample mission statement for a department of pharmaceutical services appears below:

> The mission of The University of Minnesota Hospital and Clinic, Department of Pharmaceutical Services is to provide a comprehensive range of clinical and product services which will assist in providing quality care to all patients. Specifically, the department will seek to ensure rational drug therapy and provide for a responsive and accurate drug distribution system in the inpatient and outpatient settings. These services shall foster research and provide a model for other institutions to follow. The department will provide teaching programs for practitioners, students, and the public. In these respects, the mission of the department is consistent with the mission of the hospital.

To achieve its mission, a department of pharmaceutical services will develop annual goals. These serve to guide and track accomplishments, assign responsibility, and provide clear direction. In today's practice environment, goals often include the expansion of clinical pharmacy services to improve drug therapy. As the mission of a department embraces management of all aspects of drug therapy, including ambulatory drug therapy, goals often include expanding or strengthening clinical pharmacy services provided to a hospital's clinic patient population.

ORGANIZATIONAL STRUCTURE OF THE DEPARTMENT OF PHARMACEUTICAL SERVICES

Director of Pharmaceutical Services

The director of pharmaceutical services is responsible for all pharmaceutical services delivered in the institution. This includes those provided by pharmacy department staff, pharmacy faculty, and in some cases, other health care professionals such as nurses, in the absence of a pharmacist. An example of the latter would be a nurse preparing an intravenous (IV) admixture on a nursing unit. The director is responsible for developing policies and procedures to guide the provision of pharmaceutical services and to see that they are carried out. JCAHO, the accrediting body for hospitals, stipulates requirements for pharmaceutical services in hospitals, and the *Practice Standards of ASHP* further define acceptable levels of pharmacy practice.[11,14]

Pharmaceutical services managed by the director of pharmaceutical services include both the preparation of drugs and the provision of clinical services, along with pharmaceutical teaching and research conducted in the hospital. These responsibilities extend to personnel management, management of drug expense and revenue, and ensuring appropriate quality of service.

Pharmacy Managers

The director of pharmaceutical services is also responsible for the selection of administrative staff for the department to manage day-to-day operations and the provision of services. The size and nature of a department's management staff will depend on the number of personnel in the department and the scope of services delivered. A small pharmacy department of 5-10 full-time equivalents (FTE's) may have a management staff of 1, the director. A medium-sized department of 20-40 FTE's may have 1-2 managers in addition to the director, whereas a large department of 100-150 FTE's, offering extensive pharmaceutical services, may have 7-10 managers. In general, most departments have 1 manager per 15-20 FTE's.

In larger departments, there may be multiple levels of management (see figure 3-2). For example, in addition to the director, there may be a level of associate and/or assistant directors. Reporting to these individuals may be a level of supervisors or coordinators. A smaller department may have only two levels of management, the director and either assistant directors or supervisors. Terminology applied to managers may also differ by department (see figure 3-3). For example, in some organizations, assistant or associate directors of pharmacy are simply called pharmacy managers. The organizational chart of a department of pharmaceutical services depicts management levels and the areas of responsibility of each manager.

Assistant and associate directors of pharmaceutical services represent the second level of management in many pharmacy departments. These individuals have responsibility for several departmental areas or services. For example, one assistant director may have responsibility for the IV admixture services, specialty clinical services, and ambulatory pharmacy services. A second assistant director may have responsibility for the unit dose services, general clinical services, and drug use evaluation.

As previously mentioned, in a small department, an assistant director may also have direct supervisory responsibilities, that is, be the only level of management between the director and the general staff. In medium-to-large departments, however, there is usually a level of management—the supervisors—between the assistant directors and the general staff. Supervisors, coordinators, or "line" managers are responsible for directly managing people to ensure production and distribution of drugs and provision of clinical services. Supervisors are usually responsible for one area of the department or one type of service. For example, a supervisor or coordinator may have responsibility for the ambulatory pharmacy or for general clinical pharmacy services.

Supervisors evaluate employee performance and manage issues as they arise. They often spend 50 percent or more of their time directly providing services to their area of responsibility. A clinical coordinator is a type of supervisor who manages aspects of clinical services. In departments with extensive clinical pharmacy services, all supervisors may be clinical supervisors and have responsibility for both product and clinical services for a specific part of the hospital, specific patient types, or a section of the department. For example, one supervisor may have responsibility for critical care pharmacy services, which would include a satellite pharmacy providing drug product to the critical care units and also pharmacists providing both general and specialty clinical pharmacy services to those areas. A second supervisor may have responsibility for the outpatient pharmacy and also the clinical pharmacy services delivered to the hospital's clinics and emergency room.

Examples of Organizational Structure

Departments of pharmaceutical services increasingly are becoming clinical departments with the expansion of the provision of clinical pharmacy services. This fact is prompting many departments to reevaluate organizational structures to integrate management responsibilities for both product and clinical services to maximize quality of service delivered. Departments in the early stages of clinical pharmacy development often separate management responsibility for product and clinical services. This may take the form of a department, for example, with an assistant director for clinical services and other assistant directors dividing responsibility for product services. This type of organizational structure often assists a department to more rapidly develop and justify clinical services. Departments that have well-established clinical services may find it to their benefit, from both a resource and quality-of-service standpoint, to eliminate the separation of the management of clinical pharmacy and product services.[13] Elimination of this separation may allow for a further expansion of clinical services. Figures 3-2 and 3-3 illustrate sample organizational structures for small and large pharmacy departments with well-developed clinical pharmacy services.

PERSONNEL IN A DEPARTMENT OF PHARMACEUTICAL SERVICES

Personnel in a department of pharmaceutical services can generally be divided into three categories: professional, technical, and support. Most departments of pharmaceutical services have staff of all three types. Individual State board of pharmacy rules and regulations may govern the number of technical and support personnel in relation to the number of pharmacists in a department. The activities that may be performed by nonprofessional personnel in hospital pharmacies may also be stipulated.

Professional personnel comprise all pharmacists, including general practitioners, clinical pharmacists, clinical specialists, management staff, and pharmacy residents. In some departments of pharmaceutical services, all pharmacists provide both product or dispensing services and clinical or drug therapy monitoring services. In a growing number of departments, however, pharmacists are specialized and may provide either predominantly product or predominantly clinical services. In the latter situation, these hospital pharmacists may be referred to as clinical pharmacists. Because the practice of institutional pharmacy is evolving, it is expected that in the future, all pharmacists will be clinical pharmacists or will spend the majority of their time providing direct patient care services, and that the preparation and distribution of drug product will be more highly automated and largely dependent on technical personnel.

A further specialization has occurred in some departments, where select pharmacists provide intensive, full-time clinical services to specific patient groups and are called clinical specialists. Examples include clinical pharmacy specialists in the areas of critical care, infectious disease, cardiology, neonatology, nutrition, and pediatrics.

Technical Personnel

The technical personnel category of a department of pharmaceutical services comprises pharmacy technicians. These are typically nonlicensed personnel who have received special training, which may have been provided at their place of employment or by the growing number of technical and vocational schools that offer pharmacy technician training programs.[15] The American Society of

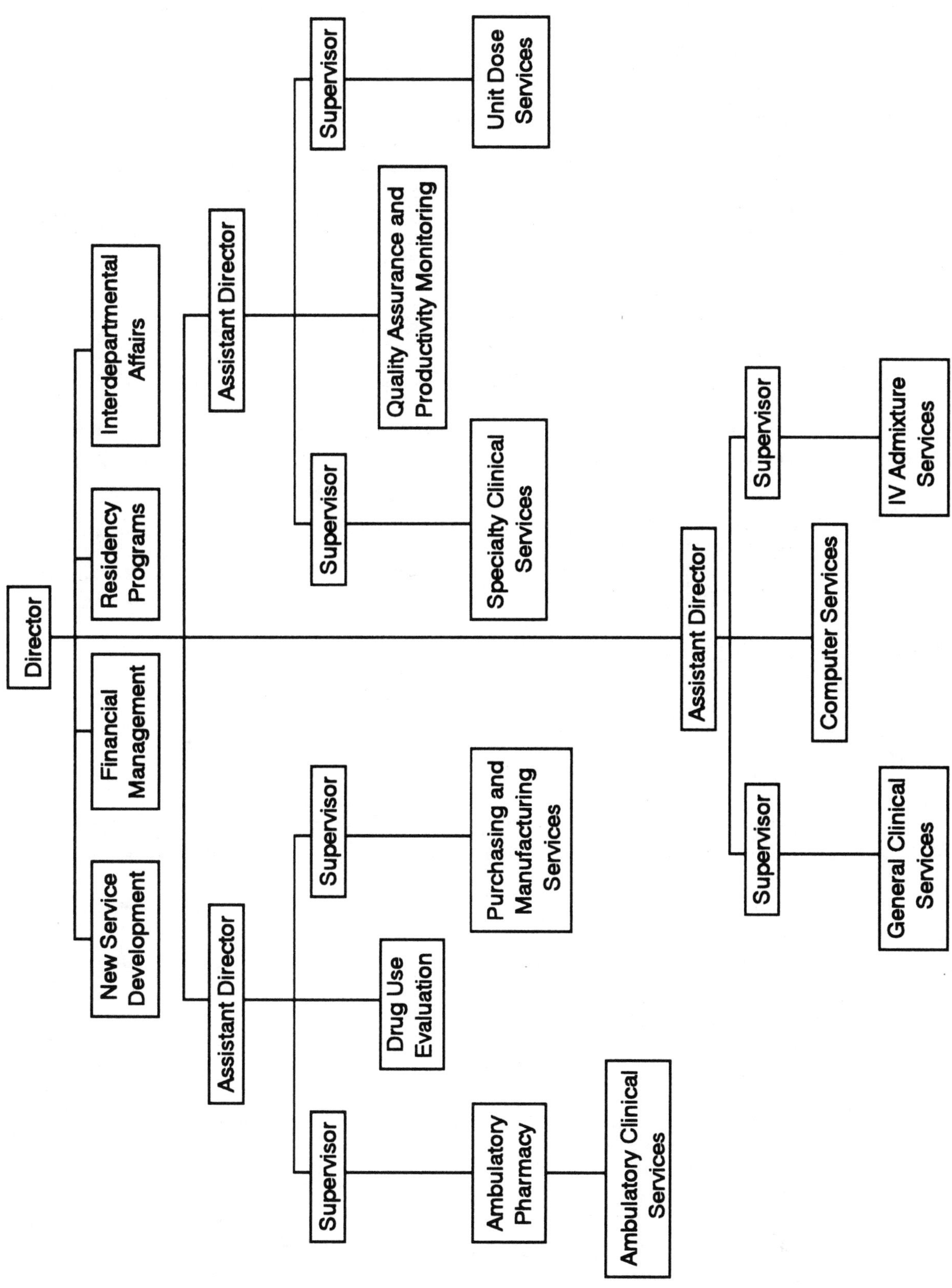

Figure 3-2. Example of an organizational chart for a large department of pharmaceutical services

Hospital Pharmacists (ASHP) accredits pharmacy technician training programs conducted in hospitals and vocational schools.[14] Although no State (at time of publication) requires certification or licensing of pharmacy technicians, two State pharmacy societies (in Michigan and Illinois) offer a technician certification exam.[15] The trend for certification of pharmacy technicians has clearly begun, as has the expansion of the technician's role to provide more product pharmaceutical services that do not require the professional judgment of a pharmacist, thus freeing the pharmacist to provide expanded clinical services. Examples of activities performed by technicians under the supervision of pharmacists (dependent on individual State board of pharmacy regulations) include the preparation of IV admixtures and the filling of unit dose medication carts.

Other support personnel in a department of pharmaceutical services may include secretaries, buyers, and clerks. These individuals generally account for less than 10 percent of total departmental personnel.

SCOPE OF PHARMACEUTICAL SERVICES PROVIDED IN INSTITUTIONS

Pharmaceutical services offered in hospitals may be categorized as product, clinical, teaching, research, and other support services. They may be further differentiated by whether they are provided to either hospitalized patients or ambulatory patients. As mentioned, in some departments of pharmaceutical services, both product and clinical services

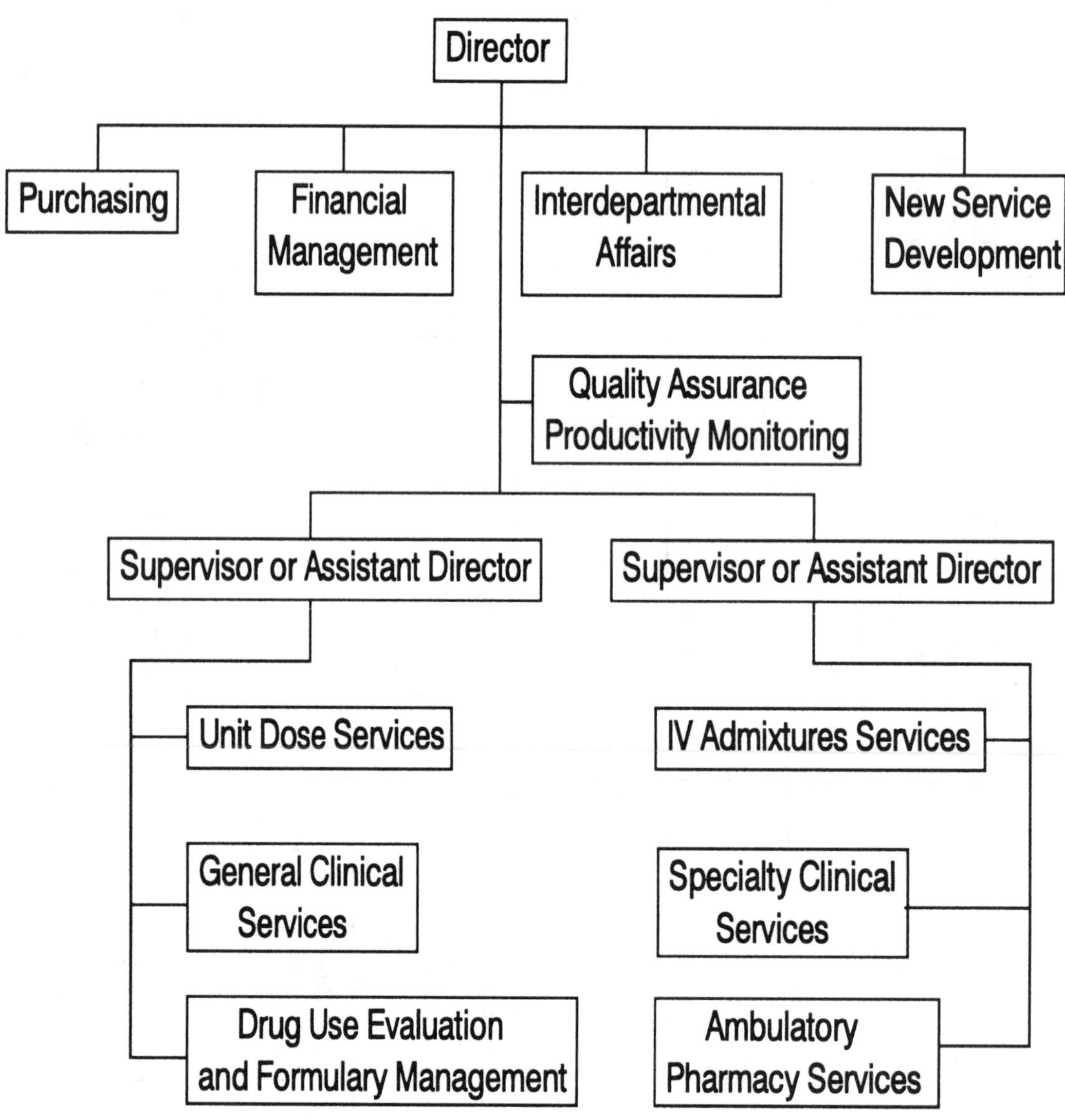

Figure 3-3. Example of an organizational chart for a small department of pharmaceutical services

are provided by all pharmacists, whereas in others specialization exists.

Product Services for Hospitalized Patients

Contemporary product pharmaceutical services for hospitalized patients include the preparation and provision of all drugs and intravenous solutions in unit use form, appropriately labeled, and delivered to the patient care area in a timely fashion. This is accomplished via unit dose and IV admixture drug distribution systems. These types of drug distribution systems minimize prescribing errors, preparation and administration errors, waste, drug inventories, and drug costs.[16-19]

In a unit dose drug distribution system, a pharmacist first reviews a direct copy of the physician's order. Before dispensing, the pharmacist evaluates the order for appropriateness of the drug for the disease state being treated, dose, route, and frequency. This also includes a review of the patient's drug profile for drug interactions, therapeutic duplication, and drug allergies. These clinical pharmacy functions are part of all unit dose drug distribution systems. Drugs are usually prepared and dispensed in a 24-hour supply, with each dose individually labeled with the drug name and dose to reduce medication errors. Pharmacy intravenous admixture services provide all IV drugs in unit of use form using aseptic preparation techniques in a laminar flow cabinet. This minimizes solution contamination, errors in preparation and labeling, errors in administration, and waste.[18,19] A more thorough description of these systems appears later in this handbook.

Unit dose and IV admixture services may be provided from central pharmacies, satellite pharmacies, mobile drug carts, or a combination thereof.[20-24] In some hospitals, satellite pharmacies have been established when adequate mechanical delivery systems for drugs do not exist, or when multiple hospital buildings preclude the timely delivery of drugs to patient care areas. Satellite pharmacies have also been established to serve intensive care units, operating rooms, emergency rooms, and day hospital units to provide the necessary level of pharmacy services required by these areas. Pharmacy computer systems are used extensively in the provision of inpatient pharmacy services. In addition, more and more hospital pharmacies are beginning to use automated drug preparation and distribution devices.[25]

Product Services for Ambulatory Patients

Frequently, hospitals operate ambulatory pharmacies to serve the medication needs of patients to be discharged from the hospital and patients seen in hospital clinics, emergency rooms, and physician office buildings, and to provide hospital employees with a prescription service. These ambulatory pharmacies may be located within the inpatient pharmacy area or in separate locations.

Services provided by ambulatory pharmacies in hospitals parallel those of community pharmacies in that pharmacists review all prescriptions for appropriateness, duplication, drug interactions, and allergies. Patient education and counseling is provided, as well as the maintenance of patient drug profiles. Hospital outpatient pharmacies may also provide over-the-counter medications and medical supplies.

Outpatient pharmacy services in hospitals may differ from those provided by community pharmacies in that more extensive clinical services can be provided, because the pharmacist has immediate access to complete patient data from both hospitalization and clinic visits. In addition, hospital outpatient pharmacies often prepare and provide drug products that are not available in community pharmacies, such as investigational drugs, select controlled substances, intravenous products, and specialty products. Advanced computer systems often linked with automated prescription-filling devices are being used increasingly by hospital ambulatory pharmacies.[25] These systems also have the capability of electronically billing third-party payers for prescriptions and interfacing with HMO and PPO systems to determine formulary status of drugs prescribed for patients who are part of these health care plans.

Clinical Services for Hospitalized Patients

Clinical pharmacy services have been growing at a rapid rate over the past 10-20 years. They are offered to ensure that drug therapy is appropriate and cost effective.[1-3,26-34] Clinical pharmacy services may be provided by pharmacists who also provide product services, or by a distinct group of pharmacists who specialize in the provision of these direct patient care services. Clinical pharmacy services at a minimum include formulary system management, drug use evaluation, maintenance of patient drug profiles, and review of every drug order for therapeutic appropriateness.[1,35] These services may be provided by pharmacists who work in a central pharmacy or in satellite pharmacies, or they may be performed by decentralized or clinical pharmacists. This level of clinical service provision is offered as part of the unit dose drug distribution system.

Many departments of pharmaceutical services offer clinical pharmacy services to inpatients beyond those described as part of the unit dose drug distribution system. These services may be provided by pharmacists who typically work in a central or satellite pharmacy but spend time outside of the pharmacy on the patient care unit. However, they are more often provided by pharmacists who spend all of their time as decentralized or clinical pharmacists.

Decentralized clinical pharmacists may be assigned to provide clinical services for a geographic area of the hospital (e.g., two nursing units), for a specific medical or surgical service (e.g., the cardiology service or the gastroenterology service), or for all patients hospital-wide on a particular therapy (e.g., total parenteral nutrition patients, patients receiving antibiotics, etc.). Services provided by decentralized clinical pharmacists include medication histories, provision of drug information, consultation in the selection and change of drug therapy, therapeutic drug monitoring (including the pharmacokinetic dosing of all appropriate drugs), selection of the most appropriate drug delivery device, accompanying the medical team on rounds, and discharge consultation.

In addition to these general clinical pharmacy services, departments of pharmaceutical services may provide various specialty clinical pharmacy services. These services are usually provided by full-time clinical pharmacy specialists and focus on patients receiving extremely intensive and complex drug therapy. For example, pharmacy clinical specialists may provide services to critical care, nutritional support, infectious disease, and transplantation services. Other pharmacy clinical specialists may provide drug information services through a formal drug information center, or manage a pharmacokinetic consultation service or a drug use evaluation service. These latter clinical specialists provide hospital-wide clinical services. The provision and organization of clinical pharmacy services offered to hospitalized patients vary and are dependent upon and integrated with the systems used to provide pharmacy product services.

Clinical Services for Ambulatory Patients

Ambulatory clinical services offered by hospital pharmacies are growing beyond those traditionally offered when prescriptions are dispensed, such as patient counseling, maintenance of patient drug profiles, and drug interaction monitoring. Ambulatory clinical pharmacists in hospitals are becoming increasingly involved in the selection and monitoring of drug therapy for patients seen in a hospital's clinics.[36-38]

In some settings, pharmacists participate in clinics to enhance or manage drug therapy. Medication counseling clinics have been established by some hospitals to see patients referred by physicians when noncompliance is suspected.[39] Some have demonstrated a dramatic improvement in disease state control when pharmacists are integrally involved in compliance enhancement.[40] Refill clinics and medication monitoring clinics, managed by pharmacists, exist to see patients when the purpose of the visit is a medication-related problem or when a refill on a prescription is required and a decision needs to be made.[41,42] Pharmacy-directed primary care clinics have also been established.[43,44] Here pharmacists see patients, as referred by physicians, to adjust drug therapy and monitor outcome. Pharmacy-directed specialty clinics have also been developed where there has been proven benefit from clinical pharmacists managing the drug therapy of select patient types. Examples include anticoagulant clinics, hypertension clinics, and others.[45-48] Usually pharmacy-directed clinics operate by protocols established by an institution's pharmacy and therapeutics committee. In addition, many departments of pharmaceutical services are becoming providers of home IV therapy.[49] This service includes both product and clinical management and may be provided solely by the hospital or in cooperation with a commercial home care vendor.

Teaching and Research

All departments of pharmaceutical services are involved in teaching. Teaching activities include in-service education to pharmacy, nursing, and medical staff regarding new pharmaceutical services and drug therapy. Many departments serve as teaching sites for pharmacy students. In addition, residencies accredited by the ASHP are offered by many departments and provide postgraduate education and training in the areas of general hospital pharmacy, clinical pharmacy, and specialty practice areas. Specialty practice residencies are offered in the areas of administration, adult internal medicine, ambulatory care, clinical pharmacokinetics, critical care, drug information, geriatrics, nutritional support, oncology, pediatrics, and psychopharmacy.

Many departments of pharmaceutical services conduct active research programs. They include the management of investigational drugs studies, research conducted to evaluate new drugs and new drug therapies, and the evaluation of drug delivery systems. Research on new types of pharmaceutical services, products used in the delivery of those services, and the effect of pharmaceutical services on the quality and cost of care may also be performed. Finally, a growing area of pharmacy research focuses on the effect of ambulatory clinical pharmacy services on patient outcome.

Pharmacy fellowships designed to teach research skills are selectively available for students who have completed a residency and desire to further their experience in this area. Fellows work with preceptor pharmacists who are actively involved in research.

Support Services

Departments of pharmaceutical services provide support functions for drug distribution and clinical services. These typically include the purchase of drugs, inventory management, manufacture of drugs or dosage forms not commercially available, repackaging of drugs, maintenance of computer systems, and various clerical activities.

FUTURE DIRECTIONS FOR INSTITUTIONAL PHARMACEUTICAL SERVICES

Departments of pharmaceutical services in hospitals strive to provide comprehensive services. Clinical pharmacy services that have been shown to have a significant impact on the quality of care by optimizing drug therapy will continue to expand. To do so, pharmacy departments will continue the process of automating the preparation and distribution of drugs.[50] In addition, the roles and responsibilities of pharmacy technicians will grow.[14] In the future, various aspects of clinical pharmacy services may become automated.

It can be argued that the department of pharmaceutical services of the future will include an automated dispensary staffed primarily by certified pharmacy technicians who prepare specialized dosage forms, supervised by a minimal number of pharmacists. All other pharmacists will be decentralized, providing clinical pharmacy services to both hospitalized and ambulatory patients.[51] Pharmacists will be involved in maintaining data bases for automated drug information systems, monitoring, and managing drug therapy.

It might be expected that, in the years to come, the majority of all pharmacists' time will be spent in the provision of clinical pharmacy services or the pharmaceutical care of their patients.

REFERENCES

1. Abramowitz PW: Controlling financial variables: Changing prescribing patterns. *Am J Hosp Pharm* 41:503-513, 1984.
2. Hatoum HT, Catizone C, et al: An eleven year review of the pharmacy literature: Documentation of the value and acceptance of clinical pharmacy. *Drug Intell Clin Pharm* 20:33-48, 1986.

3. Ambrose PJ, Smith WE, Palarea ER: A decade of experience with a clinical pharmacokinetics service. *Am J Hosp Pharm* 45:1879-1886, 1988.
4. *Hospital Statistics*, 1989-90 ed. Chicago, American Hospital Association, 1990.
5. Moore WB: CEO's plan resource shift for 1986. *Hospitals* 59:69-72, 1985.
6. Anon: Pharmacy in the twenty-first century: Results of a strategic planning conference. *Am J Hosp Pharm* 42:71-80, 1985.
7. Rakish JS, Longest BB, Darr KD: The health care delivery system. In *Managing Health Service Organizations*. Philadelphia, W.B. Saunders, 1985, pp. 27-79.
8. Hassan WE: The hospital and its organization. In *Hospital Pharmacy*. Philadelphia, Lea & Febiger, 1986, pp. 35-59.
9. Rowland HS, Rowland BL: The hospital organization. In *Hospital Management: A Guide to Departments*. Rockville, MD, Aspen, 1984, pp. 1-13.
10. *Guide to the Health Care Field*, 1989 ed. Chicago, American Hospital Association, 1990.
11. *Accreditation Manual for Hospitals 1990*. Chicago, Joint Commission on Accreditation of Health Care Organizations, 1990.
12. Anderson RW: Strategic planning for clinical services: The University of Texas M.D. Anderson Hospital and Tumor Institute. *Am J Hosp Pharm* 43:2169-2173, 1986.
13. Abramowitz PW, Scott B: Retooling pharmacy departments: Constructing the foundation for the transition to clinical practice. *Top Hosp Pharm Mgt* 9:1-17, 1989.
14. American Society of Hospital Pharmacists. *Practice Standards of ASHP 1991-92*. Bethesda, MD: American Society of Hospital Pharmacists, 1991.
15. Woller TW, Ploetz PA: Expanding the role of the pharmacy technician. *Top Hosp Pharm Mgt* 9:35-49, 1989.
16. Barker KN: Effects of an experimental medication system on medication errors. Part 1: Introduction and error studies. *Am J Hosp Pharm* 26:324-333, 1969.
17. Barker KN: Effects of an experimental medication system on medication errors. Part 2: The cost study. *Am J Hosp Pharm* 26:388-397, 1969.
18. Mitchell SR: Monitoring waste in a intravenous admixture program. *Am J Hosp Pharm* 44:106-110, 1978.
19. Sebastian G, Thielke TS: Work analysis of an admixture service. *Am J Hosp Pharm* 40:21, 49-53, 1983.
20. Castile JA, Castile RG, O'Connell EJ: Implementation and operation of a hospital pediatric satellite pharmacy. *Hosp Pharm* 15:237-240, 1980
21. Horton RG: A satellite pharmacy program in a community hospital. *Hosp Pharm* 16:74-79, 1981.
22. Caldwell RD, Tuck BA: Justification and operation of a critical-care satellite pharmacy. *Am J Hosp Pharm* 40:2141-2145, 1983.
23. Noel MW, McCoy LK, Bootman JL, et al: Management case study: Development, evaluation, and impact of mobile decentralized pharmacy services. *Top Hosp Pharm Mgt* 2:62-77, 1983.
24. Adelman DN, Friedeman L: The mobile medication cart as an adjunct to a centralized pharmacy service. *Hosp Pharm* 20:663-665, 1985.
25. Somani SM, Woller TW: Automating the drug distribution system. *Top Hosp Pharm Mgt* 9:19-34, 1989.
26. Abramowitz PW, Nold EG, Hatfield SM: Use of clinical pharmacists to reduce cefamandole, cefoxitin and ticarcillin costs. *Am J Hosp Pharm* 39:1176-1180, 1982.
27. Herfindal ET, Bernstein LR, Kishi DT: Effect of clinical pharmacy services on prescribing on an orthopedic unit. *Am J Hosp Pharm* 40:1945-1951, 1983.
28. Covinsky JO, Hambuger S, Twin EJ: A look at the educational responsibilities and cost impact of the decentralized clinical pharmacist. *Drug Intell Clin Pharm* 266-271, 1980.
29. Sveska KJ, Rome BD, Solomon DK, et al: Outcome of patients treated by an aminoglycoside pharmacokinetic dosing service. *Am J Hosp Pharm* 42:2472-2478, 1985.
30. Bertch KE, Hatoum HT, Willet MS, et al: Cost justification of clinical pharmacy services on a general surgery team: Focus on diagnosis-related group cases. *Drug Intell Clin Pharm* 22:906-911, 1988.
31. Miyagawa CL, Rivera JO: Effect of pharmacist interventions on drug therapy costs in a surgical intensive-care unit. *Am J Hosp Pharm* 43:3008-3013, 1986.
32. Hatoum HT, Hutchinson RA, Witte KW, et al: Evaluation of the contribution of clinical pharmacists: Inpatient care and cost reduction. *Drug Intell Clin Pharm* 22:252-259, 1988.
33. Claphan CE, Helper CD, Reinders TP: Economic consequences of two drug use control systems in a teaching hospital. *Am J Hosp Pharm* 45:2329-2340, 1988.
34. Herfindal ET, Bernstein LR, Kishi DT: Impact of clinical pharmacy services on prescribing on a cardiothoracic/vascular surgical unit. *Drug Intell Clin Pharm* 19:440-444, 1985.
35. Abramowitz PW, Fletcher CV: Let's expand the formulary system and renew its vigor. *Am J Hosp Pharm* 43:2834-2838, 1984.
36. Brown DJ, Helling DK, Jones ME: Evaluation of clinical pharmacist consultations in a family practice office. *Am J Hosp Pharm* 36:912-915, 1979.
37. Helling DK: Family practice pharmacy service: Part 1. *Drug Intell Clin Pharm* 15:971-977, 1981.
38. Helling DK: Family practice pharmacy service: Part 2. *Drug Intell Clin Pharm* 16:35-38, 1982.
39. Schneider P, Cable G: Compliance clinic: An opportunity for an expanded practice role for pharmacists. *Am J Hosp Pharm* 35:288-295, 1978.
40. Bond CA, Monson R: Sustained improvement in drug documentation, compliance, and disease control—a four year analysis of an ambulatory care model. *Arch Intern Med* 144:1159-1162, 1984.
41. D'Achille KM, Swanson LN, Hill WT: Pharmacist managed patient assessment and medication refill clinic. *Am J Hosp Pharm* 35:66-70, 1978.
42. Scrivens JJ Jr, Magalian P, Crazier GA: Cost effective clinical pharmacy services in a Veterans Administration drop-in clinic. *Am J Hosp Pharm* 40:1952-1953, 1983.
43. Erickson SH: Primary care by a pharmacist in an outpatient clinic. *Am J Hosp Pharm* 34:1089-1090, 1977.
44. Anderson PO, Taryle DA: Pharmacist management of ambulatory patients using formalized standards of care. *Am J Hosp Pharm* 31:254-257, 1974.
45. Reinders T, Steinke WE: Pharmacist management of anticoagulant therapy in ambulant patients. *Am J Hosp Pharm* 36:645-648, 1979.
46. Menard PJ, Kirshner BS, Kloth DD, et al: Management of the hypertensive patient by the pharmacist prescriber. *Hosp Pharm* 21:20-35, 1986.
47. Gray DR, Garabedian-Ruffalo SM, Chreitien SD: Cost-justification of a clinical pharmacist-managed anti-coagulation clinic. *Drug Intell Clin Pharm* 19:575-580, 1985.
48. Edwards R, Adams DW: Clinical pharmacy services in a pediatric ambulatory care clinic. *Drug Intell Clin Pharm* 16:939-944, 1982.
49. Chamberlain TM, Lehman ME, Groth MJ, et al: Cost analysis of a home intravenous antibiotic program. *Am J Hosp Pharm* 45:2341-2345, 1988.
50. Abramowitz PW, Daniels CE: Capturing existing resources and reallocating to clinical pharmaceutical services. *Top Hosp Pharm Mgt* 9:63-81, 1989.
51. Abramowitz PW, Mansur JM: Moving toward the provision of comprehensive ambulatory care pharmaceutical services. *Am J Hosp Pharm* 44:1155-1163, 1987.

CHAPTER 4

Marketing

MICKEY C. SMITH

Every practicing pharmacist is involved in marketing. Just as one can't *not* communicate, anyone providing a service or product to others can't *not* market. Pharmacists who are unaware of the marketing function that they perform risk doing it poorly. Acknowledgment of the importance of marketing to the practice of pharmacy will not guarantee that one will do it well, but it is certainly an important step in the proper direction.

In this chapter we will concentrate more on the philosophy of marketing pharmaceutical services in institutions than on techniques (see table 4-1). This choice is based on our judgment that marketing must be sold to pharmacists before it can be taught to them. We are way behind in this, because educators in the last couple of decades have eschewed instruction in marketing, favoring instruction in the clinical area. If we achieve nothing else here, we hope to show that, over the long term, good pharmacy *practice* (our products and services) can be more effective through good pharmacy *marketing*.

SOME DEFINITIONS

The latest definition of "marketing" from the American Marketing Association is as follows:

> Marketing is the process of planning and executing the conception, pricing, promotion, and distribution of ideas, goods, and services to create exchanges that satisfy individual and organizational objectives.[1]

A somewhat more practical definition is that of Hillestad and Berkowitz[2]:

> Marketing is the process of *understanding* customer wants and needs, *listening* to those wants and needs, and then, to whatever extent possible, *designing* appropriate programs and services to meet those wants and needs in a timely, cost-effective, competitive fashion. It is the process of molding the organization to the market, rather than convincing the market that the organization provides what they need.

Both of these definitions make it clear that in a successful marketing program, everyone benefits. Whether or not the pharmacy administrator recognizes it, he or she regularly engages in what may be called marketing activities. Marketing is a discipline that can be used not only to *attain* management objectives, but also to *identify* them. Kotler[3] defines marketing as "the effective management by an organization of its exchange relations with its various markets and publics." The central concepts underlying marketing are communication and the exchange of value for value. Marketing is more than a promotional or selling effort to increase and satisfy demand for existing products and services; rather, it seeks to identify and respond to the needs, differences, and perceptions of its clients or consumers.

Pathak[4] has described the exchange process in marketing:

> Although most definitions of exchange and marketing revolve around dyadic or restricted exchanges (two-party reciprocal relationships), exchange relationships in modern society are becoming more complicated because of specialization due to division of labor, the use of money as a medium of exchange, and the increasing number of participants. Complex exchanges (a system of mutual relationships between at least three parties) and interactive exchanges are more commonplace in today's society, especially in the pharmaceutical marketplace.
>
> Pharmaceutical marketing, as a subspeciality of marketing, can be defined as a process by which a market for pharmaceutical care is actualized. It encompasses all the activities carried out by various individuals or organizations to actualize markets for pharmaceutical care.
>
> The emphasis in pharmaceutical marketing is on pharmaceutical care, and not just on drugs. Any article, service (see table 4-1), or idea needed to anticipate and to remove gaps in pharmaceutical care should be included in the discussion of pharmaceutical marketing. The marketing of many clinical pharmaceutical services and programs is as much a part of pharmaceutical marketing as is the marketing of drug products. In other words, pharmaceutical marketing is not synonymous with, but is significantly broader than, the marketing of pharmaceuticals.
>
> The emphasis in this definition is on pharmaceutical care, indicating that the justification for the existence of pharmaceutical marketing is the patient, and not the manufacturer or the pharmacist.
>
> Any party interested in the exchange for pharmaceutical care may undertake pharmaceutical marketing activities. Hospital pharmacies, community

pharmacies, third-party insurance companies, consulting pharmacies, and many other organizations and individuals, in addition to pharmaceutical manufacturers and drug wholesalers, are involved in pharmaceutical marketing.

Table 4-1. Service marketing

Special considerations of marketers of service

1. Services cannot be stockpiled.
2. The entire service mix is usually not visible to the consumer.
3. The intangibility of services makes pricing difficult.
4. The intangibility of services makes promotion difficult.
5. The existence of a direct service organization-consumer relationship makes employee public relations skills important.
6. Services often have high costs and low reliability.
7. Peripheral services are frequently needed to supplement the basic service offering.

Basic differences between services and products

Services	Products
1. Services are often intangible. Services are acts, deeds, performances, efforts. Most services cannot be physically possessed. The value of a service is based on an experience; there is no transfer of title.	1. Products are tangible. Products are objects, things, materials. The value of a product is based on ownership; transfer of title takes place.
2. Services are usually perishable. Unused capacity cannot be stored or shifted from one time to another.	2. Products can be stored; product surpluses in one period can be applied against product shortages in another period.
3. Services are frequently inseparable. One cannot separate the quality of many services from the service provider.	3. Products can be graded or built to specifications. The quality of a product can be differentiated from a distribution channel member's quality.
4. Services may vary in quality over time. It is difficult to standardize some services because of their labor intensiveness and the involvement of the service user in diagnosing his or her service needs.	4. Products can be standardized through mass production and quality control.

MARKETING PLANNING

Successful marketing requires careful planning. Many pharmacy directors have a reasonably good system for determining and controlling expenses and mistakenly believe that this is an annual planning or market planning process. Others confuse budgeting with planning. Although budgeting and forecasting are important in the development of market plans, they are not the sole ingredients for a market plan, which, when completed, will contain answers to such questions as those shown in table 4-2.

A typical marketing planning sequence should include the following six steps:

1. Setting the mission.
2. Conducting an internal and external analysis.
3. Determining the strategy action match and marketing objectives.
4. Developing action strategies and marketing mix.
5. Integrating the plan and making revisions.
6. Providing appropriate control procedures, feedback, and integration of all plans into a unified effort.

Table 4-2. Some marketing planning questions

Where is the market?
1. Needs and demands.

Where are you now?
2. As an institution?
3. As a department?
4. As an individual?
5. With respect to the environment and competition?
6. With respect to capabilities and opportunities?

Where do you want to go?
7. Assumptions and potentials.
8. Objectives and goals.

How do you want to get there?
9. Policies and procedures and levels of initiative.
10. Strategies and programs.

When do you want to arrive?
11. Priorities and schedules.

Who is responsible?
12. Organization and delegation.

How much will it cost?
13. Budgets and resource allocations?

How will you know if you did it?
14. Feedback and review sessions.
15. Continuous monitoring.

THE MISSION

Definition of pharmacy mission has an intimate, chicken-and-egg relationship to market boundary definition. On the one hand, mission must be defined, at least in part, in terms of market scope. On the other hand, the market scope should emerge from the mission. "Mission" is a broad term that refers to the total perspectives or purpose of a pharmacy. Traditionally, the mission of a *business* corporation was framed around its product(s), and mottoes such as "Our business is textiles," "We manufacture cameras," and so on were the norm. In contrast, consider the mission statement in Glaxo Laboratories annual report (1987):

> We are in the business of providing pharmaceutical products of the highest quality that alleviate pain and suffering and enhance human health and longevity.
>
> To this end we commit all of our efforts to the discovery, development, production and marketing of medicines of the highest quality and efficacy.

The mission is neither a statement of current activities nor a random extension of current involvements. It signifies the scope and nature of the pharmacy service, not just as it is today, but as it could be in the future. The mission plays an important role in evaluating opportunities for diversification.

The mission deals with the questions: What type of services do we want to offer at some future time? What do we want to become? At any given point in time, most of the resources are frozen or locked into their current uses, and the outputs in services and/or products are, for the most part, defined by current operations. Over an interval of a few years, however, environmental changes place demands on the business for new types of resources; pharmacy management has the option of choosing the environment in which the pharmacy department will operate and acquiring commensurate new resources rather than replacing the old ones in kind. This explains the importance of defining the mission. The mission should be so defined that it has a bearing on both strengths and weaknesses.

In order to arrive at a mission statement for a pharmacy department, it is valuable to have input from the various constituencies of hospital or clinic. A difficulty in developing market-based plans in health care is the *number of constituencies* whose opinions must be assessed. Examples of these many groups are shown in figure 4-1.

INTERNAL AND EXTERNAL ANALYSIS

The first consideration in the strategic process is to recognize the individuals and groups that have an interest in the fate and nature of the pharmacy department and the extent and nature of their expectations (see figure 4-1).

In order to apply the marketing approach to its activities, the pharmacy must develop a marketing perspective: an awareness of and sensitivity to the exchange relationships it depends on for its very existence. This calls for first identifying the groups or markets with which the pharmacy director and pharmacy staff exchange values. Primary internal markets for pharmacy are the organization itself and the patient population. In a hospital, other internal markets are the medical staff, other departments' employees, volunteers, and trustees. External pharmacy markets include the community, families, visitors, suppliers, regulators, donors and supporters, professional associations, and colleagues employed elsewhere.

The exchanges between a pharmacy and its markets can be very complex and vary with each individual encounter. The values exchanged between a pharmacy staff member and the organization involve wages or salary, fringe benefits, security, social rewards, and feelings of accomplishment and responsibility in exchange for the pharmacist's time, effort, loyalty, and support of organizational objectives. Patients exchange money, approval, and gratitude for pharmacy care, relief of symptoms, pain, and anxiety, health teaching, primary preventive measures, and attentiveness.

Examination of the pharmacist-physician relationship from an exchange of values perspective is a complex exercise. Within the entire hospital organization, the physician exchanges patient referrals in return for a fully equipped workplace, service, prestige, and a number of conveniences. Pharmacy service is part of this exchange, but what the pharmacist receives of value is not as easy to define (see final section of this chapter). In addition to being consumers of services, physicians have been called marketing intermediaries, the sales force of the hospital, and competitors. The attending physician is responsible for admitting the patient, providing medical care, and writing orders for medications, treatments, and patient activities that the pharmacist carries out. Therefore, the pharmacist does not have complete control of all of his or her exchange relationships with the patient and physician. In order to apply a marketing approach to pharmacy administration, internal and external markets with which the nursing division exchanges values must be identified, segmented, and analyzed. A marketing information and research program can be designed to systematically monitor the attitudes and desires of these markets so that strategies can be developed to satisfy them.

The attitudes, perceptions, needs, and wants of the market must be monitored in some systematic way so that strategies can be developed for satisfying them. This is done by means of various types of marketing research and feedback systems that collect, process, and analyze information. The motivation for new or continuing pharmacy services should not be emotional enthusiasm but marketing information that objectively identifies the potential markets, market needs, and financial feasibility of services.

The pharmacy director must consider present and future needs to forecast volume and frequency of demands for services, and the types of programs and services desired and required by patients, physicians, and staff. He or she must

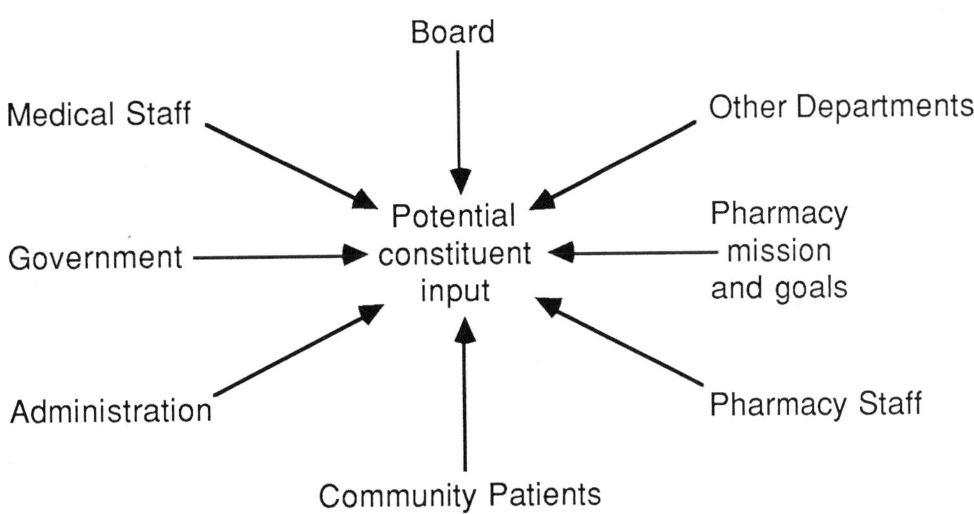

Figure 4-1. Potential constituents who influence the pharmacy's mission

project the reimbursement demands, the numbers of pharmacy personnel, and the skills and knowledge personnel will need to meet at least some of the needs, preferences, and expectations of patients, physicians, and other markets. These demands are not created by market research, but their discovery can lead to a more efficient, effective, and appropriate exchange of values.

Qualitative Studies

Markets often have perceptions of their needs that differ from the pharmacy administrator's perceptions of their desires and expectations. In the qualitative phase, the market segments are given an opportunity to verify or challenge the administrator's assumptions. Feedback can be solicited from patients, families, visitors, nurses, physicians, personnel department, patient representatives, and others.

The director can use focus group discussions to identify general attitudes toward the services provided and those that are desired by patients or to identify pharmacy staff attitudes and needs. The in-depth individual interview may be used in lieu of focus group discussions or to clarify issues raised by a focus group.

Quantitative Studies

Questionnaires and brief personal or telephone interviews are the survey techniques most often used for quantitative market research. Existing internal and external sources should be tapped before new survey research instruments are developed so that market research studies complement existing marketing information rather than duplicate it. Because quantitative research can be very costly in time and money, it is essential that the pharmacy director seek expert assistance if he or she does not have the research skills necessary to plan and execute the studies. Even with careful design and sample selection, an internal market research study may be fraught with problems. Employees' biases may affect the way they ask questions of patients. The interviewed patient is subject to bias in some responses if he or she knows who is sponsoring the research. Confusing market research with promotion activities by attempting to educate or "sell" the target market under consideration is less likely to occur if market research experts are consulted. The bias of managers protecting their own turf must also be considered in evaluating market information and research. For example, a patient evaluation form designed with several levels of choice can provide ongoing data about patients' expectations and perceptions of pharmacy services.

GOALS, OBJECTIVES, AND STRATEGIES

Goals and objectives flow from and must be consistent with the mission. There are differences of opinion about the definition of each. Goals are often described as long-term (5-15 years) accomplishments consistent with the mission. Objectives are often shorter term and should always be measurable. These terms are used interchangeably in practice, but within a department a commonly understood definition of both is essential.

Objectives form a specific expression of purpose, thus helping to remove any uncertainty about policy or about the intended purpose of any effort. Properly designed objectives permit measurement of progress and determination of whether adequate resources are being applied or whether these resources are being managed effectively. Finally, objectives facilitate the relationships between units, especially in a diversified department where the separate goals of different units (e.g., outpatient and home care) may not be consistent with some higher purpose.

Despite their overriding importance, defining objectives is far from easy. Defining goals as the future becomes the present is a time-consuming and continuous process. In practice, many pharmacy departments are run either without any commonly accepted objectives and goals or with conflicting objectives and goals. At times, the objectives may be defined in such general terms that their significance for the job is not understood.

Strategy in a pharmacy department is concerned with the basic goals and objectives of the business, the product-market matches chosen on which to compete, the major patterns of resource allocations, and the major operating policies used to relate the pharmacy to its institutional environment.

Each functional activity (e.g., marketing) makes its own unique contribution to strategy formulation at different levels. The marketing function represents the greatest degree of contact with the external environment, the environment least controllable.

In its strategic role, marketing consists of establishing a match between the department and its environment to seek solutions to problems of deciding how the chosen endeavor may be successfully run in a competitive environment by pursuing product, price, promotion, and distribution (see below) perspectives to serve target markets. Marketing provides the core element for future relationships between the department and its environment. It specifies inputs for defining objectives and helps in formulating plans to achieve them.

Strategy specifies the direction. Its intent is the evolution of the market to the advantage of the pharmacy and the parent institution. Thus, a strategy statement includes a description of the new competitive equilibrium to be created, the cause-and-effect relationships that will bring it about, and the logic to support the course of action. Planning articulates the means of implementing strategy. A strategic plan specifies the sequence and timing that will alter relationships.

MARKETING STRATEGIES

The fourth component of a marketing program is the management phase in which research information is translated into strategies and tactics that meet the markets' needs. In addition to the overall marketing strategy for the organization, subordinate strategies, or road maps, must be devised for each market segment if exchange relationships are to be managed to meet the pharmacy department's and consumers' long- and short-range objectives. Tactics are the programs used along the strategic path to accomplishing short-term objectives.

In a marketing approach to pharmacy, the target markets' needs and expectations, rather than those of the organization, guide nontechnical strategic decisions. When the actual service meets expectations, the consumer will be happy.

Marketing strategy involves decisions basic to the daily functioning of the nursing division: whom to serve, what services to offer; how to promote these services; where to serve; whom to hire; what to pay; and what to charge. Marketing strategy and tactics use combinations of the four elements known as "the four P's" of the marketing mix: product, promotion, place, and price. These elements are the tools marketers use to satisfy markets.

The key to success in understanding and applying the marketing mix is having "the right product in the right place at the right time with the right promotion"—and for the right price. Marketing research and the management elements of planning, organizing, directing, and controlling are involved in developing the marketing mix strategy in exchange relationships; the marketing objectives of the organization flow from these activities.

The definitions we use for the marketing mix components listed above are as follows:

1. *Product.* The *benefits* or positive *results* that markets derive from using the services you offer in the way you offer them.
2. *Promotion.* What markets are informed of the department's product, place, price, and how.
3. *Place.* The distribution channels and physical distribution practices through which markets use your services.
4. *Price.* The total cost that markets must bear in order to use the services offered. (These are not necessarily monetary, but may include time, inconvenience, etc.)

Elaboration on these definitions follows.

In marketing terms, a product is anything that fills a need or want and includes services, individuals, organizations, and ideas, in addition to physical objects. When the product is an idea, its exchange is called "social marketing." Health care as a product has three components: services offered, physical characteristics of the institution, and personnel. It is the personnel who are most important to the patient markets.

There are four distinct characteristics of services that should be considered in planning service marketing strategies. Services are *intangible* commodities, requiring a measure of confidence in the provider's abilities. A service is *inseparable* from its provider and is consumed as it is produced. It is *perishable* and cannot be stored until it is needed. Finally, service quality is highly *variable* depending upon the abilities, and even the moods, of the provider.

The marketing strategy should include offering services that are desired by the marketplace, remembering that a consumer values a service in direct proportion to its perceived benefits. Services also should be distinguishable from those offered by competitors. If the pharmacy administrator does not believe that the services offered compare favorably with those of the competition, the services should be improved before being promoted.

Place or distribution decisions are the second component of the marketing mix. As with the other elements of marketing strategy, place decisions are based on patient, physician, employee, and other target group preferences and not on what the pharmacy director wants to provide. The department must decide how to make its services accessible and available to the target markets. Place decisions involve what services will be offered in each location.

As part of place decisions, one should consider the concept of "atmospherics": the intentional design of space to create feelings such as well-being, safety, and competence. Some of management's attitudes toward patients, visitors, employees, physicians, trustees, and the community will be perceived by these target groups through the facilities and conveniences provided for them.

Price decisions include consideration of direct and indirect costs associated with a valued product or service. The price of a staff member to the organization involves wages, fringe benefits, recruitment and orientation costs, and some indirect costs such as managerial effort, waiting, and psychological costs. For patients, indirect costs may include discomfort, pain, anxiety, disruption of lifestyle, economic distress, costs of babysitters, and transportation. The director who can identify the total price of the exchange to both parties is more likely to achieve marketing success in the long run.

The director of pharmacy in many hospitals may be directly involved in setting fees and hospital rates, and it is very important that he or she understand how the prices for pharmacy services and pharmacy revenue centers are determined. There are three stages in setting prices. First, the price objective is determined: maximizing use or profits, cost recovery, fairness, and other goals. Second, pricing strategy must be planned based on competition, demand, or actual cost. The last stage considers whether price change is warranted and how such a change can be implemented. These stages also apply to wage and salary price decisions.

Often, the third-party payment system in the health care sector obscures the price of health services from users and providers. Third-party payers also limit the ability of health care providers to price services competitively, because penalties may be imposed when price reductions are implemented. Since physicians usually admit their patients to hospitals of the physician's choice, the voluntary exchange relationship of a free market is violated by both physicians and third-party payers.

PROMOTION

As the successful organization must do more than make attractive products and services available, promotional strategies are used to develop persuasive communication between the organization and its markets. The end result of this communication should meet the markets' needs as well as the organization's goals. Too often the promotion element of the marketing mix is thought of as "marketing" in and of itself.

An important caveat for the pharmacy administrator to remember is that "everything about the organization talks, but not all of it will promote the organization." Services, employees, facilities, actions, and attitudes communicate something about the pharmacy and the hospital organization. When these factors are recognized as sources of marketing promotion, their impact can be realistically assessed. Other forms of promotional efforts will not override the daily personal communication an organization has with its markets.

Table 4-3 provides examples of strategic questions that might be asked when considering new services.

With the basic nature of marketing previously identified as dealing with exchange, marketing management can also be interpreted as an action-oriented science consisting of principles for improving the probabilities and effectiveness of exchanges. Kotler[5] sees marketing management as representing professionalization in the carrying out of exchange relationships and defines it as:

> the analysis, planning, implementation, and control of programs designed to bring about desired exchanges with target audiences for the purpose of personal or mutual gain. It relies heavily on the adaptation and coordination of product, price, promotion, and place for achieving effective response.

Table 4-3. Questions regarding innovative services*

1. Are there market segments (such as the aged) for which you could develop a new service program?
2. Do you now have the basic capability of providing those services, or would you have to start from scratch?
3. What is your present competition, and what does it offer in terms of product, price, and place to that segment?
4. Which other organizations have a better basic capacity to provide such services (personnel, equipment, facilities, location) and might decide to do so?
5. What can you do that is better than existing and potential competition?
6. What would be the impact on your organization if you succeeded in implementing such a program? At what levels of utilization?
7. Which *internal* groups must be won over to the idea for it to succeed?
8. Which *external* groups must be won over to the idea for it to succeed?
9. How might the program be developed so as to improve the probability that internal groups will support it?
10. Can you involve potential consumers or referral agencies in developing the program?
11. Which groups or individuals might oppose the development, and for what reasons?
12. Can they be won over, or is it necessary to defeat them?
13. Which strategies can you use for either?
14. Which benefits can you promise to interested groups as a result of implementing the program, and at what costs?
15. How can you communicate most effectively to the precise segments of the market most likely to use the program?
16. Which message will be most likely to stir their interest?

*Modified from *Marketing by Objectives for Hospitals*. Germantown, MD, Aspen Systems, 1980, p 263.

The major working assumption of Kotler's view of marketing management is that desired exchanges "do not automatically come about through any process in nature. Rather they require an expenditure of time, energy, skill and supervision."

Internal hospital conflicts between and among departments arise, in part, from difficulties in the allocation of scarce resources. Through internal marketing it may be possible to temper conflict through cooperation. As Kenneth Boulding[6] has written: "There is cooperation in increasing the pie and competition in sharing it."

Many conflicts occur over issues of power or control over institutional actions, decisions, and resources. In competitive markets, the key goal in the struggle is often not just profit but a certain share of the market. There are several reasons why power and control might be sought instead of more resources[7]:

1. Power can obtain resources, often in large quantities.
2. Power is a more generalized medium than are mere resources—it may be used to obtain a wide variety of resources and other desired outcomes.
3. Power has an "ego-boosting" quality; it provides gratification of self-image, satisfaction of status need, implications of mastery, and so on.
4. Power may be used to control the actions and decisions of others, and can be used to make a wider sector of the world (market) conform to one's wishes or images of how things ought to be. In this way, it may be used to protect a privileged position with regard to resources.

Effective marketing plans can be the means to gaining and exercising power.

EVALUATION

Evaluating the results of strategic and tactical programs is part of the management phase of marketing and may demonstrate a need for altering the marketing mix. Four levels of marketing outcomes can be assessed in the evaluation program: awareness, change of attitudes, conviction, and action or behavior. The director can measure marketing effectiveness by analyzing use of services and programs, revenues and expenses, patient compliance and satisfaction, health outcomes, physician satisfaction, employee job satisfaction, turnover rates, number of unfilled positions, continuing education program attendance, and many more indicators. As program outputs are measured against marketing plans, new problems and challenges surface that need additional market research, different strategies and tactics, and further evaluation, all of which demonstrates the dynamic nature of marketing management.

Each pharmacy administrator should develop a marketing perspective and view marketing problems as a managerial responsibility. The organization has marketing problems when it fails to meet the desired exchange relationships with its markets. These problems exist when there is a gap between a target market's needs and what is offered by the pharmacy to patients, nursing staff, physicians, community, or regulating agencies. Unfortunately, pharmacy has not always viewed all of these groups as target markets. In the exchange with the patient, the fact that the patient is purchasing pharmacy service has been obscured by the way charges are billed as drug products.

The market planning model begins with an analysis of the needs, preferences, and perceptions of current and potential consumers as well as the capabilities of the organization. Marketing information and research are the basis for this analysis or audit. Specific strategies are determined for each market segment, following mission statements, goals, objectives, implementation of marketing plans, and evaluation.

A pharmacy director cannot undertake a marketing approach to pharmacy service without the support and commitment of the hospital administrator, board of trustees, staff, medical staff—the groups that are, in essence, the consumers as well as colleagues. To be committed and supportive, these groups must understand the rationale, purposes, goals, objectives, strategies, and tactics of marketing.

REFERENCES

1. AMA board approves new marketing definition. *Marketing News*, vol 21, #5, Chicago, IL, American Marketing Association, March 1, 1985, p. 1.
2. Hillestad SG, Berkowitz EN: *Health Care Marketing Plans: From Strategy to Action*. Homewood, IL, Dow Jones-Irwin, 1984.
3. Kotler P: *Marketing for Nonprofit Organizations*, 2nd ed., Englewood Cliffs, NJ, Prentice-Hall, 1982.
4. Pathak D: Introduction to Pharmaceutical Marketing. In Smith, MC, *Principles of Pharmaceutical Marketing*, Philadelphia, Lea and Febiger, 1983.
5. Kotler P: *Marketing Management: Analysis, Planning and Control*. Englewood Cliffs, NJ, Prentice-Hall, 1972.
6. Boulding, K: *Conflict and Defense: A General Theory*. New York, Harper Torchbooks, 1962.
7. Nelson SD: The concept of social conflict. Center for Research working paper. Ann Arbor, MI, 1971.

ADDITIONAL READING

Journal of Health Care Marketing. Chicago, IL, American Marketing Association.

Journal of Pharmaceutical Marketing and Management. Binghamton, NY, Haworth Press.

Klepcyk JC: Marketing a discharge prescription program. *Am J Hosp Pharm* 47:1006, 1990.

Posey LM: Making ends meet in IV therapy services. *Consult Pharm* 2:117-120, 1987.

Rockwell MM, Manchester RF: Funding and marketing of an investigational drug service. *Am J Hosp Pharm* 46:1339-1340, 1989.

Smith, MC: *Pharmaceutical Marketing: Strategy and Cases*. Binghamton, NY, Haworth Press, 1991.

Thompson DF, Kaczmarek ER, Hutchinson RA: Attitudes of pharmacists and nurses toward interprofessional relations and decentralized pharmaceutical services. *Am J Hosp Pharm* 45:345-351, 1988.

CHAPTER 5

Residency Programs in Pharmacy Practice

HERMAN L. LAZARUS and DONALD E. LETENDRE

A pharmacy residency is defined as an organized, directed, postgraduate training program in a defined area of pharmacy practice.[1] Each of these adjectives bears some comment.

1. *Organized.* A residency program is planned with specific outcome objectives in mind and structured in such a way that those objectives may be attained. Specifically, a list of competency-based learning objectives is prepared in advance for each area of training in which the resident will be expected to gain experience. Pharmacy residencies commonly consist of several discrete blocks of training, or rotations, each devoted to one particular aspect of practice. Further, a residency is structured in such a way that the competency-based objectives can be accomplished within the allotted time for the program. (The minimum length of a pharmacy residency is 12 months, full time.)

2. *Directed.* The director of pharmacy services in the facility in which the residency is conducted has ultimate responsibility for the residency program. In many instances, the director of pharmacy serves as the residency program director. However, the director may choose to appoint another pharmacist on staff to serve as residency program director; in these instances, the individual to whom coordination and oversight for the program has been delegated must be accountable to the director of pharmacy. The residency program director is responsible for ensuring that the overall program goals and specific learning objectives are met, training schedules are maintained, adequate preceptorship for each rotation is provided, and resident evaluations based on the pre-established learning objectives are routinely conducted.

3. *Postgraduate.* A pharmacy residency occurs subsequent to graduation from pharmacy school (i.e., following completion of an entry-level degree for pharmacy practice).

It is important to distinguish between a residency and other types of professional practice education and training. A residency is distinguished from externships and clerkships in that these two experiences are associated with degree requirements and typically represent the student's initial exposure to various professional practice settings. Although these experiences are designed to demonstrate the principles of pharmacy practice, they do not provide opportunities for independent judgment by the student. A residency, by contrast, is a program in which one learns to practice; it provides opportunities for a graduate pharmacist to build on his or her undergraduate clerkships and internships through responsible, independent judgment and enhanced practice competence.

A residency differs from an internship in that an internship is a training program meeting the requirements established by boards of pharmacy for licensure. The amount of internship training required subsequent to graduation varies considerably from State to State. A residency program, on the other hand, seeks to develop independent thinking and clinical competence beyond that which is required for licensure. As noted earlier, a residency is a minimum 12-month program.

Finally, a clear distinction should be made between residency and fellowship programs. As noted above, residencies exist primarily to teach one how to practice; however, a fellowship is a directed, highly individualized, postgraduate program designed to prepare the participant to become an independent researcher.[1]

The authors strongly encourage the reader to review the *Practice Standards of ASHP* for the latest residency accreditation regulations and standards.

ORIGIN AND EVOLUTION OF PHARMACY RESIDENCIES

Hospital pharmacy as a distinct form of practice began to take shape in the 1930's, paralleling the growth of the hospital industry in general. The history of this development lies outside the scope of this chapter; however, by the end of the 1930's there was considerable interest in forming a national association of hospital pharmacists. The American Society of Hospital Pharmacists (ASHP) was finally established in 1942.

Pharmacy schools in that era concentrated almost exclusively on training community practitioners, and hospital pharmacy pioneers found that they had to establish their own postgraduate apprenticeship programs to prepare pharmacists for institutional practice. Several hospital pharmacy "internships" (the term used at that time) were established in various parts of the country before the formation of ASHP. There were no standards for such training programs at that time, however, and the quality of these early internships must have varied greatly.

The need for standardized guidelines for training hospital pharmacists was identified early in ASHP's existence, and the first set of standards was published in 1948.[2]

As the demand for qualified hospital pharmacy manpower grew, it became increasingly more apparent that a program of accreditation of hospital pharmacy internships was needed. ASHP established such a program in 1962, predicated on the first accreditation standard for hospital pharmacy residency training. (This marked the first time the term "residency" was used in an official ASHP document, and this term was adopted to distinguish between an internship, which had come to be used in referring to the practical experience required for licensure, and the formal 12-month training program required in the new accreditation standard.) The hospital pharmacy residency accreditation program represented the first effort in American pharmacy practice to ensure, through external review, adherence to a minimum standard in postgraduate professional practice training programs.

Many believe that the development of residency programs has been one of the most important factors contributing to the dramatic growth in hospital pharmacy during the past 30 years. Residency preceptors, by and large, have aspired to train not merely technically competent practitioners, but also people with leadership potential. The ideal for residency training expressed by Latiolais[3] some years ago has influenced an entire generation of preceptors and residents:

> There are essentially four phases through which a new resident graduate must progress before he [or she] becomes a knowledgable hospital pharmacist...:
>
> (1) The first phase revolves around gaining experience in basic practice situations. The pharmacist learns how to perform the basic functions of everyday practice in each division of the hospital pharmacy.
>
> (2) The second phase revolves around gaining experience in learning how to coordinate the various functions and divisions within the hospital pharmacy so that a meaningful service can be provided.
>
> (3) The third phase revolves around gaining experience in learning how to coordinate this total pharmacy service with the needs of the total institution.
>
> (4) The fourth phase revolves around gaining experience in learning how to conceptualize his [or her] accumulated experiences and knowledge of practice and to transform these concepts into new and improved types of pharmaceutical services.

ACCREDITATION OF RESIDENCY PROGRAMS

Accreditation is the process by which an agency or organization evaluates and recognizes a program of study or an institution as meeting certain predetermined qualifications or standards. The accrediting body for residencies in pharmacy practice is ASHP. ASHP's accreditation program has as its objectives the following: (1) to improve the professional competence of pharmacists practicing in various health care settings and prepare pharmacists for entry into these practice settings through organized, competence-based, educational training programs; (2) to guide, assist, and recognize health care providers who wish to support the profession by operating such programs; (3) to provide criteria for the prospective resident in selecting a program by identifying those facilities that conduct accredited residency programs; and (4) to provide prospective employers a basis for determining the level of practice competence by identifying those pharmacists who have successfully completed accredited residency programs.

In 1980, ASHP adopted the "ASHP Position on Long-Range Pharmacy Manpower Needs and Residency Training,"[4] which related the residency accreditation program to manpower needs in pharmacy practice. Specific categories of professional manpower needs identified in this document are pharmacy generalists, clinical practitioners, specialized practitioners, and managers/administrators. Accordingly, ASHP has developed residency accreditation standards to evaluate programs offering training in each of these four categories. Specifically, accreditation standards exist for programs that intend to offer training in general hospital pharmacy practice (this is the standard that was first promulgated in 1962), clinical pharmacy practice, hospital pharmacy administration, and specialized clinical practice (e.g., adult internal medicine, critical care, drug information, geriatric, nuclear, nutritional support, oncology, pediatric, psychiatric, clinical pharmacokinetics, and primary care).[5-19]

The promulgation of new residency accreditation standards during the past two decades directly reflects changes in professional manpower needs. As the profession continues to mature and assumes greater responsibility for the therapeutic needs of patients, there exists a growing need for even greater numbers of pharmacists to address complex drug therapy issues. Indeed, the current general hospital standard that was approved in 1985,[5] which contains considerably more emphasis on clinical practice than the previous standard, reflects this trend. Moreover, in anticipation of these future manpower needs, attendees at the 1989 National Residency Preceptors Conference urged that the general hospital and clinical residency standards be merged.[20] Hence, a new accreditation standard for residency training in pharmacy practice, that has as its core requirements extensive training in clinical practice, is currently under development. With this new standard serving as the foundation for practice in organized health care settings, it is anticipated that completion of this type of residency will eventually be required as a prerequisite to specialized residency training. Currently, only the specialized residencies in hospital pharmacy administration and critical care pharmacy practice require completion of a general residency beforehand.

The Commission on Credentialing

The body within ASHP that has been granted responsibility for administering the accreditation program is the Commission on Credentialing. The commission comprises 10 pharmacy practitioners, 2 public members, and a staff secretary (the ASHP director of accreditation services). The commission's charges include development of accreditation standards for pharmacy residency training programs and onsite accreditation review based on those standards. The commission meets twice a year, and its agenda typically includes considering new accreditation applications, reviewing programs for reaccreditation, and assessing interim progress reports from residency preceptors, among other items.

A practitioner member of the commission, along with a representative of the ASHP Division of Accreditation Services staff, serves on accreditation site visit teams. In the case of specialized residency training programs, a specialist in the corresponding area of practice is added to the site survey team. Each commission member presents reports on programs he or she has surveyed at the next commission meeting following the survey. That surveyor's recommendation is then considered by the full commission. Commission members are appointed by the ASHP president; the normal term of appointment is 3 years.

Applying for Accreditation

The procedures for making an application for accreditation of a pharmacy residency training program are provided in the "ASHP Regulations on Accreditation of Pharmacy Residencies."[21] The application may be submitted any time after the first resident has started the training program. After all application materials have been received by the Accreditation Services Division, arrangements are made with the institution for a site evaluation by the accreditation survey team. Since survey visits are scheduled in the order of receipt of completed applications, there may be a delay of as long as 6 months or more before the site visit can be scheduled.

The Accreditation Survey

A typical accreditation site visit is completed in 2 days and includes interviews with designated individuals (e.g., hospital administrator, chairman of the pharmacy and therapeutics committee and other members of the medical staff, the director of nursing service, the director of pharmacy services, and members of the pharmacy staff, including the residents). There is also an extensive review of the documentation of the pharmacy service and the residency program and of the institution's facilities, with primary emphasis on the pharmacy department and the areas it serves. The survey is usually conducted by a two- or three-member team, as described above.

The purpose of the site evaluation is to determine the degree of compliance with the requirements of the appropriate accreditation standard. The evaluation is conducted in the spirit of offering recommendations and advice for meeting the requirements of the accreditation standard and not primarily to criticize existing shortcomings or deficiencies.

The Accreditation Survey Report

Following the site evaluation, the survey team prepares a report summarizing its findings, listing significant shortcomings, and offering specific recommendations for correcting deficiencies and for improving pharmacy services and the residency training program. The report is sent to the chief executive officer of the institution and to the director of pharmacy services for their review. They are invited to submit their written comments responding to the deficiencies and recommendations listed in the report and to correct any factual errors. The report, along with comments submitted by the institution in response to the report, are considered by the Commission on Credentialing when it acts on the accreditation application.

Reaccreditation and Interim Self-Audit

Accreditation is granted for a maximum period of 6 years; however, the Commission on Credentialing may request a site evaluation at any time if it becomes evident that there has been a major change in the residency training program. Each accredited residency program is required to submit every 2 years a status report on progress made in correcting shortcomings cited in the previous survey report. Each status report is reviewed by the Commission on Credentialing, which then makes a determination on any required followup action.

SELECTING A RESIDENCY PROGRAM

Any pharmacist or pharmacy student should give serious consideration to residency training. Because of the formal structure and concentrated nature of the training in a residency program, the resident should develop competence in a broader scope of pharmacy practice in a 1- or 2-year residency program than might be expected in several years as a staff pharmacist with a fixed assignment. For this reason, more and more directors of pharmacy prefer hiring individuals who have completed a residency program. In fact, many "positions available" listings in the ASHP Personnel Placement Service or in the classified advertising section of the *American Journal of Hospital Pharmacy* specify completion of an accredited residency as an employment prerequisite.

Types of Residencies

Pharmacy residency programs may be categorized in two ways: by practice area and by academic affiliation status. With respect to practice area, there are three broad categories of accredited residencies: general hospital pharmacy, clinical practice, and specialty practice (hospital pharmacy administration residency programs are included in this latter category).

The general hospital pharmacy residency is the most common type of residency. The objective of this program is to train competent pharmacy practitioners to provide a broad scope of pharmaceutical services (e.g., clinical services, drug distribution services, drug information, product formulation, quality control, and supportive administrative services). The resident usually spends a specific length of time or "rotates" through each of these aspects of the pharmacy service. In addition to these rotations, the resident usually spends time in one or more areas of particular interest, such as clinical services, or in some cases, limited experience is provided in pharmacies in other hospitals or organized health care settings. Some general residency programs emphasize hospital pharmacy management and administrative skills, whereas others emphasize clinical practice; however, in either case, a broad experience in hospital pharmacy practice is required.

A clinical residency emphasizes the provision of clinical services to a wide variety of patients in an organized health care setting. The Pharm.D. degree, or clinical training equivalent to that which might be expected of a recent doctor of pharmacy graduate, is usually a prerequisite for such programs. The objective is to build upon the clinical skills of pharmacists in order to make them more capable of managing the drug therapy of patients. In addition, clinical residents gain an understanding of how to plan and implement new clinical services. Although most of the resident's training will occur in the hospital, less emphasis is placed on the overall operation of a hospital pharmacy than is the case in the general residency in hospital pharmacy described above.

Specialized residency programs concentrate exclusively on one specific area of pharmacy practice. Examples of specialized residencies include: adult internal medicine, primary care, drug information, geriatrics, nuclear pharmacy, nutritional support, oncology, pediatrics, critical care, clinical pharmacokinetics, psychopharmacy, and advanced administrative pharmacy practice.

A minimum of 2,000 hours of training extended over a minimum period of 50 weeks is required in an ASHP-accredited residency program—the equivalent of 1 normal work year. Some residency programs are offered only in conjunction with an advanced degree (either a Pharm.D. or a Master of Science degree) in a college of pharmacy or graduate school. Such programs are commonly referred to as "affiliated" residencies and generally require 2 years for completion. A resident in some affiliated programs pursues the residency on a part-time basis so there will be adequate time for course work, thesis research, and other degree requirements. Many affiliated programs, however, allow the residency to be taken either before or after the postgraduate academic course work. Other residency programs ("nonaffiliated" residencies) are offered independently of an advanced degree and typically require 1 year of full-time work for completion. An applicant who already holds an advanced degree would normally choose one of these programs if he or she is interested in pursuing residency training.

A prospective resident should be able to state as clearly as possible what his or her career objectives are. For example, some may aspire to become pharmacy managers (directors of pharmacy service departments), while others may have specific interests in clinical practice or some specialized area of pharmacy. Certain residency programs are promoted on the basis of their particular strengths in one or more special areas of practice; others stress the "general practice" concept. All ASHP-accredited hospital pharmacy residencies provide a general orientation in all basic areas of institutional pharmacy practice. Some provide additional experience and training in specialized areas of practice but may require more than the minimum 2,000 hours for completion of the residency. An applicant who knows clearly what his or her own objectives are can determine through the application and interview process whether a particular program provides the type of training sought.

Residency Directory

ASHP publishes annually a *Residency Directory*. The directory is an essential item for anyone interested in applying for admission to an ASHP-accredited residency program. It provides uniform information about each accredited residency, and identifies those programs that are participating in the Resident Matching Program (explained later in this chapter). Among other things, the *Residency Directory* provides specific information about the following: name, address, and telephone number of the director of the program; program code number, which is essential in applying to a particular residency (see section on Enrolling in the Resident Matching Program); type and duration of each program; number of positions that each program has available; application deadline; date the program starts; estimated stipend (see section on Residency Stipends); fringe benefits; special features about each program; and detailed information about each facility in which the residency training program is conducted.

A copy of the *Residency Directory* is provided to anyone who enrolls in the Resident Matching Program or may be obtained for a nominal fee directly from ASHP.

Entry-Level Requirements

To be eligible to apply for a residency, an applicant must be a graduate of an American Council on Pharmaceutical Education (ACPE)-accredited college of pharmacy (or must have graduated prior to the beginning date of the residency) and should have demonstrated an interest in and aptitude for advanced training in pharmacy. Some residencies require that the applicant be licensed to practice before entering the program, although others will accept applicants who have some limited internship obligation remaining for completion of State board licensure requirements. In the case of an affiliated residency program, the applicant must satisfy the requirements of the college of pharmacy or graduate school for admission to the advanced degree program in addition to the requirements established by the institution in which the residency is offered. Completion of a Pharm.D. or M.S. degree is generally required for admission to clinical and specialty residencies. Information on specific entry requirements may be found in the annual *Residency Directory* published by ASHP.

Residency Stipends

All accredited residency programs provide the resident with a stipend, although the amount varies from program to program, depending on such factors as number of actual training hours per year, the value of any fringe benefits provided, geographic location (cost of living), and related factors. Cash stipends generally are inadequate to cover living costs for a resident with significant family support responsibilities. Furthermore, a residency, whether affiliated or nonaffiliated, requires a full-time commitment on the part of the resident and usually does not permit supplementing income through part-time employment. For these reasons, applicants with family support obligations generally must have financial resources in addition to the residency stipend on which they can rely during the residency training period. The ASHP *Residency Directory* lists in the description of each program the annual stipend paid to the resident, as well as applicable fringe benefits and prerequisites.

Enrolling in the Resident Matching Program

In 1977, ASHP initiated the Resident Matching Program. The purposes of the matching process are to bring about a free and competitive but orderly choice between residency applicants and pharmacy residencies in hospitals, to avoid unwarranted competition between hospitals, and to prevent undue pressures or coercion from being exercised on residency applicants. Except for some of the specialized clinical programs, all eligible accredited residency programs participate in the matching program. Therefore, applications will be accepted by residency programs only from pharmacy students or pharmacists who also have signed agreements to participate in the ASHP Resident Matching Program. The Resident Matching Program does not alter significantly, for either the applicant or the hospital, existing application, interview, and selection procedures, except for observing certain time deadlines for completing applications and submitting the required matching plan documents.

The ASHP Resident Matching Program is open to all qualified applicants and to all pharmacy residency training programs in hospitals accredited by ASHP. To participate, applicants must sign a form contracting to accept any residency position listed by them to which they are matched. They are free to apply or accept positions at any other hospital if they are not matched by the announced deadline. Similarly, hospitals must agree to accept any candidate whose name they have submitted and ranked and who is matched with them by the deadline. A hospital must also agree not to appoint any applicants outside of the matching plan before the announced deadline. Both the applicant and the hospital are assessed a nominal fee for participation in the Resident Matching Program. On receipt by ASHP of the applicant agreement (contract) form and the required fee, a copy of the annual *Residency Directory*, which provides a description of all accredited residencies (plus those with application for accreditation pending), will be mailed to the applicant, along with an acknowledgment letter showing the applicant's assigned code number. This number identifies the applicant in all subsequent communications with residency programs and ASHP.

Application for admission to an accredited residency is made directly to the hospital, not to ASHP. The ASHP *Residency Directory* contains information on the procedures to be followed in applying for admission to accredited residencies.

Residency Showcase

Since there are many steps involved in selecting a residency program that will best fit the individual's needs, prospective residents are encouraged to begin seeking information about residencies during their next to last year in pharmacy school. Discussions with faculty members, employers, clerkship preceptors, and others is always helpful. Perhaps the best place, however, to learn about residencies is at the ASHP Midyear Clinical Meeting, which is held each December. The Residency Showcase at the meeting routinely features more than 200 ASHP-accredited residency training programs. The annual Residency Showcase is a unique opportunity for those interested in applying to residencies, since applicants can obtain information and have discussions with most program preceptors and current residents all in one location.

REFERENCES

1. Definitions of pharmacy residencies and fellowships. *Am J Hosp Pharm* 44:1142-1144, 1987.
2. Standards for internships in hospital pharmacies. *Bull ASHP* 5:233-234, 1948.
3. Latiolais CJ: Objectives for Hospital Pharmacy Residency Training. Paper presented at the Second Special Conference on Hospital Pharmacy Residency Training, Columbus, OH, October 12-14, 1966.
4. ASHP position on long-range pharmacy manpower needs and residency training. *Am J Hosp Pharm* 37:1220, 1980.
5. ASHP accreditation standard for pharmacy residency in a hospital (with guide to interpretation). *Am J Hosp Pharm* 36:74-80, 1979.
6. ASHP accreditation standard for residency training in clinical pharmacy (with guide to interpretation). *Am J Hosp Pharm* 37:1223-1228, 1980.
7. ASHP accreditation standard for specialized pharmacy residency training (with guide to interpretation). *Am J Hosp Pharm* 37:1229-1232, 1980.
8. ASHP supplemental standard and learning objectives for residency training in drug information practice. *Am J Hosp Pharm* 39:1970-1972, 1982.
9. ASHP supplemental standard and learning objectives for residency training in geriatric pharmacy practice. *Am J Hosp Pharm* 39:1972-1974, 1982.
10. ASHP accreditation standard for residency training in nuclear pharmacy (with guide to interpretation). *Am J Hosp Pharm* 38:1964-1971, 1981.
11. ASHP supplemental standard and learning objectives for residency training in nutritional support pharmacy practice. *Am J Hosp Pharm* 38:1971-1973, 1981.
12. ASHP supplemental standard and learning objectives for residency training in oncology pharmacy practice. *Am J Hosp Pharm* 39:1214-1215, 1982.
13. ASHP supplemental standard for residency training in pediatric pharmacy practice. *Am J Hosp Pharm* 41:334-337, 1984.
14. ASHP supplemental standard and learning objectives for residency training in psychiatric pharmacy practice. *Am J Hosp Pharm* 37:1232-1234, 1980.
15. ASHP supplemental standard and learning objectives for residency training in adult internal medicine pharmacy practice. *Am J Hosp Pharm* 41:1383-1385, 1984.
16. ASHP supplemental standard and learning objectives for residency training in hospital pharmacy administration. *Am J Hosp Pharm* 45:1930-1933, 1988.
17. ASHP supplemental standard and learning objectives for residency training in clinical pharmacokinetics practice. *Am J Hosp Pharm* 45:1934-1937, 1988.
18. ASHP supplemental standard and learning objectives for residency training in critical care pharmacy practice. *Am J Hosp Pharm* 47:609-612, 1990.
19. ASHP supplemental standard and learning objectives for residency training in primary care pharmacy practice. *Am J Hosp Pharm* 47:1851-1854, 1990.
20. Proceedings of the 1989 National Residency Preceptors Conference. *Am J Hosp Pharm* 47:85-126, 1990.
21. ASHP regulations on accreditation of pharmacy residencies. *Am J Hosp Pharm* 37:1221-1223, 1980.

CHAPTER 6

Institutional Pharmacy Practice Standards

WAYNE F. CONRAD

The purposes of this chapter are to define, describe, and discuss standards for institutional pharmacy practice. The relationship of practice standards to quality of pharmaceutical care, legal aspects of institutional practice, accrediting bodies, pharmacy organizations, and pharmacy practitioners will be presented.

DEFINITIONS

Several terms are closely associated with standards of practice, including quality, quality assurance, criterion, and standard. "Quality" is an elusive and complex concept. It is a multidimensional phenomenon, differently defined depending on perspective. Stated in the most general terms, quality consists of the ability to achieve desirable objectives using legitimate means. Almost always, the objective specified is an achievable state of health, with health defined narrowly or broadly, depending on the context of the assessment. Described most narrowly, health is a measurable improvement in physical or physiological function. At its broadest, health is as inclusive as the quality of life.[1]

"Quality assurance" describes all efforts to measure, assess, ensure, and evaluate health care.[2] The word "assurance" suggests action to eliminate substandard performance and improve efficiency of the system of care.[3] In a programmatic fashion, Stolar[4] describes quality assurance as deciding what is to be done, measuring how well the job was done after completion, and then, if the results are not acceptable, undertaking corrective action to ensure that in the future they will be acceptable.

Quality is a judgment about care. Before it can be assessed, monitored, or assured, the abstract formulations of quality must be translated into more objective criteria and standards that can be used as reliable and valid measuring devices.[5]

"Criterion" is a stated expectation of what should be found if quality is optimum. It is an absolute. "Standard" is a more flexible term that expresses the degree of acceptable variation from the criterion. When no deviation is acceptable and the criterion must always be met, the standard and criterion are equivalent.

Sometimes, the criteria and standards of quality are "empirically derived," which means they are obtained by the observation of good, acceptable, or average practice. More often the criteria are "normatively derived," which means that they represent published, scientific knowledge as interpreted, and perhaps added to by its leading students and practitioners.[5]

Quality Assessment

The classic approach to quality assessment is based on the widely acknowledged classification system devised by Donabedian.[6] He categorizes all assessment efforts as either structure, process, or outcome. Structure may be defined as the facilities, equipment, services, and manpower available for care and the credentials and qualifications of the health professionals involved. Examples of structural characteristics in a pharmacy program include the presence or absence of a unit dose program, IV admixture program, or formulary system.

Process refers to the content of care. These are the activities that take place between the patient and the provider. Process measures include the procedures or steps followed in providing care. Many pharmacy quality assurance programs use process measures. Drug utilization studies and an audit of operational standards for drug distribution are examples of process assessment.[7]

"Outcome" refers to the results of care. Outcome measures encompass biological changes in disease, ability for self-care, physical function, and mobility and patient satisfaction.[8] Although most of the literature discusses outcome in terms of patient outcomes, the concept can also be applied to pharmacy services. Outcome in this case is simply the result of a set of procedures operating within a structure.[7]

Although all three care elements have individual merit as indicators of quality, the review system should also attempt to statistically identify and "validate" on an ongoing basis those elements of structure and process that are consistently associated with favorable patient outcomes. This enables more informed attempts to change practice behavior when indicated, as well as assuring the relevance of the structure and process-based criteria used in assessment.[8]

As a rule, it is best to include in any system of assessment elements of structure, process, and outcome. This allows supplementation of weakness in one approach by strength in another; it helps one interpret the findings; and if the findings do not seem to make sense, it leads to a reassessment of the study design and questioning of the accuracy of the data themselves.[9]

Donabedian[10] believes that quality assurance has two components. The first is system design, which includes all the measures that an organization uses to safeguard and promote the quality of health care. The second component is monitoring. Monitoring is the process by which performance is periodically or continuously reviewed and, when found to be deficient, first modified and then evaluated once again. System design and monitoring should be an inseparable, mutually supportive pair. Design brings about rough adjustments in performance; monitoring is responsible for fine tuning. Standards of practice are important yardsticks for both.

Use of Standards

Standards of practice are fundamental tools needed for objective quality assessment. Standards are predetermined elements against which aspects of the quality of medical care may be compared. They provide a yardstick by which quality may be measured. Standards represent an acknowledged measure of comparison for quantitative and qualitative value and can be used by members of the profession at all levels. In addition, other health care professionals, institutions, and regulatory bodies are provided with a reference of expectation of the profession. Standards increase accountability of the profession to the public by articulating, supporting, and protecting the rights of patients.[11]

Practice standards are generally viewed as those expectations which are believed to be reasonable and practical given limitations of resources and circumstances. Quality care is sometimes described in terms of minimum standards, and other times as maximum achievable goals in recognition that criteria and standards may be different.

There are several sources for the standards that affect institutional pharmacy practice. These are illustrated in table 6-1. In their broadest context, standards for professional practice include laws, regulations, and rules promulgated by government, and standards developed by accrediting bodies as well as those developed by the profession.

LEGAL STANDARDS

A number of readily identifiable standards have legal significance in the practice of institutional pharmacy. The U.S. Government, through its Food and Drug Administration (FDA), is responsible for implementing and enforcing the Federal Food, Drug, and Cosmetic Act. The FDA is responsible for the control and prevention of misbranding and adulteration of food, drugs, and cosmetics moving in interstate commerce. The FDA sets label requirements for food, drugs, and cosmetics; sets standards for investigational drug studies and for marketing new drug products; and compiles information on adverse drug reactions.[11]

Federal agencies issue enforceable standards and regulations associated with their realm of responsibility. For example, the Department of Health and Human Services, through the Health Care Financing Administration (HCFA), is responsible for the development of requirements that long-term care facilities must meet to participate in both the Medicare and Medicaid programs. These requirements vary depending upon the type of long-term care facility. Revisions in these requirements focus on actual facility performance in meeting the needs of long-term care residents rather than on provision of services designed to meet needs.[12]

The Health Care Financing Administration also develops "Federal Conditions of Participation" for hospitals to participate in the Medicare program. Each condition consists of one or more standards that define the requirements for compliance. The standards take into consideration that hospitals and departments within hospitals are subject to State and Federal laws and undergo substantial State inspection through licensure programs.[13]

State and Federal laws and regulations contain rules that must be followed in practice. The State board of pharmacy is the agency of State government responsible for regulating pharmacy practice within the State. Practitioners, institutions, and community pharmacies must obtain licenses from the board to practice pharmacy or provide pharmacy services in the State. State boards of pharmacy promulgate numerous regulations pertaining to drug dispensing and control. Pharmacy Practice Acts and accompanying rules and regulations are considered to be minimums. In some States, the State board of health licenses the hospital pharmacy separately or through a license that includes all departments of the hospital. In others, there are separate classes of pharmacy licenses, including retail, hospital, parenteral, and nuclear.[11]

ACCREDITATION

Accreditation is acknowledgment that an institution or program has met predetermined standards of quality. It is a voluntary process. The principal organization associated with accreditation of hospitals is the Joint Commission on Accreditation of Healthcare Organizations. JCAHO standards are primarily structure and process in nature and address services provided in organized health care settings. The Joint Commission has developed standards for hospitals, home care, long-term care, psychiatric and mental health care, and hospice care. The standard-setting process involves participating institutions, health care organizations, and government agencies. The standards are drafted by professionals and technical advisory committees to the accreditation programs; American Society of Hospital Pharmacists (ASHP) is consulted for the pharmacy standards.

The Joint Commission on Accreditation of Healthcare Organizations is a not-for-profit, nongovernmental corporation whose member organizations are the American College of Physicians, American College of Surgeons, American Dental Association, American Hospital Association, and American Medical Association. Compliance with JCAHO standards is voluntary; any hospital may request a survey to determine if it is compliant.[14]

The Joint Commission accredits approximately 5,000 of the 6,100 acute-care hospitals in the United States as well as 2,500 other health care facilities. To be accredited, a hospital must demonstrate that it is in substantial compliance with the applicable standards; it need not be in full compliance with all standards. Failure to comply fully with a standard may result in a type II recommendation. Noncompliance or minimal compliance may result in a type I recommendation.[15] Both types of recommendations require corrective action by the hospital. The Joint Commission will not accredit a hospital that has excessive unresolved recommendations or fails to meet certain essential standards. About one-half of hospitals receive full 3-year approval, and only about 2 percent of surveyed hospitals are denied accreditation.[16]

The Joint Commission issues a certificate of accreditation to a hospital that substantially complies with its standards. Accreditation is currently for 3 years and is not renewed automatically. To continue its accreditation beyond this period, a hospital must undergo another full survey and demonstrate substantial compliance with the current standards.

Accreditation is important for the hospital in many ways. For example, JCAHO has agreements with about 40 States in which accreditation may fulfill all or part of the State licensing requirements. Most health insurance policies only pay for care in accredited hospitals. Accredited hospitals are considered to meet Medicare and Medicaid standards for payment without undergoing a Federal inspection. Voluntary accreditation demonstrates to the public that a hospital meets certain national standards. Finally, the accreditation process provides an opportunity for hospitals to assess their strong and weak features and make improvements.[17]

Failure to meet JCAHO standards or the loss of accreditation can severely affect a hospital's prestige. The hospital may find it difficult to attract qualified physicians and other professionals, and the adverse publicity may cause patients to seek admission elsewhere. Furthermore, hospitals accredited by the JCAHO are eligible automatically for reimbursement in the Medicare program.[18]

The Joint Commission provides uniform, nationally recognized standards that define quality patient care. Many hospitals base their bylaws, policies, procedures, and quality assurance criteria on JCAHO's standards. These standards are sometimes used in court in lieu of local or community practice norms. In some instances, they have become the expected legal standards of care. Therefore, failure to meet JCAHO standards or to follow universally recognized standards of practice may open the hospital and the pharmacy to legal difficulties.[19]

The Joint Commission publishes its standards for acute-care hospitals annually in the *Accreditation Manual for Hospitals*.[20] The chapter on pharmaceutical services contains six standards with numerous subheadings that define ethical and professional pharmaceutical practices. Several important pharmacy-related functions are included in nonpharmacy standards. These include quality assurance, pharmacy and therapeutics function, drug usage evaluation (DUE), and infection control. The JCAHO standards for pharmacy practice parallel standards developed by ASHP.

Quality Assurance and DUE

According to the Joint Commission, the standards used in a quality assurance program must define a level of patient care that is both optimal and achievable, i.e., standards that are high, yet attainable with available resources. The quality assurance process must identify problems or areas for improvement of patient care. Action must be taken to resolve the problems or bring performance closer to the established standards.

Drug usage evaluation is a medical staff quality assurance activity designed to promote appropriate, safe, and effective drug use. Although DUE is officially the responsibility of the medical staff, many medical staffs request the pharmaceutical service to guide them through the process. The pharmacy may recommend drug use criteria, gather data, identify departures, and take the action directed by the medical staff.

Coe[21] has written a detailed manual to help pharmacists prepare for a JCAHO survey. (Refer to this source for more specific information regarding standards for pharmacy services.) Two JCAHO manuals, *Monitoring and Evaluation of Pharmacy Services*[22] and *Examples of Drug Usage Evaluation*,[23] may also help pharmacists understand and comply with Joint Commission standards.

Agenda for Change

During the 1980's, considerable attention began to be focused on quality of care. Because of resource limitations, altered payment incentives, and other economic pressures, quality assurance problems became major public policy issues.[24] Increasingly, hospitals, insurers, employees, unions, consumer groups, and State and Federal governments pointed to the need for evaluation systems that look beyond what care is given and how it is rendered, to evaluate the patient's health status.

Traditionally, the Joint Commission has used structure and process evaluation to accredit health care organizations. Economists and purchasers of health care favor outcome measurement. They believe this approach is better for ensuring value for the health care dollars spent, controlling the individual components of care, and increasing the likelihood that commonly accepted performance standards are used.[25]

In 1986, JCAHO announced its intention to shift from its prescriptive view (with respect to structure and process) of quality assurance to a strong emphasis on outcome measurement. Structure and process define capability to perform; the new JCAHO standards will be designed to demonstrate whether the capability is exercised and whether it results in a constructive contribution to patient outcome.[25]

Measuring outcomes will be easier in some circumstances than in others. Surgical specialties are particularly well suited to outcome assessment, since the procedure either leads to resolution of the problem or not, with or without complications. Contrast these more "black and white" outcomes of care with those for medical specialties in which a course of treatment, once defined, may or may not ever lead to a clearly identifiable outcome, where the patient's condition moves back and forth on a continuum, and where the speed or extent of response becomes the indicator of effectiveness.[25] For medicine, the criteria and standards will be field tested to ensure that they are reliable, that they require minimal interpretation or judgment about outcome,[26] and that they take into account variance in practice patterns. Over time a national data base will develop that will identify patterns of care associated with favorable outcomes. Such a data base will facilitate comparisons among hospitals and other providers with similar and relevant characteristics and use patterns.[27]

In 1989, ASHP created a working group to develop quality assurance indicators.[28] The working group's objective is to develop, for selected clinical and selected other pharmaceutical services, quality assurance indicators that, inasmuch as possible, represent quality in terms of patient and organizational outcomes. Priority emphasis is to be given to the development of indicators that may be used by JCAHO in its accreditation standards and accreditation process.[29]

The Joint Commission's intention is not to monitor clinical care singlehandedly, but rather to monitor the effectiveness with which providers of care monitor their own performance and services.[30] Surveys by the Joint Commission will continue, but they will be different; they will assess an institution's own ability to examine the details of care rendered and to determine whether that care is beneficial to patients.

Over the years, JCAHO has contributed much to the improved quality of care in hospitals. The Joint Commission is committed to streamlining its standards, focusing them on patient care process and the essential ways that health care organizations contribute to good outcomes.[31] Its new emphasis on clinical outcomes should improve its ability to evaluate health care organizations and stimulate among them greater attention to the quality of day-to-day patient care.

PHARMACY ORGANIZATIONS

The establishment and implementation of standards of practice are two of the prime functions of a professional organization. The responsibilities inherent in carrying out these functions are to establish, maintain, and improve standards; to hold members accountable for using standards; to educate the public to appreciate the standards; to protect the public from individuals who have not attained the standards or willfully do not follow them; and to protect individual members of the profession from each other.[32]

Several pharmacy organizations have been involved in developing standards of practice (table 6-1). The American Pharmaceutical Association and the American Association of Colleges of Pharmacy promulgated the "Standards of Practice for the Profession of Pharmacy" in 1979.[33] These standards describe, in generic terms, what a pharmacist does in fulfilling the basic responsibilities of the profession. They serve a useful purpose as a philosophical document. They describe a broad-based consensus among practitioners of a shift in practice emphasis from product only to embrace also patient care service focusing on appropriate use of drugs.[34]

The American Society of Consultant Pharmacists has published *Guidelines for Consultant Pharmacists Practicing in Long Term Care Facilities*.[35] These standards go beyond the role mandated by Federal and State long-term care regulations. A different approach was taken by the American College of Clinical Pharmacy with the promulgation of minimum standards of practice for institutions, which define clinical pharmacy practice as a specialized discipline in which the desired endpoint is to provide optimal patient care. The standards discuss the various approaches by which patient care may be influenced. Through delineation of responsibilities and practice areas, a clinical pharmacy program that is integrated with the clinical services of other departments in the health care setting (e.g., medicine, surgery, laboratory, nursing) can fulfill these standards. These practice standards are described as applying to all organized health care facilities that provide inpatient or outpatient care, and to all subspecialties of medical and surgical practice.[36]

Table 6-1. Major sources of standards affecting pharmacy practice

- Statutes
  - State
    - Pharmacy Practice Acts
    - Controlled Substances Acts
  - Federal
    - Alcohol Tax Law
    - Controlled Substances Act
    - Food, Drug and Cosmetic Act
    - Social Security Amendments (Medicare and Medicaid)
- Regulations
  - State
    - Board of Pharmacy
    - Education Department
    - Health Department
    - Health and Human Services
  - Federal
    - Consumer Product Safety Commission
    - Drug Enforcement Administration
    - Food and Drug Administration
    - Internal Revenue Service
    - Department of Health and Human Services
    - Health Care Financing Administration
- Accrediting Agencies
  - Joint Commission on Accreditation of Healthcare Organizations
  - ASHP Residency Program Accreditation
- Professional Organizations
  - American Society of Hospital Pharmacists
  - American College of Clinical Pharmacy
  - American Society of Consultant Pharmacists
  - American Pharmaceutical Association
  - American Association of Colleges of Pharmacy

The most comprehensive standards for institutional pharmacy practice are those formulated by ASHP. Since its formation in 1942, ASHP has exerted a leadership role in the development of standards for the profession.

ASHP practice standards consist of the statements, guidelines, therapeutic guidelines, residency accreditation regulations, and technical assistance bulletins regularly published in the *American Journal of Hospital Pharmacy*. They are compiled annually in *Practice Standards of the American Society of Hospital Pharmacists*.[37] ASHP statements are declarations of philosophy or principle. ASHP guidelines provide general advice on the implementation of pharmacy practice programs. Therapeutic guidelines are advice on rational medication use and medication use issues. Technical assistance bulletins provide specific, detailed advice on pharmacy programs. Residency accreditation regulations and standards set forth criteria to be used in the evaluation of such programs in hospitals applying for accreditation. They define qualifications of the training site, pharmacy service, and residency director in addition to qualifications of the residency training program itself.[38]

The ASHP practice standards provide a point of reference for pharmacists (and others) to use in evaluating institutional programs and services. They are developed and periodically revised by practitioners, practitioner groups, or by ASHP staff in consultation with experts. All documents must be approved by the organization's board of directors, and the statements must also be approved by the ASHP House of Delegates. Although the Joint Commission describes its standards as optimal, ASHP standards are usually more stringent, more explicit, and less subject to interpretation.[18] Over the years, the ASHP practice standards have had a significant effect on the quality of institutional pharmacy practice. Perhaps the impact is most apparent within the residency training accreditation process. Accreditation standards provide considerable program content detail and foster consistency among programs.[39] The standards for pharmacy service represent state-of-the-art pharmacy practice, and programs must meet them to become accredited. Subsequently, the ASHP Commission on Credentialing raises the level of standards as the state of the art changes, so that by the time the next survey is conducted, the program has new goals to meet, and the cycle repeats itself. The never-ending challenge to meet higher standards stimulates pharmacies with residency programs to improve pharmaceutical services.[40]

DEPARTMENTAL STANDARDS OF PRACTICE AND PERFORMANCE STANDARDS

Development and promulgation of standards by regulatory agencies and professional organizations set the tone for pharmacy practice. However, pharmacy departments should develop their own set of standards that are applicable to their individual institution. Beyond the standards enforced by a regulatory board or a voluntary association, a health care organization can create the necessary professional goals, processes, and relationships through its management system.[41] Department-specific practice standards are necessary to ensure consistent, comprehensive services for patients.[42] They serve as a foundation for a quality assurance program directed toward bringing about improved patient care.[43] They serve as important management tools in recruitment, orientation and training, and performance planning and review and in describing staff responsibilities.[44]

Standards of practice should be incorporated into the strategic planning process of pharmacy departments. They should be consistent with the philosophy, mission, and goals of the department. Practice standards should be developed with the input of those pharmacists responsible for providing care to patients. An example of a pharmacy department practice standard used at Thomas Jefferson University Hospital is included in Appendix 6-A.

Once departmental standards of practice have been developed, audits may be done to determine if the department is compliant.[45] However, individual performance standards are needed to determine how well individual pharmacists are performing their responsibilities. A performance standard is a statement of conditions that will exist when a job is satisfactorily performed. Performance standards allow the individual to know whether his or her performance is good or whether further development is needed. It has been suggested that the majority of formal appraisal systems are trait rating systems.[46] Emphasis is on personality characteristics and behavioral patterns. Performance standards, on the other hand, are known and accepted by the employee in advance and focus attention on the desired results.[7]

Performance standards must be measurable. They should be challenging, but they must also be realistic and achievable. The employee's participation in this process should aid this objective. Each responsibility in the job description may have one or more associated standards; however, in the beginning it is best to focus first on the key responsibilities. Standards can be designed to measure quality, quantity, time, or cost associated with the job responsibilities. There are several approaches to measurement of results. A standard that is based on the results the organization needs is termed an "engineered standard." One that is based on the results that have been produced previously is a "historical standard." Finally, a standard that is based on the results that others are achieving is a "comparative standard."[47,48]

FUTURE DIRECTIONS

Standards of practice form the basis for the quantitative and qualitative measure of patient care. Today's quality-conscious health care environment demands the reevaluation of current practice standards and the development of patient management strategies that maximize the likelihood of a positive clinical outcome.[49] In the future, we need to develop better-quality measurement systems and to provide the public operational data for use in selecting caregivers with demonstrable value.[50] Future standards for measuring the quality of care delivered will be more outcome oriented, more objective, and more intellectually vigorous.[24]

Improving clinical outcomes for a wide variety of disease entities depends on optimizing pharmaceutical care. Pharmacy must play a key role in developing and implementing new ways to measure and validate the effectiveness of drug use. Future standards for care should be oriented to the patient outcomes desired.

REFERENCES

1. Donabedian A: Quality assessment and assurance: Unity of purpose, diversity of means. *Inquiry* 25:173-192, 1988.
2. Stewart JE: Effects of quality assurance efforts on patient care. *Top Hosp Pharm Mgt* 3:21, 1981.
3. Jessee WF: Quality assurance systems: Why aren't there any? *Qual Rev Bull* 11:16-18, 1977.
4. Stolar M: Model quality assurance programs for hospital pharmacies. Revised ed. Bethesda, MD, American Society of Hospital Pharmacists, 1980, pp 3-9.
5. Donabedian A: Criteria and standards for quality assessment and monitoring. *Qual Rev Bull* 12:99-108, 1986.
6. Donabedian A: Explorations in quality assessment and monitoring. Vol. I: The definition of quality and approaches to its assessment. Ann Arbor, MI, Health Administration Press, 1980.
7. Hynniman CE: Quality assurance and performance standards. In *Handbook of Institutional Pharmacy Practice*, 2nd ed. Baltimore, Williams and Wilkins, 1986, pp 632-645.
8. Anon: Quality of care—council on medical service. *JAMA* 256:1032-1034, 1986.
9. Donabedian A: The quality of care—how can it be assessed? *JAMA* 260:1743-1748, 1988.
10. Donabedian A: Commentary on some studies of the quality of care. *Health Care Fin Rev* (annu suppl) 75-85, 1987.
11. O'Donnell J: Status of standards of practice in pharmacy. *J Pharm Prac* 1:11-23, 1988.

12. Anon: Drug regimen review: A process guide for pharmacists. Arlington, VA, American Society of Consultant Pharmacists and Sandoz Pharmaceuticals Corporation, 1989, pp. 1-6.
13. Coe CP: Medicare surveys. In *Preparing the Pharmacy for a Joint Commission Survey*, 2nd ed. Bethesda, MD, American Society of Hospital Pharmacists, 1987, pp. 95-99.
14. Coe CP, Louviere ML: Understanding JCAH and preparing the pharmacy. *Am J Hosp Pharm* 43:2407-2411, 1986.
15. Kosha MT: JCAH accreditation: Top trouble spots for hospitals. *Hospitals*. 34. 1989(Aug 5).
16. Williams SJ, Torrens PR: Introduction to health services. New York, John Wiley and Sons, 1988.
17. Raffel MW, Raffel NK: The U.S. health system: Origins and functions, 3rd ed. New York, John Wiley and Sons, 1989.
18. Coe CP: Joint Commission on Accreditation of Healthcare Organizations. In *Preparing the Pharmacy for a Joint Commission Survey*, 2nd ed. Bethesda, MD, American Society of Hospital Pharmacists, 1987, pp. 2-5.
19. Fink JL III: Role of JCAH standards in negligence suits. *Am J Hosp Pharm* 38:892-896, 1981.
20. Joint Commission on Accreditation of Health Care Organizations: *Accreditation Manual for Hospitals*. Chicago, Joint Commission on Accreditation of Healthcare Organizations, 1990, pp. 169-183.
21. Coe CP: *Preparing for a Joint Commission Survey*, 2nd ed. Bethesda, MD, American Society of Hospital Pharmacists, 1987.
22. Joint Commission on Accreditation of Healthcare Organizations: *Monitoring and evaluation—pharmaceutical services*. Chicago: Joint Commission on Accreditation of Healthcare Organizations, 1987.
23. Joint Commission on Accreditation of Healthcare Organizations: *Examples of Drug Usage Evaluation*. Chicago, Joint Commission on Accreditation of Healthcare Organizations, 1989.
24. O'Leary DS: Quality assessment—moving from theory to practice (Editorial). *JAMA* 260:1760, 1988.
25. Enright SM: Assessing patient outcomes. *Am J Hosp Pharm* 45:1376-1378, 1988.
26. Stolar MH: Quality assurance of pharmaceutical services: An objective-based planning strategy. *Am J Hosp Pharm* 38:209-212, 1981.
27. Clarke RL, O'Leary DS: Leaders speak out on the quality of health care delivery. *Health Finance Mgt* 41:38-44, 1987.
28. Anon: ASHP's clinical indicator group. *Curr Concepts Hosp Pharm Mgt* 13, 1989 (summer).
29. Anon: Preliminary report of the ASHP quality assurance indicators development group. *Am J Hosp Pharm* 48:1941-1947, 1991.
30. Anon: JCAH plans new series of quality indicators based on outcome, clinical standards. *Rev Fed Am Hosp* 19:26-27, 1986.
31. Ente BH: The joint commission's agenda for change. *Curr Concepts Hosp Pharm Mgt* 7-14, 1989 (summer).
32. Donabedian A: *The Nursing Audit: Profile for Excellence*. New York, Appleton-Century Crofts, 1972.
33. Kalman SH, Schlegel JF: Standards of practice for the profession of pharmacy. *Am Pharm* 19:133-137, 1979.
34. Chalmers RK: Pharmacy education and the standards of practice. Paper presented as representative of ACPE to the 1989 annual meeting of the National Association of Boards of Pharmacy. Charleston, SC, May 9, 1989.
35. American Society of Consultant Pharmacists: *Guidelines for Consultant Pharmacists Practicing in Long Term Care Facilities* Arlington, VA, American Society of Consultant Pharmacists, 1981.
36. American College of Clinical Pharmacy: Minimum practice standards for clinical pharmacy specialists with interpretation for organized health care settings. *Drug Intell Clin Pharm* 21:645-647, 1987.
37. American Society of Hospital Pharmacists: *Practice Standards of the American Society of Hospital Pharmacists 1990-91*. Bethesda, MD, American Society of Hospital Pharmacists, 1990.
38. American Society of Hospital Pharmacists: ASHP accreditation standard for hospital pharmacy residency training (with guide to interpretation). *Am J Hosp Pharm* 42:2008-2018, 1985.
39. American Society of Hospital Pharmacists: Definitions of pharmacy residencies and fellowships. *Am J Hosp Pharm* 44:1142-1144, 1987.
40. Smith JE: The future of postgraduate training programs. *Am J Hosp Pharm* 47:98-104, 1990.
41. Hepler CD, Strand LM: Opportunities and responsibilities in pharmaceutical care. *Am J Hosp Pharm* 47:533-543, 1990.
42. Strand LM, Guerrero RM, Nickman NA, et al: Integrated patient-specific model of pharmacy practice. *Am J Hosp Pharm* 47:550-554, 1990.
43. Vogel DP, Gurwich E, Hutchinson RA: The quality assurance of professional staff. *Curr Concepts Hosp Pharm Mgt* 3:8-17, 1981.
44. Neal T: Minimum standards aid performance. *Hospitals* 54:70-73, 1980.
45. Vogel DP, Gurwich E, Campazna K, et al: Pharmacy unit devises quality assurance plan. *Hospitals* 54:83-85, 1980.
46. Pickering PH: Using performance standards for employee development. *Health Services Mgt* 13:6-9, 1980.
47. Allwine TC: Performance appraisals and performance standards. *Personnel J* 61:210-213, 1982.
48. Wells RG: Guidelines for effective and defensible performance appraisal systems. *Personnel J* 61:776-782, 1982.
49. Enright SM: Disease Audits. Philadelphia, Health Services Institute, 1990.
50. McCarthy C. Coping with the constant challenge of change. *Hospitals* 60:104, 1986.

APPENDIX 6-A

Thomas Jefferson University Hospital
Decentralized Pharmacy
Clinical Practice Standards*

Goal: The following practice activities are intended to promote rational drug use, to assure safe and cost-effective therapy, and to promote clinical pharmacy practice at Thomas Jefferson University Hospital.

Standard of Practice:

Pharmacists should prioritize their daily clinical activities to assure the following outcomes of therapy:

1. Prevent potentially significant drug interactions or allergies.
2. Avoid therapeutic duplications or contraindications.
3. Resolve significant deviations from usual dose or Pharmacy and Therapeutic guidelines.
4. Assure appropriate dosing of pharmacokinetically monitored drugs based on laboratory data or patient variation.
5. Adjust doses secondary to renal failure, etc.

Drug Information (oral and/or written) and consultation will be provided to the institution's staff upon request. The Drug Information Center and Pharmacy Consult Service are available as backup resources.

Clinical pharmacists shall identify other areas of involvement based on the patient population serviced.

*Reprinted with permission, Thomas Jefferson University Hospital.

CHAPTER 7

The Policy and Procedure Manual

JAMES M. HETHCOX

Most of what I really need to know about how to live and what to do and how to be I learned in kindergarten. . . .:

Share everything.
Play fair.
Don't hit people.
Put things back where you found them.
Clean up your own mess.
Don't take things that aren't yours.
Say you're sorry when you hurt somebody.
Wash your hands before you eat.
Flush.
Warm cookies and cold milk are good for you.
Live a balanced life—learn some and think some and draw and paint and sing and dance and work every day some.
Take a nap every afternoon.
When you go out into the world, watch out for traffic, hold hands and stick together.

Be aware of wonder. . . .And then remember the Dick-and-Jane books and the first word you learned—the biggest word of all—LOOK.

Everything you need to know is in there somewhere.
The Golden Rule and love and basic sanitation.
Ecology and politics and equality and sane living.

— **Robert Fulghum**[1]

A policy and procedure manual simplistically defined is merely a compilation of written statements that present information regarding administrative and professional policy decisions and the accepted methods for implementation of those decisions. However, when properly developed and used, it is much more—it is a valuable management tool.

For an institutional pharmacy staff, the manual can be a guide to effective and efficient provision of pharmaceutical services. For the institution's administration, medical staff, and pharmacy management, the manual can be a means to promote the safe, efficient, and uniform performance of departmental functions by all personnel.

NEED FOR POLICIES AND PROCEDURES

The need for policies and procedures governing the delivery of pharmaceutical services has been clearly stated in a number of recognized standards. In the 1950 revision of the "Minimum Standard for Pharmacies in Hospitals,"[2] which was approved by the American Society of Hospital Pharmacists (ASHP), the American Pharmaceutical Association, the American Hospital Association, and the Catholic Hospital Association, the pharmacy director was charged with responsibility for initiating and developing rules and regulations regarding the operation of the pharmacy department:

> The director of pharmacy service, with approval and cooperation of the director of the hospital, shall initiate and develop rules and regulations pertaining to the administrative policies of the department... [and] with the approval and cooperation of the Pharmacy and Therapeutics Committee, shall initiate and develop rules and regulations pertaining to the professional policies of the department.

In approving a revised "Minimum Standard for Pharmacies in Institutions"[3] in 1984, the ASHP board of directors reaffirmed the importance of written policies and procedures. Pertinent points from the latter document are presented in table 7-1.

Table 7-1. Key points from the Minimum Standard for Pharmacies in Institutions[3]

Policies and procedures should be developed by the pharmacist with input from other involved hospital staff and committees. Policies and procedures should include, but not necessarily be limited to:

1. Quality of drug therapy (developed in concert with the medical staff).
2. Procurement, distribution, and control of all drugs used within the hospital with specific references made to:
   - Use of investigational drugs;
   - Provision of pharmaceutical services in the event of a disaster;
   - Activities of medical sales representatives within the hospital;
   - Control procedures to ensure that patients receive the correct drugs at the proper time;
   - Handling of drugs that are putative occupational hazards; and
   - Identification and use of medications brought into the hospital by patients.
3. Management of drug expenditures by such methods as controlled formularies; competitive bid and group purchasing; drug use review programs; and cost-effective clinical services.

An operations manual (i.e., a policy and procedure manual) governing all pharmacy functions should be prepared and continually revised to reflect changes in procedures, organization, etc. All pharmacy personnel should be familiar with the contents.

The Joint Commission on Accreditation of Healthcare Organizations (JCAHO) has also established standards for pharmaceutical services within institutions.[4] These likewise require the pharmacist's active participation in establishment of policies and procedures specific to departmental services. Relevant points from these JCAHO standards are identified in table 7-2. Moreover, JCAHO standards for other institutional services—anesthesia services, emergency services, hospital-sponsored ambulatory care services, respiratory care, and special care units—as well as for infection control and safety, suggest establishment of additional policies and procedures related to the pharmaceutical service.

In *Preparing the Pharmacy for a Joint Commission Survey,*[5] Coe provides an excellent review of policies and procedures in the JCAHO context. Especially useful is a comprehensive checklist of JCAHO-required policies and procedures. Other entities that accredit hospitals (i.e., the American Osteopathic Association) or certify hospitals (i.e., the Healthcare Financing Administration relative to Medicare) similarly have addressed the necessity of written policies and procedures. Further information is presented in the publication by Coe.

POTENTIAL BENEFITS OF A MANUAL

Incentive to develop a policy and procedure manual should be provided by recognition of the benefits potentially derived from its creation and use. Among these is more effective departmental management:

- Establishment of standards of practice in both administrative and professional activities;
- Coordination of resources (i.e., personnel, supplies, and equipment) for delivery of efficient, economical services secondary to a reduction in or an elimination of waste of time and/or materials that otherwise results from error, inexperience, and/or need for direct supervision;
- Improvement of intradepartmental communications through provision of current, reliable, and readily retrievable information and reduction in errors associated with oral transmission of policy and/or procedural information among personnel;
- Improvement in employees' security, job satisfaction, and productivity with management's statement of performance expectations;
- Rapid detection of inefficient or inferior personnel performance through evaluation against written standards; and
- Establishment of means to evaluate the quality of services.

Additionally, consistency in orienting and training new personnel can be better achieved using a policy and procedure manual as a guide. Consistent orientation and training of personnel and the provision of a readily available, current, and comprehensive manual for *all personnel to reference routinely in their daily activities* foster service uniformity.

With input from other disciplines and services, development of policies and procedures can improve interdepartmental relationships—other departments or services will be familiar with pharmacy policies and procedures and vice versa. Moreover, interdepartmental conflict can be reduced as potential policy and/or procedural differences can be identified and less contentious policies and procedures written and communicated to the respective staffs. (In this context, some institutions require that policy and/or procedure statements having a scope spanning two or more departments or services be approved as institutional—not departmental—policies and/or procedures.)

Compliance with requirements of accrediting/certifying bodies (e.g., JCAHO) as previously discussed is another important benefit. This compliance is critical relative to third-party reimbursement (e.g., Medicare) and accreditation of an institution's teaching and training programs (e.g., residency programs).

The manual documents departmental standards of practice, and with evidence of compliance with the written policies and procedures, a manual can be used to demonstrate that due care has been taken to protect patient safety. Thus, it can be an important defense element in a legal action arising from a departmental error. It is imperative, however, that the policies and procedures be *periodically reviewed, revised as necessary to reflect operational changes, and enforced.*

Table 7-2. Key points from the Standards for Pharmaceutical Services of the Joint Commission on Accreditation of Healthcare Organizations[4]

Written policies and procedures relating to the selection, distribution, and safe and effective use of drugs in the hospital are to be established by the combined effort of the director of the pharmaceutical department/service, the medical staff, the nursing department/service, and the administration and approved by the medical staff.

Written policies and procedures pertaining to the intrahospital drug distribution system and essential for patient safety and for the control, accountability, and intrahospital distribution of drugs are to be developed by the director of the pharmaceutical department/service in concert with the medical staff and, as appropriate, with representatives of other disciplines. Furthermore, these policies and procedures are to be reviewed annually, revised as necessary, and enforced. These latter policies and procedures include, but need not be limited to, those relative to:

- Labeling, including accessory, cautionary, and/or expiration labeling;
- Disposition of discontinued, outdated, or improperly labeled drugs;
- Dispensing of drugs by pharmacy personnel;
- Removal of drugs from the pharmacy when a pharmacist is not available;
- Recall of drugs;
- Reporting of drug product defects; and
- Distribution of drug samples.

Written policies and procedures governing the safe administration of drugs and biologicals are to be developed by the medical staff in cooperation with the pharmaceutical department/service, the nursing department/service, and, as necessary, representatives of other disciplines. They are to be reviewed at least annually and revised as necessary. These policies and procedures include, but need not be limited to, the following:

- Delineation of authority to write medication orders and to receive verbal medication orders;
- Delineation of authority to administer medications;
- Establishment of automatic drug stop orders;
- Establishment of cautionary measures for the safe admixture of parenteral products;
- Verification of prescriber's orders and patient's identification at time of drug administration, and documentation of administration;
- Reporting and documentation of medication errors and adverse drug reactions;
- Use and handling of medications brought into the institution by patients;
- Self-administration of medications;
- Control and use of investigational drugs;
- Use of abbreviations and symbols in writing drug orders;
- Clear statement of administration times or intervals by prescriber; and
- Dispensing of drugs prescribed for ambulatory care patient use.

The director of the pharmaceutical department/service is responsible for providing written guidelines and for approving the procedure to assure that all pharmaceutical requirements are met when any part of preparing, sterilizing, and labeling parenteral medications and solutions is performed within the hospital but not under direct pharmacy supervision.

The director of the pharmaceutical department/service is responsible for performing an annual review of all pharmaceutical policies and procedures for the purpose of establishing their consistency with current practices within the hospital.

HOW THINGS STAND

Despite the well-established value of a manual consolidating the written departmental policies and procedures, many pharmacy departments have not had a long association with such a manual. In a 1957 survey of pharmaceutical services in this Nation's hospitals as reported in *Mirror to Hospital Pharmacy*,[6] approximately one of three pharmacy departments had written procedures regarding administrative practices, and even fewer had written policies and procedures regarding professional practices. A significant majority of the departments, however, had established—but unwritten—policies and procedures concerning both administrative and professional functions. Reasons cited for the pharmacist's failure to have developed *written* policies and procedures include:

- Failure of the administrator to insist that the pharmacist develop written policies and procedures,
- Pharmacist's lack of knowledge regarding the preparation of such statements, and
- Lack of time.

Moreover, established policy and procedure manuals are not used maximally. Frequently, their contents are ambiguous or outdated, and too often such manuals serve only as "'handsome ornaments for the management bookcase,'[7] lending an aura of organization and well-ordered communication to the department."[8]

The remainder of this chapter will focus on development and maintenance of a useful policy and procedure manual. First, however, affirmation that motivation for developing a departmental policy and procedure manual should come from the department manager—not from an insistent administrator—is made. A manual developed through any other motivation seems doomed to failure.

DEVELOPMENT OF A MANUAL

Definitions

In beginning a discussion of the development of a policy and procedure manual, workable definitions of the two key terms—"policy" and "procedure"—are useful. Formally defined, a policy is "a definite course or method of action . . .in light of given conditions to guide and determine present and future decisions."[9] More simply stated, a policy is a broad, general plan that provides a framework for decision making and action. It sets boundaries around decisions by broadly defining a position or response to a situation. A policy statement addresses specifically what must be done and sometimes addresses the questions of why and when.

A procedure is formally defined as "a particular way of accomplishing something or of acting" or "a series of steps followed in a regular definite order."[9] A procedure is a "how to" statement. It addresses how that which must be done (i.e., the policy) *is* to be done. It provides an explanation of the means or method by which the policy is to be carried out. In step-by-step fashion, it outlines the task through a complete cycle assigning responsibility for each function to specific personnel. Procedures are more subject to changes in technology, regulations, etc., than are policies; therefore, procedures are more fluid and dynamic.

In combination, policy and procedure statements answer the questions:

- What must be done?
- What is the purpose?
- When should it be done?
- Where should it be done?
- Who should do it?
- How should it be done?

Administrative Versus Professional Statements

Policies and procedures are characteristically either administrative or professional. Administrative policies and procedures relate to control of resources (i.e., personnel, supplies, and equipment) and departmental relationships to administration and other departments.

Professional policies and procedures pertain to patient care, whether direct or indirect. The foci for the latter include drug procurement, preparation, and distribution; other aspects of the handling and control of drugs, both departmentally and institutionally; and clinical services.

Writing Policies and Procedures

For the pharmacy department, policy and procedure statements are directed to a very diverse audience—pharmacists, technicians, students, other support personnel (e.g., secretaries, clerks, messengers). Information in such statements should be presented concisely and in a form easily understood by each member of the audience. Language should be simple and direct; that is, words should be short and familiar. Sentences should be short, simple, declarative, and expressive of a single idea. Format—whether outline, narrative, or playscript—should be uniform.

Various suggestions have been offered as to the individual(s) best suited to write policy and procedure statements: the department manager and/or the supervisory staff, a staff member who regularly performs or immediately supervises the activity, a committee of the department, etc. Regardless: Policies and procedures should be developed in cooperation with the institution's medical staff (usually through its pharmacy and therapeutics committee), administration, and other disciplines. Staff input should be obtained in the development of policies and procedures; the comprehensiveness, acceptance, and understanding of the statements will be improved. The person(s) writing policies and procedures should have an analytical mind. Creative writing should be avoided because of the relatively fixed writing pattern desired.

It might be beneficial to establish a departmental procedure analyst or specialist whose responsibilities could include proofing, standardizing, and editing rough and final drafts; preparing illustrations and figures; circulating drafts for comment and/or approval; preventing unnecessary duplication of material; and coordinating periodic review.[10]

A word-processing package should be used to facilitate drafting, revising, and reviewing policies and procedures.

Stepwise Approach to Preparing a Manual

One should begin a manual only after much thought and planning. However, this should not be a deterrent, nor should it provide an excuse for not developing a manual. Rather, one should find encouragement in the following facts: the developmental process has been begun with initiation of the planning (perhaps before the writing of the first policy and procedure), and success can be achieved through a strategy of "divide and conquer."

The latter would suggest updating existing policies and procedures before developing new ones as well as approaching easier statements before more complex ones. Moreover, given the dynamic state of pharmacy practice in which what is suited for today may be obsolete tomorrow, a manual should be in a state of constant development.

Ginnow and King[8] have suggested an organized approach for developing an effective policy and procedure manual (table 7-3):

Table 7-3. Seven-step approach to developing a policy and procedure manual[8]

Step 1: Analyze the mission, goals, and purposes of the institution and the department and then define the purposes(s) of the manual.

Step 2: Determine the method of content organization.

Step 3: Determine the specific subjects requiring policy and procedure statements.

Step 4: Compile a draft table of contents and circulate it to staff to ensure that the material will meet the needs of the department.

Step 5: Develop a suitable referencing system.

Step 6: Develop policies and procedures regarding (1) format, (2) writing style, (3) placement of illustrations or figures, (4) distribution of manual, (5) responsibility, (6) revisions and additions, and (7) review.

Step 7: Develop other policies and procedures in accordance with those developed in Step 6.

Step 1. Analyze the mission, goals, and purposes of the institution and the department. Then define the purpose(s) of the manual. Development of a manual should follow an outline designed to accommodate the department's unique needs. These needs will be affected by organizational structure; size of physical facilities; scope of services; complexity of operations; maturity of department; and nature of staff (e.g., size, caliber, and turnover).[8] Therefore, the contents of manuals will vary considerably among institutional pharmacy departments.

Step 2. Determine the method of content organization and presentation. The content of most manuals can be divided into several primary categories. A very basic scheme consists of only three primary divisions:

1. *General information* regarding the institution's and the department's description, development, mission, philosophy, goals, and objectives.
2. *Administrative information* including, but not limited to, personnel policies and procedures, organizational relationships, job descriptions, and control procedures for departmental resources.
3. *Professional policies and procedures* (i.e., those either directly or indirectly related to patient care). Foci include, but are not limited to, compounding and manufacturing, including IV admixture preparation and other special formulation; drug distribution, including unit dose and other inpatient drug distribution; dispensing for ambulatory care patients; control and distribution of investigational drugs; control and distribution of controlled substances; drug information services; and other clinical services.

In this scheme, much of the general and administrative information—although neither policy nor procedural in nature—is included to enhance the manual's value as an orientation and training guide. Examples of such information include mission and goals of the institution and the department; current institutional and departmental objectives; purposes of specific areas of the department; organization charts of the institution and the department (see figure 7-1); job descriptions (see figure 7-2); floor plans and location guides; and description of interdepartmental relationships.

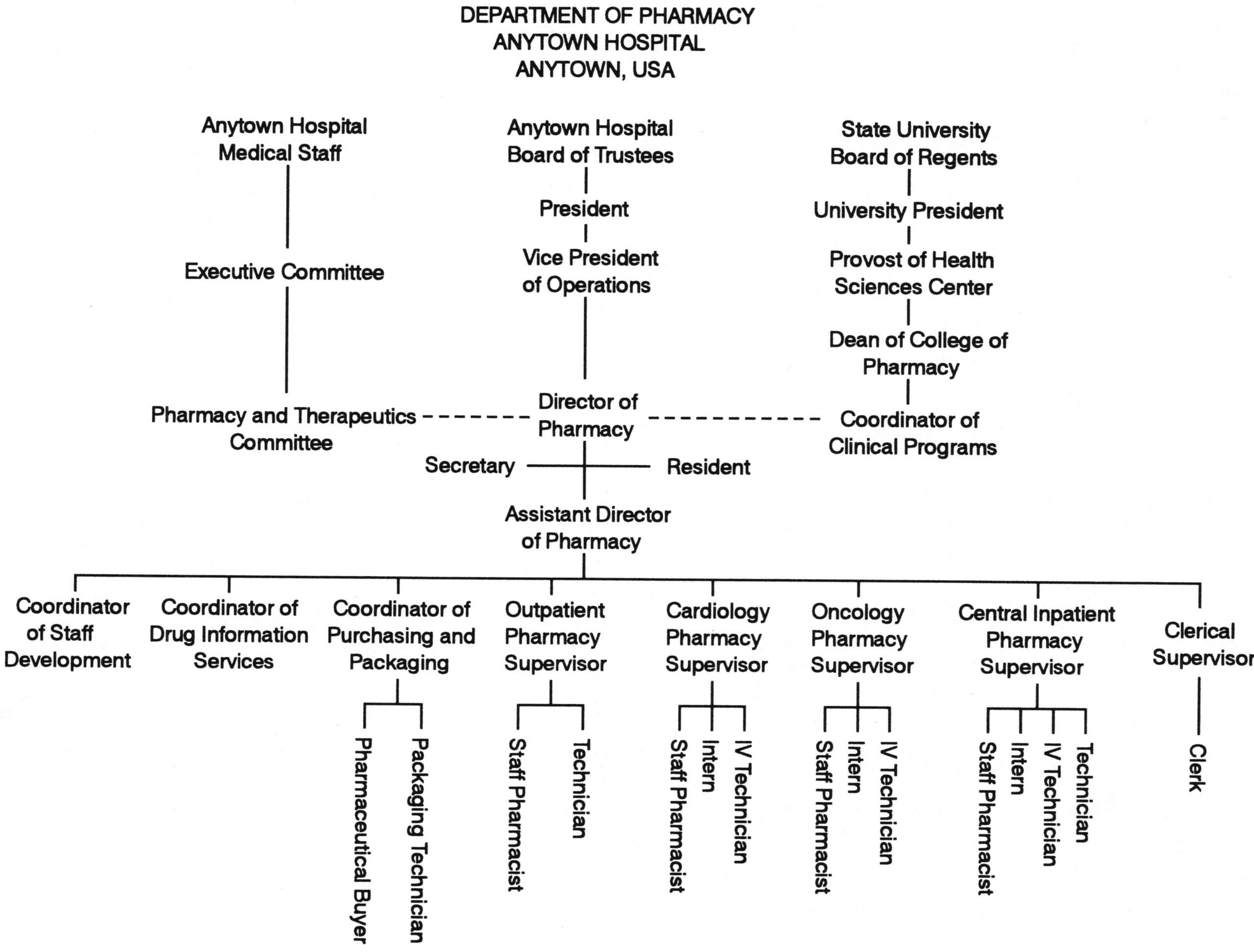

Figure 7-1. Example of organizational chart

POSITION DESCRIPTION

JOB TITLE: PHARMACIST UNIT MANAGER

POSITION NUMBER: 4740

DEPARTMENT: PHARMACY
SUPERVISOR: ASSISTANT DIRECTOR

JOB SUMMARY

The pharmacist unit manager is responsible for ensuring the effective and efficient provision of pharmaceutical care for patients in the assigned practice area. To this end, the individual must take a leadership role in planning, organizing, coordinating, directing, and controlling all unit activities. As a line manager, the individual is also required to fulfill all of the responsibilities delineated in the staff pharmacist position description related to the assigned practice area.

QUALIFICATIONS

The unit manager must have a minimum of a Bachelor of Science degree in pharmacy and be licensed as a pharmacist in the State. Proven leadership skills or potentials are required. The individual must be effective in oral and written communications as well as interpersonal relationships. The individual must possess the ability to work with automated information systems.

DUTIES AND RESPONSIBILITIES

I. Unit Operations

A. Effectively manages assigned areas by planning, organizing, coordinating, directing, and controlling all pharmacy service program elements in assigned areas.

B. Actively participates in departmental budget preparation and is responsible for expense and revenue performance for assigned cost centers.

C. Sets standards for a safe, efficiently organized and orderly practice or work environment and ensures maintenance of those standards.

D. Coordinates quality control measures and quality assurance studies for assigned areas.

E. Schedules and conducts unit staff meetings.

F. Prepares and submits productivity and other reports as required.

II. Personnel Management

A. Supervises assigned pharmacists, technicians, and other support personnel in the performance of all duties.

B. Effectively communicates with all levels of departmental and hospital staff, as well as with patients.

C. Actively participates in the development of criteria and strategies for the recruitment, selection, and retention of staff. Assists in the recruitment and selection of departmental personnel.

D. Ensures appropriate staffing for assigned practice areas or work sites through preparation of work schedules for pharmacists and technicians and arranging for coverage for staffing vacancies.

E. Ensures timely and accurate preparation and submission of attendance records for designated staff.

F. Continually appraises individual practice and work performance for assigned staff. Periodically conducts evaluation and followup as indicated.

III. Other

A. Fulfills the responsibilities of a staff pharmacist as required.

B. Establishes and integrates individual and unit goals with departmental goals and objectives, and assumes a leadership role in their realization.

C. Provides coverage for immediate supervisor as needed.

D. Assumes responsibility for all service-related activities in designated areas.

E. Performs other position-related duties as assigned by the immediate supervisor.

KNOWLEDGE, SKILLS, AND ABILITIES

I. A basic working knowledge of all practice areas of the department.

II. Currency in management and professional practice literature relevant to assigned areas.

________	________	________	________
Personnel	Incumbent	Supervisor	Dept. Head
________	________	________	________
Date	Date	Date	Date

Figure 7-2. Example of a job description

If included, organization charts should clearly reflect the department's relationship to administration and other departments as well as accurately depict departmental organization including relationships among departmental staff. All lines of authority, direct and indirect, affecting the department should be readily identified (see figure 7-1).

Ginnow and King[8] recommend that the manual include a preface (see figure 7-3) stating purpose(s) of the manual; major headings within the manual; authority of the manual; how other published instructions affect the use of the manual; explanation of the classification system (i.e., the organization of the manual and how to locate material); method for handling new material and revisions; and what is expected of users.

When possible, an alphabetical index, in addition to the table of contents, should be included to facilitate cross-referencing. The sophistication of today's word-processing software makes this task a much less formidable challenge.

Figure 7-4 provides a detailed illustration of content organization based on departmental management responsibilities.[8] Figure 7-5 illustrates, but in less detail, other schemes of varying complexity.[11-14]

Step 3. Determine the specific subjects requiring policy and procedure statements. Helpful information can be obtained from old policies and procedures; minutes of staff meetings, pharmacy and therapeutics committee meetings, interdepartmental meetings, etc.; departmental memoranda and reports; instructions on forms and equipment; job descriptions; input from staff and other departments; interviews; manuals of other departments of the institution; and manuals of other pharmacy departments.[8]

Reviewing manuals from other pharmacy departments may stimulate ideas. Additionally, ideas might be obtained from a series of sample policy and procedure statements published in *Current Concepts in Hospital Pharmacy Management* beginning with the spring 1980 issue.[15]

Specialized manuals may be used to complement the contents of the policy and procedure manual. Examples include a master formula and compounding manual and a computer operations manual.

Step 4. Compile a draft table of contents and circulate it to staff to ensure that the material will meet the needs of the department.

Step 5. Develop a suitable referencing system. The system selected must be flexible to permit additions or deletions without disruption of the previous sequence of material. Options include open numbering, closed numbering (e.g., Dewey decimal system), and alphabetical.

Step 6. Develop policies and procedures regarding format; writing style; distribution; revisions and additions; review; responsibility; and placement of illustrations or figures. (See the original report by Ginnow and King[8] for detailed examples of policies and procedures regarding the first five topics.)

Step 7. Develop other policies and procedures in accordance with the policies and procedures developed in Step 6. As noted relative to Step 3, reviewing policies and procedures from other pharmacy departments may be helpful. However, each pharmacy department is unique, and severe legal consequences could occur should another's policies and procedures be adopted without effective implementation and enforcement.

As another word of caution, many policies and procedures that may be developed by the department of pharmacy warrant explicit, extradepartmental approval prior to implementation. For example, JCAHO's Standards for Pharmaceutical Services requires that written policies and procedures relating to the selection, distribution, and safe and effective use of drugs in the hospital are to be established by the combined effort of the director of the pharmaceutical department or service, the medical staff, the nursing department or service, and the administration and *approved by the medical staff* (see table 7-2). Also, the JCAHO in its Standards for Medical Staff requires that the "pharmacy and therapeutics function [be] performed by the medical staff....[and] includes...development or approval of policies and procedures relating to the selection, distribution, handling, use, and administration of drugs and diagnostic testing materials."[4]

DISTRIBUTION OF A MANUAL

Specific policies and procedures regarding the location of all manuals, as well as the distribution of copies of new and revised policies and procedures, should be developed early. This controls the number of manuals issued and ensures that appropriate personnel receive material promptly. Also, limiting distribution reduces costs as well as difficulties in maintaining and updating manuals.

Manuals should be distributed only to individuals or areas that have a continuing and frequent requirement for them. McNairn[7] has suggested that should a manual be used less than once daily, the distribution of that copy would probably be unwarranted. Changes in interdepartmental relationships may alter the established distribution.

All departmental employees should have access to library copies available throughout the department and should be responsible for reading, understanding, and complying with the written policies and procedures.

REVIEW AND REVISION OF A MANUAL

"Even if you're on the right track, you'll get run over if you just sit there." — **Will Rogers**[16]

If the policy and procedure manual is to clarify rather than confuse, the contained information must be *current* and *reliable*. Because a pharmacy department is a dynamic rather than static entity, policies and procedures must be flexible and change accordingly. Thus, the manual must be readily revisable. A manual failing to satisfy this characteristic will become static and will not be used to its fullest. The entire contents should be reviewed or revised frequently, at least annually, "to ensure currency and conformity with new laws, rules, and regulations of government agencies...and with the standards of the Joint Commission on Accreditation of [Healthcare Organizations]."[17]

The manual should be looseleaf rather than permanently bound to facilitate entry of new materials and removal of those that are superseded. A three-ring binder rather than a post binder is recommended to permit easier insertion and deletion of materials.[8]

Policies and procedures that clearly identify the method for handling revisions in the manual should be established. These should address who can initiate change, how change is accomplished, who reviews and comments on change, and processing of revised material no longer in effect.[8]

PREFACE

I. PURPOSE

The purpose of a policy and procedure manual is to provide an authoritative source of official organizational policies, procedures, and practices, as well as to define operational responsibilities and the line of authority in the various areas within a department. The departmental *Policy and Procedure Manual* will serve:

A. As a means of standardizing and coordinating procedures
B. As a reference and guide for daily operations
C. As a means of orientation for new pharmacy personnel
D. As a central record of the departmental policies

II. MATERIALS INCLUDED IN THE MANUAL

The *Policy and Procedure Manual* is divided into five main areas:

DIVISION 01 General
DIVISION 02 Drug Distribution Division
DIVISION 03 Administration and Technology Division
DIVISION 04 Drug Information Division
DIVISION 05 Clinical Services, Education, and Research Division

The divisions are subdivided into various chapters as listed in the table of contents to cover the topics included in each division.

III. AUTHORITY OF THIS MANUAL

A. The instructions contained in this manual are official and shall be relied upon as the basis for the performance of work. It is the responsibility of each employee to be thoroughly familiar with each policy and procedure covered in the manual that affects the scope of responsibility of that employee. Questions about any specific policy or procedure should be referred to the employee's supervisor for clarification. Since all conceivable work situations cannot be anticipated by an instruction, the policies and procedures set forth in this manual shall be regarded as guides to performance under related or analogous conditions.

B. Situations may arise where conformance with the instructions in this manual may not be possible. This may be because the original instructions may not have anticipated additional factors that may be present in a given situation. Whenever such a situation arises, the supervisor is expected to exercise judgment as to whether the instruction shall be suspended pending review by the director of pharmacy or in emergency situations whether other action is required, provided there is no violation of law or fixed hospital policy. This does not mean that the supervisor may, at will, suspend the effect of instruction with which he or she may not be in agreement. This shall be regarded as an emergency authority only, and in every case of the exercise of this authority, a full written report shall be made to the director of pharmacy. This report shall justify why emergency exception to the rules was taken without prior authorization.

IV. OTHER GENERAL PUBLISHED INSTRUCTIONS

A. Other general published instructions of the Department of Pharmacy shall be within the framework of the policies and procedures of this manual or shall be supplementary to it. In the event of conflict between other published instructions and this manual, the manual shall take precedence, unless otherwise specified.

B. Occasionally, it may be necessary to issue temporary instructions that will take precedence over materials in the manual. When this is done, the temporary instruction shall clearly state the exceptions and shall include a time limit for the temporary instructions.

C. If a supervisor should issue oral or written instructions in conflict with this manual, such superseding instructions shall be followed, but it is the responsibility of the person receiving them to point out the conflict with the manual. This shall be regarded as an emergency authority only, and in every case of the exercise of this authority, a full report shall be made to the director of pharmacy. This report shall justify why emergency exception to the rules was taken without prior authorization.

V. HOW TO FIND MATERIAL

The material covered by this manual has been organized into divisions, chapters, sections, parts, and subparts. All subdivisions are numbered with Arabic numerals. A typical section designation, therefore, would be 01-20-15:

DIVISION 01 General
CHAPTER 20 Policy and Procedure Manual
SECTION 15 Distribution

When more than one page is required for a particular part or subpart, a dash and the letter "A" shall follow the first page number. The second page would be "B" and so on, as necessary. Through reference to the table of contents, one may ordinarily find all related material together. Sample forms will appear at the end of each division and will be numbered consecutively within each division.

VI. NEW MATERIAL AND REVISIONS

Chapters, sections, parts, and subparts are numbered so that additional information may be inserted without altering the numbering system; that is, originally every fifth digit was used. In most cases, a draft of proposed new material will be sent to all concerned individuals so that suggestions and recommendations can be made. All new material, as well as revisions of old material, will be placed in each volume of the manual by the secretarial staff, at which time a copy, under cover of a transmittal memorandum, where necessary, will be sent to each employee concerned, stating that the attached policy and procedure has been placed in the manuals. A copy of the *Policy and Procedure Manual* will be located in each area of the Department of Pharmacy and will be available to any departmental employee.

Figure 7-3. Example of a preface to a policy and procedure manual

DIVISION 01 General

	No.	Title
CHAPTER	05	Introduction
SECTION	05	Anytown Hospital
PART	05	General Statement
	10	Statement of Mission and Goals
	15	Maps
SECTION	10	Department of Pharmaceutical Services
PART	05	General Statement
	10	Statement of Mission and Goals
	15	Division Purposes
	20	Objectives for the Current Year
	25	Floor Plan and Location Guide
	30	Departmental Appearance
CHAPTER	10	Department of Pharmaceutical Services Organization
SECTION	05	Organization Chart
	10	Acting Authority
	15	Position Descriptions
PART	05	Drug Distribution Division
SUBPART	05	Assistant Director
	10	Inpatient Supervisor
	15	Outpatient Supervisor
	20	Staff Pharmacist
	25	Senior Data Entry Operator
	30	Pharmacy Technician
	35	Pharmacy Intern
SECTION	20	Committees
CHAPTER	15	Standards
SECTION	05	American Pharmaceutical Association Code of Ethics
	10	Joint Commission on Accreditation of Healthcare Organizations—Pharmaceutical Services
	15	American Society of Hospital Pharmacists—Minimum Standard for Pharmacies in Institutions
	20	State Board of Health—Pharmacy Standards
	25	American Society of Hospital Pharmacists—Accreditation Standard for Hospital Pharmacy Residency Training with Guide to Interpretation
	30	Minimum Expectations of a Pharmacist
	35	Hospital Code of Ethics
	40	Patient's Bill of Rights
CHAPTER	20	Policy and Procedure Manual
SECTION	05	Format
	10	Writing Style
	15	Distribution
	20	Responsibility
	25	Revisions and Additions
	30	Review
CHAPTER	25	Personnel Policies
	30	Staffing and Scheduling
	35	Security
	40	Interdepartmental Relationships
	45	Communications
	50	Safety Program—Accident Prevention
	55	Fire Emergency Plan
	60	Disaster Plan
	65	Bomb Threat
	70	Public Relations

DIVISION 02 Drug Distribution

	No.	Title
CHAPTER	05	General
	10	Central Inpatient Pharmacy Service
	15	Outpatient Pharmacy Service
	20	Satellite Pharmacies

DIVISION 03 Administration and Technology

	No.	Title
CHAPTER	05	Administration
	10	Purchasing and Inventory
	15	Quality Assurance
	20	Technology
	25	Transportation

DIVISION 04 Drug Information

	No.	Title
CHAPTER	05	Drug Information Requests
	10	Pharmacy and Therapeutics Committee
	15	Publications
	20	Investigational Drugs
	25	Library
	30	Adverse Drug Reaction Reporting Program
	35	Drug Allergy Reporting Program
	40	Drug Interaction Reporting Program

DIVISION 05 Clinical Services, Education, and Research

	No.	Title
CHAPTER	05	Clinical Services
	10	Education
	15	Research

Figure 7-4. Portion of table of contents of a policy and procedure manual: Illustration of content organization based on departmental management responsibilities[8]

The method(s) for communicating new or revised policies and/or procedures should be explicitly stated. (See item "VI. New Material and Revisions" in figure 7-3, an example of a preface to a policy and procedure manual, for one method. Figure 7-3 also illustrates methods for handling the authority of the manual (see item III) and other published instructions (see item IV).

Maintaining control of policies and procedures that are issued, revised, and/or reviewed can be accomplished through individual signatures and dates of issuance, revision, and/or review on each document, or a policy that all policies and procedures must be approved by the pharmacy director before insertion into the manual.[8]

The original date of issuance or revision can be indicated on the document. A policy requiring annual review and a central file of review dates will provide assurance of current information and necessary documentation. Copies of old policy and procedures that have been revised should be maintained on file for reference purposes.

(For additional information on developing and maintaining policy and procedure manuals, see the Additional Reading section.)

Scheme A:
- Organization
- Facilities
- Personnel
- Services and Activities

Scheme B:
- Philosophy
- General
- Administrative
- Dispensing
- Interdepartmental
- Bulk Compounding and Sterile Solutions

Scheme C:
- General
- Pharmacy Standards
- Preparation, Handling, and Dispensing of Pharmaceuticals
- Narcotics, Hypnotics, Amphetamines, Alcoholic Liquors, and Other Controlled Drugs
- Pharmacy Stores and Inventory Management
- Records and Reports

Scheme D:
- Nuclear Pharmacy Services
- Unit Dose Dispensing
- Ambulatory Care and Home Care Services
- Intravenous Admixture
- Sterile Products
- Drug Administration
- Clinical Pharmacy Services
- Drug Information and Poison Control Services
- Education and Training
- Professional Staff Development
- Residency Training Program
- Technician Selection and Training
- Computerized Pharmacy Operations
- Pharmaceutical and Clinical Research
- Assay and Quality Control
- Drug Kinetics and Bioavailability Laboratory
- Manufacturing and Packaging
- Purchasing and Inventory Control
- Departmental Services
- Investigational Drug Studies

Figure 7-5. Other schemes of content organization[11-14]

CONCLUSION

The need for written policies and procedures, the benefits afforded a department by the establishment and maintenance of a policy and procedure manual, and recommendations for the development and maintenance of a useful manual have been discussed. In closing, a final note of caution is given: The policy and procedure manual should inform and guide, not suppress professional judgment, personal initiative, or creativity.

ACKNOWLEDGMENT

The author gratefully acknowledges contributions of William K. Ginnow and Charles M. King, Jr., to "The Policy and Procedure Manual" as published in the first and second editions of *Handbook of Institutional Pharmacy Practice* (Baltimore, Williams & Wilkins).

REFERENCES

1. Fulghum R: *All I Really Need to Know I Learned in Kindergarten.* New York, Villard Books, 1989.
2. *Minimum Standard for Pharmacies in Hospitals with Guide to Application.* Washington, DC, American Society of Hospital Pharmacists, 1950.
3. ASHP guidelines: Minimum standard for pharmacies in institutions. *Am J Hosp Pharm* 42:372-375, 1985.
4. *Accreditation Manual for Hospitals, 1992.* Oakbrook Terrace, IL, Joint Commission on Accreditation of Healthcare Organizations, 1991.
5. Coe CP: *Preparing the Pharmacy for a Joint Commission Survey*, 2nd ed. Bethesda, MD, American Society of Hospital Pharmacists, 1987.
6. Francke DE, Latiolais CJ, Francke GN, et al: *Mirror to Hospital Pharmacy.* Washington, DC, American Society of Hospital Pharmacists, 1964.
7. McNairn WN: Three ways to wake up procedure manuals. *Mgt Advisor* 10:26-33, 1973.
8. Ginnow WK, King CM Jr: Revision and reorganization of a hospital pharmacy policies and procedures manual. *Am J Hosp Pharm* 35:698-704, 1978.
9. *Webster's New Collegiate Dictionary.* Springfield, MA, G&C Merriam, 1976.
10. Coughlin CW: The need for good procedures. *J Syst Mgt* 24:30-33, 1973.
11. Latiolais CJ: Pharmacy procedure manual: Policy guide and evaluation tool. *Hospitals* 33:77-78, 1959.
12. Gonzales M Sr, Reilly MJ: The preparation of a procedure manual for a hospital pharmacy. *Am J Hosp Pharm* 21:458-463, 1964.
13. Eckel FM: Developing a policy and procedure manual. *Drug Intell Clin Pharm* 1:128-131, 1967.
14. Godwin HN: Institutional patient care. In Gennaro AR (ed): *Remington's Pharmaceutical Sciences*, 17th ed. Easton, PA, Mack Publishing, 1985, pp 1702-1722.
15. The policy and procedure manual: The basis of management. *Curr Concepts Hosp Pharm Mgt* 2:7-10, 1980.
16. Byrne R: *1,911 Best Things Anybody Ever Said.* New York, Fawcett Columbine, 1988.
17. *Reference Manual on Hospital Pharmacy.* Chicago, American Hospital Association, 1970.

ADDITIONAL READING

Donnelly PR: *Guide for Developing a Hospital Administrative Policy Manual.* St. Louis, Catholic Hospital Association, 1973.

Ginnow WK, King CM Jr.: Revision and reorganization of a hospital pharmacy policies and procedures manual. *Am J Hosp Pharm* 35:698-704, 1978.

Grubb RD: *Hospital Manuals—A Guide to Development and Maintenance.* Rockville, MD, Aspen Systems, 1981.

CHAPTER 8

Drug Use Management

ARTHUR G. LIPMAN

In 1966, Brodie characterized drug use control as the mainstream of professional practice of pharmacy.[1] He defined drug use control as that system of knowledge, understanding, judgments, procedures, skills, controls, and ethics that ensures optimal safety in the use of medication. That statement is perhaps the clearest articulation of our *raison d'être*, our reason to exist. Effective management of medication acquisition, prescribing, administration, and monitoring is perhaps the most important and effective way in which pharmacists can achieve drug use control.

To manage drug use effectively in an organized health care setting, pharmacists must have appropriate policies, procedures, and programs relating to both pharmaceutical services and therapeutics within the institution. These must be both proactive and reactive; they must be both anticipatory and able to respond to the needs that arise. Effective drug use management requires that the department of pharmaceutical services continually anticipate drug needs, define and address drug information needs of the professional staff of the institution, define and address drug information needs of patients, and objectively evaluate new drugs and determine their place in therapy (figure 8-1). These services provide a basis for drug use control. They must be in place before the patient enters the system, and they provide a foundation for drug therapy monitoring and other clinical pharmacy services.

Drug needs are met through an efficient purchasing and inventory control system. Drug information needs are met through drug information and clinical pharmacy services. Effective and objective review and evaluation of pharmaceuticals and the development of policies relating to the use of the drugs in the institution are major responsibilities that have been described as the pharmacy and therapeutics function.

The Joint Commission on Accreditation of Healthcare Organizations (JCAHO, formerly the Joint Commission on Accreditation of Hospitals) mandates in the "Medical Staff" section of the *Accreditation Manual for Hospitals* that a pharmacy and therapeutics function is performed by the medical staff in cooperation with the pharmaceutical department/service, the nursing department/service, management and administrative services, and, as required, other departments and services and individuals:

> . . . the pharmacy and therapeutics monitoring function includes at least the following: (1) the development of policies and procedures relating to the selection, distribution, handling, use and administration of drugs and diagnostic testing materials; (2) the development and maintenance of a drug formulary or drug list; (3) the evaluation and, when no other such mechanism exists, the approval of protocols concerned with the use of investigational or experimental drugs; and (4) the definition and review of all significant untoward drug reactions.[2]

This pharmacy and therapeutics function could be performed by a quality control committee or even an administrative coordinator. However, due to the complexity and political sensitivity of the task, the pharmacy and therapeutics function is nearly always assigned to a medical staff committee commonly designated the pharmacy and therapeutics (P&T) committee. Other titles such as the formulary committee or pharmacy committee are sometimes used. Increasingly, hospitals that use such alternative names are changing the designation to P&T committee to more accurately describe the committee's charge.

The Joint Commission pharmacy and therapeutics monitoring mandate provides the authority for a comprehensive system of drug use management. Drug use management might be defined as the method by which pharmacists achieve drug use control. Essential to a system of drug use management is the development and operation of an effective hospital formulary system. That system provides much of the justification and authority for pharmacists to provide drug use control. Therefore, it is incumbent upon all pharmacy managers to ensure that all pharmacist and supportive personnel in the department fully understand the purpose and function of the formulary system and the role that each member of the department has in ensuring that the system is managed effectively in the interest of quality, cost-effective patient care.

Both an effective formulary system and comprehensive pharmaceutical services are essential for drug use management. Because direct responsibility for the formulary system is most commonly assigned to the P&T committee, an effective committee is essential to the department of pharmaceutical services in achieving its professional goals.

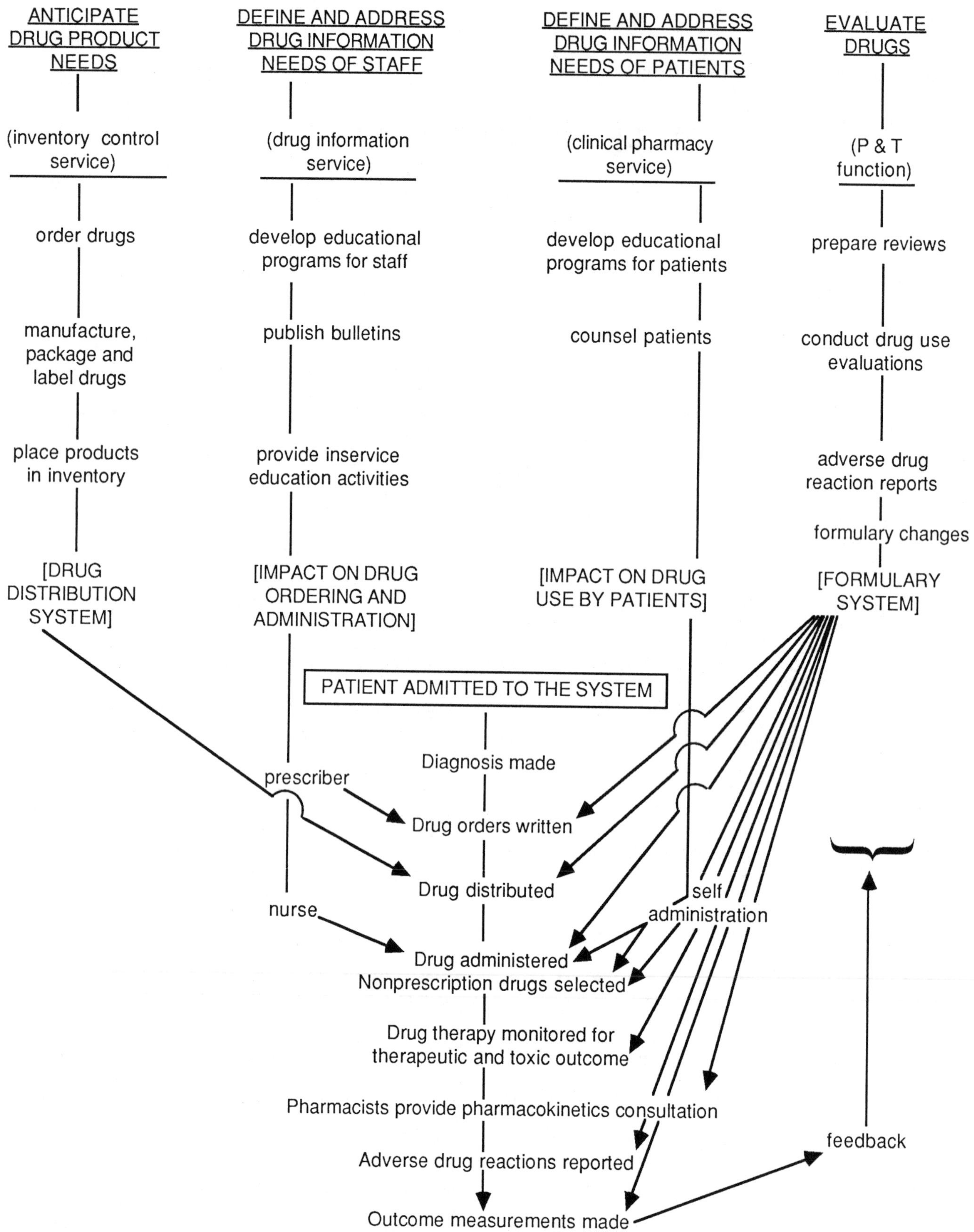

Figure 8-1. The drug use control process

THE P&T COMMITTEE

The American Society of Hospital Pharmacists (ASHP) Statement on the pharmacy and therapeutics committee defines it as "an advisory group of the medical staff and... the organizational line of communication between the medical staff and the pharmacy department."[3] To serve as the liaison between the medical staff and the department of pharmaceutical services, the P&T committee should be a strong advocate for progressive pharmaceutical services including clinical services, drug information, and an efficient drug distribution system. The chairperson of the committee should be a respected member of the medical staff who is both familiar with and an advocate for progressive pharmaceutical services. The chairperson can be the most effective political ally of the director of pharmaceutical services in dealings with both the medical staff and the hospital administration. If the committee chairperson is a pharmacist rather than a physician, the political advantage of a medical staff member's serving as advocate on behalf of pharmaceutical services is lost. The secretary of the committee should be the director of pharmaceutical services or another pharmacist appointed by the director of pharmaceutical services. The secretary sets the agenda for each meeting in collaboration with the committee chairperson.

The committee should include members from each of the major clinical departments of the medical staff; other departments that use drugs or provide data relevant to drug use, e.g., dental service and clinical laboratories; and nursing services and hospital administration. Other departments and offices might also be represented, e.g., quality assurance and risk management. If a specific pharmacist is responsible for drug information service in the hospital, that individual often sits on the committee. Guests are frequently invited to attend for educational purposes, e.g., staff pharmacists, pharmacy residents, and health professional students.

Committee members should be respected, articulate members of their departments. The chairperson and secretary of the P&T committee should review the participation and attendance of each member annually and suggest changes to the department chairpersons and chief of staff when indicated.

The P&T committee should meet on a regular schedule. Most committees find either breakfast or luncheon meetings to be most conducive to good attendance and participation. When an individual is being considered for appointment to the committee, the secretary should inform the candidate of the meeting schedule for the full year. Continuity is important for many ongoing topics. Therefore, if a nominee to the committee is unable to attend many meetings, perhaps another person should be selected. Most P&T committees meet for 60 to 90 minutes once a month.

The agenda should be prepared and distributed to the members approximately 1 week prior to each meeting. This serves as a meeting reminder and gives members an opportunity to review the topics to be discussed. Reviews of drugs being evaluated for formulary admission or deletion, policy changes, adverse drug reaction summaries, and other materials relevant to the agenda should be included. A sample agenda is shown in Appendix 8-A.

When developing the agenda, the secretary should minimize topics that can be handled administratively and maximize items that require interdisciplinary discussions. Many P&T committees use standing subcommittees that report periodically to the full committee. This is commonly done for adverse drug reaction monitoring, drug use evaluations, antibiotic resistance monitoring, and dietetic formulations. Special subcommittees may be appointed by the chairperson as necessary to develop positions on complex issues that cannot be discussed efficiently by the full committee. Such subcommittees often include specialists who do not sit on the full committee.

Most P&T committees have full authority to change the formulary and adopt drug use and pharmaceutical service policy changes. The executive committee of the medical staff usually is the institutional authority that empowers the P&T committee to do so. It is therefore important for the P&T committee secretary to ensure that the medical staff executive committee receives full copies of all P&T committee minutes. For politically sensitive issues, it may be useful for the P&T committee to request that the executive committee actively ratify the P&T committee's actions. Actions of the P&T committee are actions of the medical staff, not of the department of pharmaceutical services.

The P&T committee has an important educational responsibility to the professional staff of the institution. Most commonly, this responsibility is met through the committee's authorizing publication of a drug therapy bulletin. Under the aegis of their P&T committees, many departments of pharmaceutical services publish both general drug information bulletins and special bulletins, e.g., adverse drug reactions reports and drug use evaluation reports. The former usually appear monthly or bimonthly; the latter may be in the form of quarterly newsletters or communications to the affected hospital departments. Some committees also sponsor annual drug therapy-related lectures or seminars for the hospital staff.

THE FORMULARY AND THE FORMULARY SYSTEM

It is important that hospital staff members not confuse the formulary with the formulary system. The formulary is only one part of the system. A hospital formulary was defined more than 20 years ago by ASHP and the American Hospital Association (AHA) as "a continually revised compilation of pharmaceuticals that reflects the current clinical judgement of the medical staff."[4]

The formulary for one hospital might differ from that of another institution in the same neighborhood. This could be due to differences in staff preferences for similar drugs, antibiotic resistance patterns, or differences in the institutional case mixes.

A hospital formulary system includes the formulary, a method for staff members to request that drugs be admitted to and deleted from the formulary, programs to monitor drug use and untoward effects such as drug use evaluation and adverse drug reaction reporting activities, and provision of reference monographs and educational programs relating to the drugs on the formulary. The formulary system has been defined by ASHP and AHA as:

> a method whereby the medical staff of an institution, working though the pharmacy and therapeutics committee, evaluates, appraises, and selects from the numerous available drug entities and drug products those that are considered most useful in patient care. Only those so selected are routinely available from

the pharmacy. The formulary system is thus an important tool in assuring the quality of drug use and controlling its cost. The formulary system provides for the procuring, prescribing, dispensing and administering of drugs under either their proprietary or nonproprietary names in the instances when drugs have both names.[4]

Some hospitals claim to have an "open formulary," i.e., a system in which the formulary only recommends drugs but nonformulary drugs are routinely available. That is not a formulary system, and it is doubtful if such a system is worth the effort required to support it.

Today, formulary systems very similar to those of hospitals are used effectively by health maintenance organizations and other managed health care programs and by long-term care facilities. Formularies also are developed by some military organizations, State medical care programs, and other organized health care providers. Most of these are not analogous to hospital formularies. The formulary system of a specific health care facility normally is unique to that facility or small group of closely affiliated facilities. It is neither a governmental nor other broadly applied program. One of the important characteristics of a formulary system is that it reflects the current clinical judgment of the medical staff of the institution to which it applies. It should be flexible and dynamic.

Advantages of a Formulary System

A well-managed formulary system has three purposes that provide three benefits to the institution. The first and principal purpose of the system is to help ensure the quality and appropriateness of drug use within the institution. The second is to teach appropriate drug therapy to the staff. The third purpose is cost-effective drug therapy, not simply drug cost reductions.

The first benefit occurs because those physicians and other professional staff with the greatest subject area expertise for each drug category consult on which drugs should be routinely available for patient care. Thus, the internist who wishes to use an ophthalmic anti-infective selects from among the formulations in which the ophthalmologists have the most confidence. In this way, the formulary system provides an informal consult on drugs of choice. The formulary lists the most generally appropriate drugs, but it cannot ensure that the drugs are being used for the appropriate indications, at optimal doses, or for the appropriate durations. Therefore, a drug use evaluation program is an important component of a well-managed formulary system.

The second benefit is educational. Many thousands of drug formulations are commercially available. No single professional can know them all well enough to use all rationally. The formulary should include a reasonable number of therapeutic alternatives while being sufficiently limited that staff members can become familiar with the formulary drugs they routinely use. Staff members can be comfortable with the fact that their patients will not be denied important, new drugs if they know that those drugs will be considered for formulary admission at an appropriate time. To maintain this benefit, when new drugs are considered for formulary admission, similar agents including those previously on the formulary should be reviewed and deleted if appropriate. Not infrequently, a new drug can replace two or more older agents. A worthwhile educational benefit can result when drug class reviews are shared with the institution staff through a P&T committee-sponsored drug information bulletin.

Economic benefits to the institution accrue in several ways. With a limited formulary, the department of pharmaceutical services can maintain a more efficient purchasing and inventory control system. Maintaining a drug in stock is nearly half again as expensive as the purchase price.[5] Savings result from the department not having capital tied up in unneeded inventory and being able to buy larger quantities of fewer drugs than smaller quantities of more drugs, as is necessary with an inefficient formulary system. Obviously, when two drugs are therapeutically very similar and there is not a need for both on the formulary, the less expensive agent usually is more appropriate for the formulary. Many medical staff members may be unaware of relative drug costs. Therefore, comparative drug costs should be a feature of the drug information bulletin that supports the formulary system.

Establishing a Formulary System

The first step in establishing an effective formulary system is ensuring that the appropriate authority and scope of responsibility are described in the medical staff bylaws. When physicians join the staff, they agree to practice according to those bylaws. An explicit statement that drugs will be prescribed, dispensed, and administered according to the formulary system should appear in that document. The P&T function also should be defined in the bylaws.

Initially, the chief of staff or chairperson of the medical staff executive committee appoints the P&T committee chairperson. The chairperson should work with the director of pharmaceutical services in identifying and nominating P&T committee members to be appointed by the chief of staff and the respective department heads. All committee members should be thoroughly oriented to the authority for and function of the committee as well as the scope of pharmaceutical services provided in the institution.

The initial formulary is most easily developed by reviewing current drug use patterns and admitting most of the commonly used drugs that have established efficacy and safety, and reasonable costs. Specific, objective criteria for formulary admission should be defined *a priori.* Most commonly these are rank ordered as therapeutic, pharmaceutic, and economic considerations. Efficacy, safety, and clinical usefulness are prime considerations. If two drugs are similar in efficacy, safety, and clinical utility, then dosage form, taste, comfort on injection, and other pharmaceutic factors may be the deciding factors on which drug should be admitted to the formulary. Only after the therapeutic and pharmaceutic factors have been considered should the economic factors be weighed, lest an important, new drug be overlooked because of its budgetary impact. A well-managed formulary includes sufficient drugs for prescribing flexibility, thus allowing physicians to practice the "art" of medicine, especially in the treatment of patients with highly subjective complaints. For objective indications such as systemic infections, few if any therapeutic duplications are necessary.

Each clinical department that extensively uses the drugs within a class should be invited to comment on which drugs in the class should be admitted to the formulary. It may be wiser to admit a few extra therapeutic duplications to the initial formulary than to antagonize influential staff members by eliminating reasonable alternatives that they use regularly. Use patterns should be reviewed at least annually. At those times, the less popular therapeutic alternatives can be considered for deletion.

No effective formulary can include all of the drugs that the medical staff might reasonably use in patient care. A common reason for prescribers to request a nonformulary drug is that the patient was controlled on that agent prior to admission. It is usually unwise to change successful therapy. An efficient mechanism for obtaining nonformulary drugs should be in place. This usually is accomplished by the requesting physician's completing a nonformulary drug request form (see Appendix 8-B). Physicians often accept formulary alternatives when pharmacists contact them in a nonconfrontational manner, explain why the requested drug is not on the formulary, and suggest the formulary alternatives. Most nonformulary drugs that prescribers wish to use should be obtained as quickly as possible. Drugs with questionable efficacy, excessive adverse effect patterns, or extreme cost may be exceptions. All nonformulary drug orders should be tabulated and reviewed regularly by the P&T committee. Reasonable nonformulary drugs that are continually requested should be considered for formulary admission. When a prescriber continually requests nonformulary drugs that are less effective, less safe, or less cost effective than formulary alternatives, a member of the P&T committee should meet with the prescriber to clarify the reasons for the repeated orders. When there is not a good reason for using the nonformulary drug, the situation usually can be resolved through peer pressure. If necessary, the chief of service might be asked to assist the committee. It often is unnecessary and unwise for a pharmacist to intercede directly.

Any member of the medical staff should have the privilege of suggesting admissions to and deletions from the formulary. Some teaching hospitals require that house officers receive concurrence from the chief resident or an attending physician. Initiation of the admission or deletion review process is most commonly accomplished by the completion of a Formulary Status Evaluation Request form (see Appendix 8-C). The department of pharmaceutical services (normally the drug information service if one exists) then prepares an objective review of the literature on the drug. Most committees provide the opportunity for the person making the request to provide literature and clinical data in support of the request and to comment on the drug review before it is final. Not doing so often presents an appearance of a less than open process for considering formulary admissions. Many P&T committees invite the person making the request to attend the meeting at which the request is discussed.

Most P&T committees restrict certain drugs to specific clinical services or prescribers when the potential for less than appropriate use is high. This is not necessary for drugs that normally would not be used by physicians other than specialists in the field in which the drug is intended, e.g., toxic antineoplastic agents. Restriction of prescribing privileges within the hospital often is resented by physicians who experience no such restrictions in private practice. Therefore, restriction should be used only when the P&T committee has serious concerns about the risk-to-benefit or cost-to-benefit ratio of the drugs being generally available. Some P&T committees have eliminated restrictions and have instituted intensive drug use evaluation programs with followup education for drugs that cause concerns.

GENERIC AND THERAPEUTIC SUBSTITUTION

Generic substitution may be defined as the act of dispensing a different brand or an unbranded drug product for the drug product prescribed (i.e., chemically the same drug entity in the same dosage form, but distributed by different companies).[6] By 1985, nearly all hospital formulary systems included the provision that the brand of drug dispensed shall be selected by the department of pharmaceutical services.[7] Commonly this is authorized both by the medical staff bylaws provision that drugs will be dispensed according to the formulary system and by a written statement on the doctor's order form that specifies that generic equivalents may be dispensed. In 1989, several generic drug manufacturers were found guilty of fraud for submitting innovators' drug products as their own for bioavailability testing. As a result, the Food and Drug Administration (FDA) rescinded the licenses for some of these products and reclassifed others as lacking bioavailability comparable to the innovator products.[8] The FDA's intensive review of generic drugs revealed that most are of high quality and equal bioavailability to the innovator products. It is the responsibility of the department of pharmaceutical services to obtain and review data that ensure that generic drugs used in the institution are of reasonable quality. This includes monitoring drug recall announcements.

Therapeutic substitution now occurs in more than one-half of American hospitals for one or more specified drug groups.[9] Therapeutic substitution has been defined as a medical staff-approved procedure that provides for "automatic" dispensing of a particular drug entity in place of a therapeutically similar but chemically different drug product, unless the prescriber explicitly requests otherwise. Such substitution within a formulary system is authorized by the medical staff; it is not an independent act performed by a pharmacist. Many hospitals have chosen not to adopt such provisions. In those institutions, the pharmacists attempt to contact the prescribers and suggest the formulary alternative when nonformulary drug orders are received. Some P&T committees believe that these personal contacts provide an educational benefit of the formulary system; however, they do create additional work for the pharmacists and may place pharmacists in confrontational positions with prescribers. Therefore, the pharmacy staff should be instructed how to handle these situations tactfully.

Publication of the Formulary

The formulary per se, sometimes called the formulary catalogue or approved drug list, is published periodically by the P&T committee and must be readily available to all prescribers, pharmacists, nurses, and other health professionals within the institution. Many hospitals distribute copies to all medical staff members. Others make the formulary available in all patient care areas of the institution. Most institutions provide detailed reference monographs on drugs for use by staff in the patient care areas. This commonly is accomplished by providing the current edition of American Hospital Formulary Service *(AHFS) Drug Information.*[10] Another excellent set of drug information monographs is found in *USP DI.*[11]

The formulary may be published in either looseleaf notebook or bound volume format. The former can be updated frequently by replacing only those pages on which listings have changed. However, if the notebooks are not updated carefully, the book becomes obsolete. The latter are initially less expensive but have to be totally replaced periodically. Since most physicians define their prescribing practices according to the formulary within a short time after joining the hospital staff, it usually is not necessary for them to carry a pocket-sized formulary with them. All prescribers must be informed of changes in the formulary in a timely manner, usually accomplished by publishing the information in a drug information bulletin. Whereas formularies usually are published only every 1–2 years, bulletins commonly are published monthly.

THE FUTURE OF FORMULARY SYSTEMS

Today, most medical staffs recognize that the benefits of the formulary system outweigh the inconveniences that it creates. Good management of the system is essential for this perception to continue.

In recent years, many formulary systems have benefited from new information technology. Online computer data bases make current drug information available to all institutions.[12] Computer-based bulletin board services provide useful support to formulary systems.[13] Successful formulary management requires both objective clinical information support and good interpersonal skills.

It is important for the professional staff of the institution to recognize that the major purposes of the formulary system are to provide quality pharmaceuticals and to provide information on the most appropriate drug therapy to the staff. When formulary systems are perceived primarily as negative or restrictive programs, they cause resentment among the persons whose prerogatives are limited. If the formulary system is perceived solely as a cost-containment measure, it will not be supported by much of the medical staff. In teaching hospitals, orientation of new house staff members to the purpose and operation of the formulary system during their first days at the institution is important. All new staff members should be oriented to the system soon after joining the staff. A personal letter from the chairperson of the P&T committee welcoming new medical staff members and inviting them to share their expertise in formulary decisions can do much to diffuse resentment against the formulary system.

Five requisites for an effective formulary system have been proposed:[14] (1) true medical staff advocacy for the formulary system concept; (2) informed and timely review of drugs for formulary admission and deletion; (3) continual operationalization of the formulary system through informed professional staff; (4) flexibility in allowing use of nonformulary drugs when reasonable; and (5) perception of the formulary as a positive instrument for educational and evaluative impact on drug therapy.

Although hospital formularies have been used effectively for more than 20 years throughout the Nation, they do not enjoy universal support. The "con" argument in a published debate on the usefulness of formulary systems suggested that formularies are "a con job performed on institutional pharmacy."[15] But that position appears to have been based on the formulary's being no more than a cost-containment measure. The "pro" position attempts to present a balanced discussion of the potential benefits of a well-managed formulary system.[16] It is clear that few benefits accrue from a poorly managed formulary system. Conversely, a well-managed formulary system is an asset in drug use management.

The introduction of prospective payment systems for American health care have created a recognition that we are not a society of limitless wealth and that choices must be made in the use of health care resources. A well-defined and well-managed formulary system can be an important tool in managing drug therapy resources effectively.[17] This should be a priority for all departments of pharmaceutical services.

REFERENCES

1. Brodie DC: The Challenge to Pharmacy in Times of Change. Report of the Commission on Pharmaceutical Services to Ambulatory Patients by Hospitals and Related Facilities. Washington, DC, American Pharmaceutical Association and American Society of Hospital Pharmacists, 1966.
2. Joint Commission on Accreditation of Healthcare Organizations: *Accreditation Manual for Hospitals, 1989.* Chicago, Joint Commission on Accrediation of Healthcare Organizations, 1989.
3. American Society of Hospital Pharmacists: ASHP statement on the pharmacy and therapeutics committee. *Am J Hosp Pharm* 42:1621, 1984.
4. American Society of Hospital Pharmacists: ASHP statement on the operation of the formulary system. *Am J Hosp Pharm* 20:1384, 1983.
5. Myers CE, Pierpaoli PG, Smith MA: Measurement of formulary inclusion costs. *Hosp Formul* 16:951, 1981.
6. Anon: Weekly Pharmaceutical Reports, F-D-C Reports, Inc., 32:51-52, December 19, 1983.
7. Stolar MH: National survey of hospital pharmaceutical services, 1985. *Am J Hosp Pharm* 42:2667-2778, 1985.
8. Zellmer WE: Generic drug products (editorial). *Am J Hosp Pharm* 46:2005, 1989.
9. Stolar MH: ASHP national survey of hospital pharmaceutical services, 1987. *Am J Hosp Pharm* 45:801-818, 1988.
10. McEvoy GK (ed): *AHFS Drug Information 1989.* Bethesda, MD, American Society of Hospital Pharmacists, 1989 (published annually).
11. United States Pharmacopoeial Convention, Inc. USP DI, Vol. I, *Drug Information for the Health Care Professional.* Rockville, MD, United States Pharmacopoeial Convention, 1989 (published annually).
12. Perry CA: On-line information retrieval in pharmacy and related fields. *Am J Hosp Pharm* 43:1509-1524, 1986.
13. Selevan J: The formulary: High tech drug reviews, an electronic bulletin board for drug information and more. *Hosp Pharm* 24:652-660, 1989.
14. Pierpaoli PG: How the formulary system works. *U.S. Pharmacist* 11:H1-H8, 1986.
15. Green JA. Point: The formulary system and the emperor's new clothes. *Am J Hosp Pharm* 43:2830-2834, 1986.
16. Abramowitz PW, Fletcher CV: Counterpoint: Let's expand the formulary system and renew its vigor. *Am J Hosp Pharm* 43:2834-2838, 1986.
17. Lipman AG: Formulary system controversies in the new environment of DRGs. *Hosp Formul* 20:218-232, 1985.

APPENDIX 8-A

PHARMACY AND THERAPEUTICS COMMITTEE MEETING
Date
AGENDA

The meeting will begin at noon in the Administrative Conference Room on the second floor. Lunch will be served.

1. Call to order .... Dr. R. Williams
2. Introduction of guests .... Dr. R. Williams
3. Approval of the minutes of the October meeting .... Dr. R. Williams
   (minutes were mailed to committee members on October 22)
4. Formulary admission requests .... Dr. L. Taylor
   A. Astemizole (Hismanal[R])
      AHFS category 4:00 Antihistamine
      Dr. K. Chavez - General Medicine Clinic
      (see attached drug evaluation)
   B. Epoetin alpha (Epogen[R])
      AHFS category 20:04 Antianemia Drugs
      Dr. M. Greggs - Nephrology Service
      (see attached drug evaluation)
   C. Ranitidine (Zantac[R]) parenteral dosage form
      AHFS category 56:40 Miscellaneous
      Dr. M. Benson - Gastroenterology Service
      (see attached review of H_2 receptor blockers)
5. Review of policies and procedures .... Mr. J. Barens
   9-3 Safe handling of antineoplastic drugs
   9-17 Verbal orders
   (see attached draft revisions of these policies)
6. Quarterly report of the Adverse Drug Reaction Subcommittee .... Dr. D. Rawlings
   (see attached summary of reported ADR's)
7. Drug use evaluation data on third-generation cephalosporin use on the surgical services .... Ms. A. Mason
8. New business
9. Adjournment

Note: The next meeting will be on (date) in the Administrative Conference Room at noon.

cc:
R. Williams, M.D., Chairperson
J. Barens, M.S., R.Ph., Secretary
C. Harry, M.D.
C. Mann, M.D.
A. Lapper, Pharm.D.
S. Mack, R.N.
F. Merris, Ph.D.
V. Morton, R.N.
J. Smedley, D.D.S.
F. Reim, M.D.
D. Rawlings, M.D.
L. Taylor, Pharm.D.
S. Wong, M.H.A.
K. Yardley, M.D.

guests:
M. Benson, M.D.
M. Greggs, M.D.
K. Chavez, M.D.
A. Mason, R.Ph.

APPENDIX 8-B

UNIVERSITY HOSPITAL
UNIVERSITY OF UTAH
DEPARTMENT OF PHARMACY SERVICES

NON-FORMULARY DRUG REQUEST

STAMP PATIENT I.D. HERE

Patient's Name: ______________________ Room Number: __________

1. Drug Name: Generic: ______________________
   Trade: ______________________
2. Dosage Form and Strength: ______________________
3. Dosage Schedule: ______________________
4. Number of Doses Required: ______________________
5. Reason(s) for using this drug as opposed to other medication(s) already present on the hospital formulary:
   ____
   ____
   ____

Approval was obtained from: ______________________
(Name of Authorizing Attending or Chief Resident)

______________________ Date__________ Phone__________
(Signature of Requesting Physician or Subintern)

____
(Signature of Pharmacist) (Date)

NOTE TO THE PHYSICIAN:

The requested drug will be obtained as soon as possible; however, in some instances, several days may be required. In addition, because this is a non-formulary drug, it is necessary to charge your patient for the total quantity of medication purchased. Upon discharge if the drug is to be sent home with the patient, the medication will be dispensed with legally required labeling and packaging at no extra charge. This form should accompany the copy of the medication order sent to the pharmacy.

FOR PHARMACY USE ONLY

Date Drug Ordered: ______________________ COST: Acquisition: __________
Expected Receiving Date: ______________________ To Patient: __________
Date Received: ______________________
Emergent Need?: ______________________

UH-PH 1943/5-88

APPENDIX 8-C

REQUEST FOR FORMULARY STATUS EVALUATION

№ 158

UNIVERSITY HOSPITAL
UNIVERSITY OF UTAH
PHARMACY AND THERAPEUTICS COMMITTEE

REQUEST FOR: ______ ADMISSION ______ DELETION

1. Generic Name: ____________________

2. Trade Name: ____________________

3. Dosage form(s) and strengths desired: ____________________

____

4. Comparable products currently on the Formulary: ____________________

____

____

5. Intended therapeutic applications: ____________________

____

____

6. Reason(s) why this drug should be included on (or deleted from) the Hospital Formulary (i.e., what advantage(s) or disadvantage(s) does the requested drug have over similar Formulary drugs): ____________________

____

____

7. Should other drug(s) listed in #4 above be replaced by this newly recommended medication?

    ____ Yes ____ No

    Why? ____________________

____

____

8. References: ____________________

____

____

____

Requesting Physician: ____________________, M.D.

Division/Department: ____________________ Date: __________

Signature: ____________________ Phone: __________

Action taken by the Pharmacy and Therapeutics Committee (date): ____________________

INSTRUCTIONS:

1. This form must be typed and filled out **completely**. Any forms not completely filled out will be returned to the requesting physician.
2. The requesting physician or appointed representative **must** attend a Pharmacy and Therapeutics Committee Meeting to supply further information to the Committee.
3. A copy of this form will be sent to your Department Chairmen for their information only.
4. Please return this form to: Drug Information Center
   Department of Pharmacy Services, Room A-050
   University of Utah Hospital

CHAPTER 9

Purchasing and Inventory Management

STEPHEN J. ALLEN

INTRODUCTION

The responsibilities of the pharmacist in the arena of purchasing and inventory management appear relatively simple: acquire pharmaceuticals for patient use on a timely basis and establish an appropriate inventory of pharmaceuticals. These responsibilities are clearly delegated to the pharmacist, as the 1989 standards of the Joint Commission on Accreditation of Healthcare Organizations (JCAHO) stipulate the following: "The director of pharmacy services is responsible for maintaining an adequate drug supply and establishing specifications for the procurement of all approved drugs, chemicals and biologicals related to the practice of pharmacy."[1] With the responsibility clearly defined and the basic concept of pharmaceutical purchasing and inventory easily understood, one would expect this aspect of practice to be an area in which the pharmacist would excel. However, in a report developed by the U.S. General Accounting Office, many inadequacies pertaining to pharmaceutical purchasing practices were identified.[2] McAllister suggests that pharmacists may not perceive purchasing and inventory responsibilities as being rewarding or as demanding extensive consideration.[3] In actuality, the most important and initial clinical responsibilities of the pharmacist are an integral part of the pharmaceutical purchasing process. As the health care practitioner who is most thoroughly trained in the areas of pharmacology, therapeutics, and pharmaceutics, the pharmacist must exert the necessary influence to ensure that the highest-quality, most cost-effective agents are available when needed to treat patients.

The expectations of many disciplines and individuals in the health care system emphasize the importance of the clinical, operational, economic, legal, and societal issues associated with the pharmacist's purchasing and inventory responsibilities. Patients, physicians, and nurses desire rapid availability of the most effective therapeutic agents. Health care administrators insist upon a cost-effective system for drug procurement and inventory management. Pharmacy staff workers desire a fluid, uncomplicated process of purchasing and inventory management that does not encumber the distributive or clinical activities of the department. Financial managers, legal counsels, and risk managers seek evidence of a well-managed purchasing and inventory program that can be easily audited and minimizes the institution's liability. Finally, the government and society insist that the pharmacist employ a systematic and controlled purchasing and inventory program to prevent diversion of ethical pharmaceuticals for illicit uses.

The goals of this chapter are fourfold: (1) to provide the reader with a thorough appreciation for the impact of a well-managed purchasing and inventory management system in the institutional setting; (2) to identify the essential processes to be employed in managing a purchasing and inventory system; (3) to identify pharmaceuticals that require unique considerations within the overall purchasing and inventory system; and (4) to demonstrate the importance of computer and other technological advances that facilitate the role of the pharmacist in managing such a system.

DRUG PRODUCT SELECTION

Within the institutional setting, the pharmacy and therapeutics (P&T) committee plays the most influential and pivotal role in determining which pharmaceuticals should be purchased and maintained in stock. The American Society of Hospital Pharmacists' (ASHP) statement on the pharmacy and therapeutics committee[4] provides a detailed review of the purpose and function of a P&T committee. The P&T committee functions stipulated in the ASHP statement that drive the pharmaceutical purchasing and inventory programs are:

1. To recommend the adoption of, or assist in the formation of, policies regarding evaluation, selection and therapeutic use of drugs in hospitals.
2. To develop a formulary of drugs accepted for use in the hospital and provide for its constant revision.

In fulfilling these two responsibilities, physicians and pharmacists cooperatively identify the methods for determining how to evaluate and select those pharmaceuticals that will be used within the institution. Although policies and procedures for evaluating and selecting pharmaceuticals will vary slightly from one institution to another, most will incorporate the following provisions:

1. *Formal request for addition.* Most institutions require the completion of a request form that addresses proposed indications, alternative formulary agents, drugs that can be removed, unique characteristics, cost issues, purported advantages in effecting therapeutic outcome, and ongoing utilization criteria. Support from the requester's department chairperson

may also be required to ensure a degree of peer review prior to P&T committee evaluation.

2. *Detailed literature review.* A thorough review of the primary medical/pharmacy literature and subspecialty literature is completed by a P&T committee pharmacist or physician. A concise but thorough review that critically evaluates the literature and addresses the impact on patient management within the institution should be prepared for committee members to review prior to the meeting.
3. *Formal presentation and evaluation.* The written presentation provided to the committee should include the following categories of information: chemical and physical properties; pharmacology; pharmacokinetics; indications; clinical efficacy; safety profile; dosage and administration; compatibility and stability; comparison with existing formulary agents; and final recommendations. The assessment of the value of the proposed pharmaceutical by appropriate specialty and subspecialty medical departments should also be communicated at the time of presentation.

These three critical steps set the stage for the committee's decision process. In order to make a wise and insightful decision, McWhinney[5] suggests that the P&T committee will have to consider the following critical points: literature evaluation; clinical experience; therapeutic equivalence of chemically similar agents; cost impact within the institution; unique product properties; and unique institutional issues.

This selection and decision process is employed when new agents are considered. As pharmaceuticals are admitted to the formulary, the decisions should be communicated to the medical, nursing, and pharmacy staffs. A published formulary that is readily available and easy to use is necessary to provide a listing of available pharmaceuticals and to communicate P&T committee guidelines. The formulary should be designed to allow for periodic update inserts or be printed frequently enough to keep practitioners informed of periodic modifications.

In order to meet its charge of providing for the constant revision of the formulary, the P&T committee must establish a process for a continual review and evaluation of the currency of the products on the formulary. When new agents are requested for formulary inclusion, it is a common practice in many institutions to conduct a drug class review or therapeutic category assessment to ensure that section of the formulary reflects current medical treatment. However, reviewing categories of the formulary only when new agents are requested is insufficient. Periodic reviews that guarantee evaluation of the entire formulary over a defined period of time are required. Some institutions approach this by reviewing therapeutic categories on an assigned basis over a 1- or 2-year period. Other institutions may review the formulary by assessing current therapies of specific disease states or patient types. Regardless of the specific process of periodic review employed, it is paramount to consider the management of the selection of pharmaceuticals for the institution as an ongoing process.

Once the formulary status of a pharmaceutical has been established, it is routinely and almost exclusively the decision of the pharmacist to determine which brand of product is acquired. For the patent-protected, single-brand pharmaceutical, the primary consideration is manufacturer acceptability. The pharmacist must assess whether the manufacturer has the ability to consistently produce a quality product and operate a reliable business operation. If a manufacturer's reputation is considered questionable by the pharmacist when considering a single-source pharmaceutical, the P&T committee must incorporate this information in the decision process.

The pharmacist's role is critical in considering the purchase of a multiple-source pharmaceutical. Mehl[6] describes six major areas that must be considered: product properties; manufacturer acceptability; packaging; availability; cost; and site characteristics.

In evaluating product properties, the issue of generic equivalence must be initially considered. Generic drugs are those that are not patent protected, are chemically the same, and are available from multiple manufacturers. Generically equivalent drugs must be therapeutically and otherwise equivalent to the innovator drug and must be approved by the Food and Drug Administration (FDA). The bioavailability of a product is another important product property to be considered. Measurement of the concentration of a product in the blood at predetermined times after a single dose of drug is the method most commonly employed to determine bioavailability. When two products display equal bioavailability, they are viewed to be bioequivalent. The FDA has the responsibility for establishing standards for the safety and effectiveness of all drugs used in the United States. In fulfilling this responsibility, the FDA has worked to establish a standard to define bioequivalency and generic equivalency between pharmaceutical products. An FDA publication, *Approved Drug Products and Therapeutic Evaluations* (7th edition),[7] is an essential reference for the pharmacist in determining drug equivalency. This publication has been designed to provide detailed information on equivalency issues and is formatted to enable comparisons between different products.

The final consideration in evaluating product properties is the physical differences among pharmaceuticals. Issues such as size of the product, odor, color, and palatability may be important factors in determining patient acceptance of a particular product. It is important for the purchasing pharmacist to consider patient factors in relation to physical aspects of a pharmaceutical. Pediatric and geriatric patient populations are two distinct groups for whom physical properties of a pharmaceutical often require assessment.

Manufacturer acceptability is the second major area requiring evaluation by the pharmacist. The *ASHP Guidelines for Selecting Pharmaceutical Manufacturers and Distributors* (Appendix 9-A) is an excellent reference for evaluating a manufacturer's overall acceptance, and often serves as the blueprint for individual pharmacists or purchasing groups in establishing criteria to evaluate manufacturers. Other factors such as recall reports, FDA inspection reports, returned goods policy, personal experience, and internal institutional testing of products are examples of additional points of consideration.

Availability of products by a manufacturer must be considered in the selection process. Distribution methods by a given manufacturer need to be consistent with the overall methods and modes of purchasing used by an institution. A product available only on a direct-order basis from the manufacturer versus availability through a wholesaler may be less desirable. A product from one company that is available in only one strength may be less appealing than a more complete product line from another manufacturer. Minimum-order quantity stipulations are another example of an availability issue that must be assessed before a specific product is selected.

Packaging considerations are another critical issue in the selection process. The *ASHP Technical Assistance Bulletin on Single Unit and Unit Dose Packages of Drugs* (Appendix 9-B) provides a comprehensive set of standards for single-dose products. Package size, plastic versus glass, ease of administration, storage space, disposal and waste issues, interpretability of labeling, and color coding issues are examples of specific packaging features that warrant consideration before a specific pharmaceutical is purchased. Pharmacy distribution systems, nursing practices, and previous experiences all must be considered in relation to the packaging of each pharmaceutical purchased.

Once these issues have been assessed, the cost of a pharmaceutical should be evaluated. Upon initial consideration, a cost comparison between two pharmaceuticals appears simple. The product that costs less to acquire, with all other product issues equivalent, should be purchased. Within the institutional setting, the determination of final cost can often be difficult to identify. Volume discounts, rebates, handling costs of a purchase order, cash flow issues, wholesaler mark-up, freight costs, prepayment discounts, multidepartment contacts, and corporate contracts are examples of issues that can modify the overall cost of a pharmaceutical. The pharmacist must determine which, if any, of these factors affect the overall cost of a pharmaceutical. A close working relationship between the financial manager, materials manager, or other hospital administrative staff and the pharmacist is required to determine the importance of any of these issues in balancing pharmaceutical costs with overall institutional expenses.

Finally, the institution's operational site characteristics play a role in determining which pharmaceutical product is purchased. Political issues, systems issues, and patient population sometimes have a bearing on the pharmacist's decision process. These types of issues vary tremendously from institution to institution and sometimes make an objective decision on product selection difficult. Physician brand preference, intravenous administration system used, and unusual clinical experience reports in patients treated in one's institution are examples of such unique site characteristics. The pharmacist must evaluate these situations independently and make decisions that demonstrate thoughtful analysis and objectivity.

GROUP PURCHASING VERSUS INDEPENDENT PURCHASING

With a process established for the selection of pharmaceuticals, the next step required is the development of a system for purchasing. Two broad options are available: independent purchasing and group purchasing. In an independent purchasing program the pharmacist, independently or in conjunction with the purchasing agent, interacts with pharmaceutical companies to negotiate pharmaceutical pricing and other mutually beneficial relationships for the institution. Group purchasing involves the collaboration of multiple institutions in negotiating with pharmaceutical firms to achieve advantageous pharmaceutical pricing and other mutually beneficial relationships. The driving principle in group purchasing is that high volumes of committed purchases will enable the manufacturer to reduce the profit margin and offer more competitive pricing. Larger, prestigious institutions are more likely to conduct an independent purchasing program. However, it seems that independent pharmaceutical purchasing programs are becoming less appealing and group purchasing systems are being used by the majority of institutions in the 1990's. The advantages of group purchasing are numerous and have been clearly identified:[8,9]

- Lowest possible drug costs
- Standardization of products
- Reduction in contract labor costs for institutions
- Enhancement of member institution's purchasing program
- Enhancement of information sharing
- Enhancement of purchasing expertise
- Achievement of protracted periods of price protection
- Coordination of contracting and budgeting processes
- Reduction in duplication of purchasing efforts among institutions

Managing a pharmaceutical purchasing program that uses a group purchasing system requires a dynamic relationship among the institution, the purchasing group, and the vendor. Each participant must fulfill a series of obligations and performance factors. These performance factors have been identified by Allen (see table 9-1).[10]

Table 9-1. Multiple-group purchasing system: Participant requirements

Institutional pharmacy performance requirements

- Operate an efficient P&T committee
- Provide utilization data and packaging and labeling requirements
- Demonstrate commitment to honor group awards
- Provide feedback on vendor performance and market conditions
- Participate in purchasing group committee structure
- Contribute to procedural development and refinement for the group
- Identify products suitable for bidding
- Respond to group communications and assist in sharing information among members
- Use only one purchasing group
- Communicate as necessary with vendors

Purchasing group performance requirements

- Employ well-trained staff to operate program
- Develop an organizational and committee structure that fosters member input and participation
- Provide financial support for member attendance at committee meetings
- Develop an appropriate communication network for members
- Use automation and technology to facilitate contract listing
- Communicate routinely with members on key issues
- Develop procedures that facilitate bidding and are sensitive to changing market conditions
- Maintain an acceptable fee system for members and/or vendors, as applicable
- Pursue long-term or corporate agreements as directed by the membership
- Plan strategically for long-term group success

Vendor performance requirements

- Respond to bid solicitations on a timely basis
- Anticipate supply demands to maintain uninterrupted product supply
- Promote product line according to member institution guidelines
- Provide professional representative service to member institutions
- Refrain from counterbidding activities

Although group purchasing systems are dominant in institutional settings, independent purchasing is used to varying degrees in almost all settings. Certain pharmaceuticals may not be available through the purchasing group. Patent-protected products infrequently have preferential pricing or price protection offered through a purchasing group. Other products that do not have widespread use in all of the group's institutions may be competitively bid, or extended price protection can be sought. The pharmacist must be prepared to bid competitively, negotiate favorable pricing, or secure price protection for any products possible that are not covered under group purchasing contracts.

DETERMINATION OF THE MODE OF ACQUISITION

Once the system of purchasing has been established, the pharmacist has several modes in which pharmaceuticals can be purchased: direct purchase from the manufacturer; wholesaler purchase; prime vendor purchase; direct purchase plus wholesaler purchase; and direct purchase plus prime vendor purchase.

Direct purchase requires the completion of a purchase order by the individual institution followed by the oral or written transmission of the order to the manufacturer. If the pharmacist has authority to purchase directly within the institution, a pharmacy purchase order is completed. Usually the purchase order completion is viewed as a technical function that is completed under the supervision of the pharmacist. If the institution dictates that all purchases be processed by a central purchasing department, a purchase requisition is completed by pharmacy staff. The purchase requisition serves as the basis for the generation of the purchase order by the central purchasing staff. In either case, the purchase order or purchase requisition routinely contains the following information:

- Date of order or requisition
- Type of order, i.e., contract, routine
- Vendor number, name, and address
- Billing and shipping information
- Purchase order or requisition number
- Department name, number, and budget code
- Required date for receipt
- Line item number
- Quantity, unit of measure, and complete product description
- Unit price and total price per line item
- Special requirements or conditions
- Name and telephone number of person completing order or requisition
- Authorized signature

The primary advantage of direct purchasing is that it is devoid of add-on fees or handling costs. However, it requires a significant commitment of personnel time to complete, monitor, and maintain records, receive products, and process invoices. Greater storage capacity may be required in a direct-order system of acquisition.

Wholesaler acquisition facilitates the purchase of multiple drug products from a variety of manufacturers through a single source. The wholesaler maintains an adequate supply of product, enabling the institution to reduce stock and order items periodically. Computerization has enabled wholesalers to manage inventory and ordering efficiently, and ultimately lower the handling fees offered to institutions. Additionally, automation has permitted wholesalers to offer a range of utilization, financial, and therapeutic product reports to institutions. Wholesaler acquisition advantages to an institution are reduced order turnaround time, lower inventory and carrying costs, and reduced purchasing personnel and recordkeeping. The disadvantages are higher acquisition costs, difficulty in producing an optimal purchase order control system, occasional inabilities to supply, and unavailability of slow-moving pharmaceuticals.

A prime vendor system is an enhancement of the wholesaler mode of acquisition. A prime vendor relationship involves a formal purchasing arrangement between an institution and a drug wholesaler. A contract is established that stipulates that the institution will purchase a particular percentage of all pharmaceuticals or a specified dollar volume of purchases. In return, the institution receives a highly competitive service fee with possible performance incentives; a comprehensive utilization and ordering information system; electronic or computer order entry equipment; a committed service level and delivery schedule; emergency delivery service; and a guarantee that individual or group contract prices will be the base price for applicable items. For noncontract items, the prime vendor wholesaler charges the institution the wholesaler's actual acquisition cost, not inclusive of any cash discounts, plus the service fee. A prime vendor contract can be negotiated by the pharmacist or by the institution's purchasing group. Institutions of all sizes frequently use the prime vendor mode of acquisition because it enhances purchasing efficiency, lowers inventory storage requirements, and provides rapid information on product availability and use.

A just-in-time (JIT) purchasing program is often associated with prime vendor arrangements. The objective of this purchasing plan is to purchase frequently in quantities that meet product supply needs until the next reordering time. The effect of a JIT program is to reduce the dollars committed to pharmaceuticals sitting on shelves, thereby reducing the total pharmaceutical inventory value. The use of bar-coded product stickers, electronic order entry devices, and computerized purchase and inventory programs supplied by a prime vendor enables a pharmacy department to order frequently and have pharmaceuticals arrive shortly before they are needed for dispensing. The advantages are obvious in that inventory is reduced, the cash flow required for pharmaceuticals is lowered, and inventory storage space can be significantly reduced. The potential difficulties in operating a JIT purchasing program are the requirement for close monitoring of stock on a continuous basis, the need to devise a system that detects deviations from the norm on product use, and a consistently high level of fill rates by the prime vendor.

INVENTORY MANAGEMENT

The pharmacist also has the responsibility of determining how much inventory of pharmaceuticals should be maintained, where inventory should be located, and when inventory should be adjusted. Space allocation within a pharmacy is usually established, thereby imposing certain conditions within which one must operate. Square footage allotment, shelving configuration and design, refrigerator capacity, freezer capacity, and number of pharmacy locations all must be analyzed carefully in determining where the pharmaceutical inventory can be optimally maintained. Historical use data serve as a major determinant in calculating what amount of product should be maintained for a given time period. These data can be gathered manually by reviewing purchase order data, or more optimally, tabulated by the computer system of the hospital or hospital's prime vendor.

Inventory or carrying costs must be considered in the review of use data. By keeping pharmaceuticals on the shelf, the institution incurs costs relating to interest rates on capital, obsolescence, waste, insurance, utilities, depreciation, pilferage, etc.[11] An institution's cash-flow can be hindered if a large dollar value of pharmaceuticals is maintained on the shelves in the pharmacy. These issues must be carefully weighed to achieve the delicate balance between product availability and cost efficiency. The goal in today's health care environment is to approach a system of inventory management whereby the products, including pharmaceuticals, arrive shortly before they are used.

The pharmacist has a variety of methods to choose from in selecting a system for inventory management:

- Order book system
- Inventory record card system
- Minimum/maximum level system
- ABC inventory method
- Economic order quantity (EOQ) system
- Economic order value (EOV) system
- Computerized inventory system

These systems vary greatly in terms of simplicity, sophistication, effectiveness, and effort to operate. The order book system relies on the person dispensing a product to determine whether a product needs to be reordered. There is no standard order amount, and the system depends on the dispenser's experience and ability to predict need. The inventory record card system relies on the maintenance of an ongoing use and purchase history on a card or paper system. Staff time is required to maintain a system, and purchase amounts are based upon historical use and the frequency of ordering. The minimum/maximum level system relies on a predetermined order point and order quantity which are based on historical use. Customarily, there is a sticker on the shelf that facilitates rapid product review and order amount. Prime vendors often supply such labels with product information, blank spaces for order points, and order quantity and either bar coding or electronic order entry product numbers. Hand-held electronic order entry machines are supplied to facilitate order entry and transmission to the prime vendor via telephone or computer modem transmission. This method is employed by a large number of institutional pharmacies because it is relatively easy to operate and facilitates the order process. The ABC, EOQ, and EOV inventory methods are more sophisticated methods and are not widely employed by many institutional pharmacies.[12-14] The computerized inventory control method is the likely system of the future. Such systems are beginning to evolve as automation and technology expand. This method will likely eliminate ongoing personnel needs for inventory management, because it enables purchase orders to be automatically generated and executed under predetermined inventory management conditions that will require only periodic review and adjustment.

A physical inventory for pharmaceuticals is required for pharmacies that do not have a perpetual inventory system. Even with advances in automation, most institutional pharmacies currently do not maintain a perpetual inventory system. Consequently, a physical inventory must be performed at intervals that are acceptable to both the finance and pharmacy departments. Most pharmacies will conduct an inventory on either an annual or semiannual basis. Either the pharmacy staff or an outside contracting firm can conduct the inventory. Many pharmacies use companies that specialize in inventory management because of their speed and accuracy; these firms employ automated programs to assist in identification of the purchase price of each pharmaceutical. The exact process for conducting the inventory must be defined, accepted, and applied following approval by the finance, internal audit, and pharmacy departments. Often the pharmacy manager and an internal auditor oversee the conduct of the physical inventory.

The physical inventory value is then used to determine the average inventory and the inventory turnover rate. Determination of average inventory enables the institution to calculate the number of times pharmaceuticals are repurchased during a cycle that is customarily annual. It is calculated as follows:

$$\text{average inventory} = \frac{\text{beginning inventory} + \text{ending inventory}}{2}$$

Turnover rate makes it possible to determine how many times in a year the stock is completely used and repurchased. The turnover rate is an indicator of the efficiency with which the inventory management maintains as low a level of inventory as possible and consistently meets the demand for product. Turnover is calculated as follows:

$$\text{turnover rate} = \frac{\text{annual dollar purchases}}{2}$$

With the advent of prime vendor purchasing programs and other advances in technology affecting the purchasing industry, the annual norm for inventory turnover rates is approximately 10 turns. Some institutions that take aggressive measures to manage inventory are approaching twice this number of inventory turns.

ASSIGNMENT OF PURCHASING RESPONSIBILITIES

The ultimate responsibility for all purchasing and receiving responsibilities rests with the pharmacy manager. However, most of the routine ordering and receiving responsibilities can and should be delegated to properly trained technical staff. A pharmacy technician for purchasing can be trained to generate purchase orders, coordinate group purchasing contract data, conduct routine inventories, coordinate invoices for processing, and place electronic and computer orders with the wholesaler or prime vendor.

The pharmacy manager must establish clear guidelines for performance and monitor the functions of the purchasing pharmacy technician. Another pharmacy technician or assistant should be delegated the receiving and stocking responsibilities associated with the pharmaceutical inventory stock management. This approach optimizes the use of the pharmacist's time by ensuring that the technical functions are completed by technical staff. The pharmacy manager can then concentrate on the professional decisions and issues in the purchasing program. A quality assurance program should be established for the purchasing program to assess purchasing performance and to properly manage any drug supply programs.

RECEIPT AND CONTROL OF PHARMACEUTICALS

The receipt of pharmaceuticals must be an orderly and well-controlled process. The individual who receives the shipment of pharmaceuticals must not be the person who ordered the products. This ensures that a system of checks and balances is in place and prevents any one person from having full control over the entire process of ordering and receiving. The product received must be compared against the purchase order, and quantity, product name, product strength, and product size must be confirmed. Damaged products or products that were not shipped under proper storage conditions must be identified and reported to the pharmacist responsible for purchasing. Governmental laws pertaining to return of pharmaceuticals are stringent, and the manufacturer must be contacted immediately to arrange for an authorized return of damaged or incorrectly ordered or shipped merchandise.

Each pharmaceutical received must be checked for an expiration date. Expired products or products with expiration dates less than 30-120 days should be returned to the supplier. An organized method for stock rotation must be incorporated into the process for storage and stocking of pharmaceuticals. Expiration dates of existing stock can also be assessed at the time of receipt of new products.

Occasionally, the inability of a manufacturer or supplier to provide a pharmaceutical ordered will make it necessary to borrow or purchase small quantities of a pharmaceutical from another institution. A detailed procedure and record-keeping system must be maintained in order to provide a system of control and accountability for the loan or borrowing of pharmaceuticals. Periodic review of any loan or borrow issues should be performed in order to maintain a tight control over all pharmaceutical transactions.

PHARMACEUTICALS REQUIRING SPECIAL CONSIDERATION

Two types of pharmaceuticals require unique consideration from a purchasing and inventory control standpoint. Controlled substances and investigational drugs have specific ordering, inventory, and handling requirements. The Controlled Substances Act of 1970 stipulates detailed ordering and inventory requirements for the pharmacist.[15] All purchases for schedule II controlled substances must be executed on the Drug Enforcement Agency (DEA) Form 222 by an authorized pharmacist. Receipt must be accurately documented on the form and maintained for possible review and inspection by DEA officials. A perpetual inventory of all schedule II controlled substances should be maintained to ensure rigid control and accountability. A physical inventory is required every 2 years and must be maintained on file for 2 years by Federal requirements. Procedures should be developed that are explicit regarding the detail of ordering, receiving, storage, dispensing, inventory, recordkeeping, return, waste, and disposal requirements.

Investigational drugs also require unique ordering and handling procedures. These agents will either be used on a compassionate-use basis or under a formal protocol approved by an institution's institutional review board. In both cases, the physician investigator is responsible for initiating contact with the pharmaceutical manufacturer regarding the conditions for authorization for use. Once the authorization for use is established, it routinely becomes the responsibility of the pharmacist to identify initial order quantity, storage and receipt mechanisms, and ongoing inventory management procedures. Again, procedures for handling these agents become paramount. Procedures must be developed that address order coordination, receipt, storage, inventory and recordkeeping requirements, dispensing, monitoring of drug supplies, return of products, and any other special handling requirements. It is advisable to segregate the stock of investigational drugs from the routine pharmaceutical inventory. When possible, it may be advantageous to maintain the investigational drug supply under lock and key. Access can be limited to staff knowledgeable and trained to handle these products and the inventory.

IMPACT OF AUTOMATION AND TECHNOLOGY

At the beginning of this chapter, it was noted that pharmacists have demonstrated some failings in the management of pharmaceutical purchasing and inventory programs. The management of a manual system of pharmaceutical purchasing and inventory control is an extremely labor-intensive process that requires a significant amount of time of valuable personnel and tedious monitoring. Managing the purchasing and inventory activities described thus far, without automation, will likely result in continued inadequacies relating to these functions. However, computerization and expanding technologies can enable the pharmacist to manage these systems more simply and efficiently and expand his or her influence over drug use within the institution. Every process described in this chapter can be facilitated through computerization or other technological advances.

A sample listing of such applications follows:

- Maintenance of the institution's formulary on a microcomputer or mainframe computer system
- Computer-assisted programs to facilitate periodic review of therapeutic sections of the formulary
- Online, computer-assisted literature retrieval systems to aid in the pharmaceutical evaluation and selection process
- Computerized data base to provide institution-specific information on vendor performance
- Computerized purchase order programs that provide linkages with the institution's financial and budget performance systems
- Automatic computerized perpetual inventory and ordering system between an institution and its prime vendor
- Electronic order entry devices using numeric or bar-code systems that function via computer modem or telephone transmission

- Prime vendor or mainframe purchasing computer programs that generate vital reports on drug use, dollar purchases by therapeutic category, product availability, vendor performance, purchase history of satellite pharmacies, and fill rates

The availability of complete, comprehensive, automated systems of pharmaceutical and inventory control programs is still somewhat limited. Vendor-supplied programs and customized or purchased microcomputer programs can be used to facilitate key aspects of a purchasing and inventory program. The pharmacist must view automation and advanced technology as a necessity for the purchasing and inventory system, and must pursue every opportunity to develop a completely or partially automated system. Doing so not only will streamline the mechanical aspects of the process but will provide additional information that can link financial performance and drug use within the institution. The challenge to the pharmacist in the 1990's is to integrate the pharmaceutical purchasing performance with the evaluation of the therapeutic effectiveness of pharmaceuticals.

REFERENCES

1. Joint Commission on Accreditation of Healthcare Organizations: Pharmaceutical services. In *Accreditation Manual for Hospitals, 1989 ed.* Chicago, Joint Commission on Accreditation of Healthcare Organizations, 1989, p 72.
2. U.S. General Accounting Office: *Study of Purchasing and Materials Management Functions in Private Hospitals: Opportunities for Improving Hospital Purchasing, Inventory Management and Supply Distribution, Part I.* PSAD-79-58A, April 1979.
3. McAllister JC III: Challenges in purchasing and inventory control. *Am J Hosp Pharm* 42:1370-1373, 1985.
4. American Society of Hospital Pharmacists: ASHP statement on the pharmacy and therapeutics committee. *Am J Hosp Pharm* 41:1621, 1984.
5. McWhinney B: The pharmacy and therapeutics committee and formulary management. In *Level II ACCRUE Program, Purchasing and Inventory Control Module.* Bethesda, MD, American Society of Hospital Pharmacists, 1990, pp 48-52.
6. Mehl B: Drug product selection. In *Level II ACCRUE Program, Purchasing and Inventory Control Module.* Bethesda, MD, American Society of Hospital Pharmacists, 1990, p 62.
7. Food and Drug Administration: Approved drug products and therapeutic evaluations, 7th ed. Rockville, MD, 1987, p 1-1.
8. May BE, Herrick JD: Evaluation of drug-procurement alternatives. *Am J Hosp Pharm* 41:1373-1378, 1984.
9. Wetrich JG: Group purchasing: An overview. *Am J Hosp Pharm* 44:1581-1592, 1987.
10. Allen SJ: Drug product procurement. In *Level II ACCRUE Program, Purchasing and Inventory Control Module.* Bethesda, MD, American Society of Hospital Pharmacists, 1990, pp 107-108.
11. Hotaling WH: Inventory management. In *Level II ACCRUE Program, Purchasing and Inventory Control Module.* Bethesda, MD, American Society of Hospital Pharmacists, 1990, p 164.
12. Hughes TF: Objectives of an effective inventory control system. *Am J Hosp Pharm* 41:2078-2085, 1984.
13. Noel MW: Quantitative measurements of inventory control. *Am J Hosp Pharm* 41:2378-2383, 1984.
14. Bicket WJ, Gagnon JP: Purchasing and inventory control for hospital pharmacies. *Top Hosp Pharm Mgt* 7(2):59-74, 1987.
15. U.S. Department of Justice Drug Enforcement Administration. *Pharmacist's Manual — an Informational Outline of the Controlled Substances Act of 1970,* 5th ed. Washington, DC, April 1986.

ADDITIONAL READING

Purchasing and Inventory Control Systems and Concepts

ASHP 13-part series of articles on managing the purchasing and inventory control systems for the hospital pharmacy department:

Bair JN, Lee GF: Developing a hospital pharmacy purchasing system. *Am J Hosp Pharm* 41:1574-1578, 1984.

Buchanan EC: Planning and coordinating pharmaceutical purchasing. *Am J Hosp Pharm* 41:1829-1834, 1984.

Daniels CE: Managing the inventory control system. *Am J Hosp Pharm* 42:346-351, 1985.

Dedrick SC, Eckel FM: Assessment of vendors and drug-product selection. *Am J Hosp Pharm* 41:703-708, 1984.

Hughes TF: Objectives of an effective inventory control system. *Am J Hosp Pharm* 41:2078-2085, 1984.

Lindley C, MacKowiak J: Methods of inventory control. *Am J Hosp Pharm* 42:122-128, 1985.

May BE, Herrick JD: Evaluation of drug procurement alternatives. *Am J Hosp Pharm* 41:1373-1378, 1984.

McAllister JC III: Bid solicitation and contract negotiation. *Am J Hosp Pharm* 41:1164-1172, 1984.

McAllister JC III: Challenges in purchasing and inventory control. *Am J Hosp Pharm* 42:1370-1373, 1985.

McAllister JC III: Purchasing and inventory control systems management. *Am J Hosp Pharm* 41:310-322, 1984.

Noel MW: Quantitative measurements of inventory control. *Am J Hosp Pharm* 41:2378-2383, 1984.

Skolaut MW, McAllister JC III: Purchasing and inventory control — past, present, and future. *Am J Hosp Pharm* 41:522-525, 1984.

Soares DP: Quality assurance standards for purchasing and inventory control. *Am J Hosp Pharm* 42:610-620, 1985.

Abramowitz PW: Controlling financial variables — purchasing, inventory control and waste reduction. *Am J Hosp Pharm* 41:309-317, 1984.

Bicket WJ, Gagnon JP: Purchasing and inventory control for hospital pharmacies. *Top Hosp Pharm Mgt* 7(2):59-74, 1987.

Davern PF, Kubica AJ: Controlling drug costs: Administrative and clinical strategies. *Top Hosp Pharm Mgt* 7(2):48-58, 1987.

Lunik MC, Sherrin TP, Grauer DW: Pharmaceutical practices in large hospitals. *Top Hosp Pharm Mgt* 7(2):15-21, 1987.

McAllister JW III: Managing purchasing and inventory control functions. In Williams RB (ed): *Hospital Pharmacy Management Primer.* Bethesda, MD, American Society of Hospital Pharmacists, 1985, pp 57-77.

Roffe BD, Powell MF: Quality assurance aspects of purchasing and inventory control. *Top Hosp Pharm Mgt* 3(3):62-74, 1983.

Group Purchasing

Chawla AK, Hayas SR, Zabriske DE: Center for health affairs, Greater Cleveland Hospital Association. *Am J Hosp Pharm* 44:2498-2500, 1987.

Currey RD: The Sisters of the Third Order of St. Francis. *Am J Hosp Pharm* 44:2509-2511, 1987.

Grimes JP: Group purchasing: Evaluating groups. *Am J Hosp Pharm* 44:1794-1797, 1987.

Grimm JE: Practical aspects of selecting a pharmaceutical purchasing group. *Top Hosp Pharm Mgt* 1(1):49-59, 1981.

Grotzinger RP, Ivey MF: Hospital Shared Services of Washington State. *Am J Hosp Pharm* 44:2504-2506, 1987.

Herrick JD: Group purchasing: Vendor selection. *Am J Hosp Pharm* 44:2035-2040, 1987.

Kroll DJ, Herrick JD, Ashby DM: American Healthcare Systems. *Am J Hosp Pharm* 44:2493-2495, 1987.

Long CW: Hospital Corporation of America. *Am J Hosp Pharm* 44:2501-2503, 1987.

Olsen JC, Bray RK: Humana, Inc. *Am J Hosp Pharm* 44:2507-2509, 1987.

Powers JR: Hospital pharmacy buying groups: The perspective of a contract sales manager. *Top Hosp Pharm Mgt* 7(2):9-14, 1987.
Raehtz TR, Milewski R, Massoud N: Factors influencing prices offered to pharmaceutical purchasing groups. *Am J Hosp Pharm* 44:2073-2076, 1987.
Randle W: Voluntary purchasing groups: Commitments and concerns. *Top Hosp Pharm Mgt* 7(2):33-39, 1987.
Spitler JD: Amerinet. *Am J Hosp Pharm* 44:2496-2497, 1987.
Wetrich JG: Group purchasing: An overview. *Am J Hosp Pharm* 44:1581-1592, 1987.
Zellmer WA: Purchasing power. *Am J Hosp Pharm* 44:2491, 1987.
Zilz DA: University Hospital Consortium. *Am J Hosp Pharm* 44:2511-2513, 1987.

Prime Vendor and Wholesaler Programs

Bobbitt RA: The role of the pharmaceutical wholesaler in hospital purchasing group contracts. *Top Hosp Pharm Mgt* 7(2):22-32, 1987.
Boland DA: The prime-vendor concept: Making it work. *Am J Hosp Pharm* 41:1765, 1984.
Christensen DB, Ivey MF: Monitoring a primary wholesaler depot program. *Am J Hosp Pharm* 41:1778-1782, 1984.
Johnson LH, Herrick JD: Evaluating group purchasing through a prime vendor. *Am J Hosp Pharm* 41:1783-1788, 1984.
Lee GF, Bair JN, Piz JW: Alternative to the traditional discount method of wholesaler purchasing. *Am J Hosp Pharm* 39:1192-1194, 1982.
Minor MF: Hospital pharmacy advisory board influencing service improvements by a drug wholesaler. *Hosp Pharm* 21:674, 1986.
Olson SM, Hammel RW, Liegel AR: Feasibility of prime vendor purchasing for a state university hospital. *Am J Hosp Pharm* 42:566-570, 1985.
Yost RD, Flowers DM: New roles for wholesalers in hospital drug distribution. *Top Hosp Pharm Mgt* 7(2):84-90, 1987.

Appendix 9-A

ASHP GUIDELINES FOR SELECTING PHARMACEUTICAL MANUFACTURERS AND SUPPLIERS

Pharmacists are responsible for selecting, from the hundreds of manufacturers and suppliers of drugs, those that will enable them to fulfill an important obligation: ensuring that patients receive pharmaceuticals and related supplies of the highest quality and at the lowest cost. These guidelines are offered as an aid to the pharmacist in achieving this goal.

Obligations of the Supplier

Pharmacists may purchase with confidence the products of those suppliers meeting the criteria presented below. Other factors such as credit policies, delivery times, and the breadth of a supplier's product line must also be considered in selecting a supplier.

Technical Considerations

1. Upon request of the pharmacist (an instrument such as the ASHP Drug Product Information Request Form* is useful in this regard), the supplier should furnish
   a. Analytical control data,
   b. Sterility-testing data,
   c. Bioavailability data,
   d. Bioequivalency data,
   e. Descriptions of testing procedures for raw materials and finished products, and
   f. Any other information that may be indicative of the quality of a given finished drug product.

   Testing data developed by independent laboratories should be identified by the supplier. All information should be supplied at no charge.
2. There should be no history of recurring product recalls indicative of deficient quality control procedures.
3. The supplier should permit visits (during normal business hours) by the pharmacist to inspect its manufacturing and control procedures.
4. All drug products should conform to the requirements of *The United States Pharmacopeia—The National Formulary (USP-NF)* (the most recent edition) unless otherwise specified by the pharmacist. Items not recognized by the *USP-NF* should meet the specifications set forth by the pharmacist.
5. To the extent possible, all products should be available in single unit or unit dose packages. These packages should conform to the ASHP Technical Assistance Bulletin on Single Unit and Unit Dose Packages of Drugs.[1]
6. The name and address of the manufacturer of the final dosage form and the packager or distributor should be present on the product labeling.
7. Expiration dates should be clearly indicated on the package label and, unless stability properties warrant otherwise, should occur in January or July.
8. Therapeutic, biopharmaceutic, and toxicologic information should be available to the pharmacist on request. Toxicity information should be available around the clock.
9. Patient and staff educational materials that are important for proper use of the product should be routinely available.
10. Upon request, the supplier should furnish proof of any claims made with respect to the efficacy, safety, and superiority of its products.
11. Upon request, the supplier should furnish at no charge a reasonable quantity of its products to enable the pharmacist to evaluate the products' physical traits, including pharmaceutical elegance (appearance, absence of physical deterioration or flaws), packaging, and labeling.

Distribution Policies

1. Whenever possible, delivery of a drug product should be confined to a single lot number.
2. Unless otherwise specified or required by stability considerations, not less than a 12-month interval between a product's time of delivery and its expiration date should be present.
3. The supplier should accept for full credit (based on purchase price), without prior authorization, any unopened packages of goods returned within 12 months of the expiration date. Credits should be in cash or applied to the institution's account.
4. The supplier should ship all goods in a timely manner, freight prepaid, and enclose a packing list with each shipment. All items "out of stock" should be noted, and the anticipated availability of the item should be clearly indicated. There should be no extensive recurrence of back orders.
5. The supplier should warrant title to commodities supplied, warrant them to be free from defects and imperfections and fit for any rational use of the product, and indemnify and hold the purchaser harmless against any and all suits, claims, and expenses, including attorneys' fees, damages, and injuries or any claims by third parties relating to the products.

Marketing and Sales Policies

1. The supplier should not, without written consent, use the pharmacist's or his or her organization's name in any advertising or other promotional materials or activities.
2. The supplier should honor formulary decisions made by the organization's pharmacy and therapeutics committee, and the supplier's sales representatives should comply

*Available from ASHP, 4630 Montgomery Avenue, Bethesda, MD 20814.

Approved by the ASHP Board of Directors, November 14, 1990. Revised by the ASHP Council on Professional Affairs. Supersedes previous versions approved November 17-18, 1983, and September 22, 1989.

with the organization's regulations governing their activities.

3. The supplier should not offer cash, equipment, or merchandise to the organization or its staff as an inducement to purchase its products.
4. Discounts should be in cash or cash credit, not merchandise, and should be clearly indicated on invoices and bills, rather than consisting of end-of-year rebates or similar discount practices.
5. In entering into a contract to supply goods, the supplier should guarantee to furnish, at the price specified, any minimum amount of products so stated. If the supplier is unable to meet the supply commitment, the supplier should reimburse the institution for any excess costs incurred in obtaining the product from other sources. If, during the life of the contract, a price reduction occurs, the lower price should prevail.
6. All parties to the bidding process should respect the integrity of the process and the contracts awarded thereby.

Responsibilities of the Purchaser

It may be desirable to purchase drugs or other commodities on a competitive bid basis. The pharmacist should ensure that competitive bidding procedures conform to the guidelines below:

1. Invitations to bid should be mailed to the suppliers' home offices with copies to their local representatives (if any), unless suppliers specify otherwise.
2. Potential bidders should be given no less than three weeks to submit a bid.
3. The opening date for the bids should be specified and honored by the purchaser.
4. The language of the invitation to bid should be clear and should indicate the person (and organization address and telephone number) the bidder should contact in the event of questions or problems. Specifications should be complete with respect to products, packagings, and quantities desired.
5. If the bidding forms are used, they should contain adequate space for the bidder to enter the information requested.
6. The winning bidder should be notified in writing. Unsuccessful bidders may be informed of who won the award at what price, if they so request.
7. The quantities specified in the invitation to bid should be a reasonable estimate of requirements.
8. If the invitation to bid is offered on behalf of a group of purchasers, the individual members of the group should not engage in bidding procedures of their own and should purchase the goods in question from the winning bidder.

REFERENCE

1. American Society of Hospital Pharmacists. ASHP technical assistance bulletin on single unit and unit dose packages of drugs. *Am J Hosp Pharm* 42:378-379, 1985.

Appendix 9-B

ASHP TECHNICAL ASSISTANCE BULLETIN ON SINGLE UNIT AND UNIT DOSE PACKAGES OF DRUGS

Drug packages must fulfill four basic functions: (1) identify their contents completely and precisely; (2) protect their contents from deleterious environmental effects (e.g., photodecomposition); (3) protect their contents from deterioration due to handling (e.g., breakage and contamination); (4) permit their contents to be used quickly, easily, and safely. Modern drug distribution systems use single unit packages to a great extent and, in fact, such packages are central to the operation of unit dose systems, intravenous admixture services, and other important aspects of pharmacy practice. These guidelines have been prepared to assist pharmaceutical manufacturers and pharmacists in the development and production of single unit and unit dose packages, the use of which has been shown to have substantial benefits.

A *single unit* package is one that contains one discrete pharmaceutical dosage form, i.e., one tablet, one 2-mL volume of liquid, one 2-g mass of ointment, etc. A *unit dose* package is one that contains the particular dose of the drug ordered for the patient. A single unit package is also a *unit dose* or *single dose* package if it contains the particular dose of the drug ordered for the patient. A unit dose package could, for example, contain two tablets of a drug product.

General Considerations

Packaging Materials. Packaging materials (and the package itself) must possess the physical characteristics required to protect the contents from (as required) light, moisture, temperature, air, and handling. The material should not deteriorate during the shelf life of the contents. Packages should be of lightweight, nonbulky materials that do not produce toxic fumes when incinerated. Materials that may be recycled or are biodegradable, or both, are to be preferred over those that are not. Packaging materials should not absorb, adsorb, or otherwise deleteriously affect their contents. Information should be available to practitioners indicating the stability and compatibility of drugs with various packaging materials.

Shape and Form. Packages should be constructed so that they do not deteriorate with normal handling. They should be easy to open and use, and their use should require little or no special training or experience. Unless the package contains a drug to be added to a parenteral fluid or otherwise used in compounding a finished dosage form, it should allow the contents to be administered directly to the patient (or IPPB apparatus or fluid administration set) without any need for repackaging into another container or device (except for ampules).

Label Copy. Current Federal labeling requirements must be adhered to, with attention also given to the items below. The desired copy and format are as follows:

Nonproprietary Name
(and proprietary name if to be shown)
Dosage Form
(if special or other than oral)
Strength
Strength of Dose
and
Total Contents Delivered
(e.g., number of tablets
and their total dose)
Special Notes (e.g., refrigerate)
Expiration Date
Control Number

1. *Nonproprietary and proprietary name(s).* The nonproprietary name and the strength should be the most prominent part of the package label. It is not necessary to include the proprietary name, if any, on the package. The name of the manufacturer or distributor should appear on the package. In addition, the name of the manufacturer of the finished dosage form should be included in the product labeling. The style of type should be chosen to provide maximum legibility, contrast, and permanence.
2. *Dosage form.* Special characteristics of the dosage form should be a part of the label, e.g., extended release. Packages should be labeled as to the route of administration if other than oral, e.g., topical use. In a package containing an injection, the acceptable injectable route(s) of administration should be stated on both outer and inner packages, i.e., both on the syringe unit and carton (if any).
3. *Strength.* Strength should be stated in accordance with terminology in the *American Hospital Formulary Service.* The metric system should be used, with dosage forms formulated to provide the rounded-off figures in the USP table of approximate equivalents and expressed in the smallest whole number. Micrograms should be used through 999, then milligrams through 999, then grams. Thus, 300 mg, **not** 5 gr, nor 325 mg, nor 0.3 g; 60 mg, **not** 1 gr, nor 0.06 g, nor 64.5 mg, nor 65 mg; 400 mcg, **not** 1/150 gr, nor 0.4 mg, nor 0.0004 g; mL (milliliters) should be used instead of cc (cubic centimeters).
4. *Strength of dose and total contents delivered.* The total contents **and** total dose of the package should be indicated. Thus, a unit dose package containing a 600-mg dose as two 300-mg tablets should be labeled, "600 mg (as two 300-mg tablets)." Likewise, a 500-mg dose of a drug in a liquid containing 100-mg/mL should be labeled, "Delivers 500 mg (as 5 mL of 100-mg/mL)."
5. *Special notes.* Special notes such as conditions of storage (e.g., refrigerate), preparation (e.g., shake well or moisten), and administration (e.g., not to be chewed) that are not obvious from the dosage form designation are to be included on the label.
6. *Expiration date.* The expiration date should be prominently visible on the package. If the contents must be reconstituted prior to use, the shelf life of the final product should be indicated. Unless stability data warrant otherwise, expiration dates should fall during January and July to simplify recall procedures.
7. *Control number (lot number).* The control number should appear on the package.

Product Identification Codes. The use of product identification codes, appearing directly on the dosage form, is encouraged.

Evidence of Entry. The package should be so designed that it is evident, when the package is still intact, that it has never been entered or opened.

Specific Considerations

Oral Solids

1. *Blister package.* A blister package should:
   a. Have an opaque and nonreflective backing (flat upper surface of package) for printing.
   b. Have a blister (dome or bubble) of a transparent material that is, preferably, flat bottomed.
   c. Be easily peelable.
   d. If it contains a controlled substance, be numbered sequentially for accountability purposes.
2. *Pouch package.* A pouch package should:
   a. Have one side opaque and nonreflective for printing.
   b. Be easily deliverable, i.e., large tablets in large pouches, small tablets in small pouches.
   c. Tear from any point or from multiple locations.
   d. If it contains a controlled substance, be numbered sequentially for accountability purposes.
3. The packages should be such that contents can be delivered directly to the patient's mouth or hand.

Oral Liquids

1. The packages should be filled to deliver the labeled contents. It is recognized that overfilling will be necessary, depending on the shape of the container, the container material, and the formulation of the dosage form.
2. The label should state the contents as follows: Delivers ___mg (or g or mcg) in ___mL.
3. If reconstitution is required, the amount of vehicle to be added should be indicated. These directions may take the form of "fill to mark on container" in lieu of stating a specific volume.
4. Syringe-type containers for oral administration should not accept a needle and should be labeled "For Oral Use Only."
5. Containers should be designed to permit administration of contents directly from the package.

Injectables

1. The device should be appropriately calibrated in milliliters and scaled from the tip to the fill line. Calibrated space may be built into the device to permit addition of other drugs. The label should state the contents as follows: Delivers ___mg (or g or mcg) in ___mL.
2. An appropriate-size needle may be an integral part of the device. The needle sheath should not be the plunger. The plunger should be mechanically stable in the barrel of the syringe.
3. The device should be of such a design that it is patient ready and assembly instructions are not necessary.

4. The sheath protecting the needle should be a nonpenetrable, preferably rigid material, to protect personnel from injury. The size of the needle should be indicated.
5. The device should be of such a design that easy and visible aspiration is possible. It should be as compact as possible and of such a size that it can be easily handled.

Parenteral Solutions and Additives

1. The approximate pH and osmolarity of parenteral solutions should be stated on the label. The amount of overfill also should be noted. Electrolyte solutions should be labeled in both mEq (or millimole) and mg concentrations. Solutions commonly labeled in terms of percent concentration, e.g., dextrose, should also be labeled in w/v terms.
2. Parenteral fluid container labels should be readable when hanging and when upright or in the normal manipulative position.
3. Drugs to be mixed with parenteral infusion solutions should be packaged into convenient sizes that minimize the need for solution transfers and other manipulations.
4. Partially filled piggyback-type containers should:
   a. Be recappable with a tamper-proof closure.
   b. Have a hanger.
   c. Have volume markings.
   d. Be designed to minimize the potential for contamination during use.
   e. Contain a partial vacuum for ease of reconstitution.
5. If an administration set is included with the container, it should be compatible with all large-volume parenteral delivery systems.

Other Dosage Forms — Ophthalmics, Suppositories, Ointments, etc. Dosage forms other than those specifically discussed above should be adequately labeled to indicate their use and route of administration and should adhere to the above and other required package labeling and design criteria.

Approved by the ASHP Board of Directors, November 14-15, 1984. Revised by the ASHP Council on Clinical Affairs. Supersedes the previous version, which was approved March 31-April 1, 1977.

Reprinted from the *Am J Hosp Pharm* 42:378-379, 1985.

CHAPTER 10

Financial Management

CLYDE BUCHANAN

The health care economy is in turmoil because of policy-makers' efforts to control rapidly rising costs. Pharmacists can deal with the situation partly through better financial management. Pierpaoli[1] said that today's pharmacy managers must be "bilingual" because they must effectively relate to the hospital's corporate administration on the one hand and the hospital professional staff on the other. This chapter is written to help pharmacists and pharmacy students understand financial management as it relates to pharmacy department budgeting and financial reporting.*

HEALTH CARE INSTITUTION ACCOUNTING

Accounting is a standard system of tabulating monetary transactions and analyzing and reporting the results. Equation 1 represents the foundation on which financial accounting rests.

Equation 1

$$\text{Assets} = \text{Liabilities} + \text{Equity}$$

In this equation, assets include that which is owned (e.g., land, buildings, equipment, inventories of supplies, investments, cash, and collectible revenues). Liabilities are debts or financial obligations (e.g., outstanding bills, bond issues, principal and interest owed on borrowed money, etc.). Equity is the financial net worth (assets minus liabilities) of the institution.[2] Institutions maintain a balance sheet showing assets, liabilities, and equity. A balance sheet is a perpetual and permanent record of the financial status of the institution, for example:

Balance Sheet
MEMORIAL HOSPITAL
June 30, 1992

Assets		Liabilities and Equity	
Cash	$200,000	Accounts Payable	$ 100,000
Accounts Receivable	300,000	Long-Term Debt	7,500,000
Inventory	80,000	Equity	1,180,000
Land	200,000	Total	$8,780,000
Equipment	2,000,000		
Buildings	6,000,000		
Total	$8,780,000.		

Note that the two sides of the balance sheet reflect the two sides of the accounting equation. Any monetary transaction includes a debit and a credit (i.e., double-entry accounting) to balance both sides. For instance, purchasing a typewriter incurs a liability to pay for the typewriter and increases equipment assets by the value of the typewriter.

The general ledger is a trial (unaudited) financial balance of an institution that includes the balance sheet and various statements (reports) of revenues, expenses, and budgets. For example, an income statement summarizes revenues and expenses for a selected time period. When combined with budget figures for revenues and expenses, the income statement may be called a budget report or responsibility summary. (See further discussion under budgeting below.)

Financial Data

Pharmacy is represented in the institution's general ledger as an account (a separate department) for which monetary transactions (financial data) are recorded. The director of pharmacy is responsible for monitoring the pharmacy account. Financial reports for the pharmacy account group data into three general categories: revenues, expenses, and volumes of work (i.e., production).

Revenues

Pharmacy revenues consist primarily of patient charges, consultation fees, and research grant monies. Pharmaceutical and service (e.g., consultations) charges appear on patients' hospital bills; however, the institution receives payment as diagnosis-related group (DRG) rates, per diem rates, per capita fees, or discounted patient bills. Very few patients or third-party payers actually pay their bills as submitted to them. The difference between what patients are billed and what third parties pay is known as "allowance" or "bad debt."

Expenses

Pharmacy expenses are mainly supplies (e.g., pharmaceuticals) and personnel (e.g., pharmacists and technicians)

*Several significant ideas for this chapter originated in discussion among the authors of the ASHP Accrue Level II module *Financial Management.* Those authors include James Hethcox, Mick Hunt, Brian Dennis, and Clyde Buchanan.

salaries. These are direct expenses to the department. Indirect expenses include items such as utilities, housekeeping, hospital purchasing, and administration. Because the department does not control indirect expenses, they may not appear on pharmacy financial reports.

Direct expenses may be further subdivided as fixed or variable expenses. Fixed expenses occur unrelated to volume of work (e.g., management salaries or travel expenses). Variable expenses change in proportion to the volume of work done (e.g., pharmaceuticals and some staff personnel salaries).

Workload Volumes

Volumes consist of units of work (workload) and paid hours. Workload can be classified as revenue-producing (e.g., a charge for an injection) or non-revenue-producing (e.g., answering a drug information question). Paid hours may be productive (e.g., employee at work carrying out duties) or nonproductive (e.g., employee on paid vacation).

Although health care institutions often report workload as admissions or patient days, pharmacy itself should use workload indicators that directly reflect pharmacy work done (e.g., unit doses charged, or preferably, a weighted workload unit that also includes clinical activities). Weighted units are called relative value units (RVU's). An RVU system allots different work values to different activities. For example, a unit dose oral solid dispensed may be 1 unit; a hyperalimentation admixture, 15 units; and a pharmacokinetic consultation, 45 units. The advantage to the RVU system is that the sum of work units can be converted to hours of work done, which can be compared to paid hours of work.[3]

For reporting purposes, revenues and expenses are sorted into groups of like items (i.e., subaccounts) in a chart of accounts. Table 10-1 shows a typical chart of accounts for a pharmacy department.

Table 10-1. Pharmacy chart of accounts

Department: Pharmacy		***Account: 3-70490***
Subaccount Number	***Subaccount Name***	***Subaccount Description***
Revenues		
0600	Inpatient	Inpatient Charges and Fees
0610	Outpatient	Outpatient Charges and Fees
0630	Other Income	Research Monies, Rebates, etc.
Expenses		
Salaries		
1200	Managerial	Director, Supervisors
1300	Professional	Clinical, Operational R.Ph.'s
1400	Technical	Technicians and Messengers
1700	Clerical	Secretaries and Clerks
1900	Fringe Benefits	
Supplies (Variable)		
2100	Pharmaceuticals	Drugs and Biologicals
2200	IV Solutions	IV and Other Solutions
2300	Other Supplies	Sets, Needles, Syringes, etc.
Other Expenses (Fixed)		
2400	Communications	Phones, Pneumatic Tubes, etc.
2500	Maintenance/Repairs	Equipment and Systems
2600	Other Services	Contracted Services, Licenses
3200	Office Supplies	Paper, Ribbons, Cleaning, etc.
3400	Books/Subscriptions	Reference Books and Journals
3800	Noncapital Equipment	
6100	Travel	Educational Expenses
8400	Food/Catering	Guest Meals, Coffee, etc.
8600	Depreciation	Capital Equipment Depreciation

FINANCIAL PLANNING

Budgeting is one of the most important financial management functions. A budget is an annual plan expressed in financial terms. A budget does not represent actual money available to be spent; rather, it is an estimate of future revenues and expenses and a yardstick by which a department's financial performance may be measured.

Relation to Strategic Planning

Actually, budget preparation is one of the latter stages of strategic planning. A health care institution's mission is a broad definition of its scope and purpose. Strategic planning is the process of establishing the organization's future direction based on its mission and health care market. Strategic planning begins with a business environment assessment; continues with an analysis of strengths, weaknesses, opportunities, and threats; and results in a long-range plan for what the institution will endeavor to accomplish.

Goal Setting

Each year the institution sets a short-range (annual) plan as a step toward the long-range plan. The institution's chief executive officer (CEO) and board of directors set annual goals in general terms for the institution. This is done 6 to 9 months before the new financial (fiscal) year begins. The director of pharmacy initiates the department budgeting process by explaining institutional goals to department members. The department then develops annual goals — some related to institutional objectives, some to department-oriented objectives.

Goals should be clear, measurable, and focused on objectives of importance; they should be attainable but challenging (see example below).

Example of a Department Goal With Objectives and Measures

Goal	***Objectives***	***Measures***
To computerize outpatient dispensing. (Responsibility: ambulatory lead pharmacist)	To make refills efficient	Reduce refill time by 50%
	To automate billing	Establish billing interface by 1/92
	To reduce personnel	Transfer 0.5 FTE billing clerk

Persons who will be responsible for attaining the goals should have input into the goal-setting process. Goals that will result in greater or less revenue or expense or work volume must be reflected in the budget (see "*New Program Budgets*" on page 88).

Department goals must receive final approval by the CEO. Then the institution's chief financial officer (CFO) prepares a budget calendar, which specifies when department heads must turn in each part of their budget. The CFO also distributes a budget manual explaining how all the budget forms are to be completed. Usually, the capital equipment budget is due first, then the workload volume and expense budget, and finally budgets for new programs.

Types of Budgets

There are three basic types of budgets: the fixed budget, the flexible budget, and the zero-based budget. The fixed budget is based on workload projections. It does not change once it is final, regardless of whether workload projections are met. The flexible budget accommodates changes in workload because it changes revenues and expenses in relation to workload fluctuation.[4] The zero-based budget is developed from scratch so that all activities are analyzed for cost-effectiveness, and the top-rated programs and services are funded.[5]

BUDGETING PROCESS

Before doing any budget calculations, the manager reviews historical trends in the department and tries to anticipate any changes that will affect the budget. For example, if expensive new drugs are likely to be used to a significant extent, the manager adjusts the pharmaceutical budget accordingly.

Capital Budget

Capital budgets comprise nonconsumable equipment and building renovations that cost more than a fixed amount (e.g., $500) and have an expected life of greater than 2 years. Depending on the institution's definition, capital budgets may include rented or leased equipment and computer software as well. Some institutions require departments to set priorities on capital they request. Others set capital ceilings for each department, while others establish a capital equipment pool from which all departments draw. Coarse[6] explains the cost analysis process for capital purchasing decisions.

Fixed Budgeting Process

Following is an example of how a fixed budget is prepared. (The reader is advised to study the tables carefully.) Although each institution will have different budget report formats, the principles in the example budget are widely applicable. Flexible and zero-based budgets follow most of the same principles during their preparation.

Volume Budget

The CFO supplies the number of patient days and DRG case mix index (a reflection of the acuity of patient cases to be treated) for calendar year (CY) 1991, and the same figures projected for fiscal year (FY) 1991-2. Equation 2 forecasts the projected case mix factor for FY 1991-2.

Equation 2

$$\frac{\text{(51022 Pt Day-92)}}{\text{(52134 Pt Day-91)}} \times \frac{\text{(1.0891 Index-92)}}{\text{(1.0358 Index-91)}} = 1.029$$

The workload volume budget is based on the relative value unit. To forecast RVU's for FY 1991-2, which begins July 1, 1991, a projection is made from the number of RVU's in CY 1991. Table 10-2 shows how RVU's are forecast based on the case mix factor.

In this example, the assumption is made that all workload is directly related to patient days and case mix index. Pharmacy managers must determine which predictive factors correlate best with their actual workload.

Expense Budget

Pharmacy department expenses are determined for three categories: personnel, supplies, and other expenses.

Personnel Expenses

Personnel expenses include salaries paid plus benefits such as health, life, disability, and workers' compensation insurance. Depending on local conditions, the benefit package may represent as much as 25 percent of total salaries. The manager projects the number of paid hours based on approved positions. For each personnel subaccount (or job code), an average salary is used. Paid hours multiplied by average salaries represent the personnel salary expense, then benefits (at an incremental rate of 20 percent) are added as shown in table 10-3.

Supplies

Forecasting supply expenses involves four factors: projected units charged, cost per unit, inflation, and the case mix factor. Table 10-4 shows projected costs for supplies that are considered variable. There are several methods for projecting supply costs. This author tried six ways and found the percent change and regression time-series methods to be best for his purposes.[7]

Fixed Expenses

Nonsupply expenses are considered fixed expenses. They tend to vary only with inflation. Table 10-3 also shows projections for expenses other than personnel and supplies.

Revenue Budget

Because pharmacy charges are still made to some private payers, pharmacy managers need to know how to forecast and adjust revenue. Revenue, whether collected or not, is still part of budgets and reports for which the director of pharmacy is responsible.

Revenue can be predicted from workload forecast as shown in table 10-4; however, one must not only predict revenue but alter the charge table to generate additional revenue. The CFO required the patient revenue to be $4 million (table 10-4.) The pharmacy manager chooses dispensing fees to obtain the required revenue. Other revenue (table 10-5, Subaccount 0630) includes payments from other institutions for pharmaceuticals, any special fees collected, etc.

New Program Budgets

In justifying new or improved services, a separate budget is usually required to document the incremental increases in personnel, supplies, capital, and other expenses. This is particularly true for new personnel. This type of budget is called the "new program budget" or "incremental budget." The example of a pharmacy goal and objective for an outpatient computer system would be handled as a new program budget.

The new program budget is similar to the zero-based budget that requires a cost-benefit analysis (decision package). The new program budget should include sections on objectives, a program description, resources required, advantages, disadvantages, and a financial bottom line (see figure 10-1). McGhan and Bootman[8] provide a sophisticated reference on justifying new programs through cost-benefit analysis.

In new program budgets, institutional and department goals are followed. Even when it is tied to approved goals, the new service's chance of being funded will probably depend on its cost-benefit analysis (i.e., a positive bottom line). This will also be the yardstick by which the new service is measured once it is implemented.

Evaluation and Negotiation of the Budget Package

Completed budget forecasts are evaluated for reasonableness by comparing the new budget to actual figures from the last 2-3 years. If the new budget differs significantly from prior years' trends, the pharmacy manager must be prepared with supporting documentation to justify the budget submission. During budget negotiations, the pharmacy managers must understand the dual role of their position—that of professional pharmacist with the quality of patient care at heart and that of financial manager focused on the bottom line.

Departments are in competition for scarce resources, making the situation difficult for upper management. The pharmacy manager must also recognize the political constraints of the institution (e.g., relations with the medical staff, board of directors, and community) within which the budget must be set.

After all departments submit their budgets, the CFO and his or her staff will "roll up" the institution's budget into one package. The institutional administrators, led by the CEO and CFO, set priorities for funding based on goals and anticipated revenues. Some new program budgets are denied; departments are asked to reduce capital and discretionary expenses (e.g., travel and books), and existing programs may have to be rejustified or cut.

It is during the negotiation phase that the pharmacy manager will have to make cuts in programs, personnel, capital requests, and discretionary expenses. Pharmacy personnel should have input in making budget cuts because they will have to live with them. The pharmacy manager should make every effort to maintain his or her credibility and teamwork with upper management while being faithful to patients and personnel.

Initiation of the Budget

Eventually, the institution's budget will be approved by the board of directors, and each department will receive its final budget. The pharmacy manager should review this budget for errors and omissions (e.g., input errors such as number transpositions). There may have been many changes since the budget was last seen in the department. All errors should be reported in writing to the CFO for correction (if possible).

BUDGET MONITORING

Budgeting is a year-round process. The manager uses the final budget to monitor and control revenues and expenses.

Recordkeeping System

Because of the large volume of data involved in budget monitoring, a data-collection system is required. Following are data types that must be collected: workload units, admissions or patient days, and personnel hours. These data should be recorded at least monthly to enable budget monitoring. The goals of a data-collection system are to maximize accuracy, minimize personnel time, monitor financial performance, highlight trends, and standardize reporting periods and nomenclature.

Variance Analysis

The pharmacy manager analyzes significant variances from the budget each month. Most important to consider are pharmaceutical expenses and salaries.

Identifying Budget Variances

Table 10-5 illustrates a typical responsibility summary, which shows budget variance for the month and year to date. Variances may be favorable (i.e., improving the net margin or bottom line) or unfavorable. The first step is to decide the significance of each variance. Usually the percentage of variance from budget is found. A 5-10 percent variance in revenue or pharmaceutical expenses may be acceptable, with no further analysis required. Personnel costs should vary less than 2-3 percent from budget, because the manager exercises more control over personnel costs than over prescribing patterns that affect revenue and supply costs. The manager must also pay attention to the dollar amount of variance. A $5,000 variance in pharmaceutical costs would not be nearly as significant as a $5,000 variance in travel expenses.

Determining the Source of Variances

To investigate reasons for a variance, the pharmacy manager must look at the components that make up the variance. Salaries are composed of hours worked (a volume), salary per hour (a rate), and workload per hour (efficiency). To investigate the favorable 34.3 percent variance in clerical personnel salaries for the month ending December 31, 1991, the manager calculates actual versus budget figures for paid hours, average salary per hour, and RVU's per paid hour. This will give the manager direction for further investigations. In this example, a clerical position was open during the month.

Seasonal variances are to be expected in revenue and pharmaceutical expenses. When analyzing these variances, the manager must consider two factors: the volume of units charged or purchased and the average charge or cost per unit. The average charge or cost per unit is affected by changes in drug costs (e.g., a new bid period) or in the mix of drugs purchased (e.g., changing from ionic to nonionic contrast media). Hunt[9] has suggested monitoring revenue according to dosage form per patient day and revenue per dosage form and per number of patient days. Variances may also be due to inaccurate budgeting. This explanation should not be overlooked.

Corrective Actions

The director of pharmacy is responsible for the pharmacy department's financial performance. The budget is a primary tool used to identify any variance that must be corrected. Pharmacy management and personnel share responsibility for taking action to correct unfavorable financial situations. Primary actions to consider are reducing pharmaceutical and personnel expenses, finding other sources of revenue, and correcting an inaccurate budget.[10] Major corrective actions are proposed to upper management as a change in services (e.g., discontinuing a take-home prescription service).

FINANCIAL REPORTING

The pharmacy manager reports to his or her superior on the department's financial performance versus budget. To be effective, reports should be concise and understandable.

Monthly Report

Based on the responsibility summary, the director reports reasons for significant budget variances and corrective actions under way. The use of a personal computer is a great boon to the pharmacy manager.[11] With spreadsheet programs, the manager can collect and analyze data much more efficiently. Recognizing the value of a "picture," the manager uses charts and graphs to show trends and make points about financial data. This is easily done by integrating spreadsheet graphics into a word-processing document.

Annual Report

The director of pharmacy is responsible for the annual report. The annual report reviews all major accomplishments (and shortcomings) for the department in relation to the annual goals. It is prepared more formally, containing more text and fewer financial tables and graphics.

CONCLUSION

The budget is a financial plan negotiated by personnel at all levels in the institution. It provides a yardstick against which production and economic performance can be compared. The method of preparing the budget is less important than analyzing variances from the budget and pursuing annual goals. Reporting variances and developing strategies to handle them are critical for the pharmacy manager.

REFERENCES

1. Pierpaoli P: Management diplomacy: Myths and methods. *Am J Hosp Pharm* 44:297-304, 1987.
2. Beck DF: Principles of accounting and finance for the nonaccountant. *Health Care Supervisor* 2(1):15-26, 1984.
3. Choich R: Productivity analysis: A managerial reality. *Top Hosp Pharm Mgt* 7:23-32, 1987.
4. Coarse JF: Flexible budgeting for hospital pharmacists. *Top Hosp Pharm Mgt* 4(4):9-20, 1985.
5. Dillon RD: Zero-base budgeting: An introduction. *Hosp Fin Mgt* 31(11):10-14, 1977.
6. Coarse JF: Capital budgeting: Managing the process. *Top Hosp Pharm Mgt* 3(4):19-32, 1983.
7. Buchanan C: Selecting a method to forecast drug costs. *Top Hosp Pharm Mgt* 4(4):21-32, 1985.
8. McGhan WF, Bootman JL: The use of cost-benefit analysis in justifying clinical pharmacy services. *Top Hosp Pharm Mgt* 3(4):60-72, 1984.
9. Hunt ML: Use of financial reports in managing pharmacies. *Am J Hosp Pharm* 41:709-715, 1984.
10. Anon: ASHP technical assistance bulletin on assessing cost-containment strategies for institutional pharmacies. *Am J Hosp Pharm* 42:1583-1591, 1985.
11. Buchanan EC: Microcomputer applications in hospital pharmacy. *Top Hosp Pharm Mgt* 4(1):14-25, 1984.

ADDITIONAL READING

American Society of Hospital Pharmacists: *Financial Management* ACCRUE Level II. Bethesda, MD, American Society of Hospital Pharmacists, 1990.

Anthony RN, Young DW: *Management control in nonprofit organizations*, 4th ed., Homewood, IL, Irwin, Inc., 1988, ch 1, 3, 4, 14.

Berman HJ, Weeks LE, Kukla SF (eds): *The Financial Management of Hospitals.* Ann Arbor, MI, Health Administration Press, 1986, ch 1, 2, 5, 21.

Buchanan EC: Budgeting and financial reporting. *Top Hosp Pharm Mgt* 6(3):29-52, 1986.

Nold EG, Williams RB (eds): Reprint from financial management column *Am J Hosp Pharm* 40:1339-1341, 1983, Reprint no. 152.

Williams RB (ed): *Hospital Pharmacy Primer* Bethesda, MD, American Society of Hospital Pharmacists, 1984, pp 79-101.

MEMORIAL HOSPITAL
PHARMACY DEPARTMENT
Cost Center 3-70490

NEW PROGRAM PROPOSAL

TITLE: Outpatient Pharmacy Computer DEPARTMENT PRIORITY NO. 1

OBJECTIVES:

1. To make prescription refilling more efficient (i.e., reduce refill time by 50%).
2. To automate billing (i.e., establish interface with patient accounting by 1/92).
3. To reduce outpatient pharmacy personnel (i.e., reduce staff by full-time equivalent 0.5 [FTE] billing clerk).

DESCRIPTION OF PROGRAM: Based on proposals from three outpatient pharmacy computer system vendors, pharmacy and data-processing managers will select a system that will meet objectives. The software will be tailored to the hospital formulary and installed within 4 months after the selection is made. In-service training for pharmacy personnel and system maintenance will be provided by the vendor.

RESOURCES REQUIRED: Three desktop terminals, three printers, one network server totaling $15,000. Vendor software totaling $10,000. Yearly system maintenance estimated at $2,500. Cables and minor accessories will cost $1,000. Supplies will cost $100 per year.

ADVANTAGES: In addition to meeting the above objectives, the system will enable the outpatient pharmacy to handle 20% greater refill prescription workload without increased staff, to provide income tax records for outpatients, and to generate drug use evaluation data.

DISADVANTAGES: The system will take more space in the outpatient pharmacy; this will require rearranging the module where the billing clerk had worked. The cost of the rearrangement is negligible. The half-time billing clerk will have to be transferred or laid off.

FINANCIAL BOTTOM LINE: The system will cost $28,600 up front the first year, but due to reduction of the 0.5 FTE, the system will pay for itself in 4.5 years.

Figure 10-1. Example of a new program budget

Table 10-2. Forecast of relative value units

Account: 3-70490
Department: Pharmacy
Responsible Person: Director

Year Begin: 07/01/91
Year End: 06/30/92
Report Date: 02/12/91

Column -> Dosage Forms Column Calculation ->	A CY 1991 Units*	B Pharmacy RVU Std†	C CY 1991 RVU's (AxB)	D Case Mix Factor‡	E FY 91-92 Units (AxD)	F FY 91-92 RVU's (BxE)
UD Orals	1,255,006	1.0	1,255,006	1.029	1,291,401	1,291,401
Multidose Items	12,154	2.0	24,308	1.029	12,506	25,013
IV Adds-LVP's	12,579	3.0	37,737	1.029	12,944	38,831
IV Adds-SVP's	29,514	4.0	118,056	1.029	30,370	121,480
Hyperals	878	15.0	13,170	1.029	903	13,552
Injectables	17,756	1.0	17,756	1.029	18,271	18,271
Outpatient Rx	19,396	6.0	116,376	1.029	19,958	119,751
IV Solutions	49,985	1.0	49,985	1.029	51,435	51,435
Totals ->	1,397,268		1,632,394		1,437,789	1,679,734

*Units charged.
†Relative Value Unit (RVU) standards expressed in minutes.
‡See text for explanation.

Table 10-3. Forecast of expenses other than supplies

Account: 3-70490
Department: Pharmacy
Responsible Person: Director

Month End: 06/30/92
Year Begin: 07/01/91
Report Date: 02/12/91

Column ->	***A***	***B***	***C***	***D***	***E***	***F***	***G***	***H***
	CY 1991 Paid Hours	***CY 1991 Total Expenses***	***CY 1991 Average Salary***	***FY 91-92 Inflation Factor****	***FY 91-92 Case Mix Factor†***	***FY 91-92 Projected Hours***	***FY 91-92 Projected Salary***	***FY 91-92 Projected Expenses***
Column Calculation ->			***(B/A)***			***(AxE)***	***(CxD)***	***(FxG)***
Salaries								
Sub-Acct Description								
1200 Managerial	4,160	117,770	28.31	1.04	1.000	4,160	29.44	122,480
1300 Professional	14,768	355,170	24.05	1.04	1.029	15,196	25.01	380,089
1400 Technical	15,163	216,076	14.25	1.04	1.029	15,603	14.82	231,235
1700 Clerical	5,990	73,263	12.23	1.04	1.000	5,990	12.72	76,193
1900 Fringe Benefits	(20%)	152,456	--	1.04	--	--	--	162,000
Totals ->	40,082	914,734				40,950		971,998
Other Expenses (Fixed)	Column Calculation->							(BxD)
2400 Communications		8,058	--	1.05	--	--	--	8,461
2500 Maint./Repair		1,823	--	1.03	--	--	--	1,878
2600 Other Services		552	--	1.03	--	--	--	569
3400 Books/Subscriptions		2,016	--	1.05	--	--	--	2,117
3800 Noncapital Equipment		3,319	--	1.02	--	--	--	3,385
6100 Travel		3,614	--	1.06	--	--	--	3,831
8400 Food/Catering		753	--	1.03	--	--	--	776
8600 Depreciation		9,564	--	1.00	--	--	--	9,564
Total Other Expenses->		29,699						30,580
Total Expenses->		944,433						1,002,577

*Inflation predicted for 6 months ahead.
†See text for explanation.

Table 10-4. Forecast of supply expenses and revenue

Account: 3-70490
Department: Pharmacy
Responsible Person: Director

Year Begin: 07/01/91
Year End: 06/30/92
Report Date: 02/12/91

Column -> Dosage Forms	***A***	***B***	***C***	***D***	***E***	***F***	***G***	***H***
	CY 1991 Units*	***CY 1991 Expenses***	***CY 1991 Cost/Unit***	***Inflation Factor†***	***Case Mix Factor‡***	***FY 91-92 Expense***	***FY 91-92 Fee/Unit***	***FY 91-92 Revenue***
Column Calculation ->			***(B/A)***			***(AxCxDxE)***		***[F+(AxExG)]***
UD Orals	1,255,006	552,203	0.44	1.03	1.029	585,263	0.75	1,553,814
Multidose Items	12,154	38,285	3.15	1.02	1.029	40,183	3.00	77,703
IV Adds-LVPS's	12,579	69,939	5.56	1.03	1.029	74,127	10.00	203,564
IV Adds-SVP's	29,514	280,678	9.51	1.07	1.029	309,035	12.00	673,474
Hyperals	878	57,290	65.25	1.04	1.029	61,309	125.00	174,242
Injectables	17,756	134,235	7.56	1.04	1.029	143,653	7.50	280,685
Outpatient Rx	19,396	344,279	17.75	1.05	1.029	371,976	6.00	491,727
IV Solutions	49,985	147,457	2.95	1.00	1.029	151,733	8.00	563,213
Totals ->	1,397,268	1,624,366				1,737,280		4,018,422
Per Unit ->						1.24		2.88

*Units charged.
†Inflation predicted for 6 months ahead.
‡See text for explanation.

Table 10-5. Pharmacy department responsibility summary

Account: 3-70490
Department: Pharmacy
Responsible Person: Director

Month End: 12/31/91
Year Begin: 07/01/91
Report Date: 01/12/91

Subaccount Revenues		Current Month Budget	Actual	Variance	Var %	Year-to-Date Budget	Actual	Variance	Var %
0600	Inpatient	299,528	295,009	4,519	1.5	1,777,841	1,726,514	51,327	2.9
0610	Outpatient	40,068	39,113	955	2.4	237,823	247,153	-9,330	-3.9
0630	Other Income	6,115	5,603	512	8.4	36,296	35,145	1,151	3.2
	Gross Revenue	345,711	339,725	5,986	1.7	2,051,960	2,008,812	43,148	2.1
Work Volumes									
	RVU's	142,665	140,769	1,896	1.3	846,783	840,667	6,116	0.7
1200	Manager Pd Hr	353	352	1	0.4	2,097	2,080	17	0.8
1300	Professional Pd Hr	1,291	1,315	-24	-1.9	7,660	7,598	62	0.8
1400	Tech Pd Hrs	1,325	1,301	24	1.8	7,866	7,659	207	2.6
1700	Clerk Pd Hrs	509	334	175	34.3	3,020	2,813	207	6.8
	Total Pd Hrs	3,478	3,302	176	5.1	20,643	20,150	493	2.4
Expenses									
Salaries									
1200	Managerial	10,402	10,350	52	0.5	61,743	62,050	-307	-0.5
1300	Professional	31,372	31,998	-626	-2.0	186,206	186,504	-298	-0.2
1400	Technical	19,639	20,155	-516	-2.6	116,568	119,237	-2,669	-2.3
1700	Clerical	6,471	4,467	2,004	31.0	38,410	35,211	3,199	8.3
1900	Fringe Benefit	13,577	13,394	183	1.3	80,585	80,600	-15	0.0
	Total Salaries	81,461	80,364	1,097	1.3	483,513	483,602	-90	0.0
Supplies (Variable)									
2100	Pharmaceuticals	162,376	129,551	32,825	20.2	963,781	975,231	-11,450	-1.2
2200	IV Solutions	12,887	10,507	2.380	18.5	76,490	80,139	-3,649	-4.8
	Total Supplies	175,263	140,058	35,205	20.1	1,040,271	1,055,370	-15,099	-1.5
Other Expenses (Fixed)									
2400	Communication	684	554	130	19.1	4,062	3,401	661	16.3
2500	Maint./Repair	155	213	-58	-37.6	919	1,009	-90	-9.8
2600	Other Services	47	0	47	100.0	278	226	52	18.8
3400	Books/Subscriptions	171	157	14	8.3	1,016	1,257	-241	-23.7
3800	Noncapital Expenses	282	457	-175	-62.1	1,673	1,499	174	10.4
6100	Travel	307	998	-691	-225.1	1,822	2,118	-296	-16.3
8400	Food/Catering	64	49	15	23.4	380	391	-11	-3.0
8600	Depreciation	812	845	-33	-4.0	4,821	4,968	-147	-3.0
	Total Other Expenses	2,522	3,273	-751	-29.8	14,972	14,869	103	.07
	Total Expenses	259,247	223,695	35,552	13.7	1,538,755	1,553,841	-15,086	-1.0
	Gross Margin	84,464	116,030	-29,566	-34.2	513,205	454,971	58,234	11.3
	Adj Pat Days*	4,298	4,113	185	4.3	25,511	25,501	10	0.0
	Rev/APD*	80.43	82.60	-2.17	-2.7	80.43	78.77	1.66	2.1
	EXP/APD*	60.32	54.39	5.93	9.8	60.32	60.93	-0.62	-1.0
	Sal/Hr*	23.42	24.34	-0.92	-3.9	23.42	24.	-0.58	-2.5
	Sal/RVU*	0.57	0.57	0.00	0.0	0.57	0.58	0.00	-0.7
	RVU/PD Hr*	41.02	42.63	-1.61	-3.9	41.02	41.72	-0.70	-1.7

Adj Pat D = adjusted patient days; Rev/APD = gross revenue per adjusted patient days; Exp/APD = total expenses per adjusted patient days; Sal/Hr = total salaries/total hours paid; Sal/RVU = total salaries/total relative value units; RVU/Pd Hr = total relative value units/total paid hours.

CHAPTER 11

Product and Service Compensation

RUDOLPH CHOICH, JR.

INTRODUCTION

The significant and lasting changes in the method of health care reimbursement that occurred during the past decade—notably, from one of retrospective costs or charges to prospectively determined, fixed-rate payments based on diagnosis-related groups (DRG's)—have markedly altered the manner in which health care is provided.

The primary result has been a fundamental restructuring of the entire health care industry: rapid growth and development of health maintenance organizations (HMO's), preferred provider organizations (PPO's), exclusive provider organizations (EPO's), and other types of prepaid health care plans that seek preferential pricing and discounted fees for subscribers; corporate restructuring or corporate formation among hospitals and the development of "health care networks" that attempt to ensure a continuing patient referral base; business coalitions among hospitals, businesses, and industry; and other types of joint business ventures involving health care providers, "consumers," and insurers. All of these efforts have been undertaken for the singular purpose of reducing health care costs or reducing the rate of cost increases.

As the health care industry has been forced to diversify away from a primary focus on inpatient hospital care, a turbulent competitive environment has developed, which has also fostered a dramatic entrepreneurial spirit. Faced with the pressures of upward-spiraling health care costs—fueled in part by government-sponsored reimbursement and increasingly high labor and technology costs—hospitals are concerned about achieving adequate levels of reimbursement for the products and services that they provide while seeking alternative methods to reduce their costs and improve productivity. This has created heightened interest in developing pricing strategies that accurately document the costs associated with these products and services.

This chapter will review some of the changes that have affected hospitals' reimbursement for services and discuss various methodologies that can be used by hospital pharmacy departments to establish prices for their plethora of products and services.

REIMBURSEMENT ISSUES

In considering reimbursement issues, there are three basic but interrelated terms that should be clearly delineated: "reimbursement," "charges," and "costs." The following is a brief summary of what these three terms represent.

Reimbursement

Simply stated, "reimbursement" is nothing more than the payment that a hospital actually receives for treating a patient. In a broad context, this term is used to represent the general payment for inpatient hospital services rather than specific payment to a hospital department (e.g., pharmacy services); hospital pharmacies do not normally bill directly for products and services, but are only one of several types of charges that appear on the total hospital bill that is issued for payment. It will also become clear that the reimbursement (i.e., payment) does not always equal the total charges that appear on the patient's hospital bill, nor may it totally reflect the actual costs of providing the service. Usually, hospitals deal with multiple reimbursement systems, and the amount of reimbursement received (even for the same service) will vary, depending upon the source of reimbursement (i.e., based upon who is paying the bill).

Charge

The term "charge" (or "price") represents the established rate for specific products and services that is posted to each patient's accounts receivable (regardless of type of payer) and that is credited to the respective hospital department (e.g., hospital pharmacy) account which produced the product or service. In general, charges are the gross rates that are prospectively established by the hospital and its departments for each product and service. These charges will normally vary by department, depending upon the rate-setting method used by that department; even within a specific department (e.g., the hospital pharmacy), there may be different charges established for specific types of products or services. These product and service charges are established in order to generate a total hospital bill to be submitted for reimbursement for the various services rendered. Depending upon the contractual arrangement between the payer and the hospital, the reimbursement or payment to the hospital may differ from the established charges or prices. Note, also, that an established charge will normally be greater than the cost of providing the product or service; like any other business, hospitals must attempt to satisfy their financial requirements and generate revenue in excess of cost in order to remain competitive, replace their physical plant, and respond to the need for technological innovations and advances.

Cost

The term "cost" should logically represent all of the costs of operating the hospital: the direct and indirect costs of producing the hospital's products and services (e.g., labor, supplies, and materials), education, research and community service programs, capital equipment and facilities costs, and costs associated with credit losses, bad debts, contractual allowances, waste and obsolescence, and free service. Space here does not permit a detailed review of the various types of cost classifications or characteristics (e.g., operating versus opportunity costs, fixed versus variable costs, direct versus indirect costs). The reader is referred to other sections of this and other texts for a more thorough discussion of these cost aspects.

Nevertheless, one should note that the term "cost" rarely stands alone, but is appended with some modifier to enhance the meaning and relevance of a particular cost statistic. For example, the object being "costed" is usually first defined, and these objects are usually of two types: (1) products (outputs or services) and (2) responsibility centers (departments or large units). Next, an adjective is added to modify the "cost" term of the defined object (e.g., "direct cost" of a particular product or responsibility center). This is an attempt to more precisely define the cost in question so that it is relevant to the decision-making process, since different cost concepts are required for different decision purposes.

However, for the purpose of this discussion, it is sufficient to state that comprehensive cost analyses and cost finding are integrally related to the hospital's rate-setting process (i.e., establishing "charges" for a product or service) and its subsequent "profitability" (i.e., generating sufficient revenue to meet or exceed its economic costs). Stated another way, a hospital's financial viability is largely influenced by rate setting (i.e., setting its "charges" or prices for products and services), volume of products and services, variable costs, fixed costs, bad debts, and externally determined reimbursement formulas (e.g., a particular "cost" or "charge" component identified by the hospital may not coincide within allowable or reasonable "cost" or "charge" components that a payer incorporates into its reimbursement formula).

Historical Perspective

During the period following World War II, health care financing experienced three major transformations:

1. *Significant growth of private prepaid health insurance plans between the mid-1940's and mid-1960's.* Most notable was the rapid development and expansion of the Blue Cross plans, followed by the growth of health insurance plans offered by commercial insurance companies. This transformation period was further fueled by the Hill-Burton program, a Federal commitment to and support for hospital construction and aid to educational institutions and individuals involved with the health care professions. The result was tremendous growth in health care facilities, technology, and human resources and wholesale expansion of health insurance coverage for the general population.
2. *Establishment of the Medicare and Medicaid programs in the mid-1960's.* These programs created a philosophy and sentiment that health care was almost a "public utility" and that health care benefits were a human right to be enjoyed by all. The provision of health care via formal health care organizations experienced enormous growth in demand, use, and costs. Existing public sentiment and governmental policy, coupled with the extant cost-based or charge-based reimbursement methodologies, insulated health care organizations from the same competitive pressures that were exerted on other businesses and industries—health care services were being financed largely by governments (50 percent in the aggregate) and businesses via health insurance plans, *not* by the individual consumers of the services (i.e., the patients). This environment created insufficient incentives for health care providers to conduct themselves in a cost-conscious, consumer-sensitive manner. However, by the mid-1970's, the Federal Government was becoming increasingly alarmed over the high costs and decreased quality of health care that it was experiencing. This concern led to an expansion of the Federal bureaucracy and increased regulation of the health care industry: professional standards review organizations (PSRO's), health system agencies (HSA's), as well as hospital-focused cost-containment legislation—all in an effort to stem these upward-spiraling costs while ensuring high quality.
3. *The era of "Reaganomics"[1] ushered in by the early 1980's.* With this era came altered goals, constraints, and contingencies for the Nation's health care system. These included: (a) alternatives to regulation to promote cost containment and improved quality by competitive pressure and (b) increased roles for State and local governments and the private sector to further stimulate competition. This new era in health care began with the Omnibus Budget Reconciliation Act of 1981, which called for major reductions in Federal health care expenditures over 3 years, primarily in Medicare and Medicaid expenditures, and provided greater autonomy to State Medicaid programs to determine reimbursement formulas for providers (i.e., to prospectively set rates). Following in quick succession was the Tax Equity and Fiscal Responsibility Act of 1982 (TEFRA),[2] which subsequently led to the implementation of the DRG-based prospective payment system in October 1983. The TEFRA legislation: (a) imposed a per-case limit on hospitals' Medicare reimbursement; (b) established cost "targets" for each hospital and permitted efficient hospitals (i.e., lower-

cost hospitals) to retain 25 percent of the difference between their actual, lower costs and the target amount; (c) placed ancillary services (e.g., pharmacy services) under reimbursement limits for the first time; and, (d) mandated the Secretary of Health and Human Services to develop and present a plan to Congress for a "prospective payment system" by the end of 1982. The prospective payment system regulations implemented the Social Security Amendments of 1983 and implemented wholesale changes in the methods of reimbursing hospitals for Medicare inpatients: they brought about the demise of Medicare reimbursement based solely on retrospective costs or charges and replaced it with reimbursement predicated on a *Prospectively and Externally Determined, Fixed Rate* based on 470 diagnosis-related groups.[3,4]

Comparison of Retrospective Versus Prospective Payment Systems

Under retrospective reimbursement methods, a hospital is paid after services are rendered, and payment is based on the hospital's actual costs or established charges. The total amount of payment is directly related to the amount, or volume, of services provided during the patient stay; therefore, payments increase as more services are rendered (i.e., as more costs are incurred), and there is little or no incentive for a hospital to contain costs.

Under this reimbursement system, few arguments are ever raised against supporting a new service, a new technology, or a new procedure that could improve patient care, since all resources are viewed as virtually limitless, and there is certainly no inclination to place a "value" on human life or suffering via cost-benefit analyses. Traditionally, all third-party payers had paid hospitals by some type of retrospective cost-based or charge-based (i.e., percentage of charges) methods.

Conversely, under prospective payment methods, the total amount of reimbursement that will be paid to the hospital is generally fixed and predetermined (i.e., negotiated with the payer before a service is rendered). The basis, or service unit, for this fixed rate may vary from system to system (e.g., cost per patient day, per admission, or per case, on a capitation basis, or on amount of services rendered, etc.); however, in all cases, it establishes a reimbursement ceiling and imposes some financial risk on the hospital. Essentially, a hospital *must* provide a service at or below this fixed-rate reimbursement ceiling, or it may find itself in a deficit fiscal position. Under prospective systems, incentives to incur costs are changed to incentives to reduce costs, since the hospital may now share in any savings that accrue when services are provided at less cost than that covered by the fixed reimbursement rate.

DRG-Based Prospective Payment System

Under the Federal prospective payment system (PPS) for Medicare patients, the service unit upon which the reimbursement rate is based is a diagnosis-related group, or DRG. Each Medicare patient is classified into 1 of 470 DRG's, with each DRG having its own fixed-rate reimbursement ceiling. This single amount covers the entire occasion of service; essentially, the hospital will receive only that fixed-rate payment for any patient in a particular DRG, despite the total length of stay, the total amount of products and services provided (i.e., tests, drugs, therapies, etc.), or actual costs incurred to treat the patient.

The actual determination of the fixed reimbursement rate for each Medicare case is complex and continues to undergo periodic changes; therefore, detailed review or analysis of the rate-setting methodology is beyond the scope of this present discussion. However, it is important to note that some additional payments can be made to cover specific circumstances. These would include payment allowances for: (1) "outliers," or specific cases that have excessive lengths of stay vis-a-vis most discharges in a particular DRG, (2) capital equipment and construction costs, and, (3) some direct and indirect medical education costs experienced by teaching hospitals. There are also some special exemptions or allowances for certain types of specialty hospitals (e.g., psychiatric or pediatric facilities) and facilities that may be the only provider in a particular community or area (e.g., sole community hospitals). Note, however, that even these allowances have been subjected to continuing governmental restrictions and are being revised (usually reduced) as experience with the system continues to grow.

Although the system described above was initially applied to inpatient reimbursement for Medicare patients, other third-party payers have developed, or are developing, similar prospective, fixed-rate reimbursement systems for their subscribers, predominantly to avoid the impact of "cost-shifting" by the hospitals.

"Cost-Shifting"

In light of the foregoing discussion on prospective payment systems, it should be apparent that many of the third-party payers (e.g., Medicare, Medicaid, many Blue Cross plans, HMO's, PPO's, etc.) reimburse hospitals at a fixed rate that may be less than established charges and less than the full costs of providing the services. In their negotiated agreements with the hospitals, these payers will "disallow," or exclude, certain real costs and perhaps pay less than their fair share of the costs (i.e., they receive a "discount" from the hospital). This is now possible in the current competitive climate in health care; such plans can direct patients to hospitals that, because they wish to remain financially viable, will be willing to accept less than full reimbursement.

Conversely, self-pay patients (i.e., patients who may not be covered by some health insurance plan and/or who personally pay their own hospital bill) generally pay the hospital's full established charge rates, as do many commercial insurers, which also reimburse hospitals on some type of charge-based system. Since these latter two payers generally comprise a smaller percentage of the payer mix compared to the former payer, hospitals will attempt to recover their costs via "cost-shifting"—that is, they will set charges to the commercial insurers and self-pay patients considerably higher than the actual costs of providing the services.

As a result of cost-shifting, hospitals' established charge rates appear higher than the income that is actually produced from the services, and commercial insurance premiums are increased (as are the resulting costs to the employers that pay the majority of these premiums). The trend toward expansion of prospective payment systems (i.e., fixed-price reimbursements) will continue, particularly among commercial insurers and the employers that pay their premiums and wish to avoid cost-shifting.

It is clear that the major intent of these changes is to reduce both the price and use—and thus the total cost—of health care, especially inpatient care, and to develop equally effective but less costly alternatives (e.g., ambulatory care, home care, etc.). To remain viable, hospitals must have the flexibility and managerial skills to adapt to this continually changing environment.

PRICING

Despite this trend to prospective payment systems, hospitals must still analyze their costs. Before a hospital can determine ways to reduce its costs to a level that approximates its fixed-rate reimbursement, it must first be able to accurately identify its costs. Additionally, comprehensive cost analyses are still an appropriate means to develop equitable and defensible charge structures for their charge-based payers (e.g., commercial insurers and self-pay patients). Hospital diversification away from inpatient care also necessitates comprehensive cost analyses in order to establish competitive charges in these new business ventures. Thus, cost analysis, along with pricing strategies and rate setting (i.e., establishing charges or prices for products and services), continues to be vitally important to health care organizations.

The following sections review some of the rate-setting processes that hospitals can use and then present some of the common strategies that a hospital pharmacy department can use in establishing prices for its products and services.

General Pricing Strategies

"Pricing strategy" has been generally defined to include all activities associated with determining the price range and price changes, through time, that will support the revenue, profit objectives, and the marketing position of a service or an organization.[5] The organization must clearly define its overall business and marketing objective before it determines the price for a service. Product and service pricing should enable consumers to determine their payments in an itemized fashion, the pricing structure should be deemed equitable by the consumers, and the pricing strategy should be efficient for the organization to use.

There are four general methods that hospitals and their departments normally use in establishing their product and service rates (i.e., charges or prices), exclusive of physician charges:[6] percentage mark-up method, time rate method, routine service (or per diem rate) method, and relative value unit method. The following is a brief review of each of these methods.

Percentage Mark-Up Method

This is perhaps the oldest and simplest rate-setting method that may still be in use today, despite its many inequities. This method is most commonly applied to commodity or merchandising types of retail operations. Basically, some fixed percentage of cost is added to the commodity acquisition cost to define the price (or charge) for the product or service. Given the nature of the operations to which this method is applied (i.e, retail-type operations), the percentage mark-up is usually applied only to the purchase cost of the specific commodity or product. However, it may fail to consider adequately other operating and professional service costs or administrative overhead costs that are required to provide the product. Additionally, since the price is directly linked to the purchase cost of the product, it may encourage the use of a higher-cost product when a lower-cost product would suffice. Clearly, this method of pricing is contrary to the present societal interest in lowering health care costs.

Time Rate Method

Frequently, this method is used in departments or areas such as the operating and recovery rooms, anesthesiology, emergency services, and physical therapy. There are two basic variations of this method: (1) straight hourly rate or person-minute rate and (2) base setup charge plus time.

The former method establishes a set hourly rate for the use of a particular service (e.g., operating room suite) and simply multiplies this rate times the number of hours of service use to generate a charge. Alternatively, it may establish a set rate for ranges of time, usually in minutes (e.g., 30-60 minutes, 61-90 minutes), and charge that rate per range of time that the service was used. For example, a surgical procedure requiring the use of the operating room suite for 45 minutes would be charged at the 30-60-minute rate.

The latter variation of the time rate method establishes a fixed charge for setup and then applies an additional charge, depending on the amount of time the service was used (based on either the straight hourly rate or range of time rate). Here again, this method may not fully consider the other operating or overhead costs associated with the use of the service (e.g., supplies and equipment).

Routine Service (or Per Diem Rate) Method

This pricing strategy is normally used to establish a rate for a hospital's "room and board" accommodations and generally varies according to the type of accommodation (private, semiprivate, intensive care, routine medical/surgical, obstetrics, etc.). Computations are frequently based on factors such as fixed and variable costs associated with the accommodation and the service provided (e.g., level of nursing services), historical and projected occupancy rates, and patient mix. Like all other methods, this one may fail to consider other related costs in deriving the room rate (e.g., central supply and pharmacy).

Relative Value Unit Method

With the advent of DRG-based prospective payment systems, the concept of case mix management has received considerable attention in the health care industry. Some of the key elements associated with case mix management are: (1) volume (i.e., quantitative measure of hospital output, or the number of patients in each DRG); (2) resource consumption (i.e., the volume and type of departmental resources consumed by each DRG and the total resources, or total intermediate products and services, consumed by each DRG); (3) cost accountability and cost reduction (i.e., identification and reduction of the cost of resources consumed by each DRG plus the marginal cost of producing each DRG); and, (4) improved productivity (i.e., increased outputs which consume the same or fewer resources). Use of relative value units (RVU's) enables the hospital to develop some standardized measure for the multitude of disparate intermediate products and services (e.g., doses, meals, tests, procedures, treatments) provided to each patient by its various departments.

With this rate-setting method, each of the department's product or service outputs (i.e., its "macro" production units) is assigned an RVU that reflects the relative amount of time and/or resources consumed to provide that specific product or service. Each RVU is then multiplied by the actual number of product or service outputs and summed to determine a total weighted value (i.e., the aggregate "micro" production units). The department's total financial requirements (i.e., all operating costs plus profit expectation) to be recovered by the charge rate, divided by the total weighted values, provides a product or service unit value. When this value is multiplied by the RVU for the product or service, it provides a weighted charge rate per service. Table 11-1 provides a simplified example of how this RVU rate-setting method can be applied to specific departmental products or services.

Table 11-1. RVU rate setting example

Products or services	*Defined RVU*	*Number provided*	*Weighted value*	*Rate per RVU*	*Rate per service*
Product/Service A	50	2,000	100,000	$ .25	$ 12.50
Product/Service B	30	1,000	30,000	$ .25	$ 7.50
Product/Service C	150	500	75,000	$ .25	$ 37.50
Total weighted values			205,000		
Total financial requirements			$51,250		
Average rate per RVU			$ .25		

It is important to note that this methodology has received considerable emphasis in the health care industry today; it is integrally related to cost accounting systems and micro-costing of intermediate products and services, and it is also a key element in most workload measurement and productivity monitoring systems, both of which are of prime importance in this era of prospective reimbursement and cost containment.

It should be apparent that hospitals will use more than one of these rate-setting methods in developing their charge structure. Of crucial importance to any of these, however, is the need for comprehensive cost analysis and cost finding if the charge structure is to be equitable and defensible, and ensure adequate levels of reimbursement.

Hospital Pharmacy Pricing Strategies

The precise methods and formulas used to develop charges for hospital pharmacy products and services vary widely from institution to institution, and their derivation and application are well documented and described in the pharmacy literature.[7-11] Generally, however, they are all an adaptation or combination of the four basic methods previously described.

Additionally, it is important to recognize that, under the Medicare prospective payment system, a hospital's "final product" or its "output" is a patient case or a DRG. Hospital departments such as the pharmacy department *do not* produce final products or final outputs; they produce only *intermediate products and services* whose costs (or charges) become aggregated into the total cost of the hospital's final product, that is, its discharged patients in a specific DRG. Therefore, accurate cost accounting and accountability for each department's intermediate products and services are imperative to improve the accuracy of the total inpatient rate, or charge, for the hospital's final product.

The following is a more detailed discussion of these pricing strategies as they apply specifically to hospital pharmacy products and services for inpatients. Although these strategies are discussed separately, in order to present their conceptual basis, it is important to recognize that a combination of these pricing methods are typically used within a hospital pharmacy department.

Percentage Mark-Up Method

As stated earlier, the percentage mark-up method is one of the oldest, most common, and simplest methods of pricing used in a retail-type business. However, because of its previously stated inadequacies as a pricing strategy, it is rarely used alone in hospital pharmacy.

Simply stated, this method involves adding a defined percentage mark-up to the cost of the drug product to determine the final charge, or price, of the drug. However, this method assumes that the department's total operating costs are somehow directly proportional to only drug acquisition costs. The percentage mark-up may be fixed, with this fixed percent uniformly applied to the cost of any drug product or variable, in that a defined percent mark-up will be applied to all drug costs that fall within established cost ranges.

In the former method, a fixed percent (e.g., 10 percent) is added to the cost of any drug, regardless of its cost. For example, the charge for a $2 drug would be $2 + 10 percent = $2.20, the charge for a $25 drug would be $25 + 10 percent = $27.50, the charge for a $400 drug would be $400 + 10 percent = $440, and so on. From the consumer's standpoint, this method may be perceived to be inequitable.

The latter method is somewhat of an adaptation of the time rate method (described earlier) combined with the percent mark-up method. Under this variation, ranges of drug cost are defined (e.g., drug cost up to $5, $5-$15, $15-$25, etc.), and then some predetermined percent mark-up is added to any drug whose cost falls within one of these defined cost ranges. The percent mark-up may be direct and ascending, that is, a *higher* percent is associated with a *higher* drug cost range (e.g., drug cost up to $5, add 5 percent; $5-$15, add 10 percent; $15-$25, add 15 percent, etc.), or inverse and descending, that is, a *lower* percent is applied to the *higher* drug cost ranges (e.g., drug cost up to $5, add 15 percent, $5-$15, add 10 percent; $15-$25, add 5 percent, etc.).

Regardless of the percent mark-up used, this pricing strategy fails to consider the professional service components of pharmaceutical care and allocates these charges only according to the source of one cost component; it implies that only the cost of drugs bears a direct relationship to the department's total cost of its comprehensive pharmaceutical care. Thus, this method, aside from the inherent inequities that may be perceived by consumers, perpetuates the image of pharmaceutical services as "product" oriented and ignores the professional service components.

Per Diem Charge Method

The inherent assumption with this pricing strategy is that the aggregate costs of pharmaceutical care per day do not vary significantly among various groups or classifications of inpatients. Based on this assumption, the time and effort required to process inpatient orders for individual units or doses of drugs are unwarranted or unimportant.[12]

Typically, total historical pharmacy costs are divided by some indicator of hospital utilization (usually inpatient days) to derive a single, all-encompassing pharmacy charge for each day that a patient is in the hospital. Thus, total pharmacy operating costs are uniformly charged to all inpatients, regardless of the volume and mix of pharmaceutical care provided. Although relatively uncomplicated in its derivation and use, this pricing strategy requires ongoing monitoring of actual daily drug use and costs and subsequent comparison to the per diem charges to ensure that the pharmacy department is generating the expected revenues. If there are significant changes in the mix of patients, the volume of patients, and/or drug use patterns, the per diem charge may be inadequate and require recalibration.

It is important to note that, in its simplest form, this single daily charge represents an average charge for each day of pharmacy service provided, based on historical data about total departmental costs and hospital utilization. As such, it does not (1) identify and isolate specific components of service that may be required for comprehensive cost accounting purposes; (2) consider differences and current changes in utilization and case mix among various clinical services (e.g., critical care areas versus routine care areas); (3) equitably apportion the costs to the users of pharmacy services based on volume of use, or (4) efficiently identify the fiscal impact of newer, more costly drug technologies.

Frequently, where this pricing strategy is established, it is used in combination with one or more of the other pricing methods (e.g., the dispensing fee method described below), there may be more than one per diem rate established for various clinical service areas (e.g., obstetrics, critical care), and certain drugs or classes of drugs are handled as exceptions to the per diem method of charging.[12,13]

Dispensing Fee Method

Another commonly applied pricing strategy in hospital pharmacy is the dispensing fee method. This strategy requires the derivation of a fixed dispensing or service fee designed to cover all direct, indirect, and fixed costs of providing pharmacy services (e.g., salaries, overhead, supplies, and equipment but excluding drug costs) plus an expected profit margin.

The dispensing or service fee is typically calculated by dividing the department's total annual operating costs (excluding costs of drugs sold) plus profit margin by some indicator of total workload volume (e.g., doses, units, workload categories). The patient price, or charge, is then determined by adding this fixed fee to the actual acquisition cost for the amount of drug dispensed.

In its application, this pricing strategy is most effective when differential fees are established for various types of dosage forms (e.g., oral tablets and capsules versus parenteral doses) or for various workload categories (e.g., unit dose medications, total parenteral nutrition solutions, large-volume parenterals, small-volume parenterals). The use of multiple fees (1) provides a means to differentiate among the various workload categories by relative labor intensity and (2) enables other relevant nondistribution costs of total pharmacy services to be equitably distributed to the actual users based on volume of services provided, regardless of their relationship to the acquisition costs of the product dispensed. This pricing strategy can also be used to establish distinct professional fees for nondistribution activities (e.g., patient education, pharmacokinetic consultation services) when such services are permitted to be charged separately.[14,15]

This dispensing fee pricing strategy is more complicated and labor intensive to use than either of the two previous methods described since, in most cases, several different fees must be used to denote the different types of service or workload category provided, and the amount and cost of each drug component must be directly associated with each patient. However, it is also a more equitable and accountable method for establishing pharmacy charges, particularly if the department is able to generate itemized charges: patients' bills more appropriately reflect the total scope and the costs of pharmacy services provided; the system enables the department to more clearly distinguish among its operating costs, drug costs, and revenue from its various fees and to link these components to its workload volumes; and informed decisions and logical adjustments can be made in the fee structure as services and costs change.

Relative Value Unit Method

As noted earlier, the use of relative value units has been a commonly accepted methodology to quantify and standardize disparate product and service outputs in most workload measurement and productivity monitoring systems. With the increased cost constraints imposed by the prospective pricing system, these methods have become more closely linked with comprehensive cost accounting systems; they are now routinely used for micro-costing of a department's intermediate products and services, and they play an integral role in the development of flexible operating budgets.[16-22] As such, their application can be logically extended to the development of an RVU-based pricing structure for the pharmacy department's intermediate products and services.

A review of the precise calculations to derive the pharmacy department's weighted RVU for its intermediate product and service outputs is beyond the scope of this discussion. (The reader is referred to other sections of this text and to references cited for a detailed explanation of the RVU methodology to quantify intermediate product and service outputs.) However, this discussion will briefly summarize the application of the RVU methodology to the development of the department's pricing structure.

Once the department has clearly defined its various intermediate products and services (i.e., its "macro" production units), it assigns an RVU to each unit to convert it to a standardized "micro" production unit (or weighted RVU). Concomitantly, the cost accounting system is used to differentiate the aggregate departmental resource costs (e.g., fixed or variable labor, drug and supply costs) plus its overhead costs. These total costs plus the department's profit expectation—the department's total financial requirements—are then distributed among the "micro" intermediate product and service outputs (i.e., the total financial requirements divided by total weighted RVU) to derive a weighted charge per product or service RVU. Thereafter, this weighted charge per RVU is multiplied by the number of each RVU product or service provided to each patient to generate patient charges for that product or service (see table 11-1).

It should be evident that this pricing methodology is the most complex of those reviewed here and may require extensive use of computers to facilitate its initial derivation and application. Despite the drawbacks associated with its complexity during the development stages, once implemented, the system is relatively easy to maintain since it is largely driven by its direct linkage with the cost accounting system. As a result, subsequent changes in the rate structure can be easily accomplished, and the need for such changes becomes readily apparent and defensible. Additionally, it is the only system of those reviewed here that adequately addresses the exigent need for accurate, comprehensive cost accountability for disparate intermediate products and services in order to develop a pricing strategy that is appropriate for the present health care reimbursement environment.

SUMMARY

For the foreseeable future, the health care industry will continue to be buffeted by dissimilar, and often contradictory, reimbursement systems. Often, the only things that these reimbursement systems have in common are that (1) increasingly, the amount of payment is externally determined; (2) they are designed to reduce the payer's health care expenditures without reducing the quantity and quality of service; (3) they encompass some type of prospectively determined fixed-rate payment; and (4) they stimulate increasing regulation and bureaucracy (e.g., peer review, mandated use review, increased data compilation, etc.).

In order to survive with these seemingly paradoxical competitive pricing constraints, health care organizations must be able to effectively assess the fiscal impact of these reimbursement systems and then develop an appropriate strategic business plan based on the available resources and the need to maintain an acceptable level of quality. This virtually mandates the implementation of detailed cost accounting systems that enable them to measure profitability under different reimbursement scenarios. Thus, the underlying principles for any effective and competitive pricing strategy are comprehensive cost-volume analysis and cost control.

Hospital pharmacists may be uniquely positioned to consider both the fiscal and the clinical aspects of patient care and, in turn, support the hospital's overall business strategy. To do so, however, requires that they have an understanding of reimbursement systems and constraints, that they understand the principles of cost accountability, and that they adopt an orientation that defines the "cost effectiveness" per clinical outcome. This will enable them to identify and select innovative processes and strategies that provide the optimal health care benefit for a given level of cost from among the various alternatives available.

REFERENCES

1. Enright SM: Effect of Reaganomics on the U.S. health-care system. *Am J Hosp Pharm* 39:1169-1175, 1982.
2. Curtiss FR: Current concepts in hospital reimbursement. *Am J Hosp Pharm* 40:586-591, 1983.
3. Health Care Financing Administration: *Fed Reg* 48:39752-39890, 1983.
4. Enright SM: *Prospective Payment Regulations*. Bethesda, MD, American Society of Hospital Pharmacists, 1983.
5. Kotler P (ed): Price decisions. In *Marketing Management*. Englewood Cliffs, NJ, Prentice-Hall, 1980.
6. Herkimer AG Jr (ed): Production units and performance evaluation. In *Understanding Hospital Financial Management*. Germantown, MD, Aspen Systems, 1978.
7. Smith WE, Weiblen JW: Charging for hospital pharmaceutical services: Product cost, per diem fees, and fees for special clinical services. *Am J Hosp Pharm* 36:355-359, 1979.
8. Fish KH: Charging for hospital pharmaceutical services: Computerized system using a markup and a dose fee. *Am J Hosp Pharm* 36:360-363, 1979.
9. Dirks I, Pang FJ: Charging for hospital pharmaceutical services: Combined product-service per diem fees. *Am J Hosp Pharm* 36:363-365, 1979.
10. Wyatt BK: Charging for hospital pharmaceutical services: Flat fee based on the medication record. *Am J Hosp Pharm* 36:365-367, 1979.
11. Grauer DW: Pricing Strategies for hospital pharmacy services. *Top Hosp Pharm Mgt* 5(l):46-52, 1985.
12. Bower RM, Hepler CD: A statistical approach to per diem pharmacy pricing. *Am J Hosp Pharm* 31:1179-1188, 1974.
13. Bonchonsky JJ: Per diem pharmacy rates for inpatients. *Hosp Pharm* 6:15-23, 1971.
14. Nold EG, Pathak DS: Third party reimbursement for clinical pharmacy services: Philosophy and practice. *Am J Hosp Pharm* 34:823-826, 1977.
15. Curtiss FR: Reimbursement for clinical pharmacy services. *Top Hosp Pharm Mgt* 2(l):6-21, 1982.
16. Levin RH, Letcher KI, deLeon RF, et al: Patient care unit systems for measuring clinical and distributive pharmacy workload. *Am J Hosp Pharm* 37:53-61, 1980.
17. Roberts MJ, Kvalseth TO, Jermstad RL: Work measurement in hospital pharmacy. *Top Hosp Pharm Mgt* 2(2):1-17, 1982.
18. Choich R, Jr: Productivity analysis: A managerial reality. *Top Hosp Pharm Mgt* 7(l):23-31, 1987.
19. Suver JD, Cooper JC: Principles and methods of managerial cost accounting systems. *Am J Hosp Pharm* 45:146-152, 1988.
20. Gouveia WA, Anderson ER, Jr, Decker EL, et al: Design and implementation of a cost-accounting system in hospital pharmacy. *Am J Hosp Pharm* 45:613-620, 1988.
21. Choich R, Jr: Relationship of productivity analysis to departmental cost-accounting systems. *Am J Hosp Pharm* 45:1103-1110, 1988.
22. Carlson BR: Development and integration of cost accounting, pharmacy workload, and charging systems. *Top Hosp Pharm Mgt* 9(2):11-20, 1989.

CHAPTER 12

Cost Control

JOSEPH D. JACKSON, AILEEN M. GRIMM, and LEIGH E. HOPKINS

INTRODUCTION

The United States is at a unique juncture in history. Internationally, astounding change has occurred, and the developed world continues to evolve toward democratic systems. Politically, it is apparent that nothing will be left untouched. For most Americans, even aspects of life that were operating in an acceptable manner are being altered in response to pressures for change. Health care in the United States is one such aspect.

Although most Americans are personally satisfied with the health care they receive, doubts are often raised concerning the ability of the U.S. health care system to meet the expectations of the society. The U.S. health care system has not been operating efficiently or effectively for a number of years, despite leading the world in technological advances. Issues of accessibility, acceptability, and affordability remain.

THE U.S. HEALTH CARE SYSTEM

Total health care costs in the United States, when expressed as a percentage of the gross national product (GNP), are the highest, at more that 11 percent, of any industrialized nation in the world (figure 12-1).[1] The estimated 1990 expenditure for health care is 13.1 percent of GNP.[2] Despite this percentage, recent articles in both the lay and scientific press have made it clear that Americans are not receiving the highest quality of care for their money.[3,4] The United States has a pluralistic health care system with many payers including consumers, private insurers, health maintenance organizations, and State and Federal governmental agencies. There are also many different types of providers of health services such as private (fee-for-service) practitioners, health maintenance organizations, and public, not-for-profit and for-profit hospitals and clinics.

Exactly who pays for this care is another important piece of the health care puzzle. In the United States, the Federal Government pays less than half of the health care costs, whereas other countries' governments cover 70-90 percent (figure 12-1). Medicare, a government insurance program to cover the health care costs of the elderly and the disabled, represents the largest Federal Government contributor or payment source (figure 12-2).[5] The other large government-sponsored program is Medicaid, the health program for 27 million low-income people. The costs for the Medicaid program are jointly shared by the Federal and State governments.

In 1983, the government implemented the diagnosis-related group (DRG) program in an attempt to bring Medicare inpatient hospital costs under control. It has been the most effective cost-containment program introduced to date and has fundamentally changed reimbursement philosophy in the United States. Under DRG's, reimbursement for in-hospital care changed from retrospective billing on a cost plus overhead basis to prospectively set, fixed-rate amounts calculated on a per case basis and based upon averaged resource use. It is important to realize that, though this program has been effective in slowing the rate of growth in government costs for Medicare, the actual costs of the program have continued to rise.

Health care institutions, such as hospitals, have for years relied on the overhead component of Medicare to fund capital improvements. Under rules published in the *Federal Register* (February 28, 1991), beginning in October 1991, the methodology that governs capital payments to hospitals as a portion of Medicare expenditures will change. The changes in capital payments will be phased in over 10 years. In fiscal year 1992, for example, capital payments to hospitals will comprise a 90 percent hospital-specific rate and a 10 percent national or Federal payment rate. Each year for 10 years, the Federal payment share will rise by 10 percent until the capital payment is a nationally determined rate. Hospitals are concerned about the base rate for their share of the payments and about the long-term implications for market and facilities expansion. To maintain enhanced services, many hospitals have found it necessary to raise costs to other insurers to continue a similar rate of enhancement.

In the United States, 58 percent of the cost of health care is paid by private (nongovernmental) sources, whereas these figures are much lower for our European counterparts.[6] Private funding underscores the pluralistic nature of the U.S. health care system. As cost-containment efforts become more widespread, different patterns and approaches emerge among our private institutions in terms of their payer profiles. Commercial carriers such as John Hancock, Aetna, and Prudential are working to support standards of health care that promote efficiency. "The Blues" (Blue

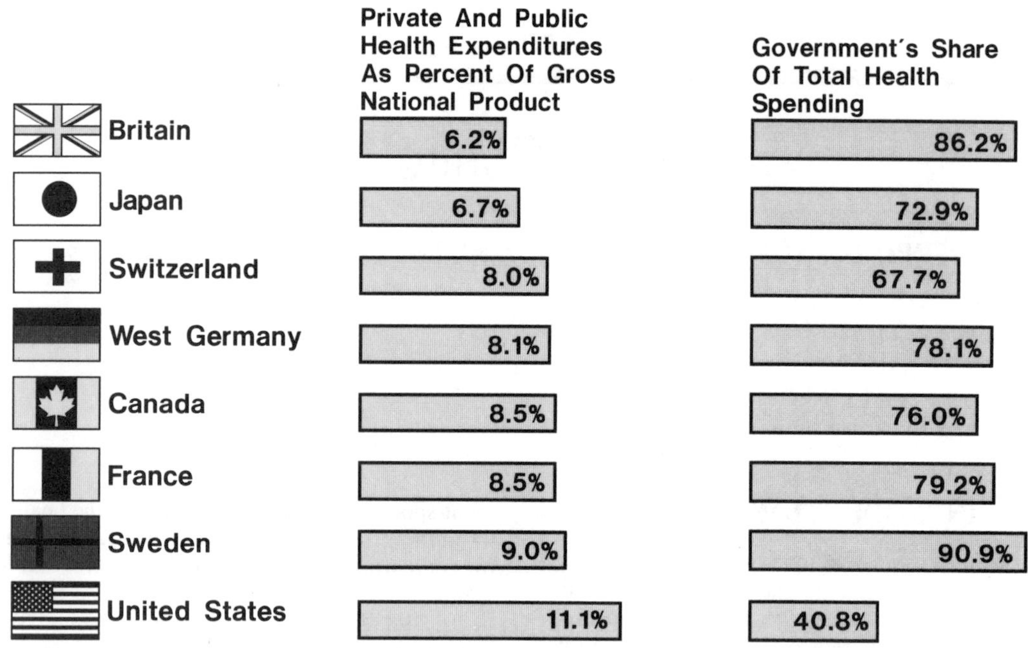

Figure 12-1. Spending on health care: A look at 8 countries (figures for 1986)

Sources: The Organisation for Economic Cooperation and Development, U.S. Department of Health and Human Services.

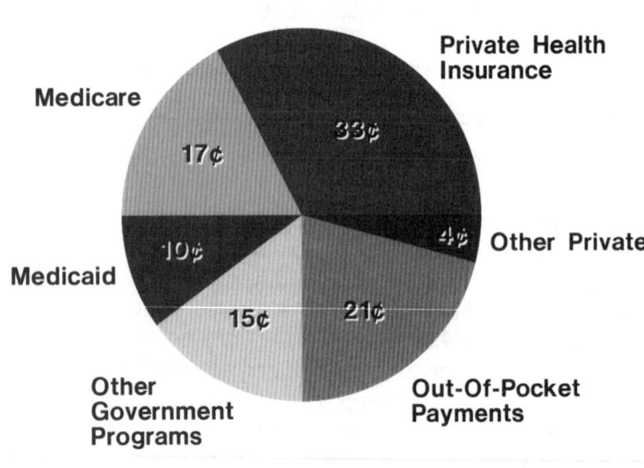

Figure 12-2. The Nation's health dollar by payment source, 1989

Source: *Health Care Financing Review*, Winter 1990.

Cross and Blue Shield) are moving toward more stringent and centralized decision-making processes. Medicare remains the most rigid of all payers in the health care sector. Medicaid, as noted with the rebate legislation, is undergoing revision.

Further examples of pluralism are extant in the managed care sector. Managed care is expected to top 60 percent of the private pay network during the 1990's. Managed care relies heavily on bureaucratic appeals processes to control delivery of health care goods and services. The following are examples of how managed health care seeks to control health care costs by limits on the delivery of goods and services.[7]

Texas Instruments — Requires physicians to seek approval before performing outpatient diagnostic procedures.

3M — Requires doctors to seek approval before performing inpatient surgery.

General Electric — Meets with doctors in communities with above-normal treatment to discourage such excesses.

General Motors — Pays bonuses to hospitals with low rates of hospital-related infections, mistakes, and inappropriate services.

Hershey — Plans to use data on treatment patterns to determine which hospitals have the lowest costs and rates of complications and deaths.

Counterbalancing efforts to cut costs are efforts to maintain benefits. Health care benefit packages have evolved into a potent strike issue in recent years, and health care benefits have become a key factor in preparing for a successful collective bargaining outcome in the Nation's top corporations. With health care costs increasingly taking center stage as labor contracts come due around the country, several major unions have banded together with influential members of the business community to address rising health care costs. In 1990, 55 unions, corporations, and medical groups formed the National Leadership Coalition for Health Care Reform to develop proposals to overhaul the Nation's health care system.[8]

It is important to distinguish in this context, however, the notion of cost containment from price containment. It would appear that the current initiative on the part of the Federal Government through the Medicaid Rebate Program is directed primarily at price containment issues, which directly affects the overall issue of cost containment. Cost-cutting efforts by the Federal Government and other health care providers, including self-insured corporations, have promoted the idea of cost shifting.

The danger for hospitals, especially private sector hospitals, is that drug companies will eliminate discounts because of the implications of the best-price provisions in the rebate law. Another significant concern is the tendency of drug companies to raise prices to offset limitations associated with the rebate program.[9] Historically, similar pricing behavior was observed with hospital and physician goods and services when the Medicare and Medicaid legislation was passed in 1965.

Action in the areas of health benefits and corporate funding for health care is due to the dramatic increase in corporate health care spending, which rose from 9 percent of profits in 1965 to 46 percent in 1988, as described in an article by Loomis,[10] aptly entitled "The Killer Cost Stalking Business." Because of the size of the corporate contribution and the consequence to profits, the private sector will undoubtedly be a major force in modifications to the health care system.

Despite the more than one-half-trillion-dollar expenditure by the public and private sectors to health care, the fact remains that approximately 37 million Americans are uninsured or underinsured with limited access to hospitals, doctors, pharmaceuticals, emergency rooms, and clinics.[11] The call to address the health care needs of these people is fast becoming a focal point of legislation in a number of States.[12]

Oregon applied for Federal Government approval for a plan to provide poor people under the Medicaid program with a basic level of care while restricting more costly care such as transplants. Oregon, because of limitations in State funding, is able to provide health care benefits under the Medicaid program only to those at 58 percent of the Federal poverty level. The Federal poverty level for a family of four is approximately $12,000 per year. Oregon's proposal would provide limited services to everyone under the Federal poverty level as opposed to the current program, which provides all services to those under 58 percent of the Federal poverty level. An unmistakable conclusion is that, until or unless the United States can somehow bring health care costs under control, access to health care for many Americans will be regulated or restricted.

The following factors are providing the foundation for significant change in the U.S. health care system: (1) the prohibitive rise in health care costs without a perceptible difference in quality, (2) an increasing portion of costs becoming the responsibility of the private sector, and (3) the large number of uninsured Americans who are not receiving even a basic level of health care.

Three additional factors promise to influence the institutions responsible for health care in the United States: (1) efforts, in process, to revise methods of paying physicians for Medicare services (see The Consolidated Omnibus Budget Reconciliation Act of 1985, or COBRA, P.L. 99-272),[13] (2) the changes in capital payment methodology, and (3) the decision by the Health Care Financing Administration (HCFA) to include evidence of cost-effectiveness as a factor in reimbursement decisions.[14] It behooves us to be cognizant of these major forces for change.

CONTRIBUTORS TO RISING COSTS: PHARMACEUTICAL INFLUENCE

Though many Americans realize that health care costs are out of control, very few have a realistic understanding of what contributes to the rising costs of care. Because of their visibility, pharmaceuticals are often labeled as major culprits in the cost of care. Although it is true that drug costs are proportionately higher than pharmacy personnel costs with respect to the pharmacy budget, in the United States pharmacy costs—drug and personnel—are only about 7 percent of the total health care dollar (figure 12-3).[5] In comparison, hospital care and physician services account for 39 percent and 19 percent of the costs of care, respectively.

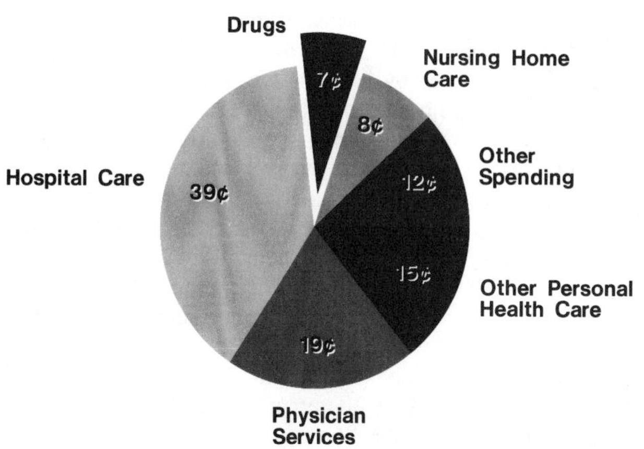

Figure 12-3. The Nation's health dollar by expenditure type, 1989

Source: *Health Care Financing Review*, Winter 1990.

Though drug costs contribute a small portion to the total health care dollar, these costs are likely to change in the near future as technology-based factors continue to evolve. In general, drug therapy represents a valuable commodity that is usually cost effective. Drug therapy, properly selected, administered, and monitored, is commonly associated with positive health outcomes for the patient. Now more than ever, the control of costs, in addition to positive medical outcomes, is a vital responsibility of the pharmacy manager. The pharmacy manager must obtain as much information as possible regarding the contributors to drug and drug-driven costs as well as savings.

By using the budgetary process rather than the legislative process, Senator David Pryor (D-AR) engineered the passage of The Medicaid Prudent Pharmaceutical Purchasing Act (MPPPA) as a provision of the Omnibus Budget Reconciliation Act (OBRA) 1990. The MPPPA is designed to return $3.4 billion in State and Federal pharmaceutical expenditures over the next 5 years by requiring manufacturers to rebate a percentage of the drug cost as a condition of coverage. To appreciate the size and scope of the program needed to accomplish this objective, a review of the major responsibilities of HCFA, the State Medicaid agencies, and the manufacturers is useful.

Under the Medicaid Rebate Law, HCFA has the responsibility to collect the rebate agreements from manufacturers in the absence of previously negotiated State-specific rebate agreements that were in effect prior to November 1990. They also have the responsibility to prepare a data file of covered drugs that includes average manufacturer price, best price, and rebate amount. This drug-specific information must be supplied by the National Drug Code (NDC) number. HCFA then provides these data to the States. They have the authority under the law to survey manufacturers to ensure that the data are accurate; significant penalties exist under the law for manufacturers that supply false information to HCFA concerning their prices. HCFA finally has the responsibility to conduct and monitor a series of mandated studies that concern aspects of pricing and drug utilization review.

States have a number of different responsibilities under the Medicaid law. They must prepare statewide summary data of drug use by NDC code number. They are required to organize invoices by manufacturer according to the use by NDC code number. Next, they submit the data and the invoices to the manufacturer while also providing the same data to HCFA. Upon receipt of the invoice, the manufacturer has 30 days to pay the invoice, and it is the State's responsibility to track the receipt of the rebate dollars from the manufacturers. The final responsibility of the State is to return the Federal Financial Participating portion of the rebate to HCFA; this portion is based upon the Federal matching share within a specific State; for example, California's share would be 50 percent, whereas Mississippi's share could be as high as 80 percent Federal with 20 percent matching funds from the State.

Manufacturers also have a series of responsibilities under the Medicaid law. First, they must sign the rebate agreement and submit it to HCFA. Quarterly, they must provide information to the HCFA concerning their average manufacturer prices and best prices. The manufacturer may elect to validate the State utilization information. Outside auditors at the local level will probably be needed to accomplish this task. When there are disputes concerning the appropriate rebate amount, it is the manufacturer's responsibility to adjudicate the dispute. This legislation puts the pharmaceutical industry on notice that in the future, it will be required to give value for money to discourage regulatory solutions to rising health care and pharmaceutical costs.

One of the unquestioned contributors to rising costs is the explosion of biotechnology products that are currently marketed or will soon be approved by the Food and Drug Administration (FDA) for general use. Dr. Frank Young, during his tenure as FDA Commissioner, stated that "biotechnology is the third revolution in pharmaceutical sciences."[15] Although the lead in research efforts to bring these products to market is being challenged by foreign competitors (e.g., Japan), the United States continues to outdistance those competitors with approximately 78 percent of genetically engineered patent volume.[16]

The biotechnology drugs provide an opportunity to evaluate changes in the per patient drug treatment cost averages over recent years. This phenomenon will also be examined with respect to the aggregate distribution of high-cost care within a DRG context.

COST DISTRIBUTIONS

Using 1984 data, Nash and Goldfarb[17] studied the cost of care of three DRG's at a university teaching hospital. The DRG's included congestive heart failure (DRG 127), pneumonia (DRG 89), and pyelonephritis (DRG 320). The sample included 265 cases with about 20 percent representing high-cost care, which was operationally defined as care costing greater than $15,000 per case. Costs were broken down by hospital service. Pharmaceutical costs as a percent of total cost are listed in table 12-1.

Table 12-1. Pharmaceuticals as percent of total cost

	Pneumonia DRG 89 n=90	*Congestive heart failure DRG 127 n=110*	*Pyelonephritis DRG 320 n=65*
High cost (>$15,000)	9.6%	5.3%	8.4%
Low cost (<$15,000)	6.8%	3.0%	7.7%

Pharmaceuticals represented approximately 6.3 percent of total costs. A Lorenz curve analysis was performed on the cases in DRG 127 (figure 12-4). Classically used to depict disparities in the relationship of population to wealth, this analysis is useful in examining how costs distribute over all of the patients in a given category or DRG.[18] Observe that 80 percent of the patients accounted for half of the total costs of DRG 127, while only 10 percent of the patients were responsible for 30 percent of the total costs. A minority of the cases had a substantial impact on costs. This is a phenomenon that has developed in conjunction of the delivery of more intensive "high-tech" medicine and the need to shorten the treatment interval because of the financial pressures of the DRG payment methodology.

Stolar[19] has described the types of data displays or drug use indicators that can be employed with these large data sets. His example uses DRG's 121 and 122, which are for acute myocardial infarction. These displays are helpful in exploring the many useful relationships that exist.

In the biotechnology drug example, similar patterns emerge in which a few cases account for large portions of

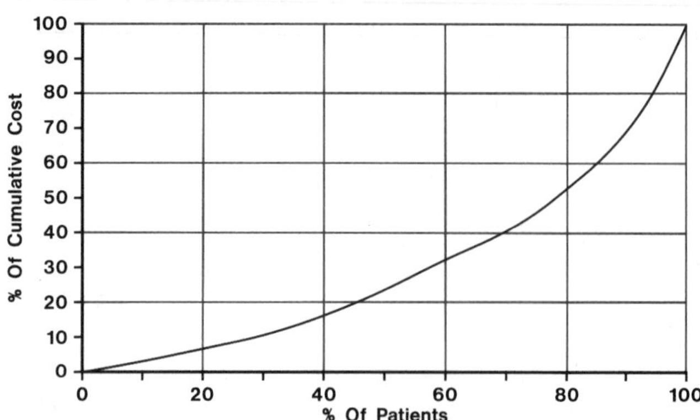

Figure 12-4. Lorenz curve, percentage of costs against percentage of patients, DRG 127

total pharmaceutical expenditures. During the 1980's, significant introductions of new biotechnology drugs have occurred. Table 12-2 lists the top drugs per patient costs from 1985 to 1988.[20] Many of the drugs on this list could be considered high-technology products. Paradoxically, the patients using these drugs are relatively few in number. Initially, the markets for high-technology drugs are narrowly defined; however, over time, new indications are established such as muromonab use in heart and liver transplants and tPA use in pulmonary embolism, deep vein thrombosis, and perhaps unstable angina. In 1988, two of the top five drugs in per patient cost were products of biotechnology.

Table 12-2. Top 5 drugs listed by cost per patient[20]

*1985**		*1986*		*1987*		*1988†*	
IVIG	$1,289	IVIG	$1,521	Muromonab	$2,192	IVIG	$2,650
Moxalactam	613	Lympho Glob	577	IVIG	1,674	Muromonab	2,570
Lympho Glob	537	Imipenem	486	Lympho Glob	1,222	tPA	2,406
Azlocillin	446	Brunarubicin	422	Brunarubicin	625	Pentamidine	874
Cyclosporin	437	Leucovorin	379	Azlocillin	522	Ribavirin	823

*18 hospitals.
†1st quarter.

In terms of pharmacy budgets, it is expected that dollars consumed by high-technology drugs will increase. Herfindal[21] of the University of California at San Francisco predicts that by 1995, 25 percent of the drug budget at San Francisco General Hospital will be consumed by products of biotechnology. The reality of the cost of these agents should not detract from their potential benefits, however. Thus, it will be increasingly important to understand the basic concepts behind and potential applications of these agents. This will, in turn, give the pharmacy manager a more rational basis on which to justify the effective use of these drugs in the appropriate disease settings.

THE FDA APPROVAL PROCESS

Another drug-related initiative that will influence the release of drugs and consequently drug costs is the evolution of the FDA drug approval process. Approximately 10 years ago, the FDA established the "fast track" category for new drugs that were considered therapeutically significant. Additionally, two new strategies, the treatment investigational new drug (Treatment IND) regulation of 1985 and the expedited approval process for life-threatening and severely debilitating illnesses of 1988 (subpart E of 21 C.F.R. 312.21), have led to an acceleration in the approval of a number of new molecular entities (NME).[22-24] There is also a parallel track program for investigational drugs. This program allows unapproved drugs to be used by patients before approval. Most of the parallel track programs have focused on the AIDS drugs.

Under the expedited approval process, the FDA plans to exhibit more of an advocacy role during the entire drug development and evaluation process (i.e., preclinical, clinical, FDA review, and postmarketing surveillance periods). To qualify for expedited approval under subpart E, a therapy must prevent or reverse a life-threatening or severely debilitating illness. Had the expedited approval process been established in 1980, the FDA estimates that 17 new drugs, 6 new biologicals, and 7 new indications would have met its criteria for vitally important therapies (VIT's).[24]

It is likely that a substantial number of agents that benefit from the expedited approval process in the future will be those of a biotechnology-derived origin. In addition, the current move by clinicians toward use of more expensive agents (i.e., VIT's approved via the expedited process) earlier in the therapeutic regimen will undoubtedly accelerate. This can only compound the problem of the high cost of care.

The expedited approval program could effectively place a large number of drugs on the market at a greatly accelerated pace, and this would represent significant improvements in the FDA drug-approval process. As mentioned previously, however, the changes in the approval process and the emergence of biotechnology as a prominent method of drug discovery and production are likely to contribute significantly to increased individual costs to the patient. The FDA deserves high praise for its efforts to expedite the approval of VIT compounds. It should be noted, however, that continuing resource limitations present significant challenges for the agency in the conduct of other functions such as non-VIT drug approvals, audits, and quality control activities.

COST ANALYSIS

The challenge, then, is to understand the benefits these drugs yield for the treatment of various diseases. It is probable that benefits gained from the availability of these agents will offset much of the concern for their costs. Economic analysis, however, is as much about benefits as it is about costs. This concept is basic to understanding health economics (table 12-3). It is also difficult to grasp and to apply in daily practice.[25]

Table 12-3. Ten basic notions of health economics[25]

1. Human wants are unlimited but resources are finite.
2. Economics is as much about benefits as it is about costs.
3. The costs of health care programs and treatments are not restricted to the hospital, or even to the health sector.
4. Choices in health care (that is, in health planning or in treatment mode) inescapably involve value judgments.
5. Many of the simple rules of market operation do not apply in the case of health care.
6. Consideration of costs is not necessarily unethical.
7. Most choices in health care relate to changes in the level or extent of a given activity; the relevant evaluation concerns these marginal changes, not the total activity.
8. The provision of health care is but one way of improving the health of the population.
9. As a community we prefer to postpone costs and to bring forward benefits.
10. Equity in health care may be desirable, but reducing inequalities usually comes at a price.

Even more important (and as difficult to grasp) is the ability to quantify the benefits of drug therapy, medical and economic. It should be noted, however, that there is substantially more evidence concerning the medical effectiveness of drugs than there is concerning other health care goods and services. The ability of pharmacy managers to assume the task of monitoring the value and the proper use of pharmaceuticals will be heavily dependent on their knowledge of the principles behind the surge in biotechnology and the methods available to conduct economic analyses.

Phillips and Hopkins[26] have examined the criteria to determine the quantifiable benefits of drug therapy: How often does the therapy work? How rapid is the patient's recovery? What are the costs of drug-driven adverse events? What are the costs of drug-driven therapeutic failure? Armed with the answers to these questions, the pharmacist should be a force for cost-effective medical management. Institutional budgets stand to benefit from this input. Automated programs such as decision analysis and applications of spreadsheet software could aid the pharmacist in understanding the relationship of therapy to budgets.[27]

Outcomes or medical effectiveness research represents an emerging scientific area of study that includes pharmacoepidemiologic and pharmacoeconomic research. The goal of this research is to understand outcomes of health care. By seeking to identify institutions with good outcomes, one can analyze the associated structures and processes used to achieve those outcomes. Thus, out of the natural experiment of all health care management, centers of excellence are identified, studied, and promoted as providing optimal care.

The Agency for Health Care Policy and Research is a Federal agency that has the primary responsibility for the implementation of the outcomes research agenda. In its March 1990 Program Note, it cited the following areas of academic expertise as being relevant to the conduct of outcomes research: clinical expertise, epidemiology, biostatistics, research design, economics, decision analysis, survey research, data management, research synthesis, and research dissemination.[28] Pharmacy managers could benefit from training in these areas.

INTRINSIC FACTORS

An important contributor to the rising cost of health care is the increasing age of our population. Americans 65 years or older represent an ever-increasing portion of the population, both in numbers and proportion (figure 12-5).[29,30] From 1900 to 1984, the population over age 65 has increased from 4 percent (3 million) to 12 percent (26 million). The fastest growing segment of this population is the 85 and older age group. This group will have increased by seven times over the 1980 to 2050 time period.

Although patients over the age of 65 currently account for only 12 percent of the population, they use approximately 30 percent of all drugs prescribed in this country.[31] The most obvious reason for this disproportionate use of pharmaceuticals is that with advancing age come multiple medical problems. It is estimated that the hospitalized elderly typically present with three to five chronic conditions per patient. Some of the most common coexisting medical conditions are listed in table 12-4.[31]

As the list suggests, the majority of these conditions require at least one drug for adequate management, making it clear that the provision of health care to these elderly is likely to be associated with considerable costs.

Table 12-4. Common coexisting medical conditions

Rank	Condition	Drug treatments*
1	Congestive heart failure	Diuretics • antiarrythmics
2	Depression	Antidepressants
3	Dementia	Antipsychotics(?)
4	Chronic renal failure	Antihypertensives • calcium • diuretics • erythropoietin
5	Angina pectoris	Nitrates • calcium antagonists
6	Degenerative joint disease	Aspirin • NSAID's • steroids
7	Gait disturbance	None
8	Urinary dysfunction	Antispasmotics
9	Constipation	Laxatives
10	Peripheral vascular disease	Pentoxifylline
11	Diabetes mellitus	Insulin • sulfonylureas
12	Chronic pain	Narcotics • NSAID's
13	Sleep disturbances	Hypnotics

*NSAID's = nonsteroidal anti-inflamatory drugs.

CHRONIC ILLNESSES

The costs of treating chronic illnesses are disproportionately expensive, and these costs are concentrated in the elderly population. Whether as a result of disease, injury, birth defect, or the very process of aging, chronic illnesses account for almost 90 percent of all illnesses in this country. Example diseases include diabetes, asthma, epilepsy, arteriosclerosis, and muscular dystrophy. As the size of the elderly population grows, increases in both the incidence and the severity of chronic illnesses are probable.

Chronic conditions receive the least monetary support from third-party payers and thus constitute the single largest problem in the management of the individual's health care costs. This is because the American health care system focuses primarily on reimbursement in the hospital or acute care setting. Fortunately, the health care system is developing new avenues of health management in the form of other providers such as surgicenters, hospices, and home care. These programs will clearly challenge the traditional reliance on the hospital for general health care. Hospitals are increasingly focused on intensive care treatment as less severely ill patients are being managed in an outpatient setting.

Another perspective on chronic disease is the observation that nine preventable chronic diseases (table 12-5) are responsible for more than half of the deaths in the United States.

These diseases are known to be largely preventable as associated risk factors include cigarette smoking, obesity, hypertension, alcohol consumption, and lack of exercise. In addition, the leading cause of premature death is injury. Despite these facts, these diseases are allocated only 3 percent of state public health dollars for their prevention and control.[32]

DRUGS AND HIGH-COST PATIENTS

The hospital is the microenvironment in which the demographic and scientific changes and trends are constantly evident in the evolving practice of health care. It is

Table 12-5. Preventable chronic diseases*

Disease	*1986 Deaths*
Heart disease	593,000
Stroke	149,000
Lung cancer	125,000
COPD†	71,000
Colorectal cancer	55,000
Breast cancer	40,000
Diabetes	37,000
Cirrhosis	26,000
Cervical cancer	4,500

*Responsible for greater than 50 percent of deaths in the United States.
†COPD = chronic obstructive pulmonary disease.
Source: *Philadelphia Inquirer*, January 20, 1990.

obvious that hospital costs are steadily increasing despite attempts by government, health care administrators, insurers, providers, and recipients to control these costs. This rapid acceleration in costs is principally a function of labor costs,[33] but other factors include more expensive drugs (i.e., biotechnology-derived products), devices, and diagnostic procedures as well as the aging population and the associated number of chronic diseases noted in this group. A further contributor, and the focus of this section, is that of high-cost patients, or "outliers." Though many hospital formularies contain approximately 1,000 drugs, it is the top 50 drugs to which are assigned the bulk of the costs—up to 75 percent of the total budget. Fully half of these drugs are sole-source agents for which bidding serves no purpose other than to establish a price. This highly skewed cost distribution within the pharmaceutical budget may be viewed as a mixed blessing. Although it allows the pharmacy manager to focus on a manageable number of line items, it relegates the bidding process to a large number of items with limited potential for major impact. Therefore, a new strategy is required that directs cost control efforts at the most visible drugs. Increasingly, visible drugs will be the

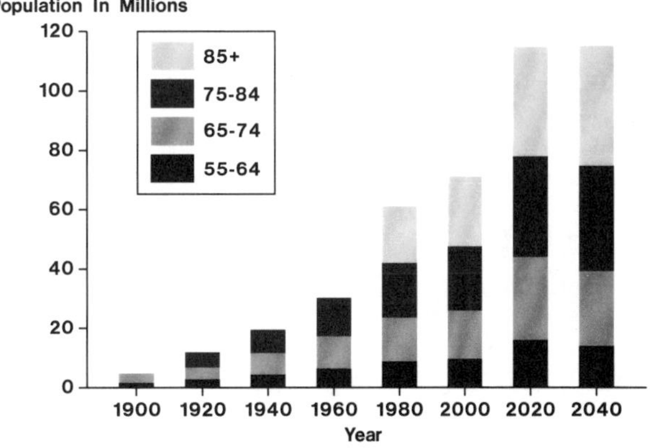

Figure 12-5. Population 55 years and over by age: 1900–2040

Source: *Current Population Reports*, Sept. 1983 and May 1984.

"high-tech" or biotechnology-derived agents whose target population is very small.

An alternate strategy in cost control may be an attempt to identify less expensive substitutes that perform in a like manner. The substitution of newer drugs with smaller doses or decreased dosing frequencies could decrease drug costs but might, if improperly evaluated and implemented, increase the risk of therapeutic failure and ultimately increase hospital costs. Therapeutic failure could be as subtle as a delay in the patient's response or as dramatic as death. The effects of therapeutic failure could be imperceptible in the hospital's microenvironment. The true picture of therapeutic failure is further confounded where the etiology of the failure is unclear. Few patients present with a single disease etiology. Patients present with different levels of disease severity and unique sets of existing comorbidities. All of these factors cloud the true impact of a potentially less effective regimen. Pharmacy managers must evaluate the comparability of similar drugs and consider aspects of therapeutic failure to determine which drugs are actually cost effective.

Although the above discussion may sound speculative, consider the following statements. Outlier patients (as defined within the DRG system) represent 5 percent of the Medicare population but consume between 35 and 45 percent of the health care (including pharmaceutical) resources in the hospital.[34] The pharmacy manager is confronted with the phenomenon of a pharmaceutical budget that constitutes only 5 to 7 percent of the total hospital budget; yet in the pharmacy's drug budget, which goes for as many as 1,000 items, approximately 50 drugs account for 75 percent of expenditures. These 50 drugs are disproportionately administered to outlier patients, which further confuses the clinical economic picture.

Because this phenomenon is potentially overwhelming, many pharmacy managers direct cost-saving efforts at the 950 drugs that consume 25 percent of the pharmaceutical budget for the majority of the inpatient population. The problem with this strategy is that while many drugs are restricted, the impact on the hospital and the pharmacy budgets is minimal. Pharmacy managers must refocus their efforts toward promotion of the effective use of the 50 most expensive drugs, perhaps through the use of prospective audit techniques. It is imperative that the sicker patients, those who account for the greatest proportion of hospital costs in the Lorenz curve example (figure 12-4), receive the most intensive pharmacy management. Intensive pharmacy management for the sicker patients has the potential to produce large returns for hospital budgets. The impact on pharmacy budgets may be less definitive in terms of cost savings.

Thus, it becomes increasingly important to develop an understanding of the outlier patient and his or her impact on health care costs. Even though it is very difficult to identify the outlier patient before or at the outset of the hospital stay, it may be possible in the future to develop risk indices or other predictive measures to prospectively identify and target high-risk patients during their hospital stay. Knowing who these patients are is an important part of the battle to decrease costs to the health care institution.

CONCLUSION

Clearly, hard choices must be made in the future, given the financial pressures in the health care system. The Oregon medical rationing plan (Oregon State bill SB-27) is an indicator of this phenomenon. Pharmacy has both the opportunity and the responsibility to conduct the research necessary to prove the value of pharmaceutical interventions. Adding the economic component will further support the value of pharmaceuticals relative to other medical and surgical interventions and represents an important opportunity for pharmacy.. Pharmacists must accept the responsibility to manage pharmaceutical resources in order to demonstrate medical and economic value. Their standing among health care leaders will be enhanced if they accept the responsibility. Under pharmacy's leadership, society should receive the drugs it needs consistent with medical and economic objectives.

REFERENCES

1. Organisation for Economic Cooperation and Development: *Financing and Delivering Health Care: A Comparative Analysis of ERCD Countries.* Paris, France, Number 4, 1987, p 11.
2. Health Care Expenditures. (Statistical Abstracts of U.S., 1989). Washington, DC, Department of Commerce, 1989.
3. Roper WL, Winkenwerder W, Hackbarth GM, et al: Effectiveness in health care: An initiative to evaluate and improve medical practice. *New Engl J Med* 319(18):1197-1202, 1988.
4. Miller A, Bradburn E, Hager H, et al: Can you afford to get sick? *Newsweek* January 30, 1989, pp 44-52.
5. Lazenby HC, Letsch SW: National health expenditures, 1989. *Health Care Fin Rev* 12(2):1-26, 1990.
6. Anon: Health care spending. *Healthweek* September 19, 1988, p 3.
7. Garland SB, Freundlich N: Insurers vs. doctors: Who knows best? *Business Week* February 18, 1991, pp 64-65.
8. Anon: Health costs. *The Washington Post* February 16, 1991, p D2.
9. "Drug Companies Hike Prices 14%-20%, ASHP Finds." *ASHP Newsletter* 24(4):2, 1991.
10. Loomis CJ: The Killer Cost Stalking Business. *Fortune* February 27, 1989, pp 58-62.
11. Thorpe KE, Siegel JE: Covering the uninsured: Interactions among public and private sector strategies. *JAMA* 262(15):2114-2118, 1989.
12. Gerry R: Moves to rational Medicaid healthcare spreading from Oregon to other states. *Physicians Financial News* 8(13):2, 1990.
13. Office of Technology Assessment: *First Report on the Physician Payment Review Commission (PPRC).* Washington, DC, Office of Technology Assessment, November 1987.
14. Pear R: Medicare to weigh cost as a factor in reimbursement. *The New York Times* April 21, 1991, p 1.
15. Young FE: A new era in drug regulation and development. Paper presented at American Medical Association/FDA Conference on Drug Regulation and Availability: Balancing the Needs of the Individual and Those of the Society. Vienna, VA, October 26, 1989.
16. Szkrybalo W: Genetic engineering patents: What they tell us about biotechnology research today. Washington, DC, Pharmaceuticals Manufacturers Association, July 1988.
17. Nash DB, Goldfarb NI: Exploring resource use in high-cost versus low-cost care: The pharmaceutical example. *DRG Monitor* 4(8):1-8, 1987.
18. Ruchlin HS, Rogers DC: *Economics and Health Care.* Springfield, IL, Charles C. Thomas Publisher, 1973, p 31.
19. Stolar MH: Developing drug-use indicators with a computerized drug database and a personal computer software package. *Am J Hosp Pharm* 44:1075-1086, 1987.
20. Enright SM: Trends: High cost drugs. *IHS Data Link Newsletter* 1(3):1-6, 1988.
21. Herfindal T: Personal communication. University of San Francisco, San Francisco, CA, January 4, 1991.
22. Kessler DA: The regulation of investigational drugs. *New Engl J Med* 320(5): 281-288, 1989.
23. Investigational New Drug, Antibiotic, and Biological Drug Product Regulations; Procedures for Drugs Intended to Treat Life-Threatening and Severely Debilitating Illnesses, 21 C.F.R. Parts 312 and 314 (Docket No. 88N-0350). *Fed Reg* (October 21) 53(204):41516-41524, 1988.
24. Food and Drug Administration Office of Planning and Evaluations: OPE Study 79: A Research Profile of Thirty Recent Therapies for the Treatment of Life-threatening and Severely-debilitating Illness. Washington, DC, October 1989, p 5.
25. Drummond M, Stoddart G, Labelle R, et al: Health economics: An introduction for clinicians. *Ann Intern Med* 107: 88-92, 1987.
26. Phillips DJ, Hopkins LE: Determining total cost-effectiveness of drug therapy (letter). *Am J Hosp Pharm* 44:67, 1987.
27. Gladen HE, Jackson JD, Jordan JT: Antibiotics, DRGs, and the personal computer: Simple techniques to estimate true cost. *Infections in Surgery* 5(10):559-569, 1986.
28. Agency for Health Care Policy and Research, U.S. Department of Health and Human Services: AHCPR Program Note; Medical Treatment Effectiveness Research. Rockville, MD, March 1990, p 5.
29. Taueber CM: *America in Transition: An Aging Society.* Current Population Reports Series P-23 (for 1900-1980), no. 128. Washington, DC, U.S. Bureau of the Census, 1983.
30. Spencer G: U.S. Bureau of the Census. *Projections of the Population of the United States, by Age, Sex, and Race: 1983 to 2080.* Current Population Reports Series P-25, no. 952. Washington DC, U.S. Bureau of the Census, May, 1984.
31. Solan G, Behney C, Herdman R: U.S. Congress Office of Technology Assessment Health Program, *Prescription Drugs and Elderly Americans: Ambulatory Use and Approaches to Coverage for Medicare.* Washington, DC, October 1987, pp 1-4.
32. Proceedings of Surgeon General's Workshop on Health Promotion and Aging, Washington, DC, March 1988.
33. Fuchs VR: The health sector's share of the gross national product. *Science* 247:534-538, 1990.
34. Reinhardt VE: *Health Care Systems in Transition.* Organization for Economic Cooperation and Development, no. 7, Paris, France, 1990, p 106.

CHAPTER 13

Relationships Between New Management Approaches and Quality in Pharmacy Practice

JAMES R. KNIGHT and PHILIP E. JOHNSTON

INTRODUCTION

In this era of spiraling costs and new technology, what is happening to the quality of health care and pharmaceutical care? Personnel reductions and other expense reductions are the initial reactions from most hospital administrators. In a goal statement for a new expense reduction program, quality is couched in terms like "acceptable quality" or "equal quality." Will goals of this type (the management style of today) enable us to manage and contain health care cost in the long run? The only success stories using this approach are institutions facing severe financial crisis, where everyone is motivated to cooperate because of their desire to survive. If we are successful in reducing expenses, what will be the resultant effect on the quality of health care and pharmacy practice?

America has a health care finance problem. Americans are likely to experience a time in the near future when adequate health care is not available to the average income person. America's health care has a management problem, too, not unlike management problems recently experienced in other American industries, where quality has diminished, growth in the standard of living has stagnated, exports have declined, and productivity growth in industry is last compared to other industrialized nations.[1] The purpose of this chapter is to contrast the traditional approaches to management, and measuring and obtaining quality, with the newer approaches promulgated by Ackoff, Deming, Juran, and others. We will demonstrate how hospital pharmacy management can be enhanced by using the most beneficial portions of each philosophy.

Table 13-1 implies that the role of the pharmacist will expand to include a cooperative responsibility for the quality of drug therapy the patient receives with the physician, the nurse, and other health care providers. Pharmacists will be working more autonomously and will be responsible for their own actions and quality of their services. This decentralized role of a pharmacist requires a management approach that fosters this type of responsibility for quality and cooperative work. Eventually, this approach will positively affect the product-related tasks of pharmacy practice as well as the patient-oriented clinical services now termed "pharmaceutical care."

The basis for America's management problems, according to W. Edwards Deming, lies in the four-decade-old management philosophy propagated by Frederick Winslow Taylor, an influential industrial engineer.[2] In Taylor's concept, control over a worker's performance was obtained through work standards and rules. He used time and motion studies to break jobs down to the simplest possible step that a worker could perform with little variation. Minimizing complexity maximized efficiency. Although this method resulted in high production volumes for low-skilled, untrained workers, this management philosophy, and others developed from this concept, such as management by objectives, did not help us address quality issues of today because management did not encourage employees to think beyond their current job. (Management by objectives focused mainly on management issues and progress, but not on the rank and file.) The employees' work is not meaningful, they do not see the "big picture" or how their job relates to the final product or service. Employees are not trained to solve problems, to focus on quality or on the end product or service. Figures 13-1 and 13-2 provide a comparison of traditional and newer management philosophies.

Today's quality professionals bear little resemblance to their turn-of-the-century predecessors. They are managers, not inspectors, they are planners, not controllers. Sensitivity to customers and competitive pressures have forced today's managers to link quality with other business needs.[3] Deming's prescription for American management is to discontinue the traditional control-oriented viewpoint. Improving management skills in the health care industry requires a focus beyond cost. Continued quality health care can be offered in American hospitals at costs lower than are present now. Managers in health care who change will cultivate employee quality orientation by involving employees in outcome decisions, and by increasing the scope of each employee's tasks and responsibilities. According to Deming, successful managers will make a commitment to continuous quality improvement that leads to customer satisfaction. In Deming's philosophy, employees will be highly skilled in their work, know how to measure the quality of their tasks statistically, and know how their work relates to the work that precedes and follows it, as well as to the total product or service. The Deming manager enables

Table 13-1. Comparison of traditional, current, and future management approaches on the role and responsibilities of a pharmacist

Role of the pharmacist:	***Traditional historical management approaches***	***Current management approach***	***Future management approach***
Relationship of the pharmacist to the physician/nurse	Receives physician's order, does not question the doctor, fills the order as written. The pharmacist is not expected to be involved in the outcome of the therapy for the patient.	Receives physician's order. Is somewhat involved in determining the appropriateness of the medication order for that patient.	Pharmacist is part of the team of professionals rendering patient care. In conjunction with the physician, nurse, and patient, the pharmacist is involved in the entire process of drug therapy from prescribing through administration and monitoring to ensure the therapeutic effect is acheived.
Primary task	Filling the prescription.	Ensures the prescription order is correct for the patient. Checks the technician's work in filling the prescription.	Ensures the drug therapy the patient receives is safe and effective and is individualized for the patient's disease or problem.
Relationship with the pharmacy technician	Pharmacist passes orders to technicians. Not concerned with their input or questions.	Pharmacist is always involved in assessing the efficiency and accuracy of technicians who process the prescription. The pharmacist depends heavily on the technician.	Pharmacist works with technicians who are responsible for assessing the quality and efficiency of the filling and delivery processes.
Pharmacy's relationship with hospital administration	Pharmacy does what it is told to do and when it should do it.	More involved with pharmacy and how the pharmacy should deliver its services. Involvement is as a clinical service, and is recognized by nursing and medicine as a clinical service.	Pharmacy will be mandated to be involved with nurses and physicians to meet the overall hospital goals, and has input on how best to achieve these goals for optimal patient outcome.
Who decides quality issues? How is quality assurance managed?	Management is responsible for setting quality goals and ensuring these goals are met.	Each department is responsible for deciding its own quality monitors per hospital and regulatory agency guidelines. A committee in each department is responsible for managing quality assurance. Departments act independently.	Quality is built into each step of the work process. The employee is taught how to monitor his or her work and makes recommendations as to how to improve the quality and efficiency of the process on a continuous basis. Focus is placed on the process of providing the product and service and the outcome of the service.

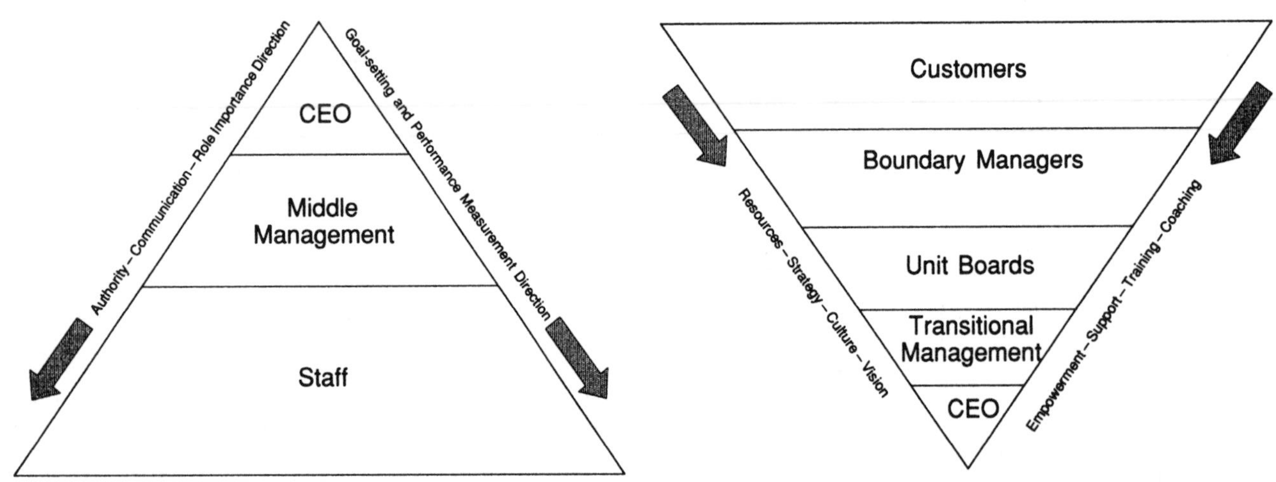

Figure 13-1. Traditional organization pyramid

Figure 13-2. Total quality management pyramid

the employees to improve their job continuously and have input beyond their immediate area of responsibility.

In the first section of the chapter, the traditional approach to improving quality through inspection is contrasted with Deming's approach to building quality into each step in the process.

In the second section, we review management approaches proposed for hospitals, with emphasis on newer management concepts that significantly improve quality. In each management concept reviewed, there is a critique of how concept presently affects quality compared with how newer management concepts impact quality. Implementing some of these new management approaches may be out of the pharmacy director's control, since these concepts depend on the CEO and others to adopt the new management approach. There are, however, several management concepts that pharmacy directors can choose to implement themselves, and for this reason, we have included circular organization[4] and work redesign.[5]

The third section of the chapter is an illustration of how a pharmacy department can change its management approach and the roles and responsibilities of its employees while expecting improvement in quality.

The chapter concludes with a projection of what the future holds for the quality of pharmacy practice under the Deming management philosophy.

CONTRASTING THE TRADITIONAL APPROACH TO QUALITY WITH THE DEMING APPROACH TO QUALITY

In chapter 61 of the second edition of this handbook, Clifford E. Hynniman[6] defined the traditional approach to quality as it is generally described in the literature. Hynniman states:

> Very simply, quality can be defined as conformance to requirements. With respect to health care, quality care can be considered the most favorable balance of benefit and risk. Quality assurance describes all efforts to measure, assess, ensure, and evaluate health care. The word "assurance" suggests action to eliminate substandard performance and improve efficiency of the system of care. The goal is to detect problem areas or individuals and weed them out. In a programmatic fashion, Stolar describes quality assurance as deciding what is to be done, measuring how well the job was done after completion, and then, if the results were not acceptable, undertaking corrective action to ensure that in the future the results will be acceptable.

Take note that traditional statements focus on improving quality through inspection. Inspection of products or service identifies defects but does not explain why they occurred or what to do about them, and it does not identify all of the quality problems. Since the defect is often discovered late in the process of preparing a product or completing a service, it is a very costly system.[2] The inspection approach depends on developing criteria, setting standards, and measuring the standard. All too often, the criteria are written to evaluate a step in the process or the end product rather than each step of the process. Improving quality through inspection frequently does not result in improved quality because of the defensive reactions individuals express when they are found to be deficient. Employees spend their time figuring out how to defend their actions or procedures rather than hearing evaluation results and participating in the development of ways to improve the quality of their actions or procedures. Traditionally, deterrence is used to improve quality, along with reward and punishment to affect employees' behavior. This approach "forces employees to care." The usual employee response to this approach is negative because it does not encourage improvement; employees are not taught, nor have they invested in analyzing what it is about their work process that could improve quality.

In the Deming philosophy quality improvement does not come through inspection of the final product or outcome of a service. In the traditional approach, some managers believe the leadership for quality assurance comes from the quality assurance department. According to Deming, a quality assurance department can only report on what has happened; it has no way to affect future performance. With Deming's methods, future performance and contributions to quality come from management, supervisors, and the professional and technical employees. Quality is built into the execution of each work step; it is part of the description of the job.

Rarely is a lack of quality the result of a deficiency in the employee.[2] Taguchi and Clausing state[7]: "Quality is a virtue of design. The 'robustness' of products is more a function of good design than on-line control..." Deming does not say that inspection is unnecessary. He states that we must cease to rely on mass inspection and work to eliminate the need for it. According to Deming, we can reach our goal when selective inspection of each step of the process will be sufficient to measure quality, particularly when those involved in the process are motivated to want higher quality, are trained to measure and evaluate their quality level, and are enabled to improve their activity in the process. Employees, therefore, need to be trusted with autonomy and empowered with authority. We will still use inspection to measure quality, but we will avoid the use of measurement as a retrospective view of performance. With Deming's tools of statistical measurement, a concurrent measurement of quality is considered state of the art. (Refer to the seven charts discussed in the section titled "The Deming Management Approach.")

According to Deming, we must stop blaming our employees for poor quality. Eighty-five percent of the causes of poor quality are attributable to problems with "systems" and only 15 percent to employees.[2] Further, he found that when an individual was assumed to be the basis for deficiency, the defect was often not the employee but a problem in the way the job was designed, or a failure of management to clearly define the purpose of the procedure, or to put the right employee in the right job. The theory underlying this approach is that quality is improved when employees understand their job, have pride in what they do, and receive positive recognition for their efforts and contributions.

Managers who are able to clarify employee jobs, refine their quality measurements, and provide methods of incorporating employee suggestions will have accomplished much, but there is more. Training employees to monitor their quality statistically, to uncover the ways to improve their work, and to regard both as highly valuable continuous processes are major components of the Deming philosophy. This requires caring, learning, and cooperation between the employee and management. When this approach is used, discovery of a problem is the first essential step to improving quality. Without defects and problems, there can be no improvement. The Deming Chain Reaction, figure 13-3,[2] provides an excellent summary of this section.

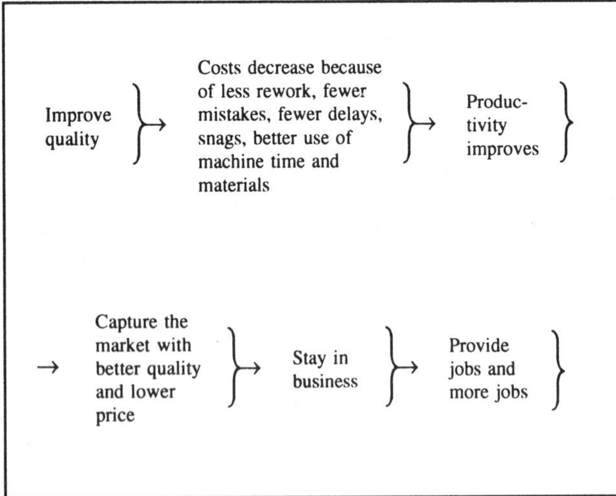

Figure 13-3. The Deming chain reaction

Source: Walton M: *The Deming Management Method.* New York, Putnam Publishing Co., 1986, p. 25.

PROPOSED MANAGEMENT APPROACHES: COMPARISON OF THEIR EFFECTS ON THE QUALITY OF PHARMACY PRACTICE

This section contains a description of the management approaches already in use, or proposed, in hospitals. The newer management concepts that significantly improve quality are emphasized. Each management concept is critiqued for its effect on quality.

Matrix Management Method

The primary purpose of a matrix structure is to increase the organization's ability to respond quickly to change or to address a specific issue.[8] The matrix method can be used on a permanent basis but is more frequently used on a temporary basis, leaving the traditional organizational structure intact. The identifying aspect of matrix organizations is that a project structure is superimposed over a traditional organizational structure. A manager is made available to coordinate the organization's response to new opportunities, or to specific issues, without the formation of a new organization. The resources for the project manager come from the departments or services that the project or issue involves. Thus, these employees learn to apply their skills across various work lines and report to two managers, their functional manager and the project manager.

A benefit of a matrix organization is that it enables a traditional organization to respond quickly to a needed change, or to address an issue that crosses many departments. Dual reporting and the requirement to share resources can cause problems for both staff and managers unless there is cooperation and a willingness to work together. The matrix concept can be an excellent training opportunity for the project manager, the functional manager, and the staff in learning the human relation skills necessary to work in this cooperative manner. The matrix management method does not improve quality, but may be used as an interim tool to facilitate employee communication and to develop better working relationships.

Product Line Management

In the product line management style, the chief executive officer chooses to organize the hospital by its services (product lines, e.g., transplant services or trauma services) rather than its functional departments (e.g., nursing, dietary, pharmacy). The overall goals of this management style are to define and manage the central components of a hospital business, to maximize profits, and to increase quality.[9] Product line management has been applied successfully to business; one example is the pharmaceutical industry. Some hospital administrators have chosen to implement product line management to attain the benefits of cost-effectiveness, expanded volume of services, coordinated services, enhanced internal controls, and improved the quality of patient care and patient satisfaction.[10]

Product line management includes positive aspects. For example, it includes use of interdisciplinary groups relevant to a specific patient type to affect patient outcome positively. On the other hand, product line management is designed to work in the hierarchical management style; therefore, the focus is not on the individual staff member to continually increase the quality of his or her work.

Zero Defects Management Approach

Zero defects is simply a method of motivating employees to do the best job possible.[11] After a kickoff program designed to motivate and indoctrinate employees, each employee signs a zero defect pledge. Management establishes acceptable deviations from a target for each process performed. Employees are trained to use statistical quality control to monitor the deviations from these targets; therefore, quality assurance is preventive as opposed to reactive (inspection and correction of the final product). The zero defect management style has several problems. Managers often set the acceptable level of deviation from the target at too broad a range, allowing decreased quality because minor variations are viewed as too expensive to correct. Others have reported that this management style has decreased in popularity because of extensive record keeping.[11] Taguchi and Clausing's[7] philosophy of quality assurance states: concentrate on resolving the quality problems your customers experience with your product or service and you will automatically resolve the quality problems within your business. Deming[2] states: do not just set a goal or target (as in zero defects); supply a method to reach a goal.

Quality Assurance Circles

Quality assurance (QA) circles are an approach in which employees and their supervisor form small problem-solving groups within their work area. This group meets once or twice a month and discusses opportunities to improve the quality of its work and other work-related issues.[11] A key requirement for the success of QA circles is that the chief executive officer, and top management, must not simply endorse but enthusiastically support QA circles and be willing to delegate the necessary authority and responsibilities to the QA circle. Without support from the top, the group will fade out of existence. This necessity was one of the major problems with QA circles when they were first introduced in the United States. Another key requirement is that the supervisor (leader) must be skilled in group facilitation; if not, a trained facilitator should be used. Similarly, employees must be trained in how to work in a group and in basic statistical problem-solving techniques. In QA circles, quality assurance is everyone's responsibility. QA circles therefore may be very productive for self-limited projects or in interim situations as a director prepares his or her personnel for change. However, QA circles are not an adequate method of managing or improving quality long term without significant administrative support.

Strategic Quality Management

Juran's[12] definition of quality includes meeting customer needs and decreasing deficiencies in products or services. Juran's philosophy is that everyone has a role in providing quality products or services. Quality planning, quality control, and quality improvement are the three main aspects of Juran's strategic quality management. Quality planning is used to identify customer needs and to define the products or services required to meet these needs. Quality control denotes measuring the actual quality results against quality goals set for that product or service, then working on differences discovered. Quality improvement emphasizes increasing the level of quality to previously unattained levels. Strategic quality management is a structured, organization-wide program by which the quality goals set by top management are incorporated into the business plan of the organization, and can be reached with the cooperation and support of everyone in the organization. Juran emphasizes that it is top management's responsibility to provide the overall leadership and control over the quality program in each organization. Juran proposes establishing a quality council. This council initiates the program and coordinates the program. In addition to the quality council, in Juran's view, there is also a need for a quality controller who provides quality reports to top management. Juran changes the reward and recognition system to align it with the progress made in departments and with individuals who identify with the strategic quality management concept and have successfully implemented quality enhancement projects. Juran believes that realigning the reward system is essential to solidify the concept and foster project after project implementation.

Juran's emphasis is similar to Deming's in that it is directed toward individuals. Juran differs from Deming in that there is less emphasis on statistical analysis, control of the program remains with management, and the focus is more on management than on quality.

Self-Managing Work Groups

Self-managing work groups, as described by Hackman and colleagues,[13] are: "intact social systems whose members have the authority to handle internal processes as they see fit, in order to generate a specific group product, service, or decision." These may be small groups, or even temporary groups, assembled to solve a problem or redesign a service or institute self-management teams. The work of the group must be productive and measurable. It is essential that management support this concept and be willing to give the group control over how it carries out its assigned work in order for this concept to be successful and improve quality of the work or process.

Self-managed work groups are very similar to matrix management groups. Employees working in self-managed work groups must be matched by personality type, and each member of the team must be sensitive to the needs of other team members.

The Circular Organization

The author of *The Circular Organization*, Russell L. Ackoff,[4] developed this concept to address three organizational issues: (1) to implement organizational democracy, (2) to increase the readiness, willingness, and ability of organizations to change, and (3) to improve the quality of work life for the employees. This management philosophy is one progressive structure a pharmacy director may adopt as an appropriate working interim step, changing from traditional management style to circular organization to the Deming philosophy.

The overall concept of *The Circular Organization* is that everyone is in a position of power. Anyone who has power over others is subject to the collective authority of these individuals. Accountability is accomplished by the integration of boards into the traditional hierarchical organizational chart. Each board is minimally made up of a manager, the immediate supervisor, and the immediate subordinates. The board's responsibilities include planning; policy making (not policy decisions); coordinating the plans and policies at the next lowest level; integrating its own plans and policies and those of the immediately lower level with those made at higher levels; and making decisions about the quality of the work life of the board members. In some companies using the circular organization, boards have the authority to evaluate the manager's leadership and support effectiveness that is necessary for the subordinates to carry out their responsibilities. If warranted, the board has the ability to vote to remove the manager from that position, not fire him or her. Few boards have found it necessary to exercise this option, as most managers listen to their subordinates and make the appropriate adjustments, when needed. Quality is enhanced under the premise that when otherwise underused employees are given the ability to make decisions concerning their work and have control over the quality of their work life, the result is increased employee productivity and work quality.

The Deming Management Approach

The best way to describe Deming's management approach is to examine his famous 14 points. Each point is annotated with Deming's interpretation.

DEMING'S 14 POINTS

1. CREATE CONSTANCY OF PURPOSE FOR THE IMPROVEMENT OF PRODUCT AND SERVICE
   - Plan for the future—continuously innovate services that benefit your customers.
   - Fund research and education—invest in research to discover needed innovations and train employees to provide these innovations.
   - Maintain equipment and furnishings and fund any product and equipment that increases productivity in the workplace.
2. ADOPT A NEW PHILOSOPHY
   - of management. Totally replace the existing traditional "top down" style of management with the Deming management method.
3. CEASE DEPENDENCE ON MASS INSPECTION
   - Desist from inspecting the final product or output of a service as a method of determining quality.
   - Quality does not come from inspection but from improving each process. Quality is built into each step of the process in the design phase.
4. END THE PRACTICE OF AWARDING BUSINESS ON PRICE TAG ALONE
   - Purchasing decisions should be made by a team of all individuals concerned.
   - Select few suppliers to deal with, ideally those that follow the 14 points in their business, and establish long-term partnerships with these suppliers.
5. IMPROVE CONSTANTLY AND FOREVER THE SYSTEM OF PRODUCTION AND SERVICE
   - Everyone in the organization, led by the chief executive officer and management, must adopt the philosophy to improve productivity and quality on a continuous basis.
6. INSTITUTE TRAINING AND RETRAINING
   - End the practice of having other employees informally train new employees.
   - Train employees for the job until no further training is beneficial.
   - Retrain employees as needed and when new services or technology is implemented.
7. INSTITUTE LEADERSHIP
   - A manager's responsibility is to find ways to enable employees to perform their duties better and better.
   - Management is responsible for the success or failure of the employees it hires.
8. DRIVE OUT FEAR
   - in organizations. Employees will not express themselves, or offer meaningful contributions, unless they are confident they will not experience any reprisals, and unless they believe their contributions and suggestions will be heard and acted upon.
   - Significant dollars are wasted as a result of the fear possessed by both managers and employees in organizations managed by the Western style of management.
9. BREAK DOWN BARRIERS BETWEEN STAFF AREAS
   - Management is responsible for the working environment, and this includes promoting harmony and teamwork between department and services.
   - This goal cannot be accomplished with the current traditional management style.
10. ELIMINATE SLOGANS, EXHORTATIONS, AND TARGETS FOR THE WORKPLACE
    - All of these give employees the feeling they can do better. If the employees already think they are doing their best, or if they know and have communicated why they cannot do their best, this approach is frustrating and demoralizing for them.
11. ELIMINATE NUMERICAL QUOTAS AND GOALS
    - For example, eliminate commands such as "reduce expenses next year by 5 percent" without providing a plan on how best to accomplish this goal.
    - Setting quotas or work standards, instead of improving productivity and quality, actually results in decreased productivity and quality. Once a standard is set, the majority of people tend to perform at average or below-average levels.
12. REMOVE BARRIERS TO PRIDE OF WORKMANSHIP
    - Focus on quality work, let employees know what is expected of them, and provide feedback on job performance in a constructive manner whenever it is needed, not just at the time of annual evaluations. Seek out and listen to employees' concerns and suggestions on how they can improve the quality of their work and act on these concerns and suggestions.
13. INSTITUTE A VIGOROUS PROGRAM OF TRAINING AND RETRAINING
    - Establish a continuing program of self-improvement for all managers and employees to acquire new knowledge and skills.
    - This concept is essential for long-term survival of a business.
14. TAKE ACTION TO ACCOMPLISH THE TRANSFORMATION
    - Everyone, managers and employees, must understand how they can continuously improve quality (the previous 13 points)
    - Management will organize and lead the transformation, a process that could take 2 to 4 years.

Deming also enumerates seven fatal diseases and obstacles, which he claims cannot be overcome without "a complete shakeup of the traditional management."[2]

A major part of the Deming management style is to train employees how to monitor the quality of their work using statistics and control charts. The seven charts are reproduced in figure 13-4, with the titles indicating their application. (For an explanation of how each chart is used, see *The Deming Management Method*, pp. 99-111.)

Although each company or service will adopt its own way to implement the Deming management philosophy, i.e., own mission statement, values, and guiding principles, this example provides an excellent adaptation of Deming's 14

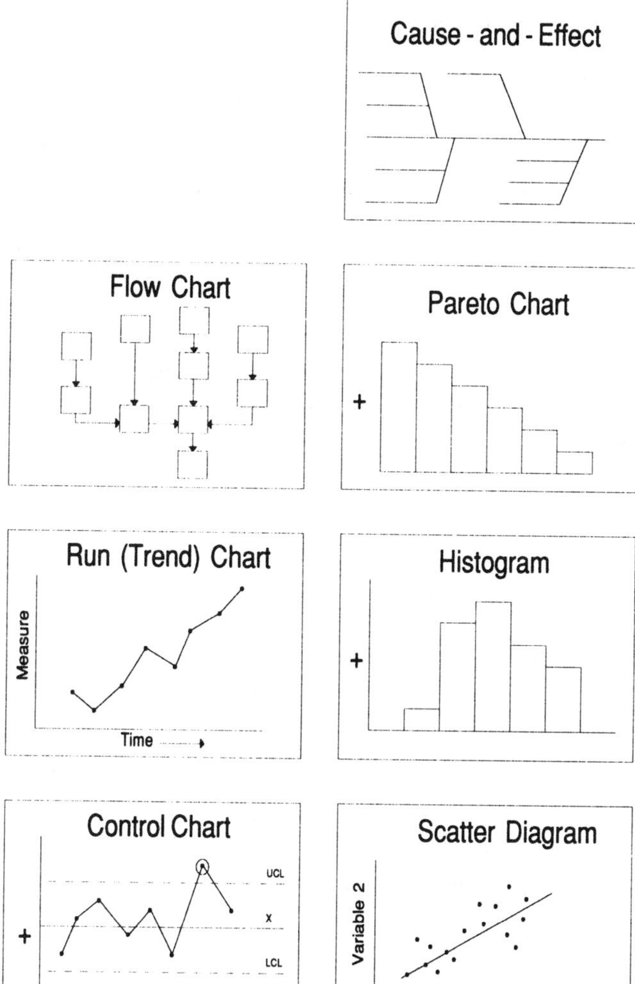

Figure 13-4. Seven helpful charts

Source: Walton M: *The Deming Management Method.* New York, Putnam Publishing Co., 1986, p. 98.

points used at Ford Motor Company. Henry Ford II formulated the following statement of mission, values, and principles.[2] It took Ford Motor Company 3 years to develop these philosophies; they are reproduced here because they offer an excellent summary to this section.

Mission Our mission is to improve continually our products and services to meet our customers' needs, allowing us to prosper as a business and to provide a reasonable return for our stockholders, the owners of our business.

Values How we accomplish our mission is as important as the mission itself. Fundamental to success for the Company are these basic values:

– People. Our people are the source of our strength. They provide our corporate intelligence and determine our reputation and vitality. Involvement and teamwork are our core human values.

– Products. Our products are the end result of our efforts, and they should be the best in serving customers worldwide. As our products are viewed, so are we viewed.

– Profits. Profits are the ultimate measure of how efficiently we provide customers with the best products for their needs. Profits are required to survive and grow.

Guiding Principles

– Quality comes first. To achieve customer satisfaction, the quality of our products and services must be our number one priority.

– Customers are the focus of everything we do. Our work must be done with our customers in mind, providing better products and services than our competition.

– Continuous improvement is essential to our success. We must strive for excellence in everything we do: in our products, in their safety and value—and in our services, our human relations, our competitiveness, and our profitability.

– Employee involvement is our way of life. We are a team. We must treat each other with trust and respect.

– Dealers and suppliers are our partners. The Company must maintain mutually beneficial relationships with dealers, suppliers and other business associates.

– Integrity is never compromised. The conduct of our Company worldwide must be pursued in a manner that is socially responsible and commands respect for its integrity and for its positive contributions to society. Our doors are open to men and women alike without discrimination and without regard to ethnic origin or personal beliefs.

WORK REDESIGN

Although work redesign is not a management philosophy, it is an important management step that may be used with several of the approaches discussed. Before the Deming management method is implemented, it should be determined if work redesign is beneficial and practical, and if so, work redesign should precede implementation of the Deming management method. The philosophy underlying work redesign is that problems between the employees and conflict over their jobs, in many instances, could be eliminated by redesigning the job.[5] In other cases, work redesign is used to tear down a procedure or job into separate work tasks or steps. The tasks or steps are analyzed, revised, and made into a new procedure or job that involves fewer tasks or steps and fewer personnel. The key premise of work redesign is that employees can be motivated if they are given the responsibility for the total job, a variety of different, meaningful, jobs, and work that contributes to the end product or service.

Table 13-2 explains the three general planning steps (questions) that must be answered to determine the applicability of work redesign to a particular task or job. In summary, refer to table 13-3, which compares various management approaches and demonstrates similarities and differences among the approaches relative to persons involved.

Once many of these management philosophies have begun to be implemented, employees experience a withdrawal from their old management philosophy. A great many questions will go through their minds: Will this new management concept really work? — What will be the impact on quality? What traditional departmental "turfs" will be eliminated? This raises another question: Who will be responsible for guiding the pharmacy profession in the institution—who will provide the leadership? Fortunately, the more pharmacists learn about the Deming management style, the quicker fears and questions subside; they become excited about the possibilities this concept holds for improving the quality of pharmaceutical care.

What will it take to transform a service to the Deming concept? It is beyond the scope of this chapter to give the reader all of the "how to" steps in implementing transformation; however, the chapter does provide the reader with sufficient background to understand what must happen for the process to be successful. (See the reference books suggested at the end of this chapter and study this material.)

Table 13-2. Deciding about redesigning work

STEP ONE: IS THERE A NEED FOR WORK REDESIGN?

1. Is there a problem or opportunity for which work redesign would be an appropriate change strategy?
2. Does the problem or opportunity centrally involve the motivation, satisfaction, or work effectiveness of the employees?
3. Might the design of the work be responsible for the observed problems or the unexploited opportunities?
4. What specific aspects of the job, as presently structured, need improving most?

STEP TWO: IS WORK REDESIGN FEASIBLE?

A. The Feasibility of Enriching Individual Jobs
   1. How ready for change are the employees whose jobs would be redesigned? Do they have appropriate knowledge and skill, growth, ability, and satisfaction with the work content?
   2. How hospitable are existing organizational systems to the needed changes? Are the technological, personnel, and control systems likely to constrain the changes that must be made to improve the jobs? If so, can these systems be made more hospitable to work redesign?
B. The Feasibility of Creating Self-Managing Work Groups
   1. Would self-managing work groups fit with the people, that is, match their skills, social development, and strengths and provide the potential for growth and satisfaction with the content of work? Are the overall climate and managerial style of the organization likely to be supportive of self-managing groups?
   2. How hospitable are existing organizational systems to the needed changes? Can intact, identifiable groups be formed that have definable products and the authority to manage their own internal processes? Are the technological, personnel, and control systems likely to constrain the creation of groups with these features? If so, can these systems be made more hospitable to self-managing work groups?

STEP THREE: CHOOSING BETWEEN INDIVIDUAL AND GROUP DESIGNS

1. If neither an individual nor a group design is feasible, do not proceed with work redesign.
2. If one alternative is feasible and the other is not, the choice is obvious.
3. If both individual and group designs are feasible, opt for the group design only if it is substantially more attractive than the best possible individual design.

AN EXAMPLE OF THE PROCESSES

Changing a hospital's or department's approach to management or quality assurance takes commitment, forethought, planning, identification of appropriate people, and time. Evolution rather than an immediate conversion of a hospital or department from traditional to more contemporary management is necessary so that people grow to trust the new approach, learn how it works, and have an opportunity to involve themselves in the process of change.

Four examples of recent changes at Vanderbilt University Hospital in the Department of Pharmaceutical Services show how change has occurred using many of the elements of the management approaches discussed previously. (The history and detail of change for each project will not be included here for brevity.) In each of the examples, notice how often key management objectives—such as quality of pharmacy care, employee satisfaction, reduced pharmacy expense, autonomy, and quality in all activities—are mentioned. Remarks included in parentheses emphasize illustrations of concepts in evolving management approach. After reading these examples, refer again to table 1 under the future management approach, which parallels the design of these examples.

Example 1: Drug Utilization Evaluation and Adverse Drug Reaction Programs

The first example is the drug utilization evaluation (DUE) and adverse drug reaction (ADR) programs. In past years, the department reviewed drug use and adverse drug reactions retrospectively. Changes in standards made by the Joint Commission on the Accreditation of Healthcare Organizations (JCAHO)[14] focus more on quality of care and improved patient outcome. This philosophy, as well as the availability of more patient data within the hospital, has motivated the department to reconstruct the DUE and ADR programs, focusing on opportunities to prevent adversities. (Constant review of services enables the discovery of new services that benefit customers.) Participating in a concurrent program, pharmacy practitioners can now affect decisions in drug selection directly during rounds by providing in-service education with patient-specific information, documenting the effect directly and measuring cost savings. (Harmony and teamwork is promoted between department and services, enabling employees to perform higher quality work.)

DUE and ADR data are collected before and after intervention, showing measures of compliance with the issue or dosing pattern or drug selection proposed in the DUE plan. In 1991, more than $500,000 was saved though use of the various cost-saving measures implemented during the same year. Presently, the DUE and ADR programs are delegated to a self-management team consisting of two physicians, two pharmacists, and a quality assurance nurse, referred to as the Therapeutic Advisory Program.

This group relies on several other persons as needed for consultation or opinion. (Peer review improves quality on a continuous basis.) The group reports to the Pharmacy and Therapeutics Committee and to the Patient Care Monitoring Committee. A basic premise of the Therapeutic Advisory Program is to approach any program with education in mind; that is, the institution should educate those it wants to influence instead of restricting freedom of drug choice or controlling the practice of medicine with written policy. (Education promotes improved drug prescribing across department and service lines.)[15]

Data on adverse drug reactions are collected through a multidisciplinary group of health care providers. Educational programs are regularly scheduled for physician groups and management personnel in medicine. Physician specialties are now using this information as a measure of quality for patient care and to monitor their own adversities. (Meeting customer needs improves quality of care.) Various "what if" questions evolve and are examined as a result of

Table 13-3. Comparison of newer management approaches with the traditional approach of management

	Matrix method	*Product line*	*QA circles*	*Circular organization*	*Strategic quality management*	*Self-managed teams*	*Deming management method*
Number one priority	Increase ability to respond to change.	Increase profits.	Increase quality.	Increase organization democracy, decrease resistance to change, and increase job satisfaction.	Increase quality, decrease waste, and increase customer satisfaction.	Increase quality and increase efficiency.	Increase quality, decrease expense, increase job satisfaction, and increase customer satisfaction.
Who is responsible for quality?	Inspector or manager?	Product line manager.	Everyone in organization.	Management with support of employees.	Team approach management and employees.	Everyone	Everyone
Role of management	No change except for the project manager concept.	Product, revenue, and quality.	Support QA circles.	Provide working environment that enables everyone to perform his or her best.	Provide quality leadership by participating on the team.	Support teams.	Provide total quality leadership and a motivating work environment.
Role of employees	To apply their skills and knowledge across various work lines and work for two bosses when required.	No change	Work cooperatively on a team to increase quality and improve working environment.	Manage themselves and have input into organization democracy.	Responsible for increased quality team participation.	Manage their own work.	Manage themselves using statistics. Monitor and continuously improve quality.
Cooperation between management and the employees	No change	No change	Increase cooperation and communication.	Cooperation and communication significantly enhanced.	Increased cooperation and communication.	Increased cooperation and communication.	Cooperation and communication significantly enhanced.
Increase in employee job satisfaction	No	No change	Yes	Yes	Yes	Yes	Yes
Long-term outlook	No	Yes	Yes	Yes	Yes	Yes	Yes
Status in Business:							
Decreased expenses	No	Yes	Yes*	Yes	Yes	Yes	Yes
Increased profit	No	Yes	Yes*	Yes	Yes	Yes	Yes
Status in hospitals	Experimental	Experimental	Experimental	Experimental	Experimental	Experimental	Experimental
Directly applicable to pharmacy	CEO decision	CEO decision	Yes*	Yes, can start at any level of organization.	Yes*	Yes*	Yes, most but not all 14 points; CEO decision required for total change.

No change = no change from current management approach.
*With approval and support from hospital administration.

findings in drug utilization and adversity patterns. (Investing in research helps to discover needed innovations.) After year 1, opinion is that this sharing of information and the educational process has decreased the occurrence and severity of adverse drug reactions experienced at Vanderbilt. (Constancy of purpose improves quality of service for the customer.)[16]

Example 2: Myelosuppression Unit

The second example is the Vanderbilt Myelosuppression Unit. Initially, a multidisciplinary team was involved in planning of the unit. The team included representatives from the medical team, nursing staff, social work, dietary, pharmacy, and environmental services. Planning consisted of meeting with architects and campus planners and discussing physical, environmental, and financially sound options (goals) for the new service. (Creation of a constancy of purpose.) Concurrently, committees were meeting to develop the operational aspects of the unit. An extensive educational plan was developed and carried out for all nurses, patient care assistants, and medical receptionists. Staff from other support services attended a 1-day training class.

To manage the service more appropriately, unit boards were created. These boards consisted of several disciplines, and were similar to self-managing groups. (A new philosophy of management was adopted, replacing the "top down" style.) These boards have now been implemented in several units of the hospital.

Interdisciplinary training followed. Skills were shared among disciplines. Employees were empowered with new skills, and they shared responsibility with others. (Training and retraining were instituted.)

Managers, most often nurses, were placed in a planning and training role, then developed as managers on a unit board or boundary management format. The manager is quite involved with service activities, but is used more as a resource than an inspector. (Institute leadership is at work, finding ways to enable employees to perform their duties.)

To further facilitate a consolidation of personnel and materials while training and cross-training continued, a service center was created. The service center consists of pharmacy, central supply, patient transport, and linen services. These services are all designed to cater to the specific needs of the customer, customizing products and services. (Barriers are broken down between staff areas, promoting harmony.)

Example 3: Quality Assurance Plan

The third example is using work redesign to revise the department quality assurance plan. For many years, only endpoint results were measured ("endpoint" refers to incident reports, time taken to fill prescription orders, etc.), and the parameters for these criteria were set by management with little involvement by the "rank and file" of the department. Personnel inside the department were made aware of deficiencies only when informed by management; therefore, any deficiency was perceived as a problem for others to solve. Personnel outside the department, except for those attending the hospital quality assurance meetings, knew very little about the department's quality assurance plan. On some occasions, criteria or standards were changed based on similar problems in other departments, e.g., security of narcotics, locking unit dose carts, etc., but in most situations, an internal audit at the end of drug handling measured the quality of service.

Changes made at Vanderbilt were given impetus recently by new JCAHO guidelines. Perceived by many to be an increased burden of record keeping and work, the 10-step process was welcomed by this department. The 10-step process requires that the quality assurance plan be structured to include a stated purpose, a designated person responsible for setting standards and standard measurements, a goal, listing of measurements, and results. A new and very important addition to the process is that conclusions and actions are offered by anyone and formulated by the group for implementation; if necessary, additional criteria and measurement standards are established (table 13-4). (The concept that quality is everyone's responsibility is promoted; promotion of a coordinated department and quality program focuses on the process rather than the end product or service.)

Table 13-4. Similarities between Vanderbilt and JCAHO "10-step" plans

Vanderbilt University Hospital	*Joint Commission on Accreditation of Healthcare Organizations*
1. Pose question or hypothesis	Assign responsibility
2. Identify rationale	Delineate scope of drug use
3. Define patient population	Identify drug to be monitored
4. Define the measures/ information to be collected	Note indications
5. Conduct analysis	Establish thresholds
6. Data base of study and start/stop dates	Collect and organize study
7. Prepare description of results	Evaluate care when threshold reached
8. Formulate recommendations	Take actions to solve problems
9. Take followup actions and document improvement	
10. Notify relevant committees (P&T, etc.)	

Vanderbilt is in transition. Initially, one primary person is assigned to a project, then a group of leaders, then the "rank and file." To make the transition to a new quality assurance plan, the first action was to identify several persons in the department who were leaders, who were cost conscious, who work in strategic patient areas, and who were assertive. These persons meet regularly not only to hear results of the past month, but also—and more important—to focus on actions to be taken in incremental steps to improve quality of various services. (Leaders focus on quality and decision and serve as role models for group members.) An umbrella statement was drafted listing the criteria to be measured for the next year. New criteria were included: (1) consistency in the quality of responses to drug information questions, (2) presence of consent forms in the charts of patients who are being treated with investigational agents, and (3) verification of appropriate laboratory monitors in home care patients. Even though these indicators of quality were "measured endpoints," they did serve as indicators of the *process*, not the endpoint, of providing patient care. Questionnaires were sent to nursing personnel to assess the department's quality of service. (Focus is on assessing the satisfaction of customers as an indication of quality services.)

Measured quality criteria is now a dynamic list at Vanderbilt, changing as necessary to assess current services properly. In addition to the progression of ideas and new parameters came a logical extension of older parameters, termed by the department as "branching logic." Results of medication errors may cause the work group to evaluate packaging, directions to the nurse, policies, or order entry processes. (Investment is made in research to determine needed innovations.) One of the best changes of the quality assurance program is that persons from different areas are part of the work group or self-assessment team, and information is disseminated to several areas of the department. (Benefits derive from promoting quality as everyone's responsibility in the department.)

Example 4: Satellite Pharmacy Distribution Services

The fourth example is a change affecting satellite pharmacy distribution services. In recent years, the hospital has made a major effort to reduce overall expense by using a prime vendor and to reduce expenses further, it is implementing a just-in-time (JIT) inventory system for pharmacy, distribution services, and other sites in the hospital. Following Deming's approach, this JIT system is developed cooperatively via a partnership with the vendor. Another unique feature of the JIT program is the role the nurse (customer) plays in defining the system requirements and monitoring the service provided to determine the nurses' satisfaction with the service. Both the hospital and the vendor strive to maximize quality and decrease operational cost in each other's areas.

Additionally, through a series of task force projects involving both hospital and vendor personnel, employees from the areas of distribution, patient transport, and pharmacy form an expanded service center called a "pharmacy service center." Pharmacy satellites are being expanded to include extra room for patient intravenous pumps, sterile supplies, central supply items, linen, and other patient care items. The concept of a hospital formulary for drugs will be expanded to cover equipment and supplies. Staff are responsible for ensuring that the most appropriate and least costly distribution and setup of such products are available on an as-needed basis to nurses (the customers). In some patient care areas supplies and/or equipment are dispensed according to standards of care written for diagnosis-specific care plans ("collaborative care pathways"). The service center will consolidate different services into one unit and foster cross-training of personnel. As a result of the consolidation of services, the employees in the service center have the same rapport with other health care workers and professionals as has already been attained by the pharmacy satellites' employees. Finally, giving these employees total responsibility for the entire process has promoted personal pride in accomplishments, motivation, spirit of teamwork, and quality of services. (Personalization increases awareness of the needs of the customer.)

In summary, each of the changes described in this section should exemplify many of the basic approaches to improved management and quality services. At the same time, several new roles for pharmacists and technicians evolve. Employee satisfaction is expected to rise, given that more advanced activities are available and time can be reallocated to more patient-oriented services. Quality assurance standards will measure quality during, instead of after, the process of providing service. We have become more aware that our customers include the patient, other health care workers, our coworkers, and administrators. We are encouraged that in many of these examples, people have already been more involved in decision making and learning the result of decisions, while learning how to identify opportunities and to take required action accordingly.

Many Vanderbilt services and operations do not have all of the characteristics of each management approach. We learn to manage as we proceed. We learn the most appropriate approach by evaluating each new project. While actively assessing newer methods of management and quality assurance, this pharmacy operates currently within a hospital management structure that is traditional. Figure 13-5 depicts Vanderbilt's present organizational design, traditional, yet including boundary management projects in coexistence. The myelosuppression unit, described earlier in this chapter, is an example of a boundary management project being used in the hospital's transition toward a more complete innovative management structure.

Figure 13-6 depicts the structure of the Vanderbilt Hospital Pharmacy, which coexists in the present hierarchical design of the hospital. The design in the pharmacy actually matches the flow of work. With this approach, goal setting, quality measurement, and communication among all employees providing service and product is improved. In this design, pharmaceutical hospital and supply vendors act as partners with pharmacy to satisfy customers. Employees at all levels are directly involved with work design and have vital information needed to enable them to supply a customized, patient-specific product or formulation. The pharmacist can manage his or her service center with greater ease, while focusing on patient-specific pharmaceutical care.

At Vanderbilt University Hospital, we began implementing three different management approaches, one after the other, to bring the staff and management team through this indoctrination process. First, we will implement Ackoff's circular organization approach. The purposes of this first phase are to foster an organizational democracy, to increase the pharmacy staff's ability to respond quickly to change, and to improve the quality of work life for our employees. Ackoff's philosophy is that anyone who has authority over a group of individuals is subject to the collective authority of those individuals. This ideology will help management realize that its primary role is to provide leadership and support to pharmacists, technicians, and other pharmacy personnel. It will enable them to perform efficiently at the best of their ability. Employees and managers will gain valuable experience in planning, policy making, and coordinating the plans and policies made by management, within their level and in conjunction with the level below them. Employees will also begin to make their own decisions regarding their quality of work life. Implementing and gaining practical experience with the circular organization will take 12 to 18 months. The results of this phase will be a change in the corporate climate relating to the roles and responsibilities of management and the staff; the change effects increased employee productivity, and increased work quality.

The first phase is implementation of a "boundary management" approach for each decentralized pharmacy. At Vanderbilt this work design is used, and those who work in this framework are considered a "unit board." The boundary management group or unit board is composed of a manager, the manager's boss, and representatives from all of the staff who report to this manager (see figure 13-6). The unit board can include other managers on a peer level with managers in boundary management. The unit board can, by consensus, change procedures that are specific to this unit and set work schedules to enable staffing and employee satisfaction; it cannot change a policy that refers to the

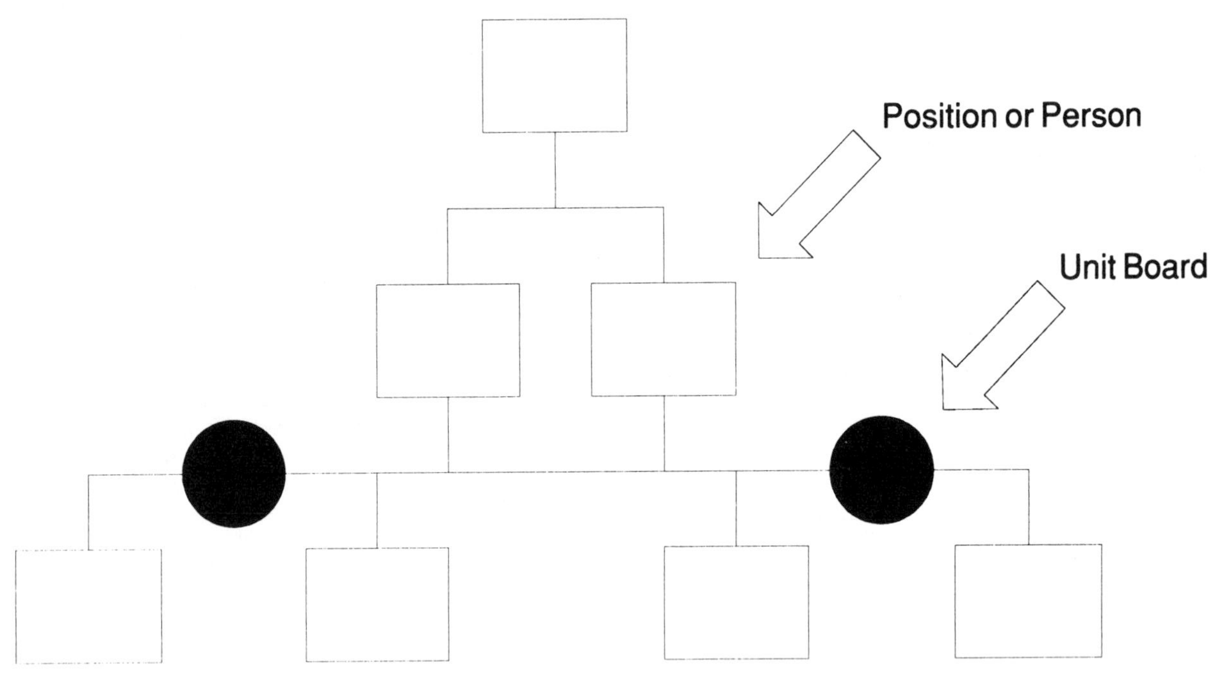

Figure 13-5. Traditional hierarchical management structure with boundary management (unit board) structure superimposed

entire hospital, or make changes that involve another unit board. By this time, the just-in-time vendor will have assumed the responsibility for the centralized dispensing functions including continuous unit dose, intravenous preparation, and home health care preparations and for delivering these services to the hospital on a JIT basis.

Our department will have only decentralized satellite pharmacies providing the doses needed immediately. The experience gained with the circular organization approach will enable both staff and managers to form self-managed work groups. The goal of this phase is to promote work groups whose members have the authority and control over their own work processes in order to provide the services required to patients, physicians, and nurses.

Managers should become boundary managers. A boundary manager is the person with overall responsibility for a service (service center) but no direct accountability for individuals performing the service. Figure 13-6 shows the boundary manager's linking to a circle with the members providing the service at the top, and the individuals at the bottom of the circle represent the individuals to whom the manager must relate in carrying out his or her responsibilities. If the boundary manager is successful in forming self-managed work groups, he or she will become a resource for these staff, and the solid line linking the manager to the circle will become a dotted line.

In this phase, staff will begin to take more responsibility for their work and to make changes in how they accomplish their work, to make it more efficient, higher quality, and personally satisfying. To accomplish this independent work ethic for the staff and advanced leadership roles for management, extensive employee and team leader training will be part of this phase. This training will provide the staff with the knowledge required to evaluate and perform analyses and to make decisions about their jobs and how they are performed, both of which will foster increased quality and productivity and decreased expense of operations. Training for boundary management is designed to ensure that the staff members understand and feel comfortable with, and are capable of performing, their leadership, supportive, and resource roles. The concept of work redesign will be employed in this phase. It is expected that it will take 12 to 18 months to implement this concept and 1 year of experience to reach the goals for this phase.

The final phase is the Deming management approach. In the previous phase, staff, boundary managers, and management will have been trained and will have gained experience with their respective roles and responsibilities and redesigning their jobs. Now, the goal is to have each employee use the Deming approach to monitor the quality and efficiency of his or her work and continuously improve it based on "customer feedback" (figure 13-7). Improving quality and productivity, satisfying the customer and employees, and meeting and exceeding their customers' needs are the primary goals of this phase. Instilling pride in workmanship and ownership of a job by each employee are also goals. The evaluation system as we know it today will have been phased out and replaced with a self-evaluation system based on "customer feedback" and day-to-day coaching and leadership from the team leaders and the entire management team. Instilling these methods will allow all our department's employees to process product orders and provide high-quality, patient-specific pharmaceutical care.

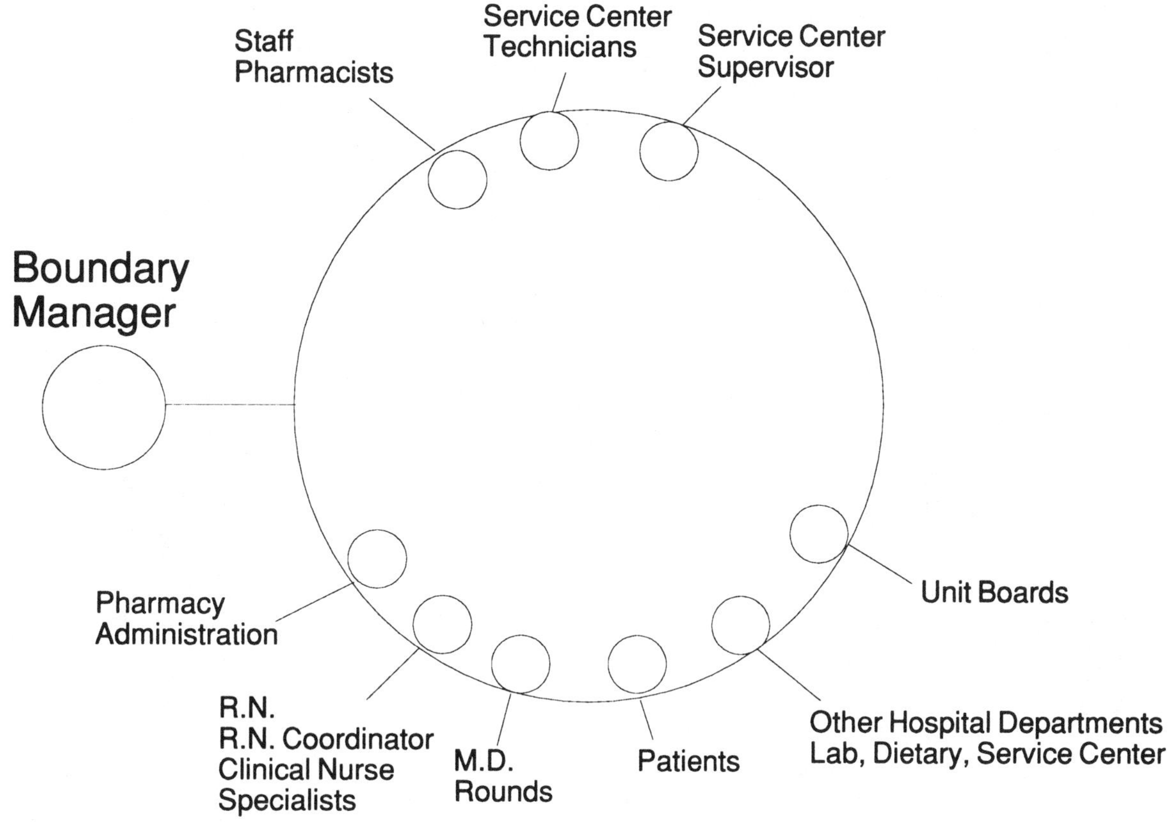

Figure 13-6. Boundary management structure for a Vanderbilt service center

SUMMARY

The American health care industry has traditionally used hierarchical "top down" management structures to produce high-quality products and services. Currently, there are many management philosophies and structures to choose from, most being products of the worldwide business changes in the 1970's and 1980's. It is generally accepted that the traditional management approach of today, which has prevailed over the past 30 years, simply will not help us meet the cost or quality challenges we face in the health care industry. The authors strongly believe that hospitals need to continue to assess what American industries, and worldwide industries, are doing to meet quality and cost challenges and determine how these approaches can be applied for use in the health care industry.

Hospitals are just beginning to experiment with the management approaches that place quality and customer and employee satisfaction as prerequisites for expense reduction. Both Deming and Juran point out that it will take 3 to 5 years for traditional managed companies to transform to their approach of continuous quality improvement. This amount of time is required to learn the concepts, implement demonstration projects, convince the employees of their new roles and opportunities, and change the corporate climate and reward system.

Successful management philosophy in the health care industry must change to a total quality management "bottom up" commitment. Customer-oriented products and services will be perceived as—and most likely will be—the best products and services available, because of competition. Customers, therefore, are not only determining trends in products and services but also determining what quality is.

In pharmacy practice, our customers include vendors, administrators, professional and technical health care workers, patients, and the public. The responsibility of each employee participating in a total quality-oriented service is to think of the ultimate needs of the customer. In pharmacy practice, this includes provision of high-quality, patient-specific pharmaceuticals and an attitude of being part of an interdisciplinary team of persons working toward a common, well-known goal consistently.

This chapter addresses several options for adopting new management structures. Most notable is the Deming method. While working to develop the Deming method, the manager can use other management structures to proceed with progressive steps, such as Ackoff's circular organization, boundary management, and unit boards.

The manager's most important role in improving the services of pharmacy to a total quality management structure will be development of a goal of continued high quality. It must also include strong communication skills, training and development skills, ability to break down barriers to communication, acceptance of ideas and changes from nonmanagers, and an attitude of openness. Trials and errors are inevitable, because these management structures are new to the health care industry; however, trials and errors are part of innovation!

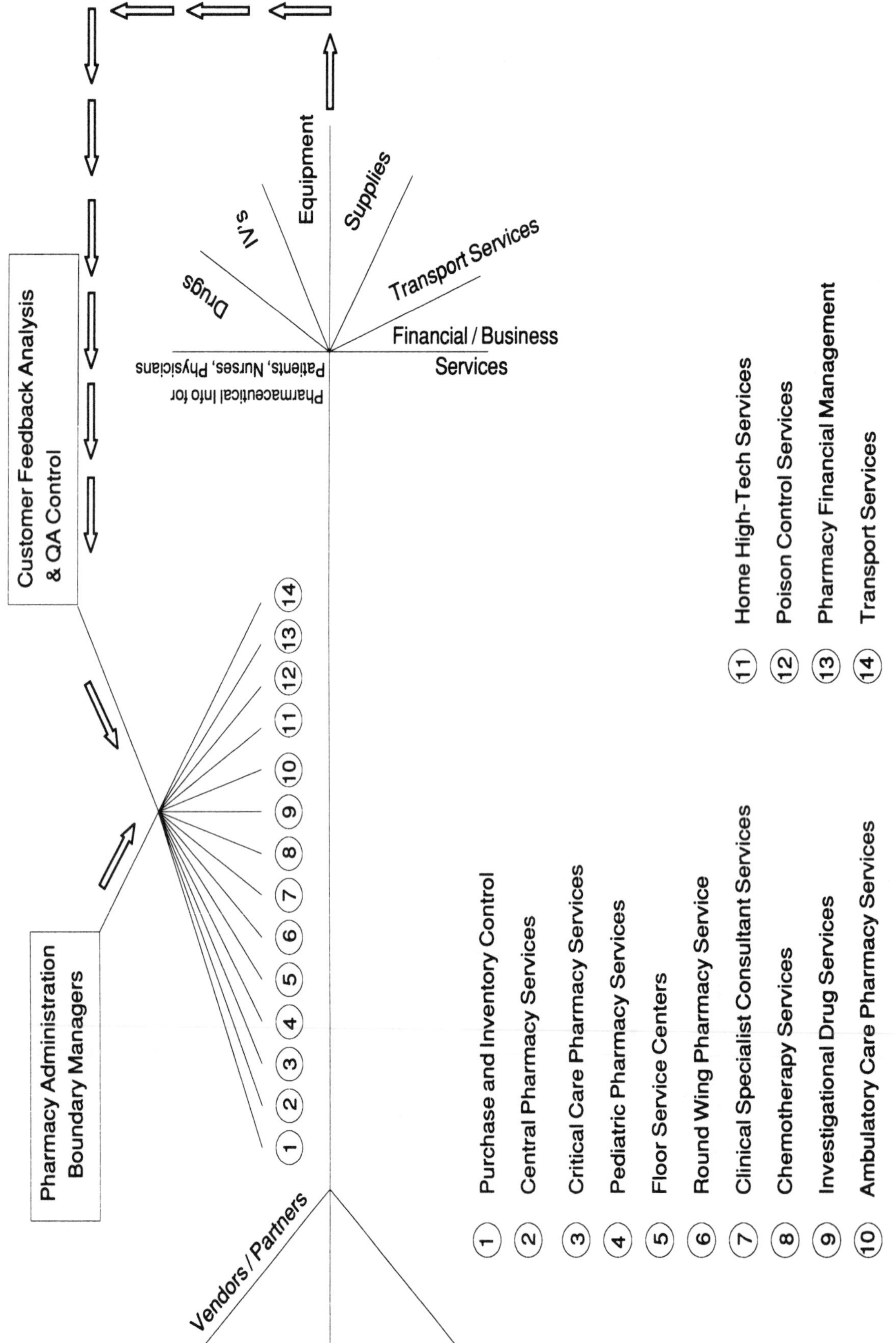

Figure 13-7. Department of pharmacy/supply/equipment/transport organizational chart

Grateful acknowledgment is made to Carol W. Meulemans for her assistance in editing and to Robert S. MacDonald for his assistance with the figures.

REFERENCES

1. Grason CJ Jr, O'Dell C: *American Business: A Two Minute Warning*. New York, The Free Press, 1988, p 7.
2. Walton M: *The Deming Management Method.* New York, Putnam Publishing Group, 1986.
3. Garvin DA: *Managing Quality: The Strategic and Competitive Edge*. New York, The Free Press, 1988.
4. Ackoff RL: The circular organization: An update. Executive summaries. *Academy of Management Executives* 3(1):11-16, 1989.
5. Hackman RJ, Oldham GR: *Work Redesign.* Reading, MA, Addison-Wesley Publishing Co., Inc, 1980.
6. Hynniman CE: Quality assurance and performance standards. In Brown TR, Smith MC (eds): *Handbook of Institutional Pharmacy Practice*. Baltimore, MD, Williams & Wilkins, 1979, pp 632-645.
7. Taguchi G, Clausing D: Robust quality. *Harvard Business Review* 65, 67, Jan-Feb 1990.
8. Durbin AJ, Ireland DR, Williams CJ: *Management and Organization.* Cincinnati, OH: South-western Publishing Co. 1989, pp 204-234.
9. MacStravic RS: Product-line administration in hospitals. *Health Care Management Review.* 11:35-43, 1986.
10. Bruhn PS, Howes DH: Service line management new opportunities for nursing executives. *JNURSADM.* 16:13-18, 1986.
11. Wadsworth HM Jr, Stephens KS, Godfrey AB: *Modern Methods for Quality Control and Improvement.* New York, Wiley, 1986.
12. Juran JM: *Juran on Leadership for Quality.* New York, The Free Press, 1989.
13. Hackman JR, Brousseau KR, Weiss JA: The interaction of task design and group performance strategies in determining group effectiveness. *Organ Behav Hum Perform* 16:350-365, 1976.
14. Joint Commission on Accreditation of Healthcare Organizations: *Accreditation Manual for Hospitals.* Chicago, Joint Commission on Accreditation of Healthcare Organizations, 1988.
15. Branch RA, Johnston PE: Therapeutic advisory program: An opportunity for clinical pharmacology. *Clin Pharm Ther* 43:223-227, 1988.
16. Johnston PE, Morrow JD, Branch RA: Use of a database computer program to identify trends in reporting adverse drug reactions. *Am J Hosp Pharm* 47:1321-1327, 1990.

CHAPTER 14

Being a Good Pharmacy Manager: The Art of Managing for Employee Success

WILLIAM N. KELLY

Managing is a complex and dynamic process. It is an art to coordinate and control the changing elements affecting the management process. What does it take to be a successful manager? Is there a pattern or formula for succeeding in such a complex environment? How can one succeed as a pharmacy manager?

Although the management environment is complex, everything comes down to people. People are our most valuable asset. They get the work done. Successful managers know how to manage for employee success. If pharmacy employees are successful, the manager and the pharmacy will also succeed.

Although it may appear that successful managers were born with innate managerial skills, most have worked very hard to become good managers by studying, observing, and learning from others. To excel in management, it is necessary to understand basic human behavior and genuinely believe that people are the key to getting the job done.

This chapter focuses on a practical approach to successfully managing people, primarily pharmacists, and building a dynamic pharmacy team. Theoretical approaches are not discussed; rather the "nuts and bolts" of managing people and getting them to achieve excellence are described. An extensive bibliography is provided at the end of the chapter for more background reading and indepth study.

PEOPLE AS MAIN FOCUS

Management begins with people—in this case, pharmacists, technicians, clerks, and secretaries. Little is accomplished without them. The best plans, elaborate equipment, and the best physical layout accomplish nothing without people. The people inside a pharmacy department and the relationships they have with each other, and outside the department, can make the department exceptional. Programs go nowhere without people. Therefore, people should be the main focus of the pharmacy manager who is striving to have an excellent program. Pharmacy managers must believe in people and effectively blend the needs of individual employees with the goals of their department and the institution. This can be a real challenge because people have feelings, prejudices, and differing needs. However, there are ways to obtain mutual success, as described by Peters and Waterman in their best-selling book, *In Search of Excellence*.

JOB SATISFACTION

With few exceptions, hospital pharmacists tend to be reasonably satisfied with their jobs. Some sources of dissatisfaction routinely identified include lack of recognition and opportunity for advancement, staffing and scheduling practices, and policies and procedures. On the other hand, it has been shown that pharmacists working in hospitals uniquely appreciate opportunities to learn, to grow, and to take on more responsibility than pharmacists working in other environments.

Studies also have consistently shown that pharmacists in clinical practice tend to be more satisfied than staff pharmacists. Why? Most agree that high job satisfaction and internal work motivation occur when people believe that they have performed a meaningful task well. Five important dimensions create this environment: skill variety, task identity, task significance, autonomy, and feedback. Pharmacists practicing in the clinical environment perceive that their jobs allow the greatest freedom and control over the work pace and that their tasks have an impact on outcomes. They have more interpersonal contact, more meaning, and more challenge. Good performance is recognized and rewarded accordingly.

On the other hand, some believe that many pharmacists are more dissatisfied with the profession than they are with their specific jobs. One explanation of this phenomenon is that drug knowledge and education have expanded more rapidly than practice has. This may be creating a "satisfaction gap," especially among younger pharmacists who find that the practice is not what they had hoped for or learned about in school. The converse of this dissatisfaction is the frustration of pharmacy managers who are dealing with recent graduates who seem to have a different value system. How can pharmacy managers get better work performance, more productivity, and better quality results from pharmacists? How do we get marginal performers to do better? How can we promote a better work ethic?

Although still not proven, it is generally believed that improved job satisfaction among pharmacists will improve job performance. Is there a defined strategy to produce a "win-win" situation? Assuming adequate compensation, what can pharmacy managers do to improve job satisfaction among pharmacists and consequently get the job done better?

GOOD PERSONNEL MANAGEMENT

Good personnel management starts at the top. This does not mean that individual pharmacy supervisors with strong personnel management skills cannot exist in a weakly led department, but generally the stronger the leadership, the stronger the personnel management. The director sets the tone and the expectation. If he or she has a high priority for good supervision and is a "people person," good management skills will be stressed. Ten key features of leadership that contribute to strong personnel management are:

1. *Leadership versus management.* It has been said that "managers do things right" and "leaders do the right things." Leaders know that people are their most valuable resource; therefore, they make quality supervision a high priority. Leaders understand and believe in people. They respect their most valuable resource.
2. *Staying in touch.* Leaders do not lose touch with their employees—not just the key employees, but employees at all levels. Good leaders listen, consider, act, provide feedback, and give credit to those who provide input.
3. *Planning: mission and vision.* Most employees feel comfortable following people who can clearly articulate a purpose and direction. These leadership skills and the resulting respect from pharmacy employees, especially the professionals, make it easier to manage those employees. The leaders need to help people focus on an agreed-upon plan to achieve the purpose and vision.
4. *Sensitivity and timing.* Assessing the current situation from a worker's standpoint, before thrusting a problem on the pharmacy staff, can make the difference between success or failure. A sensitivity to employee's feelings and other recent events also maintains integrity and a good bonding between the pharmacy staff and the pharmacy department leadership. Trusting each other cements relationships within the pharmacy team and fosters loyalty and commitment when times get tough.
5. *Pacing and focusing.* Like timing, pharmacy employees will appreciate it when the leadership does not push them too far beyond their abilities and resources or try to implement new programs or procedures too quickly. At the same time, employees need to know that managers will continually guide and encourage them toward achieving critical departmental goals.
6. *Quality and competence.* Emphasizing quality—that "we do it right the first time, all the time"—and respecting and consistently rewarding pharmacy employee competence will gain respect and loyalty from the employees pharmacists want to keep in their department.
7. *Standards.* Respect and loyalty are also gained when standards are established, uniformly followed, and enforced, especially standards of practice and supervision. Compliance with such standards will be vastly improved if those affected by the standards have a part in designing them.
8. *Good work climate.* A good work culture can make a big difference in the ease of managing pharmacy employees. Create a work environment where people feel significant, learning and competence make a difference, and the work is exciting. There is a commitment to improving service, and people are part of a community. This makes managing people easier and more pleasant. A good work culture does not just happen, but bad ones do. The power of the "grapevine" is inversely proportional to the organizational climate. In a good work culture, there is mutual respect, trust, and a sense of pride. Some other sources of work satisfaction are fair compensation, adequate benefits, job security, due process, safety, and health.
9. *Protecting workers from the bureaucracy.* Pharmacy managers need to understand and appreciate that employees feel vulnerable in the bureaucracy of an organization. Most of the pharmacy staff will have a tough enough time trying to master the rules, regulations, and policies and procedures of the pharmacy department. Pharmacy staff members will be appreciative and easier to supervise if those above them in the department "protect them" from or "take on" the hospital bureaucracy.
10. *Building a team.* Just as getting the job done requires people, having an excellent department requires building a real team. Having a team means that everyone knows his or her job, buys into mutual goals, and thrives on working together to accomplish those goals.

ORGANIZATIONAL STRUCTURE

How the pharmacy department is organized probably makes a difference in how successfully employees are managed. How a department is organized reflects its degree of respect for employee opinion and input. Some organizational designs strictly define employee categories, and the chain of command is rigidly enforced. More democratic models promote an open, participative system in which employee's ideas are always welcomed. The ideas may not always be used, but reinforcement for the input is provided and an explanation of why they will not be used is given. Such an organizational structure promotes respect for people and builds confidence and trust in the leadership. The downside is that such a system is slow and inefficient. In certain situations, there is not enough time to obtain everyone's input. However, if such situations are kept to a minimum, pharmacy workers in turn will trust departmental managers to make the best decision, especially if they feel their interests and concerns were considered.

An interesting, recently designed model for organizational structure that might work well in larger pharmacy departments is called "circular management." Circular management is unique in its ability to integrate various levels of a department effectively. Each level more closely relates to each of the two levels above and below, thus promoting a better understanding of the goals, activities, and roles of coworkers. (See bibliography and chapter 13 of this handbook for more information.)

THE IMPORTANCE OF STYLE

Numerous articles and books have been written about different management styles. The way managers conduct themselves—handle matters and project their image—has an effect on the employees under the manager's control. When pharmacy employees are asked to describe their supervisor, the adjectives used will indicate how the managers relate to their staff. Is the manager aloof or distant most of the time, or generally perceived to be warm and friendly? Does it really make a difference?

Most would agree that extreme styles are to be avoided. Inconsistent managers will confuse the employees they supervise. When asked, most employees want their leader to be honest, fair, and consistent and to lead. Employees do not always expect their supervisor to rule in their favor, as long as fairness prevails.

Supervisors and managers need to understand their own management style and recognize that each employee also has a style of communication. The burden of bringing the style of the manager and employee together falls squarely on the manager's shoulders. Managers must consciously identify styles and learn to modify their own style to communicate effectively.

In addition, exceptional pharmacy managers will show sincere interest in their employees to the degree possible. Being vigilant and sensitive to employee's needs is one of the factors that clearly separates the superior from the average manager. Managers also need to "walk the talk." In other words, it is easier to say something than to do it. The adage "action speaks louder than words" has truth and "do unto others, as you want them to do unto you" is still sound advice.

Communication is the glue that links all of this together. There is no such thing as too much good communication. Communication and work culture are often related. Poor communication will contribute to a poor work environment. In a good work environment, errors in communication will often be minimized or forgiven.

Employees like frequent and open communication in all forms. Preferred methods, however, are face to face and one on one. In addition to routine communication, feedback on issues and work performance, as well as help with the "little problems," are appreciated by employees. The best way to accomplish this is to routinely manage by walking around. Instead of attending meetings and completing paperwork, most pharmacy directors or managers would make more progress if they developed a rapport with their employees to the extent that they know their interests. Simply asking, "what can I do to help you do your job better?" then listening carefully and following through can make a big difference in employee performance. This approach shows that the manager is actually working for the employees. The contribution this makes to building a team is extraordinarily powerful.

The "bottom line" is, how interested are managers in their people? Are they developers of people or users? Do they pay attention only to the "important people"? Leaders understand that it is the "little people" who sometimes open big doors.

SUPERB SUPERVISION

We have discussed some of the critical attributes of those who are looked to for leadership within a pharmacy department, principally the pharmacy director and other managers. What about the supervisors? If there were something called "superb supervision," it would include components discussed below.

Striving Toward a Common Purpose

Are all the pharmacists committed to working toward a vision of a better practice? Does the pharmacy staff understand and believe in the goals and purpose? Can it be seen in their eyes? Their hearts? Their actions?

Developing Loyalty and Commitment

The key to developing loyalty and commitment of pharmacy employees is largely supervisory style and effectiveness in addressing employee concerns. The cornerstones of developing employee loyalty and commitment appear to be honesty, fairness, responsiveness, and recognition.

Knowing the People

The primary job of a supervisor is to accomplish as much work as possible with the assigned employees, but with respect and dignity. The exceptional supervisor will go beyond this and help develop his or her people. The most important way to do this is know them well—their strengths, weaknesses, prejudices, and especially their values. Showing sincere interest is the key to building a strong relationship with the employees.

Treating Everyone the Same . . . ?

Should professionals be supervised differently than nonprofessionals? The answer is, yes and no. Although there is a common set of workers' expectations of their employer and supervisor (the four cornerstones), pharmacists need to be supervised differently than the rest of the pharmacy staff. Professionals tend to be more independent and creative. Pharmacists respond well to flexible time schedules, quiet facilities, title variations, peer group recognition, opportunities to participate on various committees, and provide input into the overall direction for the department. Managers must continually pay attention to retention issues concerning the professional staff.

Should the more clinically oriented pharmacists be treated differently than other pharmacists? Differently, yes; more importantly, no. Lack of mutual respect for other staffmembers' unique role and contribution can prevent a department from being all that it can be. Supervisors need to promote an attitude of "how we can help each other" more. In this regard, teaching and learning are key. Manage the more clinical or more educated pharmacy employees by getting those persons to manage themselves. Guide them in such a way that they do not realize they are being managed at all, yet they feel responsible and know that they are not entirely independent.

Understanding Human Behavior

The secret of being a good supervisor is understanding human behavior. To be successful at understanding human behavior, one must like people, be a student (watch and listen), and be sensitive to others. In understanding human behavior, a basic understanding of motivation, needs, and values is important.

Motivation

There are many theories about motivating employees, (see the bibliography at the end of this chapter). The following discussion is offered as a practical approach to motivation which is based on understanding people, their needs, and their values.

The person who is the boss can make people do things by giving a direct order or threatening them, but they will usually comply with hostility. This is not motivation. Motivation is the state of wanting to do something and comes from within the individual. How do we get pharmacy employees to want to do what needs to be done? Motivation!

Employee Needs

What generally motivates employees? The answer is, rewards that satisfy various unmet needs. Such needs (in ascending order) include security, love, esteem, personal growth, achievement, responsibility, interesting and challenging work, and autonomy. Each employee will have a different set of unsatisfied needs that changes over time. The challenge for the pharmacy supervisor is to identify the unmet needs. This takes work, but it is the heart of being a good supervisor. The professional staff will generally have unmet needs at the higher level, especially esteem, professional growth, and autonomy. Managers who exert too much control will smother these needs; delegation of an appropriate responsibility with an adequate degree of support and coaching will fulfill some of these needs. Future projects are more likely to be initiated by employees who have been asked to contribute in the past. Review and recognition of their contributions and what they learned are essential parts of the process.

Other specific work-related needs include optimal elbow room, variety, feedback, maximal job meaning, support and respect, and room to grow. Attention to these needs is the essence of the Japanese model for improving efficiency, quality, and job satisfaction.

Values

Some basic values are important for everyone: respect, responsibility, consistency (fair treatment), integrity, honesty, and confidence. Each employee will hold all of these to be important, but some values will be more important than others. Supervisors must respect these basic values for all employees. Together, all six values represent dignity for the employee.

Beyond the basic values, the key to motivating employees is to examine their specific value systems. How can supervisors tell what their employees value? The answer: they probably are wearing it, driving it, living in it, spending money on it, or doing it in their free time. What is important to them? How do they relate to others? Are they independent, or do they need to associate with others much of the time?

How It Works

It is very difficult to get people to do something that serves someone else's values and needs unless they are given adequate reason to do so. The "adequate reason" must help satisfy their needs or show that there is value (to them) in doing what needs to be done. Therefore, pharmacy supervisors should think about the needs and values of the employees they supervise. Next, the supervisors must explain the value (from the employee's viewpoint) in completing the assignment. The value could be inner satisfaction (generally a need) or external rewards (generally a value).

The following example illustrates how to apply these techniques. Suppose that there is a rather tedious drug use review audit to complete. The audit will take 12 hours and will involve collecting detailed information on the overuse of tranquilizers. Select a pharmacist interested in this area, one who feels that this is a real challenge or one who wants to know more about this category of drugs. Show the pharmacist how it will help him or her, and create a "win-win" situation. What if the only available pharmacist is not interested in this project? Connect the assignment to other values. Is it possible to relieve the pharmacist of less challenging assignments, or to reward him or her (based on the pharmacist's own values and needs) for doing the assignment better than expected?

How It Does Not Work

Commitment to a pharmacy service is influenced by rewards from the work itself, compensation, benefits, the supervisor's style, growth in the job, and interaction with fellow workers. Ignoring these factors decreases morale and productivity. Demotivators contributing to this less than ideal work atmosphere include poor communication, discouragement of initiative and team spirit, neglect of rewards, "heavy-handed" policies, and lack of proper training. Symptoms of this syndrome are comments from workers such as:

"No one knows what's going on."
"Don't make waves."
"There's no way to get ahead around here."
"I had a good idea, but no one listened."
"They don't care what happens."
"Why are they doing something dumb like that."

Poor morale is a negative state of mind. Research has shown that achievement usually increases morale more often than morale increases achievement. Therefore, the key to increasing pharmacy productivity is to treat all pharmacy workers with respect and show them how getting the job done helps them achieve their values and needs.

Having Standards of Supervision

One way for a pharmacy department to consistently achieve quality supervision is to adopt standards on a consensus basis. In other words, as a department, decide what the ideal qualities of a supervisor are, then follow them. Through peer monitoring and pressure, try to hold each other accountable to the standard. Such a practice would help elevate the level of supervisory practice, employee productivity, achievement, morale, and team spirit.

Most pharmacy supervisors began as pharmacists. Pharmacists need basic skills for first-line supervision, but generally are left on their own to obtain these skills. Good performance as a pharmacist demonstrates more ability as an employee than a supervisor. The pharmacist's role has been as a player, not a captain, coach, or leader. Be sure to provide supervisory training for those who are promoted to supervisors. Share the standards with them and create an incentive for the whole management team to help the new supervisor succeed. This is frequently not an easy transition for the new supervisor, and he or she needs support and guidance.

Having Fun

Above all, it is important to have fun in the process. Why not? It makes the work much easier. Working hard and playing hard can help relieve stress and build camaraderie.

MAKING THE MAGIC WORK

Now that we have looked at job satisfaction and the roles pharmacy managers and supervisors play in making pharmacy workers feel good about themselves and their jobs, let us look at what it takes to get the work done on a day-to-day basis. How do we accomplish the end result: achieve the departmental goals and vision for a better practice?

Developing Action Plans Together

Sitting down once a year and developing a basic, yet solid, performance action plan with each employee is the key to employee and departmental success. The excuse that there is no time to do this with every employee is exactly that, an excuse. Meeting with employees and discussing the job is the very essence of effective supervision.

Although the performance action plan needs to be mutually developed, the best ideas will come from the pharmacy staff members themselves. There are four basic guidelines to follow:

1. The desired performance objectives must be set out under the major accountabilities from the pharmacy employee's job description.
2. The objectives need to focus on the end result more than on process, and many of the end results should point to major departmental goals, or, if possible, the ultimate departmental vision or "super goal."
3. The actions or objectives need to be clear, attainable, and measurable using dates, numbers, etc.
4. The performance objectives need to be mutually developed, agreed to, signed, and dated by the employee and supervisor.

In formulating the employee action plan, the supervisor should remember the unique needs and values of the employee and the needs of the department. Balancing the needs of each is the critical part of the process. In doing so, the employee pledges to work to his or her fullest capability to achieve "the expected end results," and the pharmacy supervisor pledges to help the employee be successful. There are excellent models (see bibliography) available for writing objective-focused, competency-based action plans.

Focusing on End Results and Vision

It is very easy to be consumed by day-to-day problems; however, these are just a small portion of the overall picture. Those who become bogged down by "putting out fires" will never move on to better things. The key is to doggedly resist being distracted from the main focus or vision.

Redesigning the Work

Pharmacy workers, like others, can be happy with the status quo. In many instances, the pharmacy staff will be more resistant to change than hospital administration and the medical and nursing staffs. A supervisor who redesigns the work (to move forward toward the goal) may meet resistance. However, two principles already discussed, if used properly, should minimize this problem:

1. If the departmental vision and plan have been mutually defined through open discussion and consensus, there should be little argument about what needs to be done.
2. If the individual action plans have been mutually developed, there should be little argument about who is responsible (unless the wrong person was selected initially).

Delegate decisions regarding how things will be done. Recent experiences in Japan, and now in this country, have revealed that the method is probably best determined by the employees themselves. Employees harbor tremendously important and creative ideas that need to be tapped. All they need are clear expectations, freedom to decide, and incentives (based upon their needs and values) to achieve great success. A greater democratization of the work environment has been shown to reap significant benefits. However, further study and preparation are advised before such an approach is launched, because it will mean drastic (but good) changes in the environment.

Coordinating Efforts

All efforts need to be coordinated. This is the job of the pharmacy leadership. Coordination is provided in two ways. It starts from the overall departmental vision and plan, which flows down into the action plan of each supervisor. Such downward delegation of the plan is critical to overall success. The linkage between each subsequent action plan, along with frequent checking and communication on status, orchestrates the entire process. The accountability for ensuring that the end result is properly achieved rests with the director of pharmacy.

Managing for Quality

It is becoming increasingly clear that managing only for a quality end result is not a good way to do business. The end result may be fine, but the process can be fraught with waste, inefficiency, and problems. Supervisors need to instill in the pharmacy staff the idea that "we will do it right the first time, every time." This attitude is critical to being productive and attaining goals. Supervisors must help their staff understand that better procedures and conscientious work will improve efficiency and decrease problems for everyone. Further, they must profess that this philosophy applies to everyone, and show it by being a good example.

Holding Staff Accountable

Supervisors should hold pharmacy staff accountable for their action plans, and fulfill their promise to help them be successful. They should "manage by walking around" and talking with staff to assess the progress on certain aspects of their action plans: Ask how they can help their staff, then do it. Remember, supervisors are accountable for their staff's success. If they are not successful, neither is the supervisor.

Breeding Success

There is a certain point at which the pharmacy department turns a corner and success starts coming, more in attitude at first, then eventually in movement toward a common goal. At some point it all takes off, and an air of excitement, energy, and a sense of pride will permeate the pharmacy. Suddenly challenges become fuel for future success. Such momentum seems to be derived from (1) seeing desired results, (2) working together as a true team, (3) receiving positive feedback from others—those we serve, and (4) feeling good about ourselves. Such success is contagious and breeds future success.

MANAGING FOR EMPLOYEE SUCCESS

We have been talking about supervision in general. Now we turn to the individual supervision of a single employee—the interaction that must occur between a pharmacy employee and the person to whom he or she reports.

Coaching Employees

An important part of establishing a good relationship with members of the team is developing a coaching attitude. A good coach helps each team member achieve optimum performance and reach his or her full potential, providing encouragement, inspiration, and gentle nudging to help team members do better. This attitude needs to be continual; encouragement and inspiration need to be consistently given.

Another important ingredient is feedback, mostly positive. Workers need to know their progress. They really do not know how their supervisors feel about their work unless they are told. Despite what they show on the outside, most workers need reassurance that all is well or that they need to make adjustments. It is important to be specific so that employees understand exactly how they can improve. Balancing the positive and negative is very important. Many managers focus on the negative. A good yardstick is to provide 10 positive comments for every negative one. This will go a long way toward improving the work environment.

One more point about positive comments to employees is that flattery and praise are not synonymous. Employees can detect the difference. Flattery comes from the head, and true, sincere praise comes from the heart. Most supervisors, when observing good performance, sigh, feel good, and move on without saying something nice to the person who did it. Do not let this happen.

When, where, and how should negative feedback be given? Negative, yet constructive, feedback is essential. Supervisors who do not recognize this need are probably not as effective as they can be. Correct someone as soon as possible after becoming aware of the problem. Do it when the person will be receptive to what is said, and in a place where others will not hear. No matter how serious the problem, it is essential to respect the person's dignity; therefore, all correction must be done in private. The supervisor should calmly present the facts as he or she understands them, then listen carefully. There are always two sides to every story. There may be no need to gather more facts. If the employee is clearly wrong, use a constructive teaching approach, to help minimize the power difference in the relationship and make the employee feel more at ease. Reemphasize the importance of what needs to be done and how it will serve the employee's needs. If the employee has a problem that is causing unacceptable behavior or performance, ongoing counseling may be necessary.

Managing Performance

Everyone should have a one-on-one performance review with the person to whom they report at least once each year. This is absolutely necessary to assess progress and to reward employees who are meeting or exceeding their objectives. On the other hand, saving up all positive and negative feedback to unload on the employee all at once is inappropriate. Optimally, the performance review should (1) be scheduled in advance; (2) provide an opportunity for the employee to do a "self-assessment" and think about the next year's action plan; (3) be accomplished without any interruptions; (4) be a "give and take" session; and (5) overall, be constructive. In addition, the performance review should be consistent and based on sufficient, representative, and relevant information.

If good coaching and counseling have taken place throughout the year, employees should already know where they stand and what the "formal" outcome of their performance review will be. If there are surprises, the supervisor has not done his or her job throughout the year. One good way to approach ratings is to use the written objective to hold employees accountable for their work. Another good approach is for the supervisor to ask how the employees rated themselves, then compare their response to his or her (still confidential) rating and/or those of their peers. In cases of wide variance, the employees can be asked to explain why they rated themselves the way they did, then any necessary adjustments can be made.

For poor performance, it is wise to try to identify the problem that is keeping the employee from doing well. Does the employee understand the expectation? Is the employee committed to achieving it? Does he or she know how to reach the goal? What are the barriers? If it is simply lack of commitment, the employee should be given the "yardstick"—told where he or she needs to be and is now, and that the supervisor expects the employee to achieve the objective in a given timeframe. This should be done before the actual evaluation, so the employee has time to achieve the expected result with minimal penalty.

A major portion of the evaluation should focus on the employee's new action plan. What ideas does the employee have? What is needed? What does the employee like to do? How can the supervisor help the employee do more of it? What does the employee dislike, and how can you have them do less?

To leave the performance appraisal in a positive manner, ask the pharmacy employee, "What is the one thing you did last year that makes you feel the best?" This will make the employee feel good, and will also reveal his or her value system. This step is probably where employees need to be rewarded the most, thus connecting the two important factors: work and reward.

Rewarding Employees

Employees need to be rewarded for their performance compared to the agreed-upon objectives in their action plan. Did the employee meet all of the objectives, some of them, or none of them? Did the employee exceed or far exceed them? Some managers have no merit system at their disposal to reward employees, or those who do have them need additional ways to reward exceptional performance. It is important that rewards be developed for the pharmacy employees who are doing an exceptional job. Nonmonetary rewards for pharmacy personnel include improved scheduling; continuing education opportunities; recognition; time off; favorite work; advancement; more freedom; paid professional dues; paid subscriptions to journals; prizes; fun; and personal growth. Consider each person's value system and needs, then determine an appropriate reward. Be creative and assertive. It is the supervisor's job to keep everyone moving in the same direction. Rewards are the best way to do that.

Developing Careers

The truly outstanding manager of pharmacists will go beyond basic supervision and concentrate on developing the pharmacist as a professional and as a person. In this scenario, the manager also becomes a mentor. A mentor helps a person reach his or her full potential by being intimately involved in that person's learning, growth, and development. There are several reasons for doing this: (1) That person's growth will help further the objectives of the department. (2) We should be committed to training people to further the profession. (3) That person will undoubtedly appreciate the effort, which will enhance loyalty. (4) Personal satisfaction is gained from helping someone grow.

Recently, competency-based advancement and career ladder programs have been developed in various pharmacy services. Such programs have long been overdue and can be an answer to the seemingly "dead-end job" of the staff pharmacist. Pharmacists who desire professional growth but are unable to obtain more formal education should be encouraged to pursue these career ladder programs to develop additional skills, and gain recognition and rewards.

A mentor can also help the younger pharmacist in matters of personal development, if that employee desires. Helping the pharmacists assess their strengths and weaknesses, build character and a strong ethical sense, instill virtue, and teach them how to deal appropriately with others is invaluable. Mentoring is an important strength required in pharmacy practice and education.

Counseling Employees

Effective supervision of employees involves counseling. All pharmacy supervisors must understand and accept this as a critical component of their daily responsibility. Like oil that keeps a machine running smoothly, effective employee counseling maintains a pharmacy department team and prevents the loss of responsible practitioners.

Although pharmacy supervisors must know their limits in employee counseling, they can be vigilant, sensitive, available; they can also be good listeners. The sooner problems are identified, the easier they are to solve. Pharmacy supervisors should constantly keep their eyes and ears open. Employees rarely develop problems suddenly. Most employees will use little hints, or their mood or personality will change when they are having problems. Being sensitive to these sometimes subtle changes can make a big difference. Unless the situation becomes acute, a good approach is to make sure the employee understands that the supervisor is available for discussion and support. A direct approach may scare the person, and misreading the situation can cause embarrassment. Avoid these circumstances by having an open-door policy. The employees' trust in their supervisor will be dependent on the relationship the supervisor has cultivated with them, and on his or her reputation among their peers.

Once the employee has decided to speak up, the supervisor must put all else on hold. Counsel in a manner and place that preserves the person's dignity, and listen carefully. Much has been written about the importance of listening. Active listening means giving full attention to every word; however, listening sensitively during employee counseling sessions demands even more. Some things to consider are: (1) What is the real problem? (2) What are its causes? (3) Is the employee being objective? (4) What's the other side of the story? (5) What is the emotional state of the employee? The supervisor should be attentive. Even if the supervisor is unable to provide solutions, he or she can help by listening, and allowing the person to "ventilate," and reassuring the employee that it is alright to do so. The supervisor should ask questions rather than give answers, to encourate employees to discover answers for themselves. Guaranteeing confidentiality is important.

One of the most difficult problems to counsel is employee conflicts with other employees. Do not promise the employee anything until you hear the other side of the story and consider the consequences. There will usually be some truth on both sides. Most situations should not be resolved by having someone win and someone lose. Compromises and counseling on both sides can often achieve "win-win" situations.

When counseling, the pharmacy supervisor should look for stress and burnout, especially among the professional staff and those working directly with patients, physicians, and nurses. Pharmacy directors should also observe pharmacy supervisors, who often need to fill in for staff as well as do their own job. In addition, they can become consumed by counseling other people and have no time to resolve their own difficulties. The signs and symptoms of stress and burnout are varied and are not related to specific mannerisms.

Stress management programs have proliferated. The solutions for stress and burnout vary from just lending a sympathetic ear to granting time off. Recognize stress and burnout as early as possible and deal with the actual causes rather than the symptoms. Everyone views and manages stress differently. Some things will be very stressful for one employee and not affect another. Stress management means finding ways to reduce stress or to channel it productively. Managers or supervisors must effectively handle their own stress and then help employees deal with theirs. The manager must accept the fact that a situation or event can cause stress for an individual, even if it seems insignificant from the manager's viewpoint. This demonstrates respect for the individual and acknowledges the source of the problem. Both of these must occur before the manager can assist the employee. In some situations, the manager's experience or expertise may be inadequate, and the employee should be referred for further counseling regarding stress management.

Chemical impairment of the pharmacy workforce is recognized as a potential career hazard and as a treatable condition. Sudden or continual deterioration of an employee's work habits may indicate a chemical impairment. Many excellent references are available (see bibliography) on symptoms that occur in employees who may have become chemically impaired. Some signs and symptoms include absenteeism and tardiness, decreased reliability, desire to change shifts, desire to be alone on lunch breaks, fatigue, and frequent trips to the bathroom. It is important for employees to admit their problem and to seek assistance.

Often the problem may not be the employee, but the spouse or child. This problem may hamper the pharmacy employee's work performance. Tardiness because of children or a spouse or many telephone calls to and from home may point to this problem. Pharmacy managers or supervisors need to recognize when they cannot manage the situation. Sexual harassment, financial problems, and problems with children and spouses will warrant professional counseling. Fortunately, some hospitals provide such services to their employees and family. Supervisors are obligated to know where to refer their employees and to encourage them to seek help.

DISCIPLINING EMPLOYEES

Disciplining employees is always a difficult job, but one that is needed, not only for correction, but to maintain fairness and equity on the pharmacy team. Employees will watch what is done with those who are out of line. Lack of proper discipline can cause major morale problems. Therefore, the good supervisor will always take firm but fair action whenever it is needed. Since all disciplinary action is confidential, the supervisor may be accused of being partial to some employees in spite of documentation of significant disciplinary steps. Courses are taught on this aspect of supervision, and further study is advised.

In general, several basic rules apply to disciplining when it is clear that the employee needs to be corrected. (1) Discipline in a discreet place. (2) State that the matter has been thoroughly investigated. (3) Ensure that the employee knows exactly why he or she is being disciplined. (4) Clearly define expectations with regard to future behavior. (5) Convey that it is the behavior, rather than the person, that is the problem; allow the employee an opportunity to save face. (6) Secure the employee's agreement to change. (7) Let the employee know he or she will be observed and given feedback on progress. (8) Leave the session on a good note (e.g., shake hands).

After the employee leaves, it is important for the supervisor to document the session from his or her point of view using "anecdotal notes." Future discipline resulting from lack of progress will need documentation and the signature of both parties to indicate that the counseling session occurred; this documentation is placed in the employee's permanent employee file. Without such documentation, it may be difficult to dismiss undesirable employees, thus keeping the pharmacy from being the vibrant, dynamic department that it can be. Further reading (see bibliography) on applying progressive discipline to achieve satisfactory employee performance is advised.

The majority of employees want to succeed but must clearly understand what is expected of them and have the knowledge to meet the challenge. The pharmacy supervisor must provide specific, consistent feedback, both positive and negative, to help employees reach this goal.

SUMMARY

Being a good pharmacy manager involves managing people exceptionally well. People make pharmacy programs great. There is no magic to managing people, but believing in them, coaching them, and helping them believe in themselves will provide an excellent foundation. Seldom is there more satisfaction than in helping people achieve more than they thought possible. This is a key role of the pharmacy manager.

BIBLIOGRAPHY

Leadership

Banderev KP: The emerging leader. *Top Hosp Pharm Mgt* 6:41-45, 1986.

Bennis W: *Why Leaders Can't Lead.* San Francisco, Jossey-Bass Publishers, 1989.

Calkin JD: Leadership and the effective pharmacy manager. *Top Hosp Pharm Mgt* 3:64-71, 1983.

Crosby PB: *Quality without tears.* New York, McGraw-Hill Book Co, 1984.

Hickman CR, Silva MA: *Creating excellence.* New American Library, 1984.

Lee MP: Leadership. *Top Hosp Pharm Mgt* 6:35-40, 1986.

Innovative Management Organization

Ackoff RL: The circular organization: An update. *Academy of Management Executive* III:11-16, 1989.

Management Styles

Boissoneau R: The democratically oriented pharmacy manager. *Top Hosp Pharm Mgt* 4:44-51, 1984.

Boyd M: How to really talk to another person. *Parade Magazine* 1989, pp 14-15.

Kafka VW, Schaefer JH: *Open management.* San Francisco, CA, Alchemy Books, 1975.

Peters TJ, Waterman RH Jr: *In Search of Excellence.* New York, Harper and Row, Inc., 1982.

Smith TR, Grace M: The pharmacy manager as communicator: Part II, Verbal and nonverbal communication. *Top Hosp Pharm Mgt* 3:50-63, 1983.

Job Satisfaction

Amirjahed AK, Bonser WD: Staff pharmacists' job attitudes and job performance. *Am J Hosp Pharm* 40:1198-1202, 1983.

Meyer T: Job satisfaction for supportive personnel. *Top Hosp Pharm Mgt* 5:45-51, 1985.

Quandt WG, McKercher PL, Miller DA: Job content and pharmacists' job attitude. *Am J Hosp Pharm* 39:275-279, 1982.

Rickert DR: Job design for hospital pharmacists. *Top Hosp Pharm Mgt* 7:12-17, 1987.

Stewart JE: Hospital pharmacists' job satisfaction: A review of the data. *Top Hosp Pharm Mgt* 3:1-9, 1983.

Managing People

Anon: Managing professional staff. *Management Today* (June):111-112, 1984.

Chase P: Ten nonmonetary motivators. *Top Hosp Pharm Mgt* 5:7-18, 1985.

Fichtl RE, Wilson SK, Miederhoff PA: Toward a model for the management of clinical pharmacists. *Top Hosp Pharm Mgt* 7:38-44, 1987.

Frohman AL: Mismatch problems in managing professionals. *Research Mgt* 21:20-25, 1987.

Hepler CD, Segal R: Motivating pharmacy personnel: A managerial framework. *Top Hosp Pharm Mgt* 3:10-36, 1983.

Lebell D: Managing professionals: The quiet conflict. *Personnel Mgt* 59:566-572, 584, 1980.

Lee PM: Everything comes down to people. *Top Hosp Pharm Mgt* 5:1-5, 1985.

Manning SH: Demotivation of the pharmacy technician: A preventative approach. *Top Hosp Pharm Mgt* 4:19-29, 1984.

Radica B: Managing professionals: A theoretical guide to understanding work relations. *The Dental Assistant* (July/Aug):29-30, 1988.

Smith JE, Phillips DJM: Human resource management in hospital pharmacy. *Top Hosp Pharm Mgt* 5:1-11, 1985.

Steinmetz LL, Todd HR: *First-line management—approaching supervision effectively.* Dallas, Business Publications, Inc., 1979.

White SJ, Generali JA: Motivating pharmacy employees. *Am J Hosp Pharm* 41:1361-1366, 1984.

White SJ: Personnel management for hospital pharmacists. *Am J Hosp Pharm* 41:318-319, 1984.

Coaching and Counseling Employees

Appelbaum SH: Coping with stress: Strategies for the pharmacy manager. *Top Hosp Pharm Mgt* 2:1-9, 1983.

Kendall JD: The chemically impaired pharmacist: The right approach. *Top Hosp Pharm Mgt* 7:84-92, 1987.

Miederhoff PA, Voight FB, White CE, et al: Chemically impaired pharmacists: An emerging management issue. *Top Hosp Pharm Mgt* 7:75-83, 1987.

White SJ, Scott BE: Progressive discipline. *Am J Hosp Pharm* 41:1824-1828, 1984.

Performance Management

Bair J: Peer evaluation of pharmacists' performance. *Top Hosp Pharm Mgt* 3:39-47, 1985.

Coarse JF, Kubica AJ: Objective-focused approach for appraising the performance of institutional pharmacists. *Am J Hosp Pharm* 36:1676-1682, 1979.

Guinn K: Performance management: Not just an annual appraisal. *Training Magazine* (Aug):39-42, 1987.

Ross SR: Developing performance appraisal systems. *Am J Hosp Pharm* 41:1567-1573, 1984.

Schneider PJ, Dzierba SH: Competency-based employee advancement. *Top Hosp Pharm Mgt* 3:37-45, 1983.

Schneider PJ, Fudge RP, Hafner PE, et al: Competency-based advancement program for pharmacists. *Am J Hosp Pharm* 38:1331-1334, 1981.

Smith SP, Speranza KA: Performance appraisal in New England hosp. pharmacy practice. *Top Hosp Pharm Mgt* 7:45-74, 1987.

Career Development

Boissoneau R: The developmental needs of subordinates. *Top Hosp Pharm Mgt* 5:13-17, 1985.

Gordon DW, Rich DS, Mahoney CD, et al: Human resources management and career development: A shared responsibility. *Top Hosp Pharm Mgt* 6:74-79, 1986.

Jefferson KK, Crane VS: Developing a pharmacy clinical career ladder. *Top Hosp Pharm Mgt* 6:80-84, 1986.

Meyer JD, Chrymko MM, Kelly WN: Clinical career ladders: Hamot Medical Center. *Am J Hosp Pharm* 46:2268-2271, 1989.

CHAPTER 15

Workload Analysis and Productivity Measurement

ANDREW L. WILSON

The provision of care by hospitals changed dramatically during the 1980's. Health maintenance organizations (HMO's), preferred provider organizations (PPO's), and the Federal and State governments sought to reduce expanding health care costs through fixed reimbursement to hospitals. In the past, hospitals passed on the increasing cost of salaries, equipment, drugs, and new technology through increased charges for care. Hospitals now seek to remain vital, growing organizations by seeking to contract with HMO's, PPO's, governments, and other entities by providing care at a cost less than the fixed fee from the HMO, PPO, or government. A hospital stay can be provided at this lower cost through continuing scrutiny of resources used to provide care. Methods to reduce costs include contracting for drugs and supplies, limiting salary costs, and critically analyzing delivery systems and services provided by the hospital.

Hospital pharmacy managers are a part of the continuing need to review and reduce the cost of providing health care services. Hospital pharmacy managers participate in this cost review process through a number of methods. Managing the productivity of the pharmacy department is a strategy through which a pharmacy manager can understand the cost and consumption of resources used to provide pharmacy services. An effective system for monitoring the productivity of the department allows the manager to take action and make changes in the delivery of services and consumption of resources, to improve efficiency, effectiveness, and quality of pharmaceutical care, and to monitor the effect of these changes on the cost of providing care. A productive pharmacy department is efficient and effective. Its staff wastes a minimum of time and resources in accomplishing its work.

Measurement and assessment of productivity do not establish the value of the activity performed. Managing a pharmacy to improve productivity does not determine the appropriateness of a service. Productivity measures describe operational changes to maximize the conversion of pharmacist and technician time (input) into services (output). The term "cost effective" is incorrectly used as a substitute for the term "productivity." Cost-effectiveness implies an assessment of the monetary or other value to the patient, hospital, or society. Cost-effectiveness implies that the cost is satisfactory for the results, or that the balance between the two is acceptable. Productivity and workload measures are concerned with aspects of this balance, but they do not determine the value of a service, merely the efficiency of its delivery. It is important to establish the need for or value of an activity or service independent of productivity analysis.

DEFINING PRODUCTIVITY

A specific, single definition for the term "productivity" cannot be given. Productivity can be described in many ways; in financial terms, it is the relationship between a product or service and the costs of salary, equipment, material, and other resources consumed to produce it. Productivity may also be described in terms of increased product or service output, or as a decrease in work time or money spent to produce the same output. The measurement of productivity is not an exact science. The specific measure of the productivity of a pharmacy department is a combination of the *science* of data collection and analysis and the *management art* of determining appropriate ratios and indicators to describe the results of the pharmacy's work to administrators, physicians, pharmacy staff, and others.

A broader definition of productivity is suggested by Hepler,[1] who describes productivity as the relationship between the resources consumed by an activity (input) and the goods and services produced by the activity (output). Because a hospital pharmacy service and its personnel perform a variety of tasks, the productivity of an individual pharmacist, pharmacy service, or entire pharmacy department can be described in a number of ways.

Choich[2] has concisely defined productivity as the relationship described in the ratio:

$$\text{Productivity} = \frac{\text{Output}}{\text{Input}}$$

Based on this description of the relationship, changes in productivity can occur in a number of ways:

- Output changes with no change in input;
- Output changes at a faster rate than input;
- Input changes with no change in output; and
- Input changes at a faster rate than output.

The net change in productivity, either positive or negative, is the result of the equation above. Positive changes or increases in productivity result from higher levels of output in relation to input, while decreases in productivity result from decreased levels of output in relation to input. Productivity is always described as a ratio between input and output. The particular ratio is selected or developed by a pharmacy manager based on his or her needs or the needs of the hospital to define work output and resource consumption.

DEVELOPING PRODUCTIVITY RATIOS

Managing for increased productivity requires the development of indicators that reflect changes in important individual components of the pharmacy operation, but that can also be synthesized into an overall view of the pharmacy's productivity. These indicators must be meaningful to pharmacy department managers and staff, and to senior management of the hospital or health care institution. Typically, a ratio or group of ratios is used. Sample ratios from the American Society of Hospital Pharmacists' PharmaTrend productivity system are listed in table 15-1.

Ratios used to describe productivity are of two types. *Total* or *macro* ratios are used to express the productivity of the entire pharmacy department. Ratios used to describe the productivity of a specific pharmacy service or area of the pharmacy are defined as *partial* ratios. An example of a total ratio is a hospital's calculation of its profitability by reviewing all expense and revenue for a quarter or year:

$$\text{Profitability} = \frac{\text{Revenue (\$)}}{\text{Expenses (\$)}}$$

An example of a partial ratio used by a pharmacy to evaluate productivity is doses dispensed per patient day for a month or quarter:

$$\text{Productivity} = \frac{\text{Doses}}{\text{Patient days}}$$

If this partial ratio increases over the course of several months or quarters, it suggests an increasing patient acuity, or more aggressive medical treatment of patients. The pharmacy manager may wish to perform a drug use evaluation review, or look at purchasing patterns or other ratios to determine a suitable course of action. Hospital pharmacy managers typically develop total productivity ratios by assembling the information used to calculate the partial ratios.

The absolute value of a ratio has little or no meaning. Productivity analysis consists of comparing the values of ratios or groups of ratios over time to quantify changes in the environment and to assess management actions. An absolute standard value for a ratio is generally determined after reviewing both industry averages (e.g., PharmaTrend) and the actual experience of the individual hospital pharmacy.

A productivity ratio can vary from a target or expected value for a number of reasons. In addition to a real change in the operation of the pharmacy, a ratio can experience random and systematic variations. Random variation occurs when an item is counted incorrectly or when numbers are transposed because data are entered or manipulated in the productivity system. Systematic error occurs when the individual or machine that counts the data item routinely provides a number that is inaccurate by a consistent factor. For example, a computer may routinely underreport or overreport doses dispensed by 10 percent as a result of credits made in patient bills rather than pharmacy dispensing records.

Table 15-1. PharmaTrend productivity ratios

Revenue Monitors
- Total revenue/Pharmacy patient day
- Total revenue/Admission
- Total revenue/Total drug distribution work unit
- Outpatient revenue percentage

Cost Monitors
- Total drug cost/Pharmacy patient day
- Total fluid cost/Pharmacy patient day
- Total other cost/Pharmacy patient day
- Total salary cost/Pharmacy patient day
- Total direct cost/Pharmacy patient day
- Total direct cost/Admission
- Cost-to-revenue percentage
- Salary cost/Total cost

Drug Distribution Monitors
- Total drug distribution work units/Pharmacy patient day
- Total drug distribution work units/Total drug distribution work hours
- Total drug cost/Total drug distribution work units
- Total fluid cost/Total drug distribution work units
- Total other cost/Total drug distribution work units
- Total salary cost/Total drug distribution work units
- Total direct cost/Total drug distribution work units
- Support drug distribution work hours/Total drug distribution work units
- Pharmacist drug distribution work hours/Total drug distribution work units
- Total drug distribution work hours/Total drug distribution work units
- Support-pharmacist drug distribution work hours ratio
- Total drug distribution salary cost/Total drug distribution work units
- Total drug distribution salary cost/Pharmacy patient day
- Drug distribution productivity index

Clinical Service Monitors
- Clinical service work units/Pharmacy patient day
- Clinical service work units/Admission
- Clinical work hours/Total pharmacist work hours
- Clinical salary cost/Pharmacy patient day
- Clinical salary cost/Clinical service work units
- Clinical productivity index

Research Monitors
- Research work units/Pharmacy patient day
- Research work units/Admission
- Research work hours/Total pharmacist work hours
- Research salary cost/Pharmacy patient day
- Research salary cost/Research work units
- Research productivity index

Education Monitors
- Education work hours/Pharmacy patient day
- Education work hours/Total work hours
- Education salary cost/Pharmacy patient day

Management Support Monitors
- Management support work hours/Pharmacy patient day
- Management support work hours/Total work hours
- Management support salary cost/Pharmacy patient day
- Support staff work hours/Pharmacist work hours

As a result of these two factors, productivity ratios may vary somewhat even when the actual productivity of the department remains unchanged. Pharmacy managers and hospital administrators generally agree upon an acceptable range of variance for each ratio, that is, a range of values for the ratio where the likelihood of the change resulting from chance is greater than the possibility that the new value represents a real change in pharmacy operations.

Management actions to change productivity taken by a pharmacy manager primarily comprise the control of inputs rather than outputs. A pharmacy input consists of the resources consumed to provide services: the cost of drugs, supplies, and salaries. A pharmacy output or service is the delivery of a medication, intravenous fluid, a pharmacokinetic consult, or another clinical service. The ability of a pharmacy manager to substantially increase or decrease the demand for services (output) is limited in comparison to the effect that he or she can have on resources consumed (input). As a result, most pharmacy management activities to improve productivity are focused on making better use of manpower, equipment, and supplies to meet output demands effectively.

A productivity or workload measurement system involves three elements: (1) identifying measurable input and output, (2) monitoring the ratio of output to input as an indicator of productivity, and (3) making management decisions and taking action based on the information provided by the changes in ratios over time. A hospital pharmacy department's output is the result of a combination of staff and supply input, and a mixture of both product and service output. Productivity itself is not managed, but improved productivity results from the effective review of resources used to create products and services, when combined with management action.

DETERMINING THE PURPOSE TO BE MET BY MEASURING PRODUCT PRODUCTIVITY

Developing an effective productivity measurement system requires initial analysis and planning. First, the pharmacy manager must determine the specific purposes to be served by measuring the productivity of the pharmacy service in his or her hospital. A pharmacy manager may want to measure productivity as a result of (1) a change in number of patients; (2) a change in patient case mix or acuity; (3) requirements for different services or increased output from the pharmacy; (4) a mandate from senior hospital management to improve pharmacy productivity; (5) a focus by pharmacy management on problem areas of expenditure or resource consumption; or (6) loss of pharmacy manpower or other resources available in previous years.

The data collected and ratios used are unique to each pharmacy. PharmaTrend, MoniTrend, and other packaged systems provide a representative group of ratios used consistently throughout all hospitals. Productivity ratios used in an individual hospital pharmacy may be selected from the standard ratios and developed from other information collected in the pharmacy or hospital. The specific ratios used to represent pharmacy productivity do depend on the nature of the productivity problems being addressed, on the type of information available, and on the agreements reached between the pharmacy manager and hospital administration.

SELECTING WORKLOAD INFORMATION TO COLLECT

The workload information collected should focus on indicators of pharmacy activity, both output and input. Each data element should be selected to indicate the volume or quantity of a particular item, and may be expressed in terms of time, dollars, units of service, doses, or any other relevant measure. The goal of measuring and managing productivity is not to passively measure activity, but to develop information that communicates a valid indication of the activity of the pharmacy and provides meaningful information to managers and workers, thereby allowing them to make changes in the workplace to achieve greater output for each unit of input.

The PharmaTrend manual[3] provides an exhaustive list of the information that can be collected. The workload data collected should define information, which allows managers and staff to modify the use of time and consumption of resources (input) and provision of drug products and clinical services (output) by the pharmacy. Indiscriminate collection of large amounts of data will lead to detailed, comprehensive indices of the performance of the pharmacy service, but it will require large amounts of time and effort to maintain the program itself. An ideal productivity measurement program requires limited resources to collect and review data, while providing accurate, timely, and complete information. Table 15-2 lists data elements required by PharmaTrend.

Two methods are used to set information collection priorities. First, the largest contributors of input and output are preferred over smaller contributors. For example, unit doses issued and intravenous piggybacks prepared define a greater amount of a hospital pharmacy's distributive productivity than extemporaneous compounding of dermatologicals. However, the pharmacy manager must also collect information on smaller contributors critical to the hospital or department, including high-visibility clinical pharmacy activities such as pharmacokinetic consults or code blue responses. Clinical services are often ignored in the development of productivity analysis systems. A second method that can be used to determine information collection priorities at this point is an examination of the availability of data. Data that are easily retrieved from pharmacy computer systems, and other management reports, can easily be added to productivity systems.

Examples of easily retrievable data include manpower statistics collected routinely by the payroll or personnel department, information on drug purchases and revenue generated by the pharmacy and collected by the hospital accounting department, and patient stay and census statistics collected by the admitting department. This type of information, particularly when collected as a byproduct of computer data processing, provides a reliable stream of consistent data to use in reviewing simple indices of pharmacy productivity.

Computerized data collection is always preferred because of its consistency and accuracy. In addition, it requires little or no work to maintain after the initial development. Manual systems for collecting data always take a back seat to service duties and are subject to interobserver variability, and even outright fabrication.[4]

Acquiring information from other hospital departments and from reports and information generated by the pharmacy on a systematic basis allows the pharmacy manager and staff to develop a broad understanding of the relationship between input and output. During the initial development of this information collection system, this relationship may not be well defined and managed, but the collection and review of this information will demonstrate the usual swings in productivity by describing the relationship between changes in input and output. This information will also serve as a baseline for reviewing changes in productivity as management changes are made.

It is important to maintain a consistent approach to data collection and analysis. The required result of a productivity measurement system is month-to-month, quarterly, and yearly comparisons of productivity measures. The addition and subtraction of data elements will make the internal variation in the system large enough to disguise the true variations in productivity.

A scientifically valid, 100-percent accurate system is not necessarily the result of the development process. The goal is a workable system that is not time consuming to maintain, but is sensitive to changes in product and service output and resource consumption by the pharmacy service. A functioning data collection and analysis system will provide the ability to assess:

- The workload demands placed on the pharmacy;
- The amount of time (input) spent on various departmental activities (e.g., distributive, management, and clinical functions);
- The actual costs of providing the various components of comprehensive pharmacy services;
- An index of the pharmacy's productivity; and
- The relationship of the information listed above to previous reporting periods.[2]

Through the continued use of the productivity measurement system, the pharmacy manager can assess the impact of changes in pharmacy staffing, hospital census, patient load and acuity, and other external factors on the pharmacy. A productivity measurement system is not a predictive tool, although a well-tuned, functioning system can allow concurrent and even prospective review of productivity.

It is necessary to use hospital-collected information on expenses, revenue, and manpower. Data collected outside of the pharmacy have one advantage over internally collected data: external credibility. This is not important for most aspects of the data collected for productivity review, since the primary goal of productivity analysis is to facilitate management changes within the pharmacy. Substituting internally developed data for these three areas — expenses, revenues, and manpower — in calculations creates two problems. First, it is not perceived as more accurate by hospital management in areas such as personnel or accounting. Second, the data developed by the pharmacy will not move in concert with changes described by hospital data. This disconnects the pharmacy productivity system from the hospital information system, and may even confuse pharmacy managers and staff.

In collecting data and developing ratios, standard definitions should be used within the hospital to define data elements, particularly those used for manpower and work hours. The use of standard definitions will also allow comparison of the department's statistics to national norms and workload statistics.

The basis of the productivity measurement system is the collection of information for use in the operational management of the pharmacy department. A second and equally important concern is reporting productivity measurement data to the administrator and other managers in the hospital.

Table 15-2. PharmaTrend data elements

Work Hours
- Pharmacist work hours — Drug distribution
- Pharmacist work hours — Clinical
- Pharmacist work hours — Education
- Pharmacist work hours — Research
- Pharmacist work hours — Management support
- Support staff work hours — Drug distribution
- Support staff work hours — Education
- Support staff work hours — Management support

General Statistics
- Admissions
- Inpatient days
- Transfers

Direct Costs and Revenue
- Drug costs
- Fluid costs
- Pharmacist salaries and benefits
- Support staff salaries and benefits
- Outpatient revenue
- Inpatient revenue

Clinical Interventions
- Patient care encounters
- Pharmacokinetic consults
- Chart review
- Cardiopulmonary resuscitation episodes
- Patient care rounds
- Pharmacist/Physician/Nurse information encounter
- Drug utilization review
- Nutrition support consult
- Conference lecture
- Inservice education
- Reference search — Oral
- Reference search — Written
- Pharmacy newsletter issues
- Drug information consults

Research Activities
- Research protocols initiated
- Research protocols maintained
- Research protocols audited and closed
- Investigational review board protocol review
- Protocol drug unit disbursement
- Protocol drug unit transfer/mailout

Drug Distribution Activities
- Outpatient prescription
- Sample prescription
- Over-the-counter prescription
- Compounded prescription
- Bulk compounded/repackaged batch
- Patient floor stock line item
- Unit floor stock line item
- Intradepartmental stock replacement
- Extemporaneously packaged unit dose
- Extemporaneously compounded item
- Noncompounded large-volume parenteral
- Compounded large-volume parenteral
- Time demand small-volume parenteral
- Batch prepared small-volume parenteral
- Cancer chemotherapy medication
- Parenteral nutrition formulation
- Unit dose/bulk medication
- Enteral formula
- Controlled substance issues

REPORTING PRODUCTIVITY INFORMATION

All hospitals have some type of management reporting system for costs, revenue, and manpower. Often these systems do not attempt to look at productivity on a department level. They commonly focus on overall indicators of performance for a department or group of departments, and often place pharmacy at a disadvantage because of its preponderance of supply cost over personnel cost. The system chosen or developed by a pharmacy manager should take advantage of current reporting systems, and should supplement the information already provided to hospital management.

Appropriately used productivity information can serve as an internal public relations tool in the hospital. A productivity measurement system has not lived up to its expectations if it is not used to review the performance of the pharmacy by hospital management. The indicator or indicators supplied will have to compete with those currently used in each of these areas.

The development of the portion of the program that addresses extradepartmental reporting needs is a negotiation process with the recipients of the information. Their needs or desires for information must be balanced with the complexity and labor involved in the data collection, collation, and analysis processes. The level of detail requested and the method for presenting the information are also of critical importance. A hospital administrator may wish to see only one or two global indicators of pharmacy productivity, or may require a detailed analysis of all or a portion of the pharmacy's activity. Depending on the focus of the institution, there may be a greater emphasis on financial indicators of productivity, or perhaps on indicators that reflect the level of use of pharmacy manpower. In some institutions, it may be necessary to document resources consumed and productivity by project, by product line, or even by diagnosis-related group (DRG) or diagnosis.

A major focus of productivity review in departments of pharmacy has been review of systems and indicators by outside audit firms or consultants. A well-designed work measurement system can assist in a positive outcome from an audit. An effective productivity measurement system helps in managing the pharmacy efficiently, and can be used to review and perhaps refute numbers and indicators prepared by a consultant. A poorly designed or incomplete productivity measurement system can be worse than no system at all. The system must measure clinical as well as distributive output. Data collection methods must be clean and efficient, and the results must use management reports and information generated by the financial, personnel, and general management systems of the hospital. Clinical functions are difficult to document; if manpower is documented but clinical workload is not, the pharmacy will appear less productive.

Developing a productivity measurement and management system requires careful thought and planning. Figure 15-1 illustrates the entire process of data element selection as described here. Determining what data to collect is a straightforward task when the goals of the system have been enumerated and reviewed by the pharmacy manager, hospital administrator, and the pharmacy staff.

Productivity Analysis System Development

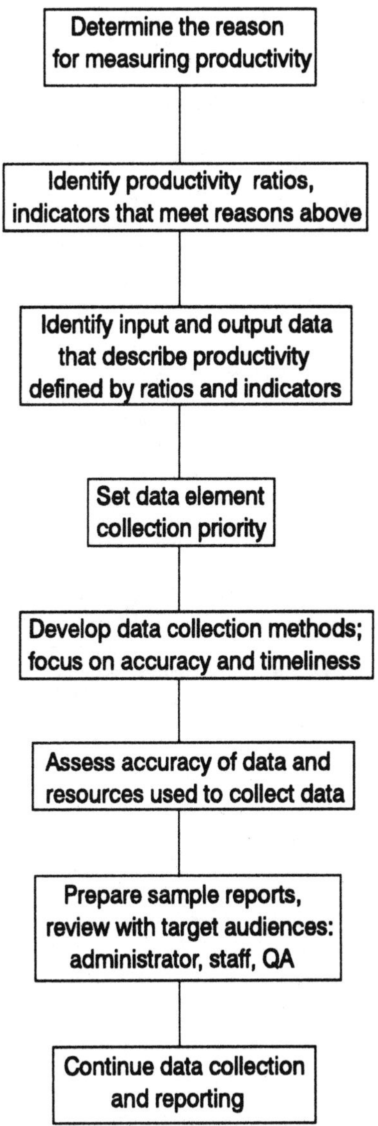

Figure 15-1. Data element selection process

The goal of this process is to create a system that is complete enough to reflect the entire range of work of the pharmacy, and is also sensitive to changes in the work output and resource consumption by the pharmacy. A judgment of the value of each activity is not a function of a productivity measurement system. The system should focus on accurate and timely documentation of resources consumed to provide pharmacy service output. Most productivity measurement systems fail based on the effort needed to collect and collate data. A critical review of the need to collect each data element, along with a consistent automated approach should provide timely and useful information. Finally, it is necessary to connect the productivity measurement system to information generated by the hospital financial, personnel, and general management systems. This will ensure the usefulness of the information in budget and service review, and in evaluations of the pharmacy by external auditors.

REFERENCES

1. Hepler CD: A primer on productivity. *Top Hosp Pharm Mgt* 1:55-68, 1981.
2. Choich R: Productivity: A managerial reality. *Top Hosp Pharm Mgt* 7:23-31, 1987.
3. PharmaTrend Advisory Group: *PharmaTrend Users Manual.* Bethesda, MD, American Society of Hospital Pharmacists, 1987.
4. Siegel J, Geier T: Workload monitoring systems for clinical pharmacy services. *Top Hosp Pharm Mgt* 7:33-48, 1987.

ADDITIONAL READING

Adams C, Tuck BA, Hunt ML: Departmental productivity reporting through computerized systems. *Top Hosp Pharm Mgt* 2:47-54, 1982.

Adams RC: PharmaTrend as a management tool: Evaluation of the program. *Am J Hosp Pharm* 46:2012-2014, 1989.

Choich R: Relationship of productivity analysis to departmental cost-accounting systems. *Am J Hosp Pharm* 45:1103-1110, 1988.

Cooper SL, Zaske DE: Seasonal variation in pharmacy work load: Implication for personnel projections. *Am J Hosp Pharm* 45:1905-1906, 1988.

Cooper SL, Zaske DE: Relationship between intensity of hospital services and work load. *Am J Hosp Pharm* 44:2267-2271, 1987.

Day DL, Mason M, Reeme PD: Using a nursing work load index to validate hospital pharmacy productivity. *Am J Hosp Pharm* 43:909-912, 1986.

Gary FK, Placko JS: Collecting IV work load data. *Am J Hosp Pharm* 43:1914, 1985.

Gouveia WA, Anderson ER, Decker EL, et al: Design and implementation of a cost accounting system in hospital pharmacy. *Am J Hosp Pharm* 45:613-620, 1988.

Hadsall RS, Gourley DR, Haggerty JA, et al: Work sampling in contemporary pharmacy practice: A multidimensional approach. *Top Hosp Pharm Mgt* 2:15-16, 1982.

Hand DL, Haas BD: PharmaTrend as a management tool: Experience with the program. *Am J Hosp Pharm* 46:2014-2018, 1989.

Hatfield SM, Alessi LS, Brown TN, el al: Documenting work load to better integrate clinical and distributive services. *Am J Hosp Pharm* 42:2175-2179, 1985.

Kienle PC: PharmaTrend as a management tool: Capturing workload data. *Am J Hosp Pharm* 46:2014-2015, 1989.

Kirschenbaum BE, Cacace L, Anderson RJ, et al: Personnel time and preparation costs for compounded versus premixed intravenous admixtures in three community hospitals. *Am J Hosp Pharm* 45:605-608, 1988.

Kubica AJ: Quantifying work load. *Am J Hosp Pharm* 44:2263, 1987.

Kvancz DA, Cummins BA, Bennett DL, et al: Evaluating pharmacist workload activities: Centralized versus mobile decentralized pharmacy service. *Top Hosp Pharm Mgt* 2:50-59, 1982.

Lundgren LM, Daniels CE: Patient acuity indicators as predictors of pharmacy work load. *Am J Hosp Pharm* 43:2453-2459, 1986.

Moss RL, Henderson RP, Burke JM, et al: Documenting the activities of clinical pharmacists. *Am J Hosp Pharm* 45:621-622, 1988.

Rascati KL, Kimberlin CL, Foley PT, et al: Multidimensional work sampling to evaluate the effects of computerization in an outpatient pharmacy. *Am J Hosp Pharm* 44:2060-2070, 1987.

Rascati KL, Kimberlin CL, McCormick WC: Work measurement in pharmacy research. *Am J Hosp Pharm* 43:2445-2452, 1986.

Reeme PD, Day DL: Number of patient days poor pharmacy work load predictor. *Am J Hosp Pharm* 42:2422-2430, 1985.

Roberts MJ, Kvalseth TO, Jermstad RL: Work management in hospital pharmacy. *Top Hosp Pharm Mgt* 2:1-17, 1982.

Robertson JA: Multidimensional work sampling: New tool for pharmacy management. *Top Hosp Pharm Mgt* 2:18-24, 1982.

Sebastian G, Thielke T: Work analysis of an IV admixture service. *Am J Hosp Pharm* 40:2150-2153, 1983.

Siegel J, Schneider PJ, Moore TD: Innovative scheduling to maintain clinical pharmacy services despite budget retrenchment. *Am J Hosp Pharm* 41:291-293, 1984.

Smith JE, Schaeffer SL, Meyer GE, et al: Pharmacy component of a hospital end-product cost accounting system. *Am J Hosp Pharm* 45:835-843, 1988.

Stirm EL, Thielke T: PharmaTrend as a management tool: Implementation in a university hospital. *Am J Hosp Pharm* 46:2019-2022, 1989.

Stolar MH: National test of a hospital pharmacy management information system. *Am J Hosp Pharm* 40:1914-1919, 1983.

Stolar MH: Description of an experimental hospital pharmacy management information system. *Am J Hosp Pharm* 40:1905-1913, 1983.

Strandberg LR, Smith MC, Sanger JM: Method for comparing hospital pharmacy staffing patterns. *Top Hosp Pharm Mgt* 2:27-39, 1982.

Thielke TS, Charlson JT, Heckethorn D: Determining drug dispensing costs for use in cost accounting systems. *Am J Hosp Pharm* 45:844-847, 1988.

Vinson BE: Adjustments of distributive and clinical pharmacy services to financial constraints. *Am J Hosp Pharm* 45:847-851, 1988.

Wellman GS, Schneider PJ, Smith GL: Activity analysis of decentralized pharmacists in a unit dose dispensing and drug administration program. *Am J Hosp Pharm* 43:1699-1702, 1986.

Wilson AL: PharmaTrend as a management tool: Introduction. *Am J Hosp Pharm* 46:2009-2012, 1989.

CHAPTER 16

Computer Technology

DAVID C. WORDELL

INTRODUCTION

In the 1960's, the first hospital pharmacy computer systems were being developed and implemented. These systems were slow, relatively cumbersome to use, and in general were crude by today's standards. Initially the growth of pharmacy systems was slow; however, as minicomputers and more powerful mainframe computers became available, the pace of development and implementation increased. In the 1970's, the pharmacy computer system industry was fairly well divided in the use of mainframes versus minicomputers. In the late 1970's, the introduction of personal computers (PC's) sent shock waves through the data processing departments and the entire computer industry. When everyone could have the power of a computer on his or her desk, the extreme dependence on the hospital data processing staff declined. In the 1980's, the number of personal computers used in hospitals increased, the power and storage capacity increased, and powerful word-processing, spreadsheet, data base, and communications software became commonplace. Another technological development that further increased the utility of personal computers was the introduction of local area networks. Although these early networks were slow by today's standards, they offered an affordable means to efficiently share data and peripherals such as printers among several PC's. Today PC's are many times more powerful than some of the mainframes and minicomputers on which the early pharmacy software was developed.

HOSPITAL PHARMACY COMPUTER SYSTEMS

The pharmacy computer systems in use today have been developed to run on mainframes, minicomputers, and microcomputers. The difference among these three types of computers is primarily related to the overall data throughput and multiuser and multitasking capabilities (defined below). Mainframe computers are generally expensive, large, and designed to handle simultaneously the processing, storage, and printing needs of a large number of users. These units typically require an environmentally stable location, a carefully filtered power source, and a commensurate support staff. Minicomputers are similar to mainframe computers but are designed for fewer users. These units are lower in cost, physically smaller, and may not require the same degree of environmental control. Smaller minicomputers may also be located within a department rather than in a central site as with large minicomputers or mainframes. Personal computers are the computers typically located on or alongside a user's desk. They are designed to run single-user applications such as word processing, spreadsheets, and data bases. Innovations in software and hardware have enabled PC's to run simultaneously several applications (multitasking) or share resources among several users (multiuser operating systems or local area networks).

Technological advances in hardware, especially with PC's, have resulted in increasingly smaller yet more powerful computers. The newest generation of PC's is in many respects more powerful than minicomputers and in some cases begins to rival mainframes. The functionality of the various systems has progressed from batch entry of pharmacy charges to interactive systems that maintain patient demographic information, medication profiles, drug use histories, and charge histories. Many systems perform drug-drug, drug-disease, and drug-allergy checking, intravenous (IV) compatibility verification, dose range checking, as well as numerous other functions.

Computerization within the pharmacy also includes substantial use of personal computers for management functions such as budgeting and expense tracking, for clinical practice such as performing pharmacokinetic calculations and literature retrieval, for bulk drug preparation through label generation or various process control devices such as unit dose strip packaging machines or IV solution pumps. Other technologies that are in use or can be implemented include bar coding, touch-sensitive screens, optical storage, light pens, optical character readers, voice recognition, automated process control devices, and computer resource sharing through local area networks.

A full-featured, well-implemented pharmacy computer system is often the backbone of a pharmacy's information processing capabilities. As shown in figure 16-1, a pharmacy system comprises several primary modules, which are inpatient order entry, outpatient prescription processing, inventory control, and secondary modules such as narcotic control (if not a part of inpatient order entry), and investigational drug tracking. Each of these modules receives, processes, stores, and "outputs" data in different ways. Input or information entered from a keyboard or received from a

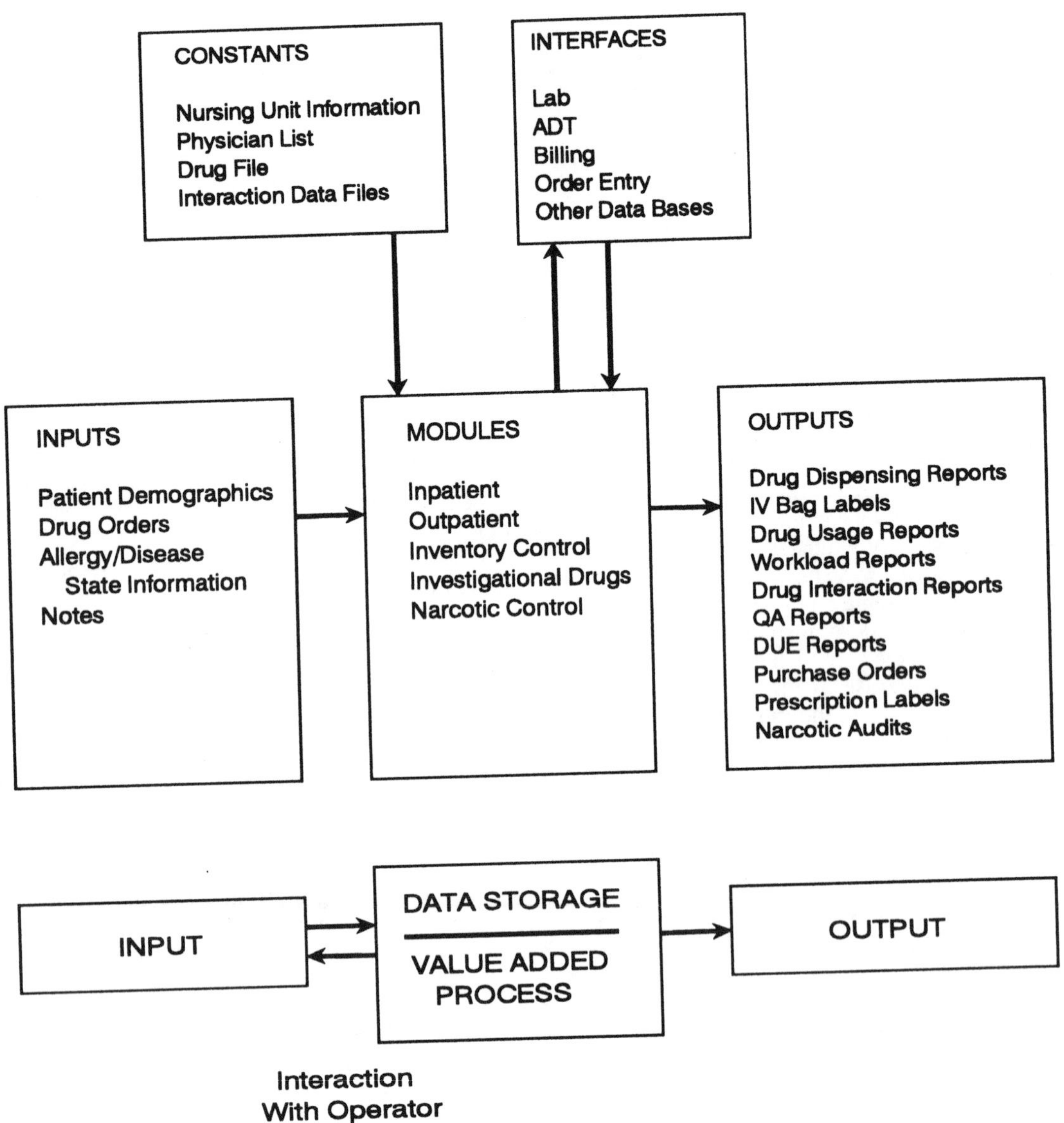

Figure 16-1. System functions

bar code reader or some other device might include demographic information such as patient name, address, date of birth, sex, social security number, height, weight, allergies; drug orders, which could include drug name, dose, route, frequency; or other pieces of information related to the practice of pharmacy.

Other data input into the system may originate from other computer systems and be transferred through interfaces. An interface is a connection between two or more computers that allows them to transfer data back and forth. The most common interfaces today are admission, discharge, transfer (ADT) information and billing information, although more and more systems are now connected to laboratory computers or to external drug product and practice information data bases related to drug use, product identification, toxicity, etc. One example of this is MicroMedex[R], which is a compilation of many clinical data bases.

Once the system has received the data it must store it for future use, output it to a printer or another computer system, or perform some process that adds value to the data. An example of the data flow is seen with order entry in which a pharmacist enters a drug order for digoxin. The system immediately compares that order to a list of patient allergies, other drugs the patient is taking, IV solutions a patient is receiving, the patient's current disease states, and the normal dose range for that drug. If the system determines the order is appropriate, it will accept the order and store it for future processing, print a label, or both. If the system identifies a potential interaction or some similar problem with the order, it will prompt the user for additional information and will interact with the user to resolve any potential risks associated with the drug order.

At some point, all systems will be called upon to generate output in one form or another. A brief list of commonly used reports is listed under outputs in figure 16-1. In generating the reports, the system will often use and integrate data from multiple sources such as patient demographics, drug orders, the master drug file, or even information from the laboratory computer. Output is not limited to printers; it can also be the transfer of billing data to the hospital financial computer system through an interface, or the selection of certain pieces of data and transfer of them to a microcomputer where they might be used in a spreadsheet.

DRUG DISTRIBUTION

Tables 16-1 and 16-2 list some of the basic functions that should be expected in an inpatient and outpatient pharmacy module. Although these two modules have many things in common and they probably share a number of data files, the flow of information in each is very different. Both modules allow manual entry or data transfer via interface of information to register a patient within the system. There should be some pieces of information that are mandatory and must be entered before registration is complete, such as gender, whereas other pieces, such as mother's maiden name, are optional and can be excluded. Once a patient is in the system, medication orders may be entered. Since this process is often the single most time-consuming function in the pharmacy, the process should be straightforward and fast. Training time should be minimal, the system should accommodate all types of orders encountered within the institution, the flow of the entry process should be conducive to correct use. If this process is slow or cumbersome, shortcuts will often be taken, resulting in a compromise in the quality of data. During order entry, the system should interact with the users to ensure that the dose and frequency of administration is within a specific range, there are no significant interactions with other drugs, disease states, laboratory or diagnostic procedures, and there are no solution incompatibilities in the case of IV drugs. The system should print labels for immediate dispensing and allow for the printing of other distribution reports at a later time. There should be predefined IV solutions, drug orders, and combinations of oral drugs and IV solutions to further enhance the order entry process.

Report generation related to drug distribution is generally limited to several reports run on a daily basis. These include unit dose pick lists, IV fill lists, unit dose update lists, IV update lists, unit dose and IV labels, and some miscellaneous output such as patient admissions, transfers and discharges, and nonformulary drug use reports.

IMPACT ON CLINICAL PRACTICE

The power of the system should extend to provide functions and support for clinical practice. Among the functions that are of value are pharmacokinetic calculations, patient monitoring capabilities, and extensive report generation capabilities. Pharmacokinetic and other dosing prediction modules have been moderately useful. In those hospitals unable to justify a clinical pharmacist staff, this function is valuable in assisting the pharmacist with dosing recommendations. In general, these modules work well in all but the very complicated patients. As with any computer program that calculates doses, the users should know what formulas are used to arrive at the dose, and what the boundaries of accuracy are.

Table 16-1. Inpatient drug distribution

I. Patient Registration/Patient Tracking
   A. Demographic information
   B. Admission, discharge, transfer (ADT) capabilities
   C. Allergies, weight, height, diagnosis, etc.
II. Internal Data Bases
   A. Drug file/IV solution file
   B. Physician file
   C. Predefined orders
   D. Nursing units/Beds
   E. Administration times, routes
   F. Drug-drug, drug-disease, drug-lab interaction data
III. Order Entry
   A. Patient identification by name or number with display of demographic data
   B. Drug selection through mnemonics, generic or trade name
   C. Dose, route, frequency
   D. Duration and scheduling
   E. Comments
   F. Order discontinue, hold, resume, or change
   G. Predefined orders
   H. Dose range checking, interaction testing
   I. Verification of orders entered by technicians
   J. IV admixture specific functions
      1. Multiple components per bag
      2. Additive sets
      3. Total parenteral nutrition
      4. Multiple solutions per bag
IV. Drug/IV Distribution Reports and Labels
   A. Unit dose cart fill and cart update lists
   B. IV solution fill lists and update lists
      1. IV labels
   C. Medication administration records
   D. IV administration records
   E. Unit dose cart and IV fill requirements lists
   F. Narcotics utilization reports
   G. Pass medication labels
V. Financial and Administrative Reports
   A. Workload and work distribution
   B. Billing and charge capture reports
VI. File Maintenance Functions
VII. Interfaces

One relative weakness of many hospital pharmacy systems is a lack of support of clinical services. The system may do an excellent job in maintaining and processing information related to a product, but most are weak in maintaining and processing information related to an activity, an outcome, or a problem. This application is currently being addressed in many systems in response to user requests.

Finally, extensive data output or reporting capabilities seem to be a requisite of the clinician. The user should be able to select and print certain predefined reports as well as easily develop, store, recall, and print custom reports. These computer systems should be able to run these reports at any time of day without slowing other processes such as order entry. Additionally, there should be an easy method to transfer data in ASCII format to disk or tape. This is of particular value in directly sharing data with other institutions, and in uploading information to data sharing services. These services provide anonymous comparison of a hospital's drug use to an aggregate of other similar hospitals.

Table 16-2. Outpatient drug distribution

I. Patient Registration/Patient Tracking
   A. Demographic information
   B. Insurance and payer information
   C. Allergies, weight, height, diagnosis, etc.
II. Internal Data Bases
   A. Drug file/IV solution file
   B. Physician file
   C. Drug-drug, drug-disease, drug-lab interaction data
   D. Payer and insurance carrier information
III. Prescription Entry and Refill
   A. Patient identification by name or number, address, or prescription number with display of demographic data
   B. Drug selection through mnemonics, generic or trade name
   C. Dose, route, frequency
   D. Duration and expiration
   E. Comments and special instructions
   F. Dose range checking, interaction testing
   G. Verification of orders entered by technicians.
   H. Price inquiry
   I. IV admixture specific functions
      1. Multiple components per bag
      2. Additive sets
      3. Total parenteral nutrition
      4. Multiple solutions per bag
IV. Drug/IV Distribution Reports and Labels
   A. Labels for dispensing containers
   B. Drug utilization reports
   C. Narcotics utilization reports
V. Financial and Administrative Reports
   A. Workload and work distribution
   B. Billing and charge capture reports
VI. File Maintenance Functions
VII. Interfaces
VIII. Third-Party Billing Functions

MANAGEMENT ASPECTS

The management staff as well as the rest of the staff must be able to generate various reports used in the day-to-day management of the department. These reports are generally related to workload, workflow, productivity, drug utilization, and drug cost. As with patient-monitoring capabilities in the above section, many systems are also weak in administrative reporting features. This may be due to a lack of use of this function, unavailability of the function, or a lack of definition of what data or reports would be of value. Although it is unlikely that all vendors will standardize their management reporting capabilities, systems should at least allow the users to define and generate their own reports. In the case of lack of definition of what data are of value, the American Society of Hospital Pharmacists (ASHP) PharmaTrend[R] program should provide a reasonable starting point.

OUTPATIENT PHARMACY

Outpatient drug distribution is very similar to inpatient distribution with differences being primarily in patient registration and order or prescription entry. With an outpatient system or module, patients may be identified by address and prescription number in addition to name and hospital number. Order entry is similar to inpatient systems but may require additional data such as insurance or payer information, and refill information.

OTHER MODULES

Additional modules available from many vendors are inventory control, narcotic control, and investigational drug control. Inventory control may be available as a module separate from other modules, or it may be closely linked to others such that the inventory is changed as individual doses of drug are dispensed to a patient. Further discussion of inventory control is beyond the scope of this chapter and may be researched through other references that specifically address this topic. Narcotic control may be available as a separate module that is linked to other modules, or the functions of this module may be incorporated within a module such as inpatient. This module must be adept in maintaining use information for each drug on a dose-by-dose basis. Additional features that are extremely important are record storage, record maintenance, and report generation in accordance with applicable State and Federal requirements.

Finally, some vendors offer software that handles the record keeping and distribution support for investigational drugs. This software will most likely vary substantially from vendor to vendor in its functionality and in its structure. Among the desired capabilities are the means to maintain data pertaining to active and inactive protocols, patients enrolled in the various studies, drugs used in the various protocols, and quantities of drug on hand. Additionally, there should be comprehensive report generation capabilities.

Overall, the computer system must be an asset to the user and promote quality and efficiency. Unfortunately, with the number of unique nonintegratable systems, this goal is sometimes difficult to attain. To illustrate this, consider the following example:

Assume the date to be the mid 1970's. Your department offers complete unit dose and IV preparation services as well as moderate drug information and clinical services. The department is not computerized, and all patient profiles are maintained on paper. The users of the drug distribution system, the pharmacists, have all the materials they need to practice at their desk or cubicle. They have the profiles, references such as Facts and Comparisons[R], a telephone, and a printout of current laboratory and census information. Over the next 5 to 10 years, a number of steps toward automation will be taken. One of the first steps toward computerization is the installation of an ADT terminal. The pharmacists now have instant access to the most current census information; however, they must get up from their "work station" and move to another location to perform this function. The second step toward computerization may have been installation of a laboratory terminal. The pharmacists now have access to the most current laboratory data, but again, they must get up from their work station to do their work. The third step in automation may have been installation of MicroMedex on another computer, most likely located in the drug information center. As with ADT and lab, the pharmacists must leave their work station to use this resource. Additional resources may include automated process control devices such as Automix^R and Micromix^R. These are IV solution compounding devices that accept computer input, interpret the data, and physically compound varying quantities of different IV solutions and additives to arrive at the final product. Even with the implementation of a pharmacy computer system, it may not be possible to integrate all the separate functions.

The result of these technological advances is that it is now more difficult for pharmacists to practice at the same level of quality. With this fragmentation of the work station, there may actually be a decrease in the quality of practice.

The key word in this illustration is "work station," which may be simply defined as the location at which a person does his or her work. *To maximize the benefits of automation, all the resources the pharmacist uses must be integrated such that multiple users can access any of the resources simultaneously from any work station.*

OBTAINING AND IMPLEMENTING A PHARMACY COMPUTER SYSTEM

In selecting a system for the first time or as a replacement for an existing system, extensive planning is required. Selection of the system involves four major processes: departmental analysis, development of the request for proposal (RFP), vendor selection, and installation and implementation.

Departmental Analysis

The first step must be a thorough analysis of the department. Each definable function performed should be scrutinized. If a particular function meets the desired goal and is done efficiently, then plan to maintain the function in its same form with the new system. If a function seems inefficient or disorganized, then look at options to improve it. This is the time to identify areas where efficiency can be improved through changes in workflow and where problems in information and product flow can be addressed through a computer system. Computerization of a department with inefficient product and information flows and no specific plans for change in conjunction with a computer system will gain little improvement in productivity and may actually lead to a worsening of the problem. Prior to completion of the analysis, the reporting or data output requirements of the various areas of the pharmacy should be reviewed. The needs of the drug distribution, clinical, and management personnel should be clearly defined. In analyzing the departmental functions, if there is no easily identifiable resolution to a problem, do not hesitate to solicit the vendors for assistance.

Request for Proposal

The second step in obtaining a system is development of the request for proposal (RFP). This document should contain the following sections: instructions to the vendor, background information pertaining to the hospital and the pharmacy, system specifications, vendor information, selection process, and cost.[1] Instructions to the vendor should clearly identify the purpose of the RFP, any timetables, the contacts within the pharmacy, and any information the vendor will require in order to respond properly to the RFP.

Background information should be of sufficient detail to provide the vendor with a general understanding of how the hospital and pharmacy operate, the various functions and services provided, and some indication of the intensity of the functions. Details might include number of beds, patient admissions per year, average length of stay, number of unit dose and IV orders processed per year, number of unit dose and IV doses dispensed per year, number of pharmacy satellites, current computerization within the department as well as the hospital, data interfaces, etc. The more complete and concise this information, the better the vendor's perspective on your department.

System specifications provide the vendor with a list of the functions pharmacy requires in a system. For a replacement system, specifications of the RFP should contain as complete a listing as possible of all the functions previously determined to be important. If there is a stipulation that the software must operate on a certain type or make of computer or interface with certain computers, this should also be included.

Background should provide the vendor with a listing of what general information you require. This may include financial data, a client or reference list, number of new installations within the past year, details of client support, installation and implementation guidelines, etc. This section should also include space for a description of proposed hardware in the absence of any constraints.

The selection process section should be a clear and concise statement on how this information will be used, how a vendor will be selected, and an approximate date when the selection will be made. Cost of the system should include all one-time and recurring costs for hardware, software, support, upgrades, and any other miscellaneous expenses.

Vendor Selection

The third step, vendor selection, should involve several subtasks. The first one is to look at each of the functions specified in the RFP and identify the personnel resources each will consume. Those functions that consume the greatest amount of resource must be accomplished with the same or a greater degree of efficiency through the new system as they are now. This information will be of value during site visits. Once all the completed proposals are received, the list of potential vendors should be narrowed to three to five finalists. In reviewing the RFP's, a vendor should be considered for disqualification if the system functionality is substantially different from your requirements, if any hardware requirements cannot be met, if the cost of the system is beyond the available budget, or for some other reason that is appropriate for vendor exclusion. A thorough reference check should be done on the remaining vendors.

Finally, site visits should be conducted. During the site visit, there should be ample time to discuss the system with the system manager or coordinator and to observe the staff using the system. Questions to ask might include: What are the backup procedures? How reliable has the system been? How much down time is there? How much training time is required for each new user? How good is support from the vendor? Is support available 24 hours per day? What are the strengths and weaknesses of the system?

In observing the system in operation, keep in mind the personnel resources of the pharmacy department. Make every effort to determine if this system provides an acceptable degree of function and efficiency for those tasks requiring the majority of personnel resources as previously determined. Finally, look at report and data output. If the data cannot be output in a manner usable to your operation, then the viability of the system should be reevaluated.

Installation and Implementation

The fourth and last step is installation and implementation. Develop an installation plan taking into account variables such as location of hardware, environmental controls, cabling, and electrical requirements as they were originally accounted for in the RFP and in cost estimates. The data processing section of most every hospital will be able to work with the vendor and the pharmacy to accomplish this task.

Develop an implementation plan in conjunction with the vendor. At a minimum, this will initially entail training of a system coordinator or a contact person knowledgeable about the system, building files (e.g., drug file, physician file, room/bed master, etc.), and training the users. In accomplishing this, establish realistic completion dates for each step but be willing to extend the implementation schedule when commonsense dictates. This phase of implementation is the most important and should be done carefully and completely before proceeding.

The final phase of implementation is entering patient data into the system and bringing individual nursing units online. There are many thoughts on how this should be accomplished. One school of thought dictates 100-percent implementation of all nursing units and all system functions at one time. This method will minimize the confusion associated with maintaining two systems; however, there is no margin for delay if problems are encountered. At the other end of the implementation spectrum is the "slow but steady" approach in which one nursing unit at a time is brought online every 1 to 3 weeks until all are implemented. This method also has its pros and cons. Although it provides considerable margin for problem resolution, there is often a great deal of stress, confusion, and overextension of resources in operating two systems.

Between these two extremes is a reasonably conservative method of implementation based on a 10/20-percent/70-percent breakdown of the beds. Initially 10 percent of the hospital's beds (usually one or two nursing units) are brought online. While this small number of beds are being serviced through the new system, there is time for the staff to become comfortable with the system. Additionally, there is an opportunity to make sure there are no serious problems. This will usually take 2 to 4 weeks. At this point, an additional 20 percent of the beds can be added to the new system. While staff members may have been comfortable with the system before, now they must become efficient with its use. Once this has been accomplished with no major problems, the remainder of the beds may be brought online fairly quickly.

There is no single best method. Each department must determine which method is best suited for its installation.

MICROCOMPUTERS IN HOSPITAL PHARMACY PRACTICE

The use of microcomputers in hospital pharmacy has increased tremendously over the past decade. The first microcomputers were not very powerful by today's standards, and there was little in the way of software. Today most microcomputers are IBM PC's, PC compatible, or Apple Macintoshes. The power of these computers allows them to be used in a local area network as a complete pharmacy system or as a stand-alone work station used in support of a pharmacy computer system. Use of microcomputers or PC's is divided among six primary areas:

1. *Word processing*. This function may be the most commonly used PC application. Uses, aside from routine correspondence, might include maintenance of the departmental policy and procedure manual and formulary, development of miscellaneous forms, and preparation of form letters. Another prevalent use is preparation of manuscripts for publication. This chapter, for example, was prepared almost entirely using a word-processing program rather than a pencil and paper.
2. *Spreadsheets*. A spreadsheet is very simply defined as a checkerboard, or large matrix of blocks or cells. The user can place data, either numeric or text, in any cell or group of cells. Data in the cells may be sorted or formatted in numerous ways, may be displayed in various graphical representations, and may be stored and printed. Mathematical operations may be performed against any group of two or more cells. The most common uses are budgeting and financial modeling,[2] basic pharmacokinetics, work-load tracking and measurement, rudimentary statistical analysis, quality assurance activities, data drug utilization evaluations[3] or drug utilization reviews, and total parenteral nutrition (TPN) calculations.[4,5]
3. *Data base managers*. A card file containing the business cards of sales representatives is an example of a data base. The entire card file is the data base or file. Each card in the file is a record, and each piece of information on a card is a field (i.e., a name). Within the realm of computers, there are two types of data base programs: flat file and relational. The card file just described is an example of a flat file data base structured such that each record exists independent of others. With a relational data base, information from several records in various files is linked together or related. Although a record may visually appear to contain all the data fields displayed, it may actually be composed of many different fields from records in the same data base or in other data bases. Which type of data base manager used is best determined by the specific application. Examples of uses are development and maintenance of a formulary, maintenance of a departmental personnel file, tracking of expenditures, controlled substance and investigational drug tracking, monitoring of adverse drug reactions,[6] and maintenance of a reference list. Note that some of the functions listed here can also be performed using other types of software such as a word processor.

4. *Desktop publishing.* This is a fairly new use of personal computers, since the application requires a relatively powerful computer. This application allows users to create documents that appear as if they were typeset and professionally printed rather than produced on a PC using a word-processing program. Some current uses within pharmacy include printing a formulary, newsletters, or other documents requiring a typeset appearance. Use of desktop publishing in pharmacy will probably increase in the next few years.
5. *Communications programs.* Computer-to-computer communication is an extremely valuable resource. Other computers containing data bases such as Medline, International Pharmaceutical Abstracts, or Drug Information FullText are just a few of hundreds currently available. Access to these external data bases is critical to most drug information centers as well as to a pharmacy's clinical and management staff.
6. *Programming of languages.* Within the profession of pharmacy, there seems to be a never-ending ingenuity for the development of computer programs. Pharmacists have written programs to calculate drug dosing and dilutions, to print labels, to randomize drug studies, and to perform myriad other tasks. Most of these programs are written in Basic, although other computer languages such as C, Assembler, COBOL, Pascal, and Fortran are used.
7. *Other functions.* There are a number of miscellaneous functions for PC's. Computer-assisted learning is steadily growing in use for pharmaceutical education on an undergraduate level as well as in training licensed pharmacists, for example, in drug therapy for situations such as cardiac resuscitation, or to update pharmacists regarding newly released drugs.

   The use of microcomputers to perform therapeutic predictions is widespread. Programs for this function are available commercially or from drug companies, and in many pharmacies they have been developed by a member of the staff using a programming language such as Basic or a spreadsheet program such as Lotus 1-2-3^{R}.

   Statistical analysis software is also used by many pharmacists. These programs excel in performing repetitive mathematical calculations, such as evaluating data for various comparisons or correlations. Some examples of this type of software include SPSSpc+ and STATPAC, although there are numerous others.

   Finally, there are a large number of memory resident applications that may run on a computer in the background while another program is in use. Some examples of these might be pop-up calendars, telephone dialers, and notepads.

CURRENT AND NEW TECHNOLOGY

A great deal of current and new technology may be easily used. Although some technologies are merely interesting with only limited practical value, others are readily accessible and offer substantial benefit and are discussed below.

Bar Coding

This offers tremendous improvements in efficiency and accuracy in data input.[7,8] Traditional implementation of bar coding is in the area of inventory control[9] and charge capture. Further use of this technology will likely be in the areas of clinical practice to assist in data collection and to verify the accuracy of unit dose cassettes prior to delivery to a nursing station.[10] This technology may find use in capture of patient monitoring data.

Touch Screens

This use is currently used only on a small scale in pharmacy. The most likely areas of use are in making selections from a menu and when there is repetitive pressing of a limited number of keys. In drug distribution, there is application in performing on-screen cart fills. Other nondistributive functions are in the areas of computer-assisted instruction and patient education.

Light Pens

This technology may be a viable supplement to and in some uses a replacement for the keyboard. It is used in many comprehensive hospital information systems for physician order entry.

Optical Character Recognition

Through this process, typed or printed pages of text are scanned, and each character is identified and written to a text file. This process is useful when large numbers of typed pages, such as a formulary or policy and procedure manual, must be transferred from a typed page to a word-processing program. Should this technology develop to a point where handwritten pages can be recognized by a computer system, there would be a substantial benefit to pharmacy.

Voice Recognition

As this technology matures such that computers can recognize consistent speech patterns as a person would use in normal conversation, many hours in front of a keyboard could be eliminated. Eventually, keyboard input may be all but eliminated; however, this process is still very immature. Some current applications include creation of documents on a word processor or entry of certain data into a data base manager. To date, this technology is still fairly expensive, and its acquisition should be carefully evaluated.

Optical Storage

As with any clinical department in a hospital, the computer system in the pharmacy department will accumulate vast quantities of data. At some point, data must be purged from the system and stored on some form of media. This may be another hard disk, floppy disks, streaming tape, nine-track tape, optical disk, or microfiche. Although any of these media can be used, optical storage offers advantages of low storage cost per megabyte, large capacity (400 megabyte to more than 1 gigabyte), stability of 10 years, and online availability of the archived data. Through use of large capacity storage such as this, an entire year of archival data can be stored on a single disk not much larger than a standard 5 1/4-inch floppy disk.

Automated Packaging

Manually packaging or repackaging oral solids and liquids into unit-of-use packaging involves both physical packaging and labeling of the dose. Systems have existed that will package a dose of a drug and print a label directly onto the package or container. Although the packaging itself is relatively fast, preparation of the label template is time consuming. Computerization of this process now combines automated packaging and computer generated labeling all in one step.

Automated Unit Dose Apportionment

Replenishing unit dose cassettes involves significant personnel resources on a daily basis and is prone to error by the nature of the process. This process may be automated such that oral solid drugs for each patient would be packaged and labeled automatically.[11] The remaining function would then be placing the strip of packaged drugs into a patient's medication cassette and adding the appropriate oral liquids and other drugs.

Process Control Devices

Intravenous TPN solutions are for the most part compounded manually. Through devices such as the Automix and Micromix, and a connection to a PC, the preparation of these solutions becomes automated. One limitation of this technology as well as automated packaging, is that some of these are still currently single-user, stand-alone systems and cannot be integrated with other computer systems used in the pharmacy.

Local Area Networks (LAN)

In addition to use as a backbone for a pharmacy computer system, LANs are also of value for simple resource sharing.[12] Some examples might include word-processing and data base applications, sharing printers and modems, and accessing common resources such as MicroMedex.

Facsimile Machines

Although these units are not typically thought of as computer equipment, they may be used as remote printers. A facsimile (FAX) board can be installed in a PC, and reports may be transferred to a single FAX machine or a group of FAX machines similar to a mailing list.

Author's Note:

When work was initially begun on this chapter, the most powerful Intel® microprocessor was the 80386, running at 25 MHz. Processors running at 33 MHz were still under evaluation. Since then, an entire new generation of microprocessors has come to market. Currently, PC's utilizing an 80486 processor running at 50 MHz are available.

Software development, as in the past, will continue to follow changes in hardware.

Selection of the appropriate generation of hardware and software must be made utilizing logic similar to that used in determining which generation of antibiotic is appropriate.

REFERENCES

1. Enright SA: Developing the request for proposal. *Top Hosp Pharm Mgt* 9:1-8, 1989.
2. Stolar MH: Use of spreadsheet software for short-range forecasting of pharmacy management data. *Am J Hosp Pharm* 45:326-332, 1988.
3. Burnakis TG: Facilitating drug-use evaluation with spreadsheet software. *Am J Hosp Pharm* 46:84-88, 1989.
4. Mitrans FP, Der MM, Baptista RJ: Customizing a spreadsheet program to perform calculations and generate reports for home tpn formulations. ASHP Annual Meeting 46:P-111D, 1989.
5. Cines D, Brown M, Green L: Spreadsheet for oncology parenteral nutrition formulations. Development of a rational, consistent approach to ordering and preparing oncology parenteral nutrition formulas. ASHP Annual Meeting 46:P-20D, 1989.
6. Johnston PE, Branch RA: Using a computerized tracking program to monitor, report and predict adverse drug reactions. ASHP Annual Meeting 46:PS-4, 1989.
7. Nold EG, Williams TC: Bar codes and their potential applications in hospital pharmacy. *Am J Hosp Pharm* 42:2722-2732, 1985.
8. Szandzik EG: Bar code technology and hospital pharmacy practice. *J Pharm Tech* (Sep-Oct):182-187, 1988.
9. Hughes TW: Automating the purchasing and inventory control functions. *Am J Hosp Pharm* 42:1101-1107, 1985.
10. Hokanson JA, Keith MR, Guernsey BG, et al: Potential use of bar codes to implement automated dispensing quality assurance programs. *Hosp Pharm* 20:327-329,333,337, 1985.
11. Prater MA: The automatic tablet counting machine, a step into the future. *J Pharm Tech* (Sep-Oct):188-191, 1988.
12. Wordell DC: Distributed processing for pharmacy and drug information at the Hospital of the University of Pennsylvania. *Top Hosp Pharm Mgt* 9:17-36, 1989.

CHAPTER 17

Facility Planning and Design

KENNETH N. BARKER, ELIZABETH L. ALLAN, ALEX C. LIN and ROBERT E. PEARSON

This chapter describes the facility planning process, along with the role of the pharmacist in this process. The purpose is to prepare the reader for participation in a facilities planning program, so that he or she can then apply this process to the enormous amount of detail involved, whether for a new facility or remodeling.

This chapter does not offer "standard plans," because experience has shown that such plans do not sufficiently recognize the variation in hospitals and their local needs. The use of "standard plans" discourages pharmacy planning founded on a thorough in-house study of future needs, functions, and operations that would yield a true picture of the facilities needed.

Topics to be addressed include the factors affecting facility needs, the hospital facility development process, current pharmacy planning and use of space, functional programming, the architectural design process, the process of designing for efficiency and flexibility, human factors in pharmacy, the satellite pharmacy, and implementation.

SIGNIFICANCE

Consider this. *If a major mistake is made in planning the pharmacy, all pharmacy staff members will have to get up and face it, and work in it, every day of their professional lives.*

One precept of architecture is that "form follows function." The wisdom of this is seen most clearly in its violation, i.e., when obsolete buildings and fixtures limit the efficiency and effectiveness with which functions can be performed and patients served. The advent of the Federal Government's prospective pricing program and the encouragement of competition have placed greater emphasis on the need for efficiency in operations than ever before. Capital investments such as buildings or remodelings that offer the prospect of lower operating costs in the short run are in demand. Increased attention is being given to the design of facilities. This is good news for the pharmacy that is inefficient now and whose administrative pharmacists understand the planning process and can effectively justify the changes needed.

FACTORS AFFECTING FACILITY NEEDS

External Factors

The factors affecting the facility needs of an institution are many and varied. Those external to the individual departments include the following:

- Changes in government or third-party reimbursement systems may directly affect planning priorities and resources.
- The current focus on cost containment in hospitals may limit the adoption of new health care technologies, and thus change equipment requirements.
- Changes in laws, regulations, codes, and standards are important. For example, the number of legend drugs for which prescription-only requirements are eliminated ("switched to over-the-counter") may change drug storage and control procedures.
- Changes in the hospital's patient mix due to aging and degree of illness are of great importance.
- Competition for patients via a demonstrated emphasis on the quality and personalization of care manifested in layout and design of patient areas is receiving increasing attention. Offering new services demanded by patients must be considered. Bed capacity and projected occupancy rates are vital to know. Hospital programs and services may need to be added or expanded, e.g., ambulatory and home health care services.
- Computerization can drastically change the work systems of the individual department. Increased hospital attention to productivity measures may result in unfavorable comparisons with comparable pharmacies, prompting changes.
- Patterns of drug prescription use may result in a decrease in drug prescriptions, thereby decreasing storage needs. The rise or decline in alternative therapies may affect drug use, as when drugs replace surgical procedures. The development of new dosage delivery systems, e.g., implanted devices, may create a need for pharmacy space dedicated to the storage of the many new high-tech medical devices involved in drug administration. Trends in

other departments can have an important effect on many aspects of drug storage and distribution. Any change in hospital mechanical service systems, such as the decision to add (or shut down) a pneumatic tube system, can affect pharmacy greatly.

- Concern for drug-related crime may warrant special security concerns.

Internal Factors

Factors internal to the pharmacy department that influence facility needs include decisions about the functions to be performed, such as whether a pharmacokinetics laboratory will be added, and the hours of operation. For example, the decision to expand to 24-hour service may necessitate a pharmacy design capable of being operated by a single pharmacist working alone on the night shift, with attendant concerns for the safety of the pharmacist and the security of areas away from view. Changes in work systems, such as the decision to recentralize the distribution process, may result in the need to close satellite pharmacies on the patient care units and expand the central pharmacy area. Automation, as in the form of computerized accounting, label typing, and automated dispensing and intravenous (IV) compounding machines, obviously will have considerable impact in terms of the rearrangement of workflow and consequent changes in facilities. Changes in the use of personnel might result in the substitution of auxiliaries for professionals in some cases, necessitating new checking procedures and the need for new "checking stations." Personnel additions obviously must be accommodated in terms of additional work stations, chairs, air-conditioning capacity, etc. Increased emphasis on continuing education and on-the-job training may necessitate special teaching and training areas, which may be shared. A change in hospital policy regarding the investment in inventory to be maintained can drastically change the reserve storage needed. And, finally, new equipment, such as a new special hood for chemotherapy, will place new demands on utilities and air-conditioning.

All of the above demonstrate the considerable interaction between what is happening in or to the hospital and the physical facility in which it happens.

HOSPITAL FACILITY DEVELOPMENT PROCESS

Planning for hospitals is in a period of great turmoil today. Because the trend is for hospitals to be reimbursed at a flat rate for any given disease state, there is great incentive to redesign inpatient areas for maximal efficiency and for hospitals to specialize in the areas in which they are most efficient, e.g., cardiac care, while dropping other inpatient services entirely. At the same time, the competition for patients has also placed heavy emphasis on making all patient facilities inviting and attractive to patients. With no lid yet on outpatient charges and a considerable financial incentive for minimizing a patient's inpatient stay, great economic pressure is thus exerted on hospitals to substitute outpatient care for inpatient care wherever possible. The result, at the departmental level, is that many department heads face instructions to cut back on plans (reduce space) related to inpatient services while developing plans for the expansion of outpatient services (e.g., outpatient dispensing, home health care services).

A separate issue is the availability of capital. Many hospitals are torn between the need to renovate for efficiency and the need to offer expanded ambulatory care services for survival under prospective pricing, but they implement neither because of the problem of raising capital. In summary, it is a difficult time to build or renovate a hospital or outpatient facility, but the need for changes is compelling hospitals into such construction projects.

The planning of the pharmacy must proceed as part of the process of designing the rest of the facility because of the relationships described above. It is essential for the director of pharmacy to understand the facility development process if he or she is to have any influence on it, and see that the needs of the pharmacy department are given their proper due, in the proper place, and at the proper time.

The hospital facility development process may be outlined as follows:

1. Marketing plan developed, to identify demand for future services by examining patient mix, services in demand, and income to be generated.
2. Competition examined, from both other hospitals and alternative modes of treatment, such as freestanding ambulatory care centers.
3. Existing facility resources evaluated, a process that may heavily influence whether to renovate or build anew.
4. Financial capability evaluated, focusing primarily on the question of raising capital, a problem made more complex by recent government programs.
5. Environmental constraints evaluated, including regulations, legal codes, and local politics.
6. "Framework for planning" statement developed, to include hospital mission and role statement, activity projections, priorities, organization plan, schedule, and monitoring and evaluation procedures.

All of these concerns are considered as the hospital periodically reformulates its "framework for planning" statement, which is the cornerstone of any specific facility planning project.

The facility planning process, which typically consumes 2-3 years and sometimes longer, includes the stages shown below.

Steps in Facility Planning Process

1. Master facilities plan developed, which sets forth the implications of the hospital strategic plan in terms of the facilities needed to accommodate all planned activities, along with a timeline to show when facility needs will occur. Each department should have its own master facilities plan to complement its strategic plan.
2. Analysis of existing facility resources compiled, including "as-built" plans, space inventory room by room, equipment list showing age and replacement value, site surveys, assessment of structural, mechanical, and electrical systems, code conformity, and traffic patterns.
3. Functional program compiled, including block diagrams that show department components, flow and traffic relationships, phases in development, new versus renovated space, gross cost estimate, state-

ment of assumptions and priorities, and a series of alternative schematic plans.

4. Architectural schematic plans drawn, showing layout and design of departments and relationships plus workflow of staff, materials, and patients (includes a brief description of fixtures, mechanical and electrical systems, and a cost estimate).
5. Architectural design developed, adding all other architectural details, including the last review by the users.
6. Construction contract documents drawn up, including final drawings for regulatory approval and bidding plus the final cost estimate.
7. Construction begun, including demolition, construction, equipment ordering, and inspection.
8. Occupancy implemented, including installation of equipment, orientation of staff, moving, evaluation, and followup.

As the major processes described above move along, it is not difficult to see why a department traditionally thought of as "small" (8 percent of the typical hospital operating budget) may find that it exerts little control or influence over its own destiny. This need not happen if pharmacists understand the process and the opportunities it affords them for influence. For example, the pharmacist can begin by taking every opportunity to assert that, from the facilities planning standpoint, the "pharmacy function" includes control of all medications and related information in the hospital and extends far beyond the walls of the pharmacy to include nursing unit design, decisions about hospital communication, transportation, and security systems, etc.

CURRENT PHARMACY PLANNING AND SPACE UTILIZATION

Facilities Surveys

The 1989 edition of the *Lilly Hospital Pharmacy Survey*,[1] sent to directors of hospital pharmacies and yielding a response rate of about 37 percent (2,048 pharmacies), found that the average hospital had a slightly smaller central pharmacy area than in the previous year, down from 7.5 square feet per bed to 7.1 square feet.

A national survey in 1982 by Alexander and Barker[2] based on a stratified random sample of hospitals with a response rate of 45.6 percent (843) showed that the pharmacies in the most common types of hospitals (general medical surgical, nonprofit, short term) occupied about 7 square feet per bed. Pharmacies in government hospitals of all kinds had the most space, whereas pharmacies in for-profit hospitals had only a little more than half the space of the not-for-profit hospitals (see table 17-1). For every hospital type, little correlation between bed size and total pharmacy space was noted. This finding was not as surprising as it may sound, because as hospitals grow in size, new functions are added, while the original functions may not require additional space as a result of economies of scale.[2]

It is impossible to evaluate the adequacy of current space allocations in hospital pharmacies without knowing the services they are attempting to provide and the work systems and personnel to be accommodated.

Table 17-1. Space per bed (gross sq. ft.) in nonprofit, for-profit, and government hospitals[2]

Hospital type*	Nonprofit	For-profit	Government	
			Non-Federal	Federal
GMS, T	7.0	5.3	8.0	--
LT	4.0	2.7	3.7	--
PSYCH	5.9	2.1	3.1	--
Overall mean	6.9	5.0	7.0	10.6

*GMS, T = general medical/surgical, short-term; LT = long-term; and PSYCH = psychiatric.

The recommended approach to determining pharmacy space needs is the functional planning approach (see below), based on an inhouse evaluation of individual hospital needs, rather than the method of relying on comparisons with other pharmacies and other hospitals.

Planning Process

Too often the pharmacist's input in the planning process is minimal. The administrator may inform the pharmacist at the last minute about the location and the space that have already been determined for the pharmacy. The pharmacist is then shown a proposed plan, which already has been drawn up by the architect. Another undesirable approach is to contact commercial vendors of pharmacy fixtures and ask them to submit the design for the pharmacy. (In recent years, the number of vendors offering hospital pharmacy design services has decreased.) Such firms can be very helpful *after* needs have been defined, i.e., after the functional program has been written. Otherwise, the designs proposed may feature unneeded quantities of the particular line of fixtures the vendor sells.

The planning approach recommended is called "functional planning." This is an organized and systematic approach based on the architectural principle that states "form follows function." The implication is that a hospital, along with each department, should be planning from the inside out--with its functional requirements dictating the arrangement, the characteristics, and even the appearance of its final structure.

The planning team should include the hospital administrator, the architect, and consultants, plus the department heads. The administrator's role is to define the hospital's goals and to allocate resources. The pharmacist's role is to set forth the objectives and work methods the pharmacy will use in pursuit of the hospital's goals. The architect's role is to translate all of this into architectural plans.

The specific responsibilities of the pharmacist on the planning team are to (1) set forth the objectives, functions, and methods (work systems) of the pharmacy department; (2) prepare the functional program for the department; and (3) serve as the ultimate authority for overseeing compliance with professional and legal standards.

The specific steps in planning a pharmacy facility using the functional planning process are shown below. The part of the planning process known as "functional programming" encompasses steps A through H. Architectural design overlaps functional programming and includes steps G through J.

Steps in Functional Planning

Steps	Primary Responsibility
A. Identify hospital purpose and goals	Administrator
B. Derive pharmacy goals and objectives	Pharmacist
C. Identify functions	Pharmacist
D. Determine workflow	Pharmacist
E. Identify work areas	Pharmacist
F. Specify requirements for each work area re: 1. Workload 2. Equipment and fixtures 3. Storage 4. Personnel 5. Materials handling 6. Communications 7. Services 8. Security 9. Utilities 10. Environment	Pharmacist
G. Find optimal arrangement for work areas	Pharmacist and Architect
H. Find optimal location	Pharmacist and Architect
I. Develop trial schematics (total space calculable here)	Pharmacist and Architect
J. Develop architectural design	Architect

The functional program will be in the form of a written report, which summarizes the requirements of the pharmacy in quantitative and qualitative terms, i.e., in words and numbers. It does not get into the drawing of plans, which comes after the functional program has been completed.

The purpose of the functional program is to describe individual pharmacy operations and the demands (i.e., performance requirements) of each on the facility. During the next phase--architectural design--the architect will translate these needs into physical space, equipment, and furnishings.

FUNCTIONAL PROGRAMMING

The functional program usually begins with a formal statement of the purpose, goals, and specific objectives of the pharmacy service for the future and then lists the specific functions to be performed. Long-range goals, including those for future growth and expansion plus a timetable for their implementation over the next 5-10 years, should be included. All of the above should appear in a separate "master facilities plan" document for the department, along with a written description of the implications for the facilities needed and a timetable.

Functions

A function is defined as "a system of one or more tasks, to serve a stated purpose." Some typical pharmacy functions include reviewing and editing orders; dispensing unit doses to inpatients; compounding of IV admixtures; purchasing; storage; and administration (the terminology used may differ from one pharmacy to another).

The key point is that an effort should be made to identify every specific function to be performed in the new facility, along with the methods and the systems to be used. For example, the type of drug distribution system to be used and whether or not satellites will be built should be known. If such decisions have not been made, then little further progress is possible until they are. (A systems analysis may be advisable, to take advantage of the opportunity to design a new system and the new facilities together for optimum efficiency of performance. Designing a new facility for an inefficient system may have the undesirable long-term effect of "designed-in inefficiency.") Facilities can and should be designed to be flexible (and how to do this is addressed later), but good predictions about future work systems are essential to contain costs.

Workflow Analysis to Identify Work Area

Workflow analysis is performed to examine what the workflow will be in order to identify all of the tasks along the way. In the new plan, each and every task must have a place where it can be performed, and that place must be properly equipped and have the proper environment. Such places are designated work areas (general and specific). This is a systematic approach to ensure that the plans provide a work area for each and every task.

Workflow analysis for the purpose of facilities design is significantly different from that for systems analysis, for example, in that the focus is limited to only those items having implications for facilities.

The analysis is begun by examining each function to be performed and the workflow involved. Workflow is defined as "the sequence of activities in response to a work order," such as a physician's medication order. The way to begin is to identify each different work order (i.e., anything that causes work to begin), such as a requisition received for filling, or even a printout indicating that inventory is low and that a purchase order should be initiated.

The way this approach generates a basic list of work areas is illustrated below. In this example, the procedure for the filling of an IV admixture order is listed on the left-hand side. Then, proceeding down the right side, the idea is to stop at each step and try to picture mentally the physical activity that will take place in that step and then give each workplace in that mental picture a generic name, such as "typing station" or "hood." In this way, a list of all of the work areas needed is generated.

Task	Work Area
1. Work order received	Pass-through window
2. Label prepared	Terminal
3. Solution, additives, and supplies obtained	Active storage solutions Active storage additives Active storage supplies

4. Assembled/checked in hood	Hood
5. Put in pass-through refrigerator	Refrigerator
6. Waste items discarded	Waste receptacle

A work area is defined as "a place where work of a similar nature is performed." A work area may be only a desk, a counter, or one section of a long counter, the corner of a room, or the whole room itself. Some work areas typically found in a hospital pharmacy are presented below, where they are organized into general and specific work areas:

A. Dispensing to outpatients
   1. Waiting
   2. Receiving and dispensing
   3. Terminal
   4. Medication profile
   5. Filling counter
   6. Communications and references
   7. Weighing
   8. Heating and stirring
   9. Sink
   10. Counseling room
   11. Waste receptacle

Once all of the work areas needed are identified, it is possible to proceed. The next step calls for the examination of each of these work areas to identify and specify for each the workload, personnel, inventory, and equipment to be accommodated, services and utilities needed, etc.

It will be advantageous to group the work areas to the degree possible. For example, the functional programming specifications for the several specific work areas contained in one small office can usually be combined and considered together under the general work area title for the entire office. This would not be the case in an IV admixture center, for example, where the laminar flow hood would have special utility requirements.

Workload Analysis

The most important determinants of the space requirements of a hospital pharmacy performing a given set of functions are (1) workload, (2) equipment and fixtures, (3) storage needs, and (4) personnel to be accommodated.

It is useful to differentiate between the extrinsic workload, which is the demand on the pharmacy from outside the department, and the intrinsic workload, which is that generated from within, as when a drug is prepackaged, creating a need for a label to be typed.

To estimate the workload (whether extrinsic or intrinsic) for any work area, the work units must first be identified. Some typical work units in a hospital pharmacy include the number of physicians' medication orders received for processing, the number of drug information requests, and the number of batches of drugs to be prepackaged. Such workloads may be analyzed and reported according to the volume per day; the distribution by hour of the day; or the distribution across a sufficient number of days to include the normal cycles and fluctuations that have implications for facility design.

A convenient way to collect workload data is to arrange to have every form time-date stamped as it is processed, for tabulation later. Often such data are already being collected for departmental reports. Otherwise, direct observation may be needed to count and record work units during typical time periods.

When a new facility is planned where none previously existed, the best approach is to begin by examining data from an institution of similar size and with similar programs and services.

Current workload data must be adjusted to reflect changes expected in the future. Formulas for forecasting the extrinsic workload of the pharmacy, based on the past and present number of patient days, for example, are available.[3] Adjustments should be made for important trends, asking questions such as these: Does the hospital plan to increase or decrease bed capacity? Will patient mix change? (This can *greatly* affect the pharmacy workload.) Is the hospital planning to discontinue certain programs, such as obstetrics, or to add others, such as home health care? Will recent medical staff decisions change the number or types of medications ordered in the future?

The study of expected workload will reveal, for example, whether the IV admixture center will require one hood or two and how many typewriters or printers will be needed. Without such information, the final plans might not include a workplace for these extra items of equipment.

Equipment and Fixtures

The cost of equipment may be the single most important cost associated with a new facility. It not only may constitute the greatest portion of the total initial expenditure, but also will be a determining factor in the day-to-day operating expenses of the facility for the long run.

The selection of the equipment for the pharmacy department should be based on an analysis of the work that the equipment is needed to do. Questions relating to how the work will be done, e.g., the degree of computerization and automation, must be addressed. If some equipment will be built into purchased fixtures, this also must be known.

The solution is to study the nature of the work at each work area, the volume involved, and the methods to be used. Based on this information, an initial equipment list can be generated. Then, published lists can be consulted for items overlooked.[3,4] The purchasing agent will be a source of information about standard items such as office equipment.

A high initial cost should not be a deterrent to the consideration of equipment that has a favorable net effect on operating costs for the long run. A method for determining the most cost-effective alternative is "life cycle costing."[3] The use of consultants is helpful and justified in the selection of expensive equipment for more complex operations, such as computer applications and unit dose packaging.

In composing the equipment list, it is important to distinguish between fixed and movable equipment. Fixed equipment is that which requires installation and becomes attached to the building. For example, many fume hoods are fixed equipment. Movable equipment includes furniture, carts, and typewriters. A separate list is important, because fixed equipment often is included in the hospital construction contract, whereas movable equipment may be bid separately.

The physical environment needed to accommodate each piece of equipment must be considered. For example, there may be a need for extra space around the sides to give access for repairs and maintenance. Some equipment manufacturers will even supply a template to show the access space requirements for each equipment item. Space must be provided for the operator to stand or sit and for the storage of supplies and accessories. Temporary storage space for incoming materials and outgoing products is needed. Trash cans and areas for waste materials are sometimes overlooked.

General characteristics to be sought in all equipment are standardization throughout the pharmacy (and hospital), compatibility with existing equipment, modularity, and flexibility. Each of these points will be addressed later.

Remember: every item of equipment ordered is going to have to be put somewhere, and the best time to provide a place for it is at the time the facility is being planned.

Storage

Storage fixtures may or may not appear on the final equipment list, as they may be treated as part of construction. However, they should be treated as equipment in the functional program to ensure that they receive proper consideration.

To estimate the type and amount of storage space needed, it is best to actually measure the amount of space currently occupied by all inventory, supplies, etc. The space now occupied by current stock should be measured with a tape measure shelf by shelf and drawer by drawer, so that the planner can form an accurate mental picture of the block of space needed to accommodate the contents. Then the average height, width, and depth needed for all of the stock on one shelf, for example, should be estimated. These data then should be broken down by class and summarized in terms of linear front feet, square feet, and cubic feet. Although such measurements will be approximate, this approach has the important advantage of avoiding the distortion that comes from the common approach of measuring the outside dimensions of existing shelving units, which too often are no longer optimal for the items stored there. When such data are collected by operating personnel, these persons can be instructed to adjust their estimates to reflect the latest developments, including departmental objectives regarding inventory levels.

The results obtained should be presented in the functional program in the form shown in table 17-2.

Table 17-2. IV reserve storage

		Shelf space needed for current stock levels	
Class and type	***Linear ft.***	***Square ft.***	***Cubic ft.***
IV's and administration sets	198	444	1,274
Floor space — pallets	12	42	108
Total	210	486	1,382

Storage requirements may be organized and reported according to the classes of storage as listed below:

A. Frequency of use
   1. Most used
   2. Less used
   3. Deep reserve
B. Environmental requirements
   1. Air-conditioning
   2. Refrigeration
   3. Freezing
   4. Protected from light
C. Security requirements
   1. Controlled drugs (by schedule)
   2. Alcoholic beverages
D. Special
   1. Disinfectant-proof
   2. Autoclave-proof

The compilation of these data in this way makes it possible to enlist the skills of the architects, consultants, fixture vendors, and other outside experts to suggest solutions beyond the storage fixtures traditionally seen in pharmacies. There has been a great need for improvements, and the recent economic pressures to reduce space use everywhere has resulted in many new and innovative approaches, all requiring a three-dimensional analysis of space requirements.

The active storage areas of the pharmacy usually include one or more cart-filling station, arranged in U-shaped alcoves. However, in some centralized operations, carts may also be filled on an assembly-line basis, cafeteria style. Unit dose dispensing systems generally require about 25 percent more storage space than other systems.

The arrangement of stock should give first priority to placing all of the fast-moving stock together near the front to minimize pharmacy travel time. Traditionally, most pharmacies have organized their stock by dosage form, i.e., all oral solids together, all oral liquids, injections, etc. Though this allows for economy of shelf space, the value of pharmacy labor wasted is likely to be much greater.

Shelving that is open and adjustable is often quite adequate, versatile, and inexpensive. Cabinets and drawers cost considerably more and are generally less efficient to use. Angled adjustable shelving provides gravity feed. These can be designed to be replenished from the rear to minimize drug stock deterioration.

Rotary files for fingertip retrieval of the most used drugs have been used in some pharmacies. However, such rotary files are usually efficient only when no more than two persons are involved in filling prescriptions from the same file. Beyond that point, the one-at-a-time access feature of this type of storage reduces its efficiency.

For bulk storage, rail-mounted shelving is recommended for its space-saving features, since fewer aisle spaces are needed.

Regarding refrigeration, unit dose dispensing systems require a greater amount of refrigerated storage for injectables and liquids. The commercial reach-in type, such as that used in food stores, is preferred by many because it eliminates the time involved in opening and closing doors.

For reserve and bulk refrigerated storage, prefabricated cold rooms are available and can be made secure for controlled drugs.

Deep reserve storage items, such as IV solutions in cartons, often are kept on pallets or on "fork-lift serviceable" steel shelving in a locked room that may be remote from the pharmacy.

"Just-in-time" purchasing policies can have a profound effect on the need for reserve storage. Hospital plans in this regard should be determined (see also chapter 9 of this handbook).

With respect to the storage of controlled drugs, the trend is to emphasize sophisticated electronic alarm systems, rather than sturdier vaults and safes. The regional agent of the Drug Enforcement Administration (DEA) should be contacted for an interpretation of the current regulations and requirements.[5]

The problem of storing flammables is familiar to the architect, and the architect should be the one responsible for complying with all applicable codes and regulations, which vary from State to State. Many hospital pharmacies no longer have their own flammables room. Sealed containers of alcohol eliminate the need in some cases and, in other cases, the hospital may provide a flammables room for use by all. In the case of shared storage facilities, the means for adequate security over pharmacy-controlled items may need to be provided.

Personnel

The personnel to be accommodated in the pharmacy are another factor of major importance in the design of a new facility.

The architect will need to have documented the number of persons who will be in each area during normal work times as well as peak work periods, to be able to provide adequate working space, the proper number of chairs, the necessary air-conditioning capacity, etc. The architect should be supplied the expected staffing pattern, as well as the hours of operation. The expected presence of individuals being *trained* should not be overlooked.

Communications

Communication systems needed by the pharmacy should be analyzed, with thought given not only to telephone systems but also to telecommunication needs, facsimile reproduction, bulletin boards, and access to all hospital-wide systems.

The pharmacy telephone systems should provide separate telephone numbers for business and professional calls, with calls related to patient care answered by a pharmacist directly. Dispensing areas should be designed so that the pharmacist can talk privately on the phone without being overheard. Telecommunication, facsimile, and computer terminals will have special requirements regarding location, space, and utilities that must be checked with the manufacturer.

Materials Handling

The hospital will likely provide central materials-handling systems such as service elevators, dumbwaiters, pneumatic tubes, or messenger service for use throughout the hospital for all departments. When planning this system, the architect should be reminded that the pharmacy will be a major user, for both drug products and documents, sending and receiving more units (in unit dose systems) than any other department. The architect should also be advised that pharmacy has some unique, special requirements such as a rapid response for stat orders and security for controlled drugs during transit. Documented for the architect should be the volume of this workload, its distribution by time of day, and size and weight of the largest and smallest units to be transported.

Before a costly and complicated automated transportation system is recommended, the advantages of manual cart delivery and messenger service should not be overlooked. These offer a relatively maintenance-free system, featuring carriers with built-in, highly versatile "computers" (the human brain) for observation, control, recording inventory, feedback, and on-the-spot problem solving. Also, the cost of expanding such systems is minimal.

Care should be taken that all carts will pass through all doors, including elevator doors and passageways, and that they will roll satisfactorily on the type of flooring anticipated.

Services From Other Departments

Services from other departments on which the pharmacy may depend must be identified so that the architect can locate them as close to the pharmacy as possible. Such services include centralized purchasing, centralized receiving, library, cashier and waiting areas for outpatients, and access to autoclaves.

Security

The hospital pharmacist must deal with security problems at a variety of levels, including the detailed requirements for the various classes of controlled drugs; the regulations for alcohol and alcoholic beverages; the regulations regarding prescription and nonprescription drugs; and concern for the confidentiality of patient information--all in addition to the normal security for the protection of the employees and property.

Security considerations may include limiting the number of doors and other means of access to storage areas, the reinforcement of door and wall materials (e.g., requiring that walls be built to extend vertically from slab to slab), the quality and types of door locks, electronic controls, and the control of keys (e.g., no master keys).

Visual surveillance of all doors and high-security areas may be needed if the pharmacy is to be staffed by one person at night. Automatic door locks, bullet-proof glass, and special alarm systems are being installed in an increasing number of pharmacies.

However, there is concern that such devices too often interfere with the pharmacist-patient interaction, which is important in providing optimal pharmacy services.

Utilities and Environmental Controls

The functional program prepared by the pharmacist should give particular attention to the requirements of the special work areas unique to pharmacy. The typical architect can anticipate the requirements of a normal office, for example, but not for an IV admixture center. The architect should also be alerted to the need for emergency power for the refrigerators, freezers, laminar air flow hoods, and the security alarm systems.

Arrangement of Work Areas

Once all work areas are known and the individual requirements have been identified, the next step is to analyze and recommend how they should be arranged in relation to each other. Factors to be considered include the flow of products and information, points of input and output, access to fixed or shared equipment (e.g., dumbwaiter), joint use of personnel and equipment, need for visual supervision, and the desire to minimize travel and delay time between work areas.

Those general work areas that probably should not be physically separated are order review, distribution, and extemporaneous compounding and packaging. General work areas that may be separated if adequate communications and transportation can be provided are administration, batch compounding and packaging, and deep reserve storage.

The desired location of the work areas with respect to corridors and elevators should be recorded. For large complex facilities, there are systematic, quantitative methods for calculating the best arrangement of work areas.[6,7] Such a quantitative reanalysis involves the determination of personnel and material flows between the work areas. A "From-To" chart (see figure 17-1) can be used in estimating the flow, or travel frequencies, of personnel and material between each pair of work areas. The evaluation of travel frequencies can be based on either workflow analyses or observation. The results of the travel frequency analyses can be ranked and classified into five closeness ratings (see figure 17-2). A second code system that describes the reasons for each relationship is also used in the chart.

The qualitative analysis is used to account for factors other than the relationships of workflow. Such factors include managerial decisions (e.g., decisions made for security reasons).

In addition to the previous five closeness ratings, undesirable (symbol: X) may be used to indicate occasions when two work areas should be segregated. For example, it is undesirable to locate the controlled drug distribution area adjacent to the main entrance.

A work area relationship diagram can be used in facilitating the layout design (see figure 17-3). The squares (work areas) are shifted around until a "neat" layout (fewer lines crossing) is obtained. The next step is to adjust the design by considering the physical constraints (i.e., location of entrance, physical shape) of the pharmacy and size of each work area. The result of this process is sometimes called a "bubble diagram" (see figure 17-4).

RENDERING THE FUNCTIONAL PROGRAM

The functional program is a written report, composed mostly of tables and diagrams, summarizing the data collected. The architect's first task is to interpret this material and translate it into visual concepts and physical forms. Therefore, every effort to help the architect through a concise presentation that pinpoints and summarizes the key information will be greatly appreciated.

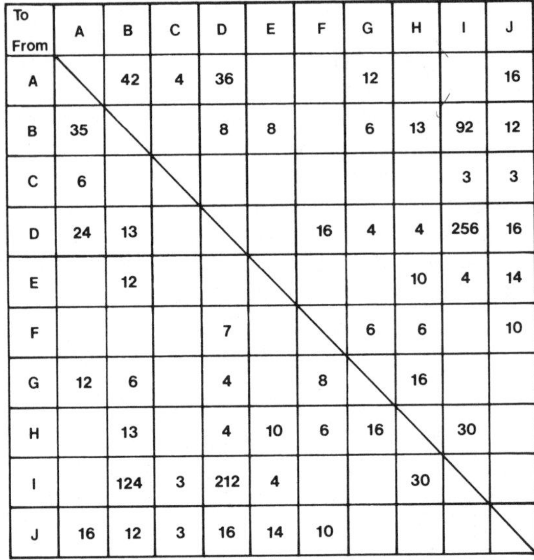

To / From	A	B	C	D	E	F	G	H	I	J
A		42	4	36			12			16
B	35			8	8		6	13	92	12
C	6								3	3
D	24	13				16	4	4	256	16
E		12						10	4	14
F				7			6	6		10
G	12	6		4		8		16		
H		13		4	10	6	16		30	
I		124	3	212	4			30		
J	16	12	3	16	14	10				

Legend: A. Entrance, Main
B. Central Drug Distribution
C. Controlled Drug Distribution
D. Central IV Admixture Compounding and Distribution
E. Production, Non-sterile Products
F. Production, Sterile Products
G. Receiving (into pharmacy)
H. Storeroom
I. Dispatching Center
J. Lockers and Lounge

Figure 17-1. From-To chart showing number of trips per day between each work area

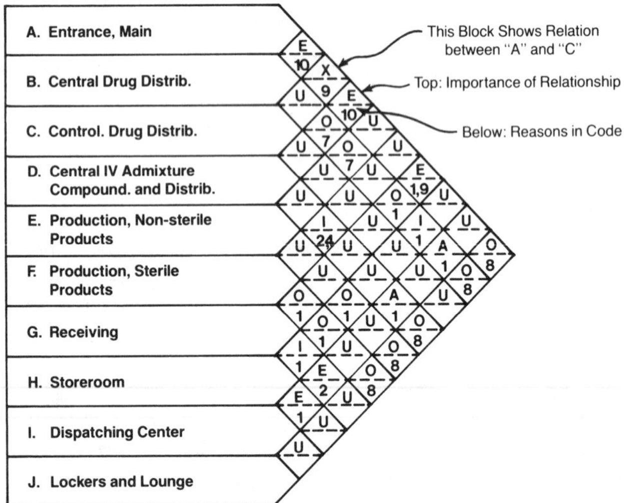

Code	Reason
1	Flow of materials
2	Common personnel
3	Common equipment
4	Supervision
5	Personal contact
6	Common records
7	Communications
8	Spec. management
9	Security
10	Interdepart. trips

Rating	Definition
A	Absolutely necessary
E	Especially Important
I	Important
O	Ordinary closeness OK
U	Unimportant
X	Undesirable

Figure 17-2. Work area relationship chart

The table of contents for a typical functional program may include:

1. Purpose of the department
2. Functions
3. Workflow diagrams
4. List of general and specific work areas
5. Workload analysis
6. Furniture and equipment list
7. Storage requirements
8. Other work area requirements
9. Arrangement of work areas

Space considerations should begin with the categorization of all pharmacy space into five major types: primary activity, support, administrative, educational, or research. (Note: Some planners include education and research under administration.)

The recommended approach is first to locate the primary activity spaces, e.g., dispensing, and then locate the appropriate support and administrative spaces. Support space would include all reserve drug storage areas, for example.

The next step may be as simple as drawing the bubble diagram shown in figure 17-4. Another approach is to put the name of each general work area on a separate circle cut out of paper and then move these around to find the best arrangement.

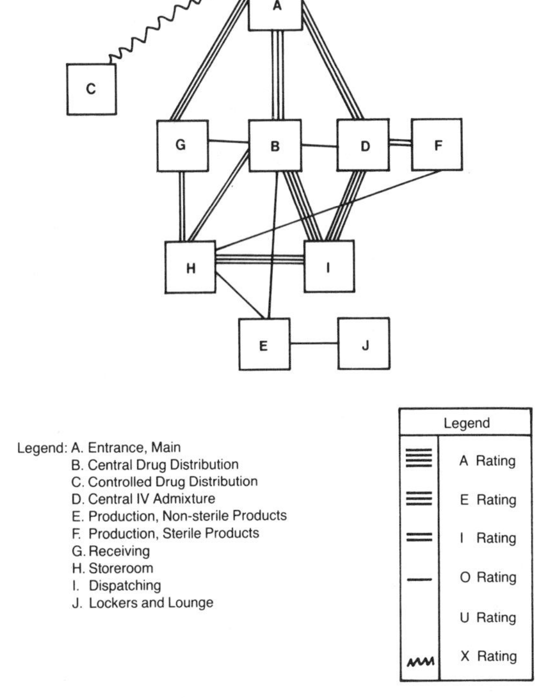

Figure 17-3. Work area relationship diagram

ARCHITECTURAL DESIGN PROCESS

Role of the Architect

From the architect's viewpoint, the creative part of a facilities design project represents only about 20 percent of total effort, but it is "the fun part." This is important to know, because it suggests that the best time to capture the architect's personal (and creative) interest in a project is at the very beginning of the design process. If given the opportunity to truly understand the department, the architect can significantly improve the effectiveness of that department through his or her designs.

The design of any facility, from the viewpoint of the architect, involves three major factors: utility, amenity, and expression. "Utility" simply means it is functional and efficient. A good functional program is the key to helping the architect address this factor. The term "amenity" refers to satisfying the human requirements for the people who will work there. Chief concerns are ease of access and movement, personal comfort, and safety and health protection. The term "expression" means the symbolic aspects or image the facility should project to others when they see it. For example, if the appearance of a dispensing window is to encourage patient counseling, its design should convey the message that an important pharmacist-patient communication occurs here, the privacy of which must be protected.

A collaborative approach between the architect and the pharmacist can produce designs that encourage the pharmacist to use the best professional practices and that discourage poor practice. For example, to promote personal contact between the pharmacist and patient, the normal positions of the pharmacist and of the ambulatory patient can be designed for their encounter to place them face to face in proximity (without a clerk between them, and without a place for a reluctant pharmacist to "hide").

Space

How much total space will the pharmacy need, and where should it be located? These will be among the *first* questions to which answers will be sought by the planning team. However, a good answer requires the comprehensive analysis of pharmacy needs described here, which are then modified and integrated with the needs of other departments by the hospital architect.

To estimate the pharmacy space required, the architect will study the functional program and add space for halls and internal passageways. He or she will consider the shape and location of available space in the hospital plan. Then the architect will develop a set of proposed schematic drawings for all to consider. Once the planning team agrees on one, then pharmacy space needs are finally determined by measuring the space that plan occupies.

The above description is the best approach and one that, unfortunately, is not always realized. Too often hospital consultants or architectural firms attempt to use "standard" space allocation formulas without proper attention to the needs of a particular pharmacy function in a particular setting. Hospital pharmacy functions and services are changing dramatically as new roles emerge for the pharmacist; these changes cannot be ignored. Some hospital systems have tried to standardize departmental space needs without success.

LOCATION

The question of the location of the pharmacy should be brought to the attention of the architect and the planning team at the earliest time. This is because it is too common for the pharmacy to be thought of as a department that can

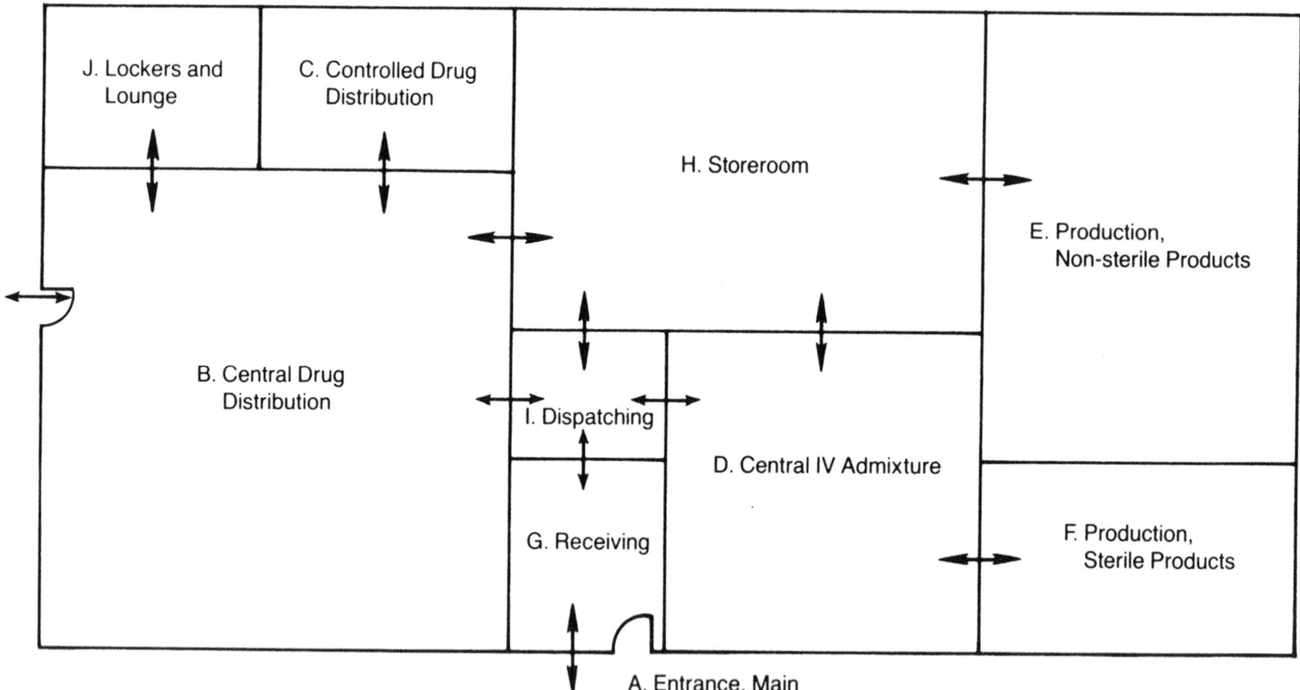

Figure 17-4. Bubble diagram

be located "almost anywhere," and it is therefore given a low priority in the competition for prime locations.

The location of the inpatient pharmacy distribution areas must provide ready and full access to the hospital's materials-handling systems (see previous discussion). When pharmacy satellites are involved, service to those satellites must be adequate and fast. Therefore, it is common to locate the inpatient pharmacy close to the central core of elevators and dumbwaiters, the only exception being if automated horizontal conveyors or automated carts will be used.

If outpatients are to be served, the outpatient pharmacy dispensing area should be located somewhere along the normal patient traffic flow, perhaps sharing the same waiting room and cashier with the rest of the outpatient clinics. This consideration often necessitates separating the outpatient pharmacy from the inpatient pharmacy, which occurs more frequently as the number of hospital beds increases.

The location of a drug information center (or any area designed to encourage physician "drop-ins") will need to be located on a route heavily traveled by physicians, such as near the hospital library or a medical staff lounge.

The location of pharmacy satellites varies widely, depending on the specific functions they serve. The ideal location for a general satellite serving a general medical or surgical service is adjacent to or directly opposite the nurses' station (most current satellites are located some distance away only because they were not part of the original plan). All satellites whose function is to dispense drugs in unit dose form to the users should be located to allow face-to-face communications with them, to ensure that the projected benefits of the use of satellites are obtained (see chapters 18 and 38).

Satellites designed exclusively for clinical pharmacy services should ideally be accessible from both the nurses' station and the physicians' work areas.

Satellites designed to serve other pharmacy satellites, such as IV admixture production units located in two or three sites throughout a multilevel hospital, should be located to maximize access to the hospital materials-handling systems.

Administrative offices may be separate from the inpatient and outpatient pharmacies. Bulk and reserve inventory can be maintained in remote locations provided the pharmacy controls all access to drug storage areas.

DESIGNING FOR EFFICIENCY

Work Systems

Designing a pharmacy for efficiency includes beginning with an efficient work system that is developed by using a task-oriented approach to design and three-dimensional ("3-D") space planning.

Efficiency is simply the ratio of output (e.g., unit doses dispensed) per resources input (e.g., labor, space). One of the most effective ways to achieve efficiency is to reexamine work systems at the beginning of the planning process and then design the facility for optimal performance of the new improved systems.

Systems analyses typically begin with flow-charting to look for tasks that can be combined, eliminated, or automated.[8] Queuing theory and computer-simulation models of pharmacy operations can be used to identify mathematically the (theoretically) most efficient operation,[9,10] although this can become quite complex.

To illustrate the application of queuing theory, its use has shown that the assembly-line method of dispensing, used mostly by military pharmacies, where the task of dispensing is broken down in various elements performed by various personnel in different locations, is efficient only where strict scheduling is possible. The most efficient way to provide service for orders that arrive at random and that require varying periods of time to dispense is to have this done in one place by one person (like McDonald's).

A systems change that can have a great impact on efficiency and on facilities needs is the alteration of the use of personnel, e.g., as when the work of a professional is redesigned and part of it delegated to an auxiliary worker.[11,12] For this reason staffing studies, if planned, should always precede facilities design.

Systems changes that have been shown to improve the efficiency of the pharmacy given the proper facility for their performance include prepackaging, standardization of quantities issued, minimization of the variety of inventory items (as possible via a formulary system), mechanization, automation, and improved use of personnel.

Task-Oriented Design

In the task-oriented design approach, a facility is viewed as a series of interrelated task centers, and the design of each general work area is based on the specific task to be performed there.

This approach contributes to efficiency through the reduction of the number of steps it takes to complete a task. Obviously, if the time consumed by such travel can be minimized, the work will be more efficient. Consider the distance traveled in an outpatient pharmacy in which the pharmacist must go to the door to receive the prescription, return to get a label typed, put the label on, travel to obtain an empty container, travel to obtain the drug, return the stock bottle, and then deliver the prescription to the door. The travel time involved can be evaluated mathematically by multiplying the number of trips times the distance per trip.

Perhaps the most obvious application of this approach is the separating of the most-used stock from the lesser used stock and the grouping of the former close at hand. The dispensing workplace should be designed to facilitate such a stock arrangement, instead of grouping drug stock by dosage forms. Modular boxes can be used for ampules and other small items.

Minimizing motion is another way to improve efficiency through the use of a task-oriented approach. This begins with the recognition of the geometry and mechanics of human movement and proceeds to design the workplace to "fit" the human[13] (see chapter 3). The natural boundaries for human movement are circular, e.g., the hand rotating around a stationary wrist, the forearm rotating around a stationary elbow, and the extended arm and trunk rotating around the waist. Most equipment and building materials are rectangular, but rectangles do not fit the human body very efficiently, since some areas are harder to reach than other areas. The consequences are increased fatigue, lower productivity, and more mistakes. Task-oriented pharmacy fixtures are commercially available.[14]

HUMAN FACTORS IN PHARMACY

Human factors engineering (ergonomics) is a specialty within industrial engineering that focuses on the design of facilities, tasks, and work environments so that they match human capacities and limitations.[15] Recognizing that humans have limited reach distances and that the environment affects performance can lead to improvements in worker efficiency, accuracy, and job satisfaction.

Appropriate lighting levels for pharmacy work areas range from 50 to 150 footcandles. Such levels are necessary for accurate and efficient visualization of written documents and working on video display terminals (VDT's).[16] Increasing the lighting level from 100 to 146 footcandles was associated with a significantly lower dispensing error rate in a high-volume outpatient pharmacy.[17]

When sound levels rise above 70 decibels, which is the same level as a typical conversation, it becomes difficult to carry on a comprehensible conversation. Label printers, telephones, loudspeakers, and other sources of sound may exceed the 70-decibel level. Unpredictable, uncontrollable, or irregular noises can have an adverse impact on worker performance.[18] Therefore, the design of the facility should protect against excessive noise levels as well as annoying sounds.

Counters that are too low require workers to lean over, which may lead to back problems; counters that are too high require workers to hold their arms higher than their normal relaxed position, leading to muscle fatigue. Chair heights that are not adjustable can impair blood circulation to the lower leg, which results in discomfort. Inadequate leg room has resulted in significantly more complaints of sore shoulders, neck, and back pain.[19]

Research-based recommendations regarding the design of a computer terminal work station are available.[20] The following guidelines are offered.

1. *Adjustability.* The heights of the keyboard (24-34 inches above floor), screen (35-50 inches from floor to top of screen), and chair (15-21 inches above floor) should all be adjustable within the ranges noted in order to accommodate the majority of workers.[19] A chair developed for VDT work stations has been described.[20] The screen should be placed so that it is 10-25 degrees below the horizontal plane (line drawn from eyes parallel to ground). This is considered the normal line of sight and will prevent neck strain. The angles of the chair's backrest and VDT should both be adjustable.[19,20]
2. *Minimum glare.* Place the VDT so that sunlight and light from other sources cannot be seen on the screen. Glare can be severe enough to prevent reading text accurately—and can also lead to worker discomfort. The surrounding walls and furniture should be of a dark color.[20]
3. *Lighting levels.* For the work area surrounding the VDT, the lighting level should be at least 50 footcandles.

Three-Dimensional Space Planning

The 3-D approach to space planning is important for efficiency and use of space. Every wasted square foot of floor space is expensive to build and will cost many dollars per year to maintain.

Storage needs should be calculated and supplied to the architect and consultants in terms of three dimensions—linear front feet, square feet, and cubic feet—to provide the maximal flexibility to explore space-saving solutions.

An alternative to the use of additional floor space for storage is, for example, vertical space, such as storage on suspended balconies to use the otherwise unusable space near the ceilings in storage rooms. Rail-mounted shelving is efficient and easy to use. The efficiency comes from the elimination of aisles between the shelves. Aisles can then be "moved" wherever needed by simply pushing apart particular shelves, offering access to the item needed.

A third approach, particularly important in the pharmacy where many small items are stocked, is to make maximal use of the space at the back of each shelf and between the shelves. The area for picking of unit doses should be compressed, to minimize travel and motion. To accomplish this, the storage containers for unit dose packages should be designed to take up a minimum of the front-of-the-shelf space; long, thin, modular boxes are ideal for this. The use of relatively shallow shelves that are easily adjustable is recommended so that shelves can be placed as close together as possible to conserve space.

DESIGNING FOR FLEXIBILITY

The practice of hospital pharmacy is in a period of great change, with considerable uncertainty about the future. This places a high priority on designing to "build in" flexibility throughout. A recommended approach involves a growth plan, the core concept, and the use of flexible fixtures. Flexible fixtures are those that are modular, interchangeable, movable, and self-contained.

Growth Plan

There should be a growth plan for the pharmacy that provides zones of transition, or space buffers, between the pharmacy and the space external to it. For horizontal expansion, the zone of transition may be an easily movable storage room located in the expansion path. Vertical expansion to another floor is also possible via stairway and elevator, but that is usually more disruptive of workflow and internal control.

Such transition zones should be outlined in the comprehensive master facility plan for the hospital, and it behooves the pharmacist to achieve recognition of his or her needs in this regard.

The development of the pharmacy growth plan should begin by analyzing future needs at the individual work area level. This is because an increased workload does not affect work areas uniformly. For example, a second computer terminal may be needed before a second laminar flow hood, and both may be needed before a second refrigerator. The goal is a growth plan that is essentially unidirectional.

Core Concept

The core concept facilitates unidirectional growth by calling for all fixed items to be placed where they will not have to be moved. Examples of such items include plumbing, dumbwaiter, and pneumatic tube stations.

Flexible Fixtures

Truly flexible fixtures should be expandable as the workload increases and should be adaptable to changes in work methods. To achieve these goals, fixtures should be modular, to allow additional units to be ordered and inserted as the workload increases. Such units may be rearranged as work methods change and to allow the substitution of new upgraded component sections to replace those that have become outmoded or obsolete.

Fixtures should be not difficult to finish and repair, and should be easily adjustable. For example, the storage of drugs in modular boxes on adjustable shelves is preferable to casework, cabinets, and drawers. Likewise, prefabricated expandable cool rooms give greater flexibility than large refrigerators.

Fixtures, including storage shelving, should be movable, although expensive castor and lift systems are not justified for one or two moves per year. Built-in fixtures and custom-built casework should be avoided.

Fixtures should be designed for grouping in self-contained task centers for the performance of a particular task in any location to which it may be moved. For example, an ambulatory care pharmacy with two outpatient dispensing task centers should be capable of being separated and each moved to a different outpatient clinic if needed as workload expands.

THE SATELLITE PHARMACY

Satellite pharmacy facilities will be given special attention because they have a number of unique design needs.

The data in table 17-3 report the number of beds served and size of the satellite for different types of pharmacy areas, revealing no obvious relationship. It should be noted that the square footage listed may or may not be ideal. It has been recommended that a satellite should serve no fewer than 85 beds[4] of the same "medical type."[30] Fricker and Davis[31] have published information on satellite sizes with additional information about functions performed. Alexander and Barker[2] reported the results of a national survey that identified the *total* amount of space allotted to satellites (see table 17-4). The design of a satellite, as with any area of the department, should be based on a functional program for a particular hospital and nursing unit.

Functions

Functions typically found in satellite pharmacies include:

1. First-dose distribution: orals, IV's
2. Routine drug distribution (cart-filling)
3. Compounding parenteral agents
4. Drug therapy monitoring
5. Order review, editing, and computer entry
6. Provision of drug information to professionals
7. Cardiopulmonary resuscitation (CPR) team participation
8. Distribution, controlled substances
9. Consultation with physicians, nurses (remote or in satellite)

Table 17-3. Space used by satellite pharmacies of various types

Type of satellite	*Square feet*	*Number of beds served*
General	200-300	100 beds[21]
Medical/surgical	375	50-98[22]
Acute care	320	120[23]
Long-term care and psychiatric	400	250[23]
Oncology, inpatient/outpatient	200	Not reported[24]
Critical care	218	82[25]
Surgery, recovery room	500	19 OR suites–RR[26]
Surgery	70	22 OR suites[27]
Surgery, recovery room	250	Not reported[28]
Surgery	(avg. 223, range 40-700)	Not reported[29]

Table 17-4. Total space allocated to inpatient satellite pharmacies[2]

*Type of hospital**	*Responses*	*Number of Mean ± S.D. (sq. ft.)*
GMS, nonprofit, short-term	31	1,005 (± 1,559)
GMS, for profit, short-term	2	110 (± 14)
GMS, government, short-term	15	1,358 (± 1,812)

*GMS = general medical/surgical.

After the workflows for each function is determined, a list of work areas can be generated. The major work areas required may include the following:

1. Order receipt
2. Order processing and preparation
3. Compounding, parenteral agents
4. Storage, active
5. Storage, reserve
6. Dispatching
7. Clinical services area

Special design needs and problems for satellite facilities include the following:

1. The number of functions may be restricted by the amount of space available. Many satellites were formerly patient rooms.
2. If drug distribution is a function, fast and reliable transportation from the central pharmacy for drugs and supplies is essential, especially in smaller satellites with limited storage space. This is particularly true where slow response times led to the implementation of some satellites in the first place.[30]
3. Space should be provided for "visiting" professionals, if increased interaction is desired. A convenient, but quiet, area will promote this type of interaction.
4. For a delivery mechanism between satellite and nursing unit, the advantages and disadvantages of pneumatic tube systems or some other method of transportation should be considered.

A unique interprofessional image opportunity is created by the satellite pharmacy's design, since it is a highly visible pharmacy area. The image of the department should be reflected in every aspect of the design, from "looking efficient" to providing adequate storage space (preventing clutter and disorganization), to selecting an interior design that emphasizes professionalism and welcomes interaction with other professionals.

IMPLEMENTATION

Preparation

The implementation of the next facilities planning project should begin the day after a facility is occupied. This statement makes the point that facilities planning should be a continuous process. The ideal plan for the facility should be a constantly evolving concept that is periodically fixed and translated into architectural plans and physical structures whenever the opportunity arises. This viewpoint is essential if the pharmacist is to cope effectively with the short deadlines so often encountered. For example, as noted previously, the first thing asked of the pharmacist will be to recommend the space and location of the new pharmacy, which is not known until the very end of the functional planning process.

Recommended references include the out-of-print Department of Health and Human Services publication, *Planning for Hospital Pharmacies,*[4] still available in many pharmacy school libraries; the manual, *Evaluation and Space Programming Methodology Series Number 10: Pharmacy,*[3] published by Chi Systems, Inc., and a pharmacy design bibliography.[32] Auburn University School of Pharmacy has a research program involving the design of pharmacy facilities.

Pharmacists should visit other hospital pharmacy departments, but be selective. They should pick those less than 10 years old or those that have been remodeled recently, and those providing the kinds of services (or performing the kinds of functions) that they expect their own facility to provide. In particular, they should look for those where substantial planning was involved and the plan was carried out. Some bad examples (which will not be difficult to find) should be included; researchers have found they often learn more from failures than from successes.

Politics of Pharmacy Expansion

Once the need for new or modified facilities has become apparent to the pharmacist, he or she faces the task of convincing those whose support will be needed, beginning with the administration. Occasionally this is easy, as when a new facility is being built, but most of the time it is not. Even when it is, careful planning is needed so that the pharmacist can defend his or her space later when cutbacks threaten.

King[33] has recommended the following approaches for competing for space with other departments:

> You must evaluate the situation very carefully and ask several questions. Who will ultimately make the space allocation? The administrator? The administrator with the advice and influence of others? If so, who? A committee? If so, who is on that committee? How much power or influence does [each member] have over the decision-makers? What can yet be done to insure the balance of influence is in your favor? Will the decisions regarding space

allocation be made on an objective or a subjective basis? It may be that specific, positive steps will be required to assure your position in the political process, or it may be that your position is already secure once the total situation is analyzed.

In any case, it is important to be assured that your plans for programs and future services have already been discussed and approval has been documented by administration and others involved. You are in a stronger position if the approved plans for these services justify the requirement for additional space rather than developing proposals for services after the space is apparently available.

Having support from various groups from within the hospital such as administration, nursing and medical staff for the projected program is important, and knowing the space requirement for each specific program is important. In this way if a total space requested is not made available, the projections regarding which programs will have to be cut can be provided before making final space assignments.

Knowing the projected space requirements of the other departments competing for the same area and the known space available will be helpful so as to be aware that cuts will be necessary in the overall program. Knowing whether these decisions will be made on a subjective or objective basis is important to your planning strategy. It may be necessary to incorporate space for Future Achievable Tasks (FAT). If it is apparent that a cut in requested space is necessary, it may take place without a great deal of sacrifice to programs projected for the near future provided the cut can be made from space for future achievable tasks or FAT.

Timetable

Some 2-3 years may elapse between the initial planning and occupancy of the pharmacy. The timing of most of the major deadlines, as the project moves from one stage to the next, will be established by the planning committee. It is essential to know these dates, and to be on the mailing list for updates and changes.

Personnel Involvement

Whenever a new work area is being designed, the people who will be working in the area should be asked for suggestions and should be allowed to review the final design. They will be able to offer many practical suggestions to help design a more efficient workplace. This also helps to promote a more positive attitude toward the new facility.

A program for orientation of employees to the new facility should be undertaken. When major projects are involved, this may include not only printed materials, lectures, and review of the plans but actual simulation by "walking through" the new work systems planned for the new facility.

It seems to be human nature for personnel to expect new facilities to work perfectly and to solve all previous problems. They never do, of course, and it is typical for a negative reaction to surface right after the first few days of occupancy. The solution is to warn employees of this phenomenon in advance, to promote more realistic expectations. Then, provide a mechanism to note and acknowledge problems as they occur and make employees feel confident that these problems are being addressed. A simple device is a log book in which problems can be noted by the employees as they occur each day. At the end of the day, the supervisor should read and initial each entry, to signal to the employee that the problem has been noted. Some problems can be resolved by bringing them back to the group and challenging its members to find a way to "make the facility work better under the unexpected circumstances." Given a supportive environment, novel solutions to seemingly insurmountable problems often emerge.

REFERENCES

1. Flohrs WJ (ed): Lilly Hospital Pharmacy Survey, 1989. Indianapolis, IN, Eli Lilly and Company, 1989.
2. Alexander VB, Barker KN: National survey of pharmacy facilities: Space allocations and functions. *Am J Hosp Pharm* 43:324-330, 1986.
3. *Evaluation and Space Programming Methodology Series No. 10: Pharmacy.* Ann Arbor, MI, Chi Systems, 1979.
4. Barker KN: *Planning for Hospital Pharmacy Facilities.* HEW Publication No. FRA 74-4003. Rockville, MD, U.S. Department of Health, Education, and Welfare, Health Resources Administration, Health Care Facilities Service, 1974.
5. American Society of Hospital Pharmacists. ASHP guidelines for institutional use of controlled substances. *Am J Hosp Pharm* 31:582-588, 1974.
6. Francis RL, White JA: Facility layout and location — an analytical approach. Englewood Cliffs, NJ, Prentice-Hall, 1974.
7. Muther R: *Systematic Layout Planning.* Boston, MA, Cahners Publishing, 1974.
8. Barker KN, Harris JA, Webster DB, et al: Consultant evaluation of a hospital medication system: Synthesis of the new system. *Am J Hosp Pharm* 41:2016-2021, 1984.
9. Johnson RE, Myers JE, Egan DM: A resource planning model for outpatient pharmacy operations. *Am J Hosp Pharm* 29:411-418, 1972.
10. Myers JE, Johnson RE, Egan DM: A computer simulation of outpatient pharmacy operations. *Inquiry* 9:40-47, 1972.
11. Barker KN, Smith M, Winters E: A study of the work of the pharmacist and the potential use of auxiliaries. *Am J Hosp Pharm* 29:35-53, 1972.
12. Dostal MM, Daniels CE, Roberts MJ, et al: Pharmacist activities under alternative staffing arrangements. *Am J Hosp Pharm* 39:2098-2101, 1982.
13. Hepler CD: Work analysis and time study. In Brown TR, Smith MC (eds): *Handbook of Institutional Pharmacy Practice*, 2nd ed. Baltimore, MD, Williams & Wilkins, 1987, p 77.
14. Swensson ES: An innovative design in hospital pharmacy facilities. *Am J Hosp Pharm* 28:442-446, 1971.
15. Chapanis A: *Man-Machine Engineering.* Monterey, CA, Brooks/Cole Publishing, 1965, p 8.
16. Niebel BW: *Motion and Time Study,* 7th ed. Homewood, IL, Richard D. Irwin, 1982, p 229.
17. Buchanan TL, Barker KN, Gibson, JT, et al: Illumination and errors in dispensing. *Am J Hosp Pharm* 48:2137-2145, 1991.
18. Holahan CJ: *Environmental Psychology.* New York, Random House, 1982, pp 133-137, 143-144, .
19. Grandjean E: The design of workstations. In Grandjean E: *Fitting the Task to the Man: A Textbook of Occupational Ergonomics*, 4th ed. New York, Taylor & Francis, 1988.

20. Sanders MS, McCormick EJ: *Human Factors in Engineering and Design*, 6th ed. New York, McGraw-Hill Book Company, 1987, pp 354-358.
21. Smith WE, Mackewicz DW: Decentralized pharmacy services. In Brown TR, Smith MC (eds): *Handbook of Institutional Pharmacy Practice*, 2nd ed. Baltimore, MD, Williams & Wilkins, 1987, p 587.
22. Suzuki NT: The ideal satellite pharmacy. *Hosp Pharm* 22:163-164, 1987.
23. Horton RG: A satellite pharmacy program in a community hospital. *Hosp Pharm* 16:74-79, 1981.
24. Eddlemon JK, Hayman JN, Breland BD: Establishment and operation of an oncology satellite pharmacy. *Am J Hosp Pharm* 41:2045-2048, 1984.
25. Caldwell RD, Tuck BA: Justification and operation of a critical-care satellite pharmacy. *Am J Hosp Pharm* 40:2141-2145, 1983.
26. Keicher PA, McAllister JC III: Comprehensive pharmaceutical services in the surgical suite and recovery room. *Am J Hosp Pharm* 42:2454-2462, 1985.
27. Buchanan EC, Gaither MW: Development of an operating room pharmacy substation on a restricted budget. *Am J Hosp Pharm* 43:1719-1722, 1986.
28. Opoien D: Establishment of surgery satellite pharmacy services in a large community hospital. *Hosp Pharm* 19:485-490, 1984.
29. Nevius L: OR satellite pharmacies: Demographics, services and implementation. *Hosp Pharm* 22:33-38, 1978.
30. Barker KN, Pearson RE: Medication distribution systems. In Brown TR, Smith MC (eds): *Handbook of Institutional Pharmacy Practice*, 2nd ed. Baltimore, MD, Williams & Wilkins, 1987.
31. Fricker MP, Davis NM: Space requirements for pharmaceutical functions in selected non-university hospitals. *Hosp Pharm* 18:645-647, 650-652, 655-659, 662-664, 1983.
32. Pearson RE, Barker KN: Pharmacy design: A basic bibliography — 1989. *Hosp Pharm* 24:301, 1989.
33. King CM: Planning facility expansion for pharmacy (letter). *Am J Hosp Pharm* 39:36-37, 1982.

CHAPTER 18

Medication Distribution Systems

HAROLD J. BLACK and STEVEN P. NELSON

Pharmacy is responsible for the safe and effective use of medications throughout the entire hospital. This responsibility includes product selection, procurement, storage, preparation for administration, and distribution to the patient care units. Pharmacy is also responsible for ensuring that appropriate prescribing takes place and that guidelines are in place to guarantee that medications are properly administered to the patient and recorded in the patient's medical record. Thus, pharmacy is accountable for ensuring that all elements of the entire medication cycle are managed properly.

The responsibility of the pharmacist has changed dramatically during the past 25 years from the role of "product dispenser" to one of expanding clinical responsibility that encompasses the entire gamut of medication therapy. Pharmacists were once completely isolated from patient care areas where medications were being prescribed, prepared, and administered. As recently as 15 years ago most pharmacists never saw or had the opportunity to react to the actual medication order written by the physician. Instead, pharmacists repackaged bulk supplies of medications ordered by requisition from nurses, who were the ultimate interpreters of all medication orders and prepared the medications for administration to the patient. The pharmacist had virtually no opportunity to use his or her extensive education to enhance the quality and safety of drug therapy by checking to see that all medication orders were appropriate and consistent with the patient's condition and organ function indices.

The 1960's marked the beginning of significant changes in the medication distribution systems used by health care institutions as a few hospitals across the Nation experimented with a concept under which the pharmacist assumed the responsibility for preparing all doses of medication for patients and routinely monitored the appropriateness of all prescribed drug therapy. This was the genesis of the unit dose drug distribution system. Changes in medication distribution continue to unfold today: increasing automation, the blurring of select elements of professional and technical staff roles, and the call for even greater pharmacy involvement in medication therapy decisions. These issues and several others will require critical examination and innovative planning to improve medication therapy in the hospital by devising further advancements in drug distribution, dissemination of drug information, drug order evaluation, physician intervention methods, and education.

This chapter focuses on those distributive activities that transpire between the time a medication order is written until the prepared dosage is delivered by pharmacy to the nurse, physician, or other health care professional for administration to the patient. It additionally describes how newer methods of drug distribution have actually created the opportunity and demand for clinical pharmacy practice and placed the pharmacist on the health care team as an integral member.

BACKGROUND

Historical Overview

Prior to the development of modern distribution systems during the past quarter century, most drug dispensing in the hospital originated from a central pharmacy, typically located in the basement. The scope of pharmacy services was very limited, as was the pharmacy space allocation and staffing complement. The medication cycle—the sequence of events that transpired from the writing of a drug order by the physician to the eventual administration of the medication to the patient—depicted pharmacy as a relatively minor participant in drug therapy matters. The pharmacy's signal functions were the compounding, repackaging, and relabeling of multiple-dose supplies of medications into containers for subsequent dispensing and storage on a patient care unit (PCU).

One of two distribution methods was employed by pharmacy departments to deliver medications to PCU's for later administration to patients. The more commonly used method was the "floorstock system." With this system, the pharmacist dispensed multiple-dose, bulk supplies of drugs to the PCU, where nurses prepared all doses of medication intended for administration to the patient. This also included the compounding of intravenous admixtures. The supplies of medications sent to the PCU were not labeled for a specific patient and could therefore be used for several doses for numerous patients. It was not uncommon for 150 to 200 medications to be stored in a "minipharmacy" found on each PCU. The pharmacist saw only transcribed drug requisitions sent by nursing personnel, who were responsible for most steps of the medication cycle, including receipt of the original medication order from the physician, interpretation, transcription to a medication administration record, and acquisition of the drug from pharmacy in bulk form. This system delegated drug order interpretation, drug inventory, and drug preparation on the PCU to the nurse.

Another distribution method used by some hospitals was the "patient prescription system." This medication dispensing system had a few advantages over the floorstock system but included many of the same weaknesses. In this system, the physician wrote a prescription order, the nurse transcribed this order onto a medication administration profile and generated a drug order for pharmacy, the pharmacist dispensed a 2- to 5-day supply of medication, and the nurse maintained the bottles in stock and used a reminder system to determine when the medication was to be administered. As with the floorstock system, the nurse was required to "dish up" oral medications into medication cups, measure liquid doses, and prepare or measure injectable doses. Although this arrangement allowed the pharmacist to review the patient's prescription before the medication was administered, it did not provide an opportunity for the pharmacist to review relevant information about the patient, including diagnosis, allergies, other active medication orders, and organ function. This system did not provide sufficient information necessary to devise a medication profile. Thus, the pharmacist did not have the opportunity to effectively monitor drug therapy and influence optimal prescribing. The nurse rather than the pharmacist continued to play the major role in drug preparation and drug order evaluation.

The Unit Dose System

In response to a perception that the pharmacist was educated and capable of providing professional services to a greater extent than that permitted by then existing medication distribution systems in the medication cycle, the University of Iowa Hospitals and Clinics and the University of Arkansas Medical Center in the middle 1960's designed, implemented, and measured several indicants associated with a concept known as the "unit dose drug distribution system."[1,2] Funding was provided by the U.S. Public Health Service. The fundamental difference between the unit dose system and older, traditional distribution methods is the more active role of the pharmacist in the medication cycle with the patient reaping the benefits of a trained medication practitioner responsible for the medication cycle and the return of the nurse to patient care responsibilities. This altered chain of events in the new medication cycle enabled the pharmacist to review an actual copy of the physician-generated medication order, oversee all medication preparation steps, and maintain patient-specific drug profiles that detail allergy, organ function indices, and patient response data. The pharmacist-physician interactive role began to emerge, as a direct result of these changes in the distribution system. Additionally, the U.S. General Accounting Office has referred to the 1971 study conducted by Black and Upham[3] and concluded that the unit dose system is the most cost effective of all pharmacy distribution systems when the entire spectrum of drug delivery activities within a hospital is considered.

Unit Dose System Components

Perhaps the most profound alteration of drug distribution produced by the unit dose system is the feature that allowed the pharmacist to review a copy of all medication orders written by the physician prior to dispensing medications. This single feature has triggered the success of the unit dose system and has given birth to clinical pharmacy practice. Because the pharmacist reviews the actual medication order, intervention to avert inappropriate drug prescribing and to influence improved drug therapy can occur before medications are administered to the patient. Various methods have been developed to allow for pharmacist review of all patient-specific drug orders. Some hospitals require the pharmacist to transcribe the contents of the original physician order to pharmacy records used for later dispensing activities.[4] Other institutions use facsimile (or FAX) devices to transmit copies of the order from the PCU to the pharmacy.[5]

A Midwest teaching hospital uses a structured, multi-ply medication order form which requires that medication orders be written within columns labeled for drug name, dose, route of administration and interval (see figure 18-1). Thus, the prescriber actually creates the medication preparation and dispensing record for the pharmacist as a byproduct of writing each medication order. Accuracy and efficiency are vastly improved because no transcription by pharmacy is required. As the prescriber writes a medication order, a carbon copy of the original is simultaneously created and then forwarded to the pharmacist for review. The order form provides additional benefit when used as an inventory control document that allows pharmacy personnel to record all doses of medication sent from the pharmacy to the PCU. Additionally, a form of this type can play a crucial role in the transition from the traditional, paper-intensive system to a fully automated medication order entry system, because it simplifies the order entry process. Because of the form structure, pharmacy and nursing personnel can interpret and manage medication orders more efficiently and accurately under a manual system, and as one or both of these disciplines enter medication orders via a computer terminal, the form simplifies that process. Eventually the need for a manually prepared medication order form will be eliminated as all prescribers enter medication orders directly into a computer terminal. The computer will then generate any documents required by nursing, pharmacy, and the permanent medical record.

Medication order processing under the unit dose system involves several steps designed to permit multiple checks of each dose of medication before it is administered to the patient. A copy of the original medication order form (prepared by the physician) is forwarded to the pharmacy, where the pharmacist reviews and edits the medication order form and compares each entry against previous drug orders and the information maintained in a patient-specific medication profile. If a problem with an order is encountered, the pharmacist directly intervenes with the prescriber to suggest more appropriate alternatives. Next, a pharmacy technician prepares the medication needed during the forthcoming 24-hour period according to protocols that differentiate the various sequences (see table 18-1). The pharmacist checks each corresponding dose of medication previously prepared by the technician for accuracy and authorizes these medications to be delivered to the PCU. The majority of medications are dispensed via a specially designed medication administration cart, which is positioned on the PCU until the prescribed administration time. After the physician writes

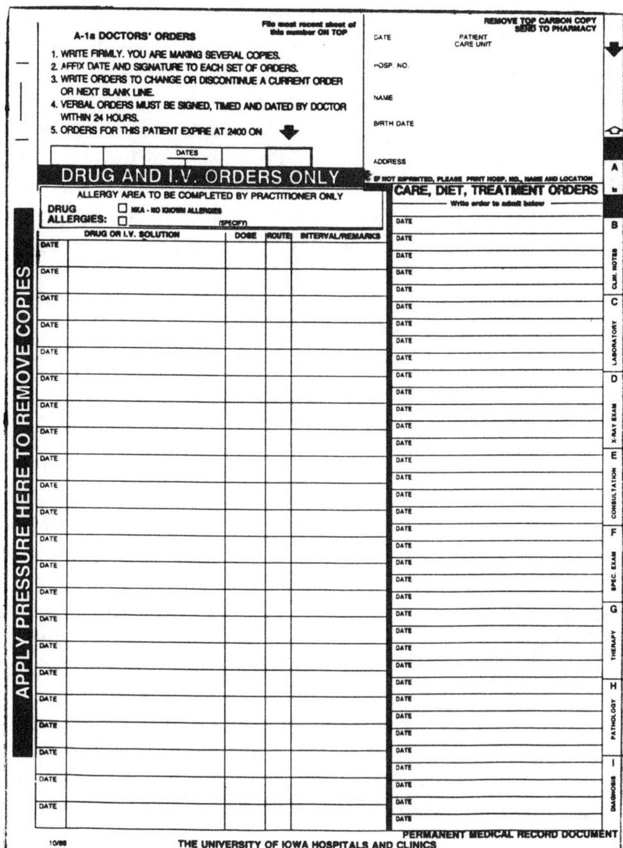

A-1a DOCTORS' ORDERS

File most recent sheet of this number ON TOP

1. WRITE FIRMLY. YOU ARE MAKING SEVERAL COPIES.
2. AFFIX DATE AND SIGNATURE TO EACH SET OF ORDERS.
3. WRITE ORDERS TO CHANGE OR DISCONTINUE A CURRENT ORDER OR NEXT BLANK LINE.
4. VERBAL ORDERS MUST BE SIGNED, TIMED AND DATED BY DOCTOR WITHIN 24 HOURS.
5. ORDERS FOR THIS PATIENT EXPIRE AT 2400 ON

DATES

REMOVE TOP CARBON COPY SEND TO PHARMACY

DATE | PATIENT CARE UNIT

HOSP. NO.

NAME

BIRTH DATE

ADDRESS

IF NOT IMPRINTED, PLEASE PRINT HOSP. NO., NAME AND LOCATION

DRUG AND I.V. ORDERS ONLY

ALLERGY AREA TO BE COMPLETED BY PRACTITIONER ONLY

DRUG ALLERGIES: ☐ NKA - NO KNOWN ALLERGIES ☐ ______ (SPECIFY)

DATE	DRUG OR I.V. SOLUTION	DOSE	ROUTE	INTERVAL/REMARKS
DATE				

CARE, DIET, TREATMENT ORDERS

Write order to admit below

DATE

APPLY PRESSURE HERE TO REMOVE COPIES

A B CLIN. NOTES C LABORATORY D X-RAY EXAM E CONSULTATION F SPEC. EXAM G THERAPY H PATHOLOGY I DIAGNOSIS

PERMANENT MEDICAL RECORD DOCUMENT

10/90 THE UNIVERSITY OF IOWA HOSPITALS AND CLINICS

Figure 18-1. Structured inpatient medication order form, which is completed by the prescriber. Carbon copies sent to pharmacy serve as pharmacy's medication preparation and dispensing record.

the chart order, all medication orders are transcribed by the nurse onto a medication administration record (MAR). The MAR form is a companion to the medication order form, and thus it can be functionally structured in a manner similar to that document to enhance consistency and accuracy. The order written on the MAR should create a duplicate copy so that in addition to providing evidence that medication doses were given to the patient, this record can provide a method to charge the patient for medication actually received, thus avoiding the need to issue credits. Before administering each dose, the nurse compares the medication label on the drug product with the appropriate MAR entry. The nurse then administers the dose to the patient and records the fulfillment of the order on the MAR.

The physical concept of the unit dose distribution program is unit dose packaging (sometimes referred to as "unit-of-use" packaging), that is, the placement of each dose of medication into a separate package that bears a label listing drug name, strength or concentration, lot or batch number, and expiration date. Rather than dispense multiple-dose bulk containers of several drugs to a PCU that may potentially be used for several patients, unit dose distribution employs single unit-of-use containers for each dose of a medication (whether oral solid, oral liquid, respiratory therapy, or injectable) that is dispensed. Use of

Table 18-1. Medication delivery methods used by a tertiary level care center.

Medication delivery from pharmacy to PCU *Medication category*	*How medication is delivered to PCU*
1. Stable scheduled medications	24-hr. supply in patient-specific bin on med cart
2. Unstable scheduled medications	Automatic delivery to PCU 1 hr. before admin. time
3. Scheduled IV/TPN solutions	Automatic delivery to PCU 1 hr. before admin. time
4. PRN ("as needed") medications	Limited supply in patient-specific bin on med cart; limited floorstock supply; delivered by pharmacy in response to request from PCU
5. Controlled substances	Limited patient-specific supply secured on med cart; limited floorstock supply
6. Demand or "STAT" medications	Delivered by pharmacy in response to request from PCU
7. Emergency medications	Emergency drug kits located on PCU; delivered by pharmacy in response to request from PCU
8. Investigational medications	Per dispensing protocol

such packaging allows the pharmacy to dispense only those doses needed by a particular patient during a designated period of time (usually 24 hours). Most drugs are now available in unit dose packaging from commercial manufacturers. Other medications that require repackaging by the pharmacy are prepared using equipment and procedures that ensure drug integrity and patient safety.[6] The greatest impact of unit dose packaging is in creating the opportunity to deploy trained pharmacy technicians for the preparation of medication for administration plus the other mechanical elements of the medication cycle. The use of carefully supervised technicians frees the pharmacist from many of the manual dispensing tasks and enables him or her to devote more time to other responsibilities.

Once dispensed from the pharmacy and delivered to the PCU, the medication is securely stored on a unit dose medication administration cart (or med cart), a unique piece of equipment that was conceived and developed in the 1960's to effectively implement unit dose drug distribution. This lockable cart, with its series of sliding drawers and removable trays, can be accessed only by authorized personnel. It houses a series of patient-labeled bins arranged in room and bed sequence, each holding a 24-hour supply of medication for the designated patient. The cart also features storage space for auxiliary supplies, a flat surface area that serves as workspace, and wheels or casters that allow it to be moved from patient to patient during medication administration activities. In most instances, there is one supply of medication for each patient in a med cart stationed on the PCU, while at the same time, there is another holding or transfer cart in the pharmacy being filled with the next day's supply of medications. On a routine basis (usually once daily) at a predetermined time, the replacement supply is taken to the PCU, the bins that held the previous day's doses are returned to the pharmacy, and the replenishment procedure begins anew. The cart fill process is usually performed by pharmacy technicians, who review all previously processed orders and then place a specified amount of medication into each patient's medication bin located on the med cart. The pharmacist later checks the contents of each bin to ensure agreement with the orders. Many pharmacy departments have streamlined the cart fill process by using an assembly-line approach and automated technology. The increased productivity of assembly-line filling is accomplished through the implementation of computer order entry and the subsequent creation of computerized fill lists detailing patient name, all scheduled medications that are ordered, and the number of dosage units needed for the following 24-hour period. This filling method can reduce cart fill time and increase accuracy.[7]

Medications that are needed on demand or prior to the time when the med cart is scheduled to be replenished must be delivered to the PCU via different mechanisms. Delivery of such medications may be prompted via a newly written medication order or a written communication form that the nurse initiates to request ordered medications (e.g., PRN or "as needed" items) from the pharmacy. Depending upon the physical configuration of facilities, many institutions use conveyance equipment such as a pneumatic tube carrier system to deliver these medications to sites physically distant from the pharmacy. Other hospitals have implemented a pharmacy courier system that is designed to routinely pick up new orders and deliver medications needed before the med cart is replenished. The courier service extends from pharmacy to each PCU and usually operates every 30 minutes during day and evening hours. In either case, all doses are placed in unit dose packaging and designated for use on a particular patient.

Unit dose distribution may be enhanced when selected stable medications are delivered to the PCU by other methods. Certain categories of medication, particularly those with unpredictable use, are frequently handled separately from most drugs that are dispensed from the pharmacy via the med cart. PRN medications have been provided to the nurse on the PCU in a variety of ways. These have included (1) fulfillment of specific-need requests sent to pharmacy by the nurse, (2) automatic placement of a predetermined supply of PRN medication into the patient's drug bin located on the med cart and, (3) placement of select floorstock supplies of medication on the PCU. Specific-need requests are time consuming for both the nurse and pharmacy personnel and can delay timely administration of the drug to the patient. Daily placement of PRN medication into the patient's drug bin is inefficient because the doses are often repeatedly returned to the pharmacy unused, credited, and sent out again with the following day's supply of medications.[8,9] These inefficient methods of dispensing PRN medications have led many pharmacy departments to use a modified floorstock system on PCUs to complement unit dose drug distribution, thus creating handling efficiencies.[10] Limited floorstock supplies of medications with low toxicity potential (e.g., liquid antacids or laxative agents) are placed onto the med cart so that the nurse can quickly and easily administer a dose when needed by the patient. Although not assigned to a particular patient, these supplies are contained in unit dose packaging, and their rate of use is monitored closely by the pharmacy. Pharmacy, nursing, and most important, the patient benefit from this slightly altered concept of unit dose distribution.

Controlled substances are also frequently handled separately from other medications as a consequence of the record-keeping and storage requirements of Federal and State laws. These agents, namely Drug Enforcement Agency (DEA) Schedule II, III, IV, and V drugs, have a substantial potential for abuse and must, therefore, be securely stored in the pharmacy and on the PCU where only authorized personnel have access. To deter the misuse of these agents, pharmacies frequently employ sophisticated accountability systems that use structured issuance records and perpetual supply inventories.[11,12] The medication order cycle remains unaltered, for the physician orders controlled substances as he or she would any other medication, the nurse transcribes the order onto the MAR, and the pharmacist reviews a copy of the order and compares it with the patient's drug profile.

These medications are in most cases stable products that do not require special storage to maintain drug integrity; in fact, most controlled substances are now prepared commercially in unit dose packaging. Many pharmacies have created distribution systems for controlled substances that employ limited floorstock storage in a secure area of the PCU, structured accountability forms, and a daily audit of the controlled substances inventory kept on the PCU. Pharmacy technicians may be assigned to make rounds to all PCU's on a routine basis to replenish floorstock supplies and participate jointly with nursing personnel in performing daily inventories. The use of such modified floorstock systems for the distribution of controlled substances decreases pharmacy labor expenditures significantly while providing needed security and having minimal impact upon nursing time. However, studies have shown that distribution of controlled substances, even with modified floorstock systems, requires a significant pharmacy and nursing labor expenditure in order to provide needed security.[13,14]

Another exception to the standard unit dose method of dispensing all medications in ready-to-administer form at the time of need involves emergency medications used in the case of a "code blue." A code blue indicates that a person has experienced cardiac and/or respiratory failure and requires immediate emergency treatment, which often includes drug therapy. Because of the short amount of time that elapses before irreversible brain damage occurs (approximately 4-6 minutes), medications needed for resuscitation efforts must be instantly available to the code team. To avoid loss of time in preparation and delivery of such drugs from the pharmacy to the code site, most pharmacy departments provide preassembled emergency drug kits or trays to all PCU's of the hospital. The kits contain selected emergency drugs (approved by medical, nursing, and pharmacy specialists) in ready-to-administer form. Alternatively, some hospitals assign a pharmacist to the code blue team and when alerted, the pharmacist selects medications from the emergency drug kit and participates in drug therapy decisions and in recording drug administration.[15] Whether or not a pharmacist participates on the team, pharmacy is responsible for maintaining the content of the emergency kit and associated controls.

UNIT DOSE SYSTEM DESIGN

When an institution makes a decision to implement unit dose dispensing, it must determine the scope of pharmacy services that will be provided. The longstanding philosophy of the authors on unit dose systems is set forth in a 1984 publication that evaluated the impact of this medication delivery system.[16] The authors define a "unit dose system" as one that includes clinical pharmacy services along with drug distribution activities; that is, the two components go hand in hand. If the scope is essentially confined to drug distribution activities, it may be classified as a "unit dose packaging and distribution program." This requires only that pharmacy prepare doses of medication, use unit dose packaging, and deliver patient-specific supplies of medication to the PCU on a routine basis. This system includes negligible clinical pharmacy services.

A unit dose system, on the other hand, requires greater personnel resources, includes a higher level of job content for pharmacy staff, and has a greater impact upon the quality of medication therapy. The key component of the system has been the requirement that clinical pharmacy services be included with unit dose medication distribution. Therefore, in addition to having responsibility for medication preparation as provided by a unit dose packaging and distribution program, the pharmacist also takes on the larger role of drug therapy expert. The pharmacist reviews each medication order and evaluates its appropriateness, performs baseline drug therapy monitoring to ensure that all prescribed drug regimens are compatible with patient condition and existing organ function, and educates other members of the health care team about the proper use and administration of all drugs. These vital activities of the unit dose system constitute the core of clinical pharmacy practice.

The next decision is to determine whether unit dose dispensing will emanate from a central location, or if one or more decentralized pharmacy satellites will be established. This decision will be based upon such factors as institution size, space availability, medical and nursing staff considerations, personnel, and other resource availability. For larger hospitals, the decentralized approach accommodates the "unit dose system" concept with its attending clinical pharmacy elements.

Centralization

Centralized unit dose services are generally provided from a single, self-contained location within the hospital. The pharmacy receives copies of all medication orders, and all medications are prepared, packaged, and dispensed using unit dose packaging and distribution methods. Complete unit dose services with baseline drug monitoring and education services may be provided depending upon staffing availability and financial resources. Centralization of services may be especially useful to hospitals with limited space, small size, or vertical design such that a central location still permits quick and easy access to all patient care areas. Centralization may have the additional advantage of requiring a smaller technical and professional staff than that necessary to operate a more widely dispersed decentralized service.[17]

Decentralization

A decentralized unit dose distribution system operates from two or more dispensing locations commonly called "pharmacy satellites." These satellites, which at a minimum provide pharmacist order review and first dose dispensing, act as the base from which clinical pharmacy services are provided by a unit dose system. In larger hospitals with several satellites, it is not efficient to duplicate all pharmacy activities at each dispensing site. In order to support the drug distribution functions of the satellites and concentrate those activities that are most efficiently performed using large-scale production, there often exists a central support pharmacy, which is staffed with a specially trained cadre of pharmacists and pharmacy technicians. The central pharmacy provides services such as unit dose medication cart fill, medication repackaging, intravenous admixture compounding, and controlled substances distribution. The products prepared at this location are then transferred to the satellites, where they are readied for final delivery to the PCU. Thus, the pharmacist stationed in the satellite is in an ideal position to oversee both the distributive and clinical aspects of medication therapy used within the hospital.[18,19] Of course, staffing-to-bed ratios must be adequate to provide the time for the pharmacist to practice clinically.

The type of facility from which decentralized unit dose services are provided will vary depending upon space and personnel availability, medical and nursing staff requirements, and level of service to be provided. The most common facility is the stationary pharmacy satellite (200 to 300 square feet), which is typically placed near one or more PCU's, serves from 60 to 120 patients, and generally provides service 16 hours a day.

In general, the staffing requirements for a typical decentralized satellite include one or two pharmacists and two pharmacy technicians per each day and evening shift; staffing is normally reduced during night hours (approximately 11:00 p.m. until 7:00 a.m.), when workload decreases. Actual staffing needs will be influenced by the acuity index of the particular patient population, spectrum of clinical services to be provided, and presence or absence of centralized pharmacy support services. Space requirements are affected by the scope of distribution services to be provided from the satellite (i.e., provision of only first dose versus complete distribution service), and by the type of patient population being served.

Specialized pharmacy satellites may be established when particular service objectives are identified relative to specific clinical services such as pediatrics,[20] oncology,[21] critical care,[22] emergency room,[23] and the operating room.[24] Again, the resources available to the pharmacy department must be carefully evaluated to ensure that the necessary staff, equipment, supplies, and drug and therapeutic information resources are available to achieve the service objective.

Some institutions provide decentralized unit dose services via a mobile pharmacy cart system.[25] The mobile cart, which is transported from one PCU to another, may be operated by both professional and technical personnel and can usually offer first dose service and baseline drug monitoring during specific times of day. Lack of space for a permanently based pharmacy facility is a frequently cited factor for using a mobile cart to implement these services.

PERSONNEL RESPONSIBILITIES

Professional Staff

The functions and responsibilities of pharmacists and nurses in the operation of a hospital drug delivery system have changed dramatically with the development of the unit dose system. The floorstock and patient prescription systems required nurses to perform many medication-related activities that are now the responsibility of pharmacists. Pharmacists formerly had few responsibilities beyond drug compounding, packaging, and labeling duties. Now, with the implementation of the unit dose system, many of the activities once performed by nurses have been assumed by pharmacy personnel. Pharmacists and pharmacy technicians perform most medication-related functions so that nurses can be more involved in other direct patient care activities. In the study conducted by Black and Upham,[3] it was determined that the implementation of a unit dose system allowed the savings in nursing labor attributable to one pharmacy satellite serving 130 general medicine beds to be equivalent to 5.5 full-time registered nurse positions. This system requires more pharmacists but fewer nurses. The patient is the winner in this tradeoff, because the expertise of the pharmacist is brought to bear on medication therapy and the nurse is more available to provide nursing care.

The evolution of the unit dose system has dramatically changed the pharmacist's responsibilities from simple, recurring mechanical duties to professional service responsibility for the hospital's complete medication order cycle. Medication order review and prospective monitoring of all drug therapy, activities once seen as revolutionary but now accepted as routine, have positioned the pharmacist as a major participant in the medication order cycle. The pharmacist has become a highly visible member of the health care team who is responsible for the quality of all medication-related activities from the time the drug is purchased to the time it is administered to the patient, and to the assessment of outcomes of therapy. This increased presence in the patient care setting has subsequently allowed for the development of extensive clinical pharmacy practices and demonstrated that the hospital pharmacist can, in a cost-effective manner, provide both quality distributive and clinical pharmacy services.

Pharmacy Technicians

A new category of health care providers was created with the establishment of the unit dose drug distribution system, the pharmacy technician. This occurred because advanced unit dose medication packaging and labeling allows for nonpharmacist staff to perform most of the manipulative tasks associated with drug preparation and delivery, functions that were formerly performed by professional staff under traditional distribution systems. Technician work is supervised and checked by a pharmacist, thus providing a double-check, a safety feature not available when one person prepared and immediately administered a dose. Additionally, unit dose packaging provides further conservation of pharmacist time because the pharmacist can make a final check in lieu of several in-process checks.

Pharmacy technicians are typically trained for 6 to 20 weeks by the employing department; this program is then followed by additional on-the-job training. Competence is subsequently certified after the individual demonstrates proficiency in medication preparation and successfully completes a written examination. The accreditation of select technician training programs has begun. There is also a movement taking place to form technician associations in concert with State hospital pharmacy societies. This alliance may culminate in the establishment of higher standards of practice and training for technicians.

The technician has assumed most duties related to medication preparation and delivery, but the pharmacist supervises all work completed and ensures the integrity and safety of each dose dispensed. Because most of the time-consuming tasks of drug preparation have been delegated to technicians, the pharmacist has been freed to pursue other opportunities, most notably the development and expansion of clinical pharmacy practice.

EVALUATION OF UNIT DOSE SERVICES

While implementation of a unit dose system has been a boon to the practice of hospital pharmacy and given the pharmacist the opportunity to more fully apply his or her education and training, one must critically evaluate the benefits of this program to modern health care in general. In many instances, such an evaluation would focus on cost analysis. However, it is also important to examine the aspect of improved patient care. In reality these issues are intertwined, for improved patient care can lead to decreased hospitalization and, during these days of prospective payment systems, decreased costs.[26]

Actual cost savings realized with a unit dose system are frequently based upon decreased expenditures for drugs and nursing personnel time associated with medication-related activities. Although the cost of purchasing and/or preparing unit dose medications is higher than that encountered in a traditional distribution system, this cost is somewhat offset by the reduction of drug inventories necessary to stock each PCU under a unit dose system. Smaller inventories on each PCU lead to reduced drug wastage, as does the packaging per se, because of the ability to return unused doses to stock. Nursing personnel requirements in medication-related activities can be reduced and/or existing staff reassigned to other patient care duties. The use of supervised pharmacy technicians has been shown to be a very cost-effective way to contain labor costs. The unit dose system can actually enhance revenue by decreasing the number of lost charges. Following the implementation of a restructured medication administration record, a Midwest teaching hospital witnessed a 12 percent improvement in medication charting accuracy, which at that time translated into an annual increase in revenue of over $1 million.[3]

Replacement of traditional medication distribution systems with unit dose services adds the safety elements of labeling to the point of administration, plus a double-check of every dose by pharmacy and nursing. Thus, a reduction in medication errors usually occurs following the implementation of a unit dose system, and this is a fact cited most often as the basis for implementation. Comparisons showing medication error rates for traditional versus unit dose distribution systems have demonstrated results favoring the latter.[27]

Perhaps the greatest positive impact that a unit dose system can have upon patient care is the subsequent enhancement of overall clinical pharmacy service. It is with this fact in mind that the unit dose system should be most closely examined.

ENHANCEMENT OF CLINICAL ROLE

Although drug distribution is a major responsibility for any hospital pharmacy service, pharmacy management must not confuse the drug distribution program and clinical pharmacy services and assume that one without the other is adequate. Unit dose packaging and distribution programs have permitted the pharmacist to accept greater responsibility for the drug products that are used in the hospital, but it is the unit dose system that has led to greater use of the pharmacist's drug therapy expertise and, in turn, improved patient care. With this system in place, the pharmacist assumes responsibility not only for delivering a carefully prepared drug product to the patient in a safe, accurate, and timely manner, but also for prospectively monitoring all prescribed drug therapy to assess appropriateness of dose, suitability of therapy in light of the patient's condition, cost-effectiveness of therapy, and the potential for drug interactions. These combined activities form the foundation of clinical pharmacy practice.

The most revolutionary component of the unit dose system was, and remains today, pharmacist review of all medication orders written by the physician. This one activity allows the pharmacist to evaluate the appropriateness of a medication order and, when required, intervene with the prescriber to ensure that optimum therapy is provided. The system can also be used to prevent drug interactions and minimize or identify adverse drug reactions that could compromise patient safety and well-being. Additionally, the pharmacist can compare all medication orders against a patient-specific medication profile (see figure 18-2) consisting of a patient problem list, allergies, age, weight, laboratory indices, and interactions with other members of the patient's health care team. Such a profile allows specific categories of patients to be followed more closely if their underlying condition or drug therapy may put them at greater risk of experiencing adverse reactions and drug toxicity. Basic patient demographics and current laboratory data are often available in the pharmacy via a video display terminal, which allows the pharmacist easy access to the most up-to-date patient information. Hence, ongoing, baseline monitoring of the patient's medication profile permits the pharmacist to use his or her extensive education and judgment to enhance the patient's drug therapy, and consequently, overall health care.

Ideally, a medication delivery system should be designed in a manner that places the pharmacist near the patient care setting where the decisions about drug therapy are being made. Such a presence can be used to influence prescribing decisions before an order is written. Lines of communication are strengthened between physicians and nurses and the pharmacist, and with experience, other health care professionals come to view the pharmacist as a primary source of drug information and seek his or her assistance when confronted with drug therapy problems. But before communication channels can be augmented and prescribing habits influenced, the pharmacist must demonstrate the technical ability to get the medication to the patient in an efficient and orderly manner.

PATIENT-SPECIFIC MEDICATION PROFILE

Patient Name:
Hospital Number:
Age/Sex: PCU
Admission Date:
Contact Physician:
Pharmacist:

Patient Drug Therapy Information
Allergies:
DATE/wt. (kg) DATE/wt. (kg)
Ht (cm)
IBW

Prior Drug Therapy
☐ Smoker ☐ Non-Smoker

Admission Problem List
(1)
(2)
(3)
(4)
(5)
(6)
(7)

Adverse Drug Reactions

Problems During Admission
(1) (4)
(2) (5)
(3) (6)

Baseline Laboratory Tests
DATE ALP LDH BILI AST BUN CRT

Additional Laboratory Information
DATE

Drug Serum Level Data
DATE Drug Dose/Schedule Level DATE Drug Dose/Schedule Level

Monitoring Plan
Problem Approach

Document Requested Medication History and/or Discharge Counseling on Reverse.

THE UNIVERSITY OF IOWA HOSPITALS AND CLINICS

Figure 18-2. Patient-specific medication profile, which is maintained by the pharmacist. The reverse side is used to record all interventions (and subsequent outcomes) with other health care professionals plus clinical workload data used to monitor productivity.

EVOLUTION OF OTHER PHARMACY ACTIVITIES

Patient Care Services

The implementation of modern drug distribution systems and expanded clinical activities have provided the stimulus for the development and growth of other pharmacy services that augment the drug delivery process. Some of these activities have been implemented as a result of outside forces (e.g., government bodies and professional organizations) that influence how health care providers should "provide," whereas other services have been created in response to the growing societal demands upon health care in general and pharmacy in particular.

In order to provide a complete medication delivery program, hospital pharmacies may now distribute medication-related "products" in addition to the drugs themselves. Several pharmacy departments in larger metropolitan or teaching hospitals have installed drug information centers that may include a poison control center. These centers have developed schemes for the organized distribution of practical drug information to health care practitioners and, in many cases, the public at large. Pharmacies may also provide an investigational drug division or investigational pharmacists who work directly with physicians to design ways to distribute, administer, and critically evaluate the effectiveness and safety of experimental drug agents. In addition to dispensing these medications in the traditional sense, the pharmacy is helping to distribute the knowledge gathered from the early use of these new agents. The pharmacy departments in a small number of hospitals coordinate all activities associated with medication administration to the patient, but the use of this type of service has remained very limited.

Quality Assurance

Pharmacy, like most other professions, has developed quality assurance standards to ensure that the products and services provided to patients are the best possible and do truly enhance patient care. The activities performed in the course of medication preparation and distribution are routinely monitored using predetermined criteria to guarantee that assigned standards of performance are met.[28] Quality assurance is used to evaluate the performance of several distributive activities, including:

1. Unit dose medication cart filling/checking
2. Creating/updating patient medication profiles
3. Prepackaging unit dose medications
4. Compounding parenteral admixtures
5. Reviewing medication administration records

Routine monitoring of these activities identifies existing or potential problems in the medication distribution process and allows the pharmacist to determine what course of action is necessary to correct the problem. Thus, quality assurance is the tool that hospital pharmacy uses to police its own operation.

Productivity Monitoring

Pharmacy managers have devised programs to document all product and nonproduct contributions to patient care and monitor the total quantity of services that pharmacy personnel provide. Only with such a productivity monitoring system in place can inefficiencies be pinpointed, resources reallocated, and services improved. Many institutions now participate in the PharmaTrend® productivity monitoring system, which is designed to measure several aspects of pharmacy services—distributive and clinical— and can be used by pharmacy administration in defense of current structures and services or as evidence of the need to expand. Furthermore, the data derived from PharmaTrend reports are very specific and can be used to quantify the workforce necessary to serve each PCU. Such specificity allows management to reallocate resources to those areas of greatest need and subsequently enhance quality and efficiency.

New Technologies

In order to more efficiently manage these new services and further reduce the pharmacist's involvement with those mechanical, nonjudgmental aspects of drug distribution, hospital pharmacies have participated in the development and implementation of several new labor-saving technologies. Automation and technological growth have been most notable in the areas of information management, medication order entry, automated drug dispensing, sterile fluid transfer, and inventory control.[29]

Installation of an information management system has become a priority for most hospitals, and pharmacy departments have taken an active part in the development and implementation of the system to ensure that the maximum payoff is realized for both distribution and clinical services.[30] Computerized information sharing can now provide the physician, nurse, and pharmacist with the most up-to-date patient information and assist with data assessment and use. Advanced information systems should at least be able to provide the user with patient medical history, current laboratory data, and medication profile data. Systems have also been developed to organize and store information relating to billing and revenue, inventory management, quality assurance data, and productivity. Applications continue as health care services move toward paper-free communication systems.

Automation has led to the development of computerized drug order entry systems. Such systems are typically used to prepare a cart fill list separate from the patient profile to facilitate the filling of a unit dose medication cart. Currently, order entry into the computer is usually performed by pharmacy or nursing personnel and is, in effect, electronic transcription of the physician's handwritten medication order. Eventually, prescribers may place all drug orders directly into the computer and further simplify the process. Clinical features have also been built into these systems so that when new orders are entered into the computer, the pharmacist is alerted to potential drug interactions, solution incompatibilities, and special dispensing warnings.

Several types of automated dispensing devices have been invented and marketed. One product has been developed to automatically dispense oral medications to be used when filling a unit dose medication cart.[31] This machine will accept a fill list that may be downloaded from a mainframe computer system into a personal computer, which in turn controls the dispensing device. The machine then packages solid oral medications contained in canisters into packaging materials that are labeled with the drug name, strength, expiration date, lot number, and other desired information. The sequence of packaging is usually by patient name, which may also be included on the label. Error rates with these systems have been claimed to be significantly less than with traditional manual operations.[31]

Other devices have been marketed that can dispense medications directly to authorized personnel working on a PCU. One such instrument is an automated dispensing module that can deliver doses of controlled substances to anesthesia personnel.[29] Only authorized staff with assigned entry codes have access to the medications contained in the module stationed in an operating suite. Thus, the machine not only aids in the distribution of these agents but also increases accountability while limiting the potential for drug diversion.

Automation of sterile fluid transfer and parenteral solution compounding is a newer technology gaining acceptance by pharmacy operations with extensive parenteral nutrition programs.[29] These systems employ a computer software package, a fluid transfer device, and "pipetting" equipment that automatically measures and injects additive solutions into parenteral admixtures. The advantage of an automated system is increased productivity, because staff are freed from many of the time-consuming, labor-intensive steps required to prepare these solutions manually and are therefore able to perform other tasks.

Bar code technology has been used extensively in retail settings; it has also shown some application in hospital inventory control and is being evaluated for facilitating the documentation of dispensing, administration, and charging of medications.[32] This technology employs bar codes, a series of lines or bars with varying width that represent a numerical code which, when electronically scanned, corresponds to an assigned product. Bar code scanning has the potential to increase productivity and reduce the "paper flow" currently used to record all medication dispensing transactions.

THE FUTURE

Medication delivery systems will continue to change and evolve during the coming years as hospital pharmacy departments rise to meet new challenges. The pharmacist must effectively integrate shifting resources, changing personnel roles, expanding technology, and new clinical services into one package that provides superior patient care. It will not be enough to buy pharmaceuticals in unit dose packaging and place them on the PCU while turning the balance of pharmacy practice over to nursing. Pharmacy leaders must acknowledge that the ever-increasing complexity of drug therapy requires that pharmacy play a larger part in the provision of health care so that therapeutic misadventures are avoided and medication therapies that are prescribed do truly improve the patient's quality of life. But before any pharmacy service can enhance patient care through the expansion of clinical services that guide medication therapies, it must first demonstrate that it can safely and competently deliver those medications.

REFERENCES

1. Black HJ, Tester WW: Decentralized pharmacy operations utilizing the unit dose concept. *Am J Hosp Pharm* 21:344-350, 1964.
2. Barker KN, Heller WM, Brennan JJ, et al: The development of a centralized unit dose dispensing system. *Am J Hosp Pharm* 20:568-579, 1963.
3. Black HJ, Upham R: *Impact of Unit Dose Pharmacy Service on the Time Involvement of Registered Nurses with Medication Activities*. Iowa City, University of Iowa, 1971.
4. Davis NM: Patient profile draws the whole picture. *J Am Hosp Assoc* 45:110-122, 1971.
5. Newberg DF, Stevens J: Reduction in order turnaround time, telephone calls, and trips to the pharmacy by means of facsimile transceivers. *Hosp Pharm* 23:128-129,138, 1988.
6. Patel JA, Curtis EG, Phillips GL: Quality control guidelines for single unit packaging of parenterals in the hospital pharmacy. *Am J Hosp Pharm* 29:947-951, 1972.
7. McGovern D: Print, prepare, check, and deliver a 24-hour supply of unit dose medication for 600 patients in one hour. *Hosp Pharm* 16:193-206, 1981.
8. Baker GE: Reducing the handling of p.r.n. doses in a unit dose drug distribution system. *Am J Hosp Pharm* 44:2255-2256, 1987.
9. Woller TW, Kreling DH, Ploetz PA: Quantifying unused orders for as-needed medications. *Am J Hosp Pharm* 44:1347-1352, 1987.
10. McCollum GK, Poe WP: An effective method of handling PRN orders to reduce labor and improve efficiency. Paper presented at ASHP Annual Meeting, Nashville, TN, 1989.
11. Somani SM, Giese RM, Roberts AW: Design of a revised controlled substances distribution system. *Am J Hosp Pharm* 39:612-618, 1982.
12. Woller TW, Roberts MJ, Ploetz PA: Recording schedule II drug use in a decentralized drug distribution system. *Am J Hosp Pharm* 44:349-353, 1987.
13. Prosnick JJ: Evaluation of a hospital controlled substances distribution system. *Am J Hosp Pharm* 32:606-609, 1975.
14. Norvell MJ, McAllister JC, Bailey E: Cost analysis of drug distribution for controlled substances. *Am J Hosp Pharm* 40:801-807, 1983.
15. Batenhorst RL, Clifton GD, Booth DC, et al: Evaluation of 516 cardiopulmonary resuscitation attempts. *Am J Hosp Pharm* 42:2478-2483, 1985.
16. Black HJ: Unit dose drug distribution: A 20-year perspective. *Am J Hospital Pharm* 41:2086-2088, 1984.
17. John GW, Burkhart VD, Lamy PP: Pharmacy personnel activities and costs in decentralized and centralized unit dose drug distribution systems. *Am J Hosp Pharm* 33:38-43, 1976.
18. Clapham CE, Hepler CD, Reinders TP: Economic consequences of two drug-use control systems in a teaching hospital. *Am J Hosp Pharm* 45:2329-2340, 1988.
19. Kelly WN, Meyer JD, Flatley CJ: Cost analysis of a satellite pharmacy. *Am J Hosp Pharm* 43:1929-1930, 1986.
20. Tisdale JE: Justifying a pediatric critical-care satellite pharmacy by medication-error reporting. *Am J Hosp Pharm* 43:368-371, 1986.
21. Sauer KA, Nowak MM, Coons SJ, et al: Justification and implementation of a cancer center pharmacy satellite. *Am J Hosp Pharm* 46:1389-1392, 1989.
22. Caldwell RD, Tuck BA: Justification and operation of a critical-care satellite pharmacy. *Am J Hosp Pharm* 40:2141-2145, 1983.
23. Powell MF, Soloman DK, McEachen RA: Twenty-four hour emergency pharmaceutical services. *Am J Hosp Pharm* 42:831-835, 1985.
24. Vogel DP, Barone J, Penn F: Ideas for action: The operating room pharmacy satellite. *Top Hosp Pharm Mgt* 6(2):63-81, 1986.
25. Cummins BA, Krancz DA, Bennett DL, et al: Implementation of mobile decentralized pharmaceutical services in a community teaching hospital. *Am J Hosp Pharm* 44:318-324, 1987.
26. Davern PF, Kubica AJ: Controlling drug costs: Administrative and clinical strategies. *Top Hosp Pharm Mgt* 4:49-59, 1984.
27. Hynniman CE, Conrad WF, Urch WA, et al: A comparison of medication errors under the University of Kentucky and traditional drug distribution systems in four hospitals. *Am J Hosp Pharm* 27:803-814, 1970.
28. Demers RF, Moore TD: Pharmacy's role in quality assurance of medication administration. *Top Hosp Pharm Mgt* 7(4):45-54, 1988.
29. Somani SM, Woller TW: Automating the drug distribution system. *Top Hosp Pharm Mgt* 9(l):19-34, 1989.
30. Daniels CE, Somani SM: The automation of information in pharmacy. *Top Hosp Pharm Mgt* 9(l):51-61, 1989.
31. Jones DG, Crane VS, Trussell RG: Automated medication dispensing: The ATC 212 system. *Hosp Pharm* 24:604-610, 1989.
32. Barry GA, Bass GE, Eddlemon JK, et al: Bar-code technology for documenting administration of large-volume intravenous solutions. *Am J Hosp Pharm* 46:282-287, 1989.

ADDITIONAL READING

American Society of Hospital Pharmacists: *Source Book on Unit Dose Drug Distribution Systems*. Bethesda, MD, American Society of Hospital Pharmacists, 1978.

ASHP Guidelines: Minimum standard for pharmacies in institutions. *Am J Hosp Pharm* 42:372-375, 1985.

ASHP statement on unit dose drug distribution. *Am J Hosp Pharm* 46:2346, 1989.

ASHP technical assistance bulletin on hospital drug distribution and control. *Am J Hosp Pharm* 37:1097-1103, 1980.

ASHP technical assistance bulletin on single unit dose packages of drugs. *Am J Hosp Pharm* 42:378-379, 1985.

ASHP technical assistance bulletin on repackaging oral solids and liquids in single unit and unit dose packages. *Am J Hosp Pharm* 40:451-452, 1983.

Black BL: *Resource Book on Progressive Pharmaceutical Services*. Bethesda, MD, American Society of Hospital Pharmacists, 1986.

Rascati KL: Brief review of the literature on decentralized drug distribution in hospitals. *Am J Hosp Pharm* 45:639-641, 1988.

Stolar MH: ASHP national survey of hospital pharmaceutical services, 1987. *Am J Hosp Pharm* 45:801-818, 1988.

Summerfield MR: Unit dose drug distribution: A basic bibliography. *Hosp Pharm* 24:673, 1989.

CHAPTER 19

Intravenous Admixture Systems

ALLEN J. VAIDA and CHRISTINE GABOS

Hospital pharmacists have been involved with the preparation of parenteral dosage forms for several decades. What began primarily as the compounding of sterile intravenous, intrathecal, ophthalmic, and irrigating solutions that were not available commercially has evolved into highly sophisticated intravenous (IV) admixture programs centralized in the pharmacy.

The word "parenteral" is derived from the Greek words "para" and "enteron," meaning outside the intestine.[1] Parenteral medications are administered by injection into veins and through subcutaneous tissues. The first needle and syringe was made from a quill attached to an animal bladder. A plunger-type syringe designed to aid in the administration of injectable drugs was eventually developed. Unfortunately, the lack of aseptic techniques and sterile, pure drugs caused parenteral therapy to fall into disfavor until the 19th century.

Animal studies encouraged scientists to pursue research in parenteral therapy as a drug delivery method. Through the efforts of Pasteur, Lister, Koch, Jenner, Hunter, and Seibert, aseptic technique, bacteriologic filtration methods, and pyrogen-free diluents were developed. It was through their research, as well as the work of other scientists, that injectable sterile solutions gained recognition by the National Formulary and U.S. Pharmacopoeia (USP) publications.[1]

It is estimated that more than 40 percent of hospital inpatients receive intravenous therapy.[2] This percentage will continue to rise as the need to contain health care costs encourages hospitals to admit only those patients in need of advanced technological support. A major component of this support will be the need for intravenous therapy to replace fluids and electrolytes, provide nutrition, and administer medications.

Parenteral therapy can also be provided to the patient in his or her home. Many hospital pharmacy departments are actively involved in compounding intravenous solutions and medications that are administered to patients in an outpatient setting. These developments have positioned pharmacists as the parenteral therapy experts. Today's pharmacy graduates are expected to know how to compound parenteral solutions to meet a patient's clinical needs. Pharmacists must also be aware of both the stability and compatibility of drugs administered by the intravenous route. In addition to learning the basic techniques for compounding oral, rectal, and topical dosage forms, today's pharmacist is also expected to be proficient in compounding parenteral dosages and to ensure that they are administered and monitored correctly.

This chapter presents the fundamentals of a pharmacy-directed intravenous admixture program and information about several types of IV admixture systems. An "admixture system" refers to sterile intravenous solutions that are prepared by using one or more medications or electrolytes and will be administered via the parenteral route. In addition to intravenous solutions, an admixture system may also encompass irrigation, ophthalmic, and intrathecal solutions. It is not possible in this chapter to cover all types of systems and new technological advances; therefore, references are listed for more extensive reading on contamination, compatibility, quality control, preparation, and administration of parenteral products. Other chapters in this text should also be consulted for specifics on policies and procedures, purchasing and inventory management, productivity, and specialized parenteral therapy.

STARTING A PROGRAM

Rationale

Most of pharmacy's initial involvement in parenteral therapy involved the compounding of solutions that were not available commercially. Pharmacy departments established compounding areas where the preparation and testing of intravenous solutions was conducted. In 1971 the Food and Drug Administration along with the USP established the National Coordinating Committee on Large Volume Parenterals (NCCLVP). The committee was initially established to identify problems associated with large volume parenterals (LVPs) in hospitals.[3] It also developed procedures to be used by hospital personnel for preparing and administering LVPs.[4] Although the committee no longer exists, it did develop several important standards of practice that are still in use today. The NCCLVP:

1. Recommended methods for compounding intravenous admixtures in hospitals,
2. Established a system for the surveillance and reporting of problems with LVP's in hospitals,[5]
3. Proposed test methods for particulate matter in LVP's,
4. Set forth recommendations for labeling of LVP's,[6] and

5. Recommended procedures for in-use testing of LVP's suspected of contamination or of producing a reaction in a patient.[7]

Although the NCCLVP no longer exists, committees for hospital accreditation (e.g., American Osteopathic Association, Joint Commission On Accreditation of Healthcare Organizations) have established standards of practice for pharmaceutical services. In order for hospital pharmacies to maintain their accreditation, they must operate within the guidelines established by these organizations.

Today's hospital pharmacy department may still perform some intravenous manufacturing, but the majority of parenteral products are prepared using commercially available medications and diluent solutions. The responsibility has remained with pharmacy due, in part, to reasons discussed below.

Contamination

The pharmacy must maintain a clean area out of the direct flow of traffic with a vertical or horizontal laminar air-flow hood to prepare intravenous admixtures. This is of great importance for minimizing the chance of contamination.

Compatibility

The pharmacist can control both the IV solutions that are used and the medications that can be combined in the solutions. A pharmacist's education should prepare him or her to deal with problems of physical, chemical, and therapeutic incompatibilities, and to design suitable alternatives when these problems arise.

Stability

Drug stability information must be readily accessible to the pharmacist in order to determine optimum conditions for drug storage prior to and after preparation. The stability of a drug at ideal storage conditions (e.g., of temperature and light) will help to establish a reasonable expiration date for the product. In addition to issues of stability, pharmacy also needs to consider issues of product sterility and overall integrity, which will be discussed later in this chapter.

Cost

Pharmacy can prepare parenteral medications more economically than individual nurses on a patient unit. The overall cost of drug and diluent procurement, storage, preparation time, and waste is less in a pharmacy-based admixture program.[8] Intravenous programs that are under the direction of nursing require coordination of effort to obtain drugs from pharmacy as well as diluent solutions from central supply. The ingredients must then be mixed on the patient units prior to administration. In the pharmacy, frequently administered medications can be obtained in bulk containers (e.g., 40-g vials of medications), which decreases drug procurement cost, and can be prepared in batches, which decreases both labor and waste. Nursing time associated with the preparation of medications for administration to patients is minimized. In so doing, it is possible to translate this reduction in time into either an actual cost saving to the institution or to provide the nursing staff greater opportunity to assume more non-medication-related time in patient care. Additionally, the amount of unused and wasted parenterals is likely to decrease when a pharmacy IV admixture program is used. Once the pharmacist receives an order or prescription to discontinue an IV product, unused doses can be quickly retrieved from the patient care area. Since pharmacy is directing the redistribution of unused doses, waste can be reduced.

Errors

The potential for medication error is reduced in a pharmacy-based admixture program. Pharmacists are educated to perform medication calculations, which are extremely important in parenteral therapy dosages, especially in nutrition and chemotherapy admixtures. It has been shown that pharmacists are less likely than other health professionals to make an error in pharmaceutical calculations.[9,10] In addition, standardized dosing charts, showing precalculated drug doses and dilutions, contained in the admixture area can also reduce the potential of error.

Quality

Pharmacy-based intravenous admixture programs allow for increased quality control measures. Proper policies for inspecting solutions prior to and after preparation are an integral part of pharmacy-based programs. Pharmacy policy and procedures governing IV admixtures can be enforced more efficiently in centralized and decentralized pharmacy-directed admixture programs. Compatibility, sterility, and labeling of admixtures are addressed in a typical pharmacy control system.

Process

First, upon profiling the original medication order, the pharmacist will determine if dosage, diluent, volume of diluent, and rate of administration are correct. For many admixtures, the diluent, volume, and rate will be determined by pharmacy. Next, the label will be checked against the original order. The final solution with additives will then be checked against the label to ensure that the proper dose has been prepared. Ideally, this check system will involve at least two different pharmacy personnel. Pharmacists and pharmacy technicians are trained to "read the label three times"[11] to ensure that orders and prescriptions are filled correctly.

Total Pharmaceutical Care

In a hospital setting, many patients may be receiving the majority, if not all, of their medications by the parenteral route. Intravenous therapy may be used on patients for part of or sometimes for their entire hospital stay. In order to affect a patient monitoring program for medications, it is necessary to centralize the preparation of all medications as well as the record-keeping function so that appropriate review can be accomplished.

Safety

In pharmacy-based admixture programs with properly established policies and procedures, the overall safety of intravenous therapy is enhanced. The Joint Commission on Accreditation of Healthcare Organizations (JCAHO) holds the director of pharmacy services responsible for "preparing, sterilizing and labeling parenteral medications and solutions that are manufactured in the hospital."[12] JCAHO further states that "the compounding and admixture of large-volume parenterals is ordinarily the responsibility of a qualified pharmacist."[12]

COMPONENTS OF AN IV ADMIXTURE PROGRAM

Preparation Area

Ideally, parenteral products should be prepared in a separate room in the pharmacy. This area is usually referred to as the "clean" room. The size of this room will vary according to space limitations and the individual institution's bed size, which will dictate the number of products to be prepared. The number of individuals who will be preparing parenteral products and the equipment necessary will also determine the amount of space needed. When contemplating the development of an admixture program, expanding an existing program, or revising a current system, the State board of pharmacy and department of health regulations should be reviewed. Some States may mandate minimum square footage and facilities that are required. Table 19-1 provides several recommendations regarding the preparation area for parenteral products.[12-15]

Table 19-1. Preparation area*

- Tiled, washable floor covered with a coat of vinyl or epoxy sealant to provide a continuous surface
- Hand-washing facilities
- Laminar air-flow hoods: horizontal and/or vertical air-flow
- Refrigerator
- Preparation equipment: needles, syringes, alcohol prep pads, gloves, masks, gowns, receptacles for disposables, small-volume parenterals, diluents, and solutions
- Good lighting
- Adequate counter space
- Restricted area or minimized traffic flow
- Prohibition of smoking, beverages, food, and unauthorized personnel

*Some references recommend that only sterile equipment be kept in the preparation area.

Although the preparation of some types of admixtures (e.g., thawing frozen premixed admixtures) does not require a clean room, one should not compromise on obtaining adequate space for an admixture area. The physical appearance of the preparation area may be viewed as a measure of the quality of the products produced.

Policies and Procedures

Guidelines for preparing parenteral products should be outlined in the pharmacy's policy and procedure manual (see also Chapter 7 of this handbook). Detailed information regarding the preparation, labeling, storage, and expiration dating of parenteral products should be readily available in the pharmacy. These policies help to provide quality control for the parenteral products that are prepared and dispensed by the pharmacy.

Stability

Expiration dating for parenteral products is established through rigorous stability testing by the pharmaceutical manufacturer. Analytical and qualitative methods are used to test products stored under different environmental conditions (e.g., varying temperature and lighting conditions). Pharmaceutical scientists or independent investigators may also perform these tests on compounded parenteral products to obtain stability information about a drug once it has been added to an intravenous solution (e.g., 5 percent dextrose in water, 0.9 percent sodium chloride) or mixed with another drug.

It should be kept in mind that the stability of the active ingredient in parenteral products may be affected by the container it is placed in, environmental conditions (e.g., light, temperature), the diluent used to administer the product, or other drugs that may be mixed with the product. Also, issues concerning stability and sterility should not be confused. Although a compounded parenteral product may be stable for several days to weeks, sterility issues must also be considered. The pharmacy's parenteral policy and procedure should set forth specific expiration dating for parenteral products based on published stability and sterility data.

Incompatibility

Drug and product incompatibilities may be categorized as being physical, chemical, or therapeutic in nature.[16] Physical compatibility problems occur when two or more products that are mixed together produce a visible change in the resulting solution (e.g., precipitate, haze, unexpected color change) upon mixing. Chemical incompatibilities may or may not produce a visible change in the final product. A chemical compatibility problem usually results in the deterioration or inactivation of an active ingredient. Finally, therapeutic incompatibilities may arise due to a drug-drug or drug-disease interaction that may result in potentiation of the drug's therapeutic effect, drug toxicity, or deterioration of the drug's pharmacologic effect. Pharmacists must be able to use their knowledge of chemistry, pharmacology, and pharmacotherapeutics to recognize and prevent physical, chemical, and therapeutic incompatibilities.

Aseptic Technique

"Aseptic technique" is the term that is frequently used to describe the method for handling sterile products. A sterile parenteral dosage form is free from living microorganisms, particulate matter, and pyrogens.

Compounded intravenous products are prepared using sterile drugs and diluents. Aseptic technique refers to the ability of personnel who prepare these IV solutions to handle these products in the clean environment of a laminar or vertical air-flow hood without introducing viable microorganisms into the product.[1] Sterile syringes, needles, drugs, and diluents are used in the preparation of compounded intravenous solutions. When used properly, a well-lit, operating air-flow hood provides the optimal environment for parenteral product preparation.

Thorough hand-washing is the first essential step in aseptic technique. An antimicrobial soap may be used for this purpose. Although it is not possible to sterilize the skin, sterile gloves may be used. However, the one disadvantage to wearing gloves is that they give a false sense of security. With or without gloves, the same aseptic techniques must be used to prepare parenteral products in order to avoid "touch contamination." Touch contamination can happen quickly and easily if personnel are not careful when preparing parenterals. For example, the plunger of a syringe that comes in contact with a person's hands should not be reused, because the potential exists for the plunger to come in contact with the inner barrel of the syringe, leaving skin contaminants or other particulate matter behind.

All intravenous compounding carries the risk of bacterial contamination. Aseptic technique, the use of laminar airflow, and maintenance of the IV laboratory help to minimize bacterial contamination. Freezing or refrigerating intravenous solutions also helps to prevent bacterial growth. This is especially important for compounded total parenteral nutrition (TPN) solutions.

IV Profiling

When an order or prescription is received for a parenteral product, it must be reviewed against the patient's current medication profile. Both manual and computerized patient profiles allow the pharmacist to determine if there are any compatibility or stability problems prior to preparing the product. Likewise, he or she can check for therapeutic duplications and easily clarify problems with the physician. Information regarding the processing of an IV order can be found later in this chapter.

Labeling and Check Systems

Proper labeling of IV admixtures is extremely important. Once an additive has been injected into an IV bag or bottle, the contents must be identified immediately. Each IV container should be labeled with the information contained in table 19-2.

Continuous infusion IV's may require additional record keeping. The pharmacy will want to keep abreast of patient IV needs so that the solutions are prepared and available for the patient unit immediately prior to use. Many pharmacies use parenteral profile cards to assist pharmacy personnel in tracking patient IV needs. An example of a parenteral profile card is shown in figure 19-1. The patient's name and room number (or nursing unit) are recorded along with the type of intravenous solution and additive the patient is receiving. The IV bag sequence number, date, and time of therapy are tracked daily; the infusion rate is also listed. A space is provided on the card to record the time that the IV is needed. The person who prepares the IV solution and the pharmacist who checks the solution both initial the card.

In addition to the contents of the IV solution, the integrity of the containers should also be checked. Pharmacy-prepared IV solutions must be checked for leaks in bags, cracks in bottles, particulate matter, cloudiness, and accuracy of compounding at least two or three times by the person who prepares them as well as by the pharmacist who dispenses the item to the patient unit. Plastic IV bags should be checked for leaks by applying pressure and squeezing the upper end of the bag. This will quickly reveal puncture holes. Glass bottles should also be checked for particular matter (e.g., cores) and cracks. Although often taken for granted, the pharmacist's initials on the final product indicate to the person who is administering the drug that the integrity and the quality of the product are suitable for administration and that the label information is accurate.

Table 19-2. Labeling and checking system

It is suggested that the following information be placed on all IV admixtures immediately following preparation:

- Patient name, identification number, and room number
- Bottle sequence number
- Name and amount of drug added
- Name and volume of admixture solution
- Approximate final total volume of the admixture (e.g., for chemotherapeutic admixtures)
- Prescribed flow rate (mL/hour)
- Date and time of scheduled administration
- Date and time of preparation
- Expiration date
- Initials of the person who prepares and/or checks the IV admixture
- Ancillary labeling: supplemental instructions and precautions

Large-Volume Parenteral Profile

IV No.	Start Date	Therapy Dates	Solution	Additives	Rate	Time RPn	and Techs	Initials
Room	Name			Solution / Additives				

Figure 19-1. A sample of one type of intravenous patient profile card is shown here. Important information can be recorded on this card in order to keep track of a patient's intravenous fluid needs.

Quality Assurance and Control

A system of checks and balances, aseptic environment, and the pharmacist's access to both the patient's medication profile and the final product provide more stringent quality control over parenteral therapy.

The majority of sterile products used in hospital pharmacy today are commercially prepared. Sterility testing, therefore, will not be a usual component of intravenous admixture programs. Some pharmacy departments may still perform sterility testing to check the compounding techniques of their IV admixture personnel. Current recommendations are to culture intravenous fluids only if a patient's infection may be related to their use.[17]

Routine inspection of all laminar air-flow hoods must also be performed. Often, pharmaceutical purchasing groups will have contracts with vendors for the testing of hoods. Routine hood maintenance (e.g., filter replacement) should be arranged through the hospital maintenance or plant inspection department. (See reference 19 at the end of this chapter for information on maintenance of vertical air-flow hoods.) Filtering devices should be available in the parenteral preparation area. Occasionally, admixtures that are not commercially available may have to be prepared from the powdered form. An example would be highly concentrated solutions of morphine for use in pain control. In these instances, passing the dissolved drug through a 0.22-micron or 0.45-micron filter will be necessary. Membrane filters may be located within the IV administration set; however, they are not routinely used in all hospitals. Although they provide an excellent means for trapping particulate matter before it enters the vein, filters may also adsorb or absorb drug. Drugs that should not be filtered include parenteral suspensions, blood and blood products, amphotericin B, insulin, 10-percent and 20-percent fat emulsions, mithramycin, nitroglycerin, and vincristine.[18]

The intravenous preparation program should be included in the pharmacy's overall quality assurance program. As mentioned above, a thorough pharmacist check system of all admixtures must be established. The finished product must be checked for particulate matter, color, compatibility of ingredients, and integrity of the container (e.g., leaks or cracks). A check of the label, additives, flow rates, and administration times should also be performed before the product is considered to be acceptable for use. In an IV admixture service that produces a large number of products, this check system should become second nature to the pharmacist.

It must be emphasized that when the pharmacist's initials are attached to the product, the above steps are always considered to have been completed. Once the product leaves the pharmacy, nurses must also be aware that they are involved in the check process. Before the drug is administered to the patient, the label must be checked against the medication administration record and the product should once again be checked for color, particulate matter, expiration date, and container integrity. If the person who administers the drug has any questions, these should be relayed immediately to the pharmacist who initialed the IV container.

A typical IV order for a patient would entail the following activities:

1. A pharmacy copy of the physician's original order is prepared, containing the patient's name, room number, IV fluid, additive(s), and flow rate.
2. The prescription order is entered into the patient's profile by a pharmacist who checks for drug interactions, proper dose, compatibility of ingredients, duplication of medication (includes medications ordered by the oral route), allergies, length of therapy compared to automatic stop order policies, and other patient therapies.
3. A label is prepared and checked against the original order.
4. The parenteral product is prepared by a pharmacist or by an experienced technician, depending on State law.
5. The prepared product is then checked against the label and original order by a pharmacist. Dosage, ingredients, auxiliary labels, compatibility, route, rate, absence of particulate matter, discoloration, and container integrity are verified. Usually, each IV dose is numbered in consecutive order.
6. Upon delivery of the IV product to the patient unit, the solution is once again checked by the person who will be administering the drug.
7. Whenever possible, IV admixtures should be refrigerated until shortly prior to use. If it is not used within 24 hours, it should be returned to pharmacy to be redistributed or destroyed.

As can be appreciated, within this system a number of checks are involved. Ideally, a pharmacist, a technician, and a nurse are involved in checking a parenteral product before it is administered to the patient. Even if one of the people involved in the check system is not available, if a system of multiple checks is maintained, an error may still be avoided.

Other important aspects of an intravenous admixture program, from a quality standpoint are listed in table 19-3. Although not all-inclusive, this list should stimulate awareness of pharmacy's involvement regarding the preparation of parenteral products.

Table 19-3. Additional components of quality assurance of an admixture service

An experienced intravenous therapy team. These persons (usually nurses) may be involved in starting and maintaining intravenous lines and administration of medications (especially chemotherapy).

A nursing orientation program discussing pharmacy involvement in the hospital's admixture program. A periodic update of this program should be conducted for all nursing personnel.

Periodic review of all hospital incident reports dealing with intravenous medications.

Pharmacy involvement in the hospital standards committee whenever products for parenteral therapy are reviewed.

An integrated quality assurance plan to identify:

- Appropriate use of parenteral rather than oral medications
- Proper rates and intervals of parenteral medication administration
- Incidence of phlebitis and extravasation
- Integration of therapeutic drug monitoring with the administration of parenteral medications

Auxiliary Labels

Once an intravenous admixture program is operating, additional medication labeling needs become readily apparent. Unfortunately, the majority of time, this need arises after a potential medication error occurs on the patient-care area.

It is recommended that when admixture programs in hospitals are reviewed, special attention should be paid to ancillary labels which are used on the intravenous products. These auxiliary labels help to enhance patient safety. Some examples of these labels are listed in table 19-4. Many of these labels elicit more attention than placing the same warning or reminder on the regular solution label.

Table 19-4. Auxiliary labels*

Note dosage strength —	to be placed on concentrated solutions which are double or triple the strengths that are normally used (these types of solutions may be used on patients who are fluid restricted)
Must activate before use —	to be placed on unactivated ADD-Vantage® solutions
Protect from light	
Do not refrigerate — Do not allow to freeze	
Caution: Chemotherapeutic agent — Dispose of properly	
Caution: Vesicant/Tissue irritant	
For epidural use only	

*Some of the labels listed above must be specially ordered.

Equipment

Emphasis should be placed on laminar air-flow hoods, refrigeration, and references, as discussed below.

Laminar air-flow hoods

Although laminar air-flow hoods may give a false sense of security to the personnel involved in preparation of parenteral products, they constitute an important component of an admixture program. These devices use high-efficiency particulate air (HEPA) filtration, which may be in a horizontal flow, convergent flow, or a vertical flow. The horizontal or laminar air-flow hood filters ambient air via the HEPA filters, thus removing particulate matter and airborne microorganisms greater than or equal to 0.3 microns. The velocity of air flow through the HEPA filters should be maintained at 90 ± 20 feet per minute. Laminar air-flow hoods should supply class 100 air described in Federal Standard 209B.[19] It should be noted that these hoods do not sterilize an environment, but rather maintain an environment in a clean state as it has been established. Proper aseptic techniques must be strictly adhered to when an air-flow hood is used for preparing IV admixtures.

Air-flow hoods should be inspected every 6 months for leaks by the manufacturer or by a hood certifier. Dioctyl phthalate (DOP) smoke is used to perform the inspection. DOP smoke has a particle size of approximately 0.3 microns. If the smoke passes through the filter, this may be indicative of a leak or problem with the HEPA filter.[1]

The advantages of a laminar air-flow hood are that the area within the hood may be maintained free of microorganisms and particulate matter even if the hood is used on a satellite pharmacy that may not have a separate clean room.

The type of hood used will depend on the medications that are prepared. A vertical air-flow biological safety cabinet (figure 19-2) should be used for preparing cancer chemotherapeutic and other hazardous agents. A horizontal hood is not adequate for the preparation of these products, because contaminants generated in the hood are blown directly at the worker. Biological safety cabinets provide an environment suitable for the handling of sterile drugs without endangering the worker.

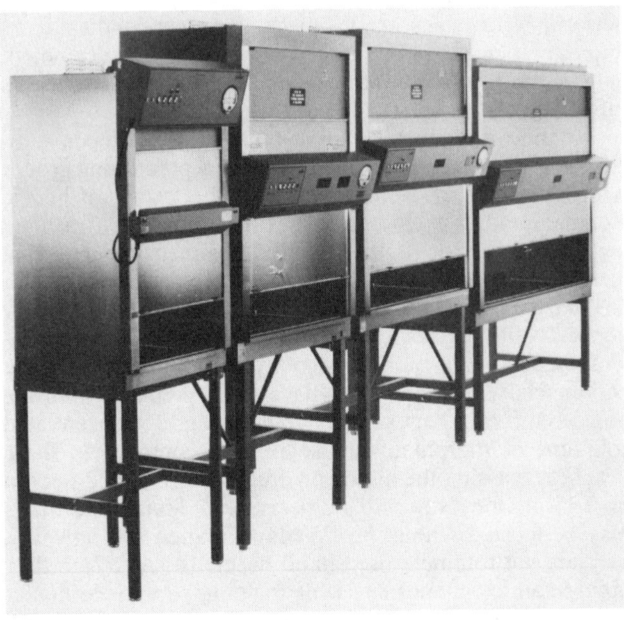

Figure 19-2. An example of one type of vertical air-flow hood is shown here.

It is important to remember that the integrity of all sterile products must be kept intact during the compounding process. Aseptic technique must be used in preparing intravenous admixtures to avoid contamination by particulate matter, pyrogens, bacteria, and yeast.

The parenteral laboratory must be kept clean, and work surfaces should be disinfected routinely throughout the day. Personnel should also be instructed in proper hand-washing techniques to minimize microbial contamination. "Touch contamination" must also be avoided during parenteral compounding.

Refrigeration

Adequate refrigeration is essential to an admixture program. Most compounded parenterals need to be refrigerated for optimal stability; the introduction of a needle into a sterile product is associated with risk of contamination. Microbial growth is retarded under refrigeration. Drugs themselves are often more stable under refrigeration than at room temperature. If premixed frozen products are purchased, one or more freezer units will be needed as well. Pharmacies that prepare parenterals in batches will usually freeze these products for extended expiration dating whenever possible. The patient care unit is another area in which refrigeration will be needed or expanded. Some IV preparations made and dispensed by pharmacy should be refrigerated on the patient unit until shortly before use.

References

Adequate reference materials are an essential component of an IV admixture program. The latest edition of the *Handbook on Injectable Drugs*, published by the American Society of Hospital Pharmacists,[20] is one of the most widely used references. Well-referenced compatibility and stability charts are also necessary in an intravenous preparation area.

Many of these charts are supplied by the manufacturers of parenteral medications.

The time spent on the preparation of several institution-specific charts is well worth the endeavor. Standardized compounding charts facilitate the preparation of parenteral products by listing precalculated doses, concentration, and administration rates.

These charts may include the following information:

- Amount and type of diluent to add to a lyophilized (powdered) medication and the resulting concentration;
- The recommended final diluent (e.g., 5 percent dextrose in water; 0.9 percent, 0.45 percent sodium chloride, etc.) and the concentration to be used for optimal stability for each particular medication;
- Lists of specific medications with the volume of drug required to prepare commonly used dosages;
- Expiration dates for compounded medication, frozen products that are thawed, and medications prepackaged in syringes; and
- Standardized diluents and concentrations used in the institution.

If the pharmacy is on a computerized patient profile system, the majority of this information can be added directly to the drug profile. This information will help the pharmacist at the time that the order is entered to properly identify the solution and final quantity. Examples of several of the above aids are listed in tables 19-5 and 19-5A.

Table 19-5. Examples of charts for admixture preparation

Drug	Size	Diluent	Amount to add	Approximate final diluted concentration	Expiration date (days)
Cefazolin	250 mg	Bacterio-	2 mL	125 mg/mL	10*r
	500 mg	static	2 mL	250 mg/mL	10 r
	1 g	water	2.5 mL	400 mg/mL	10 r
	10 g		45 mL	1,000 mg/mL	10 r
Nafcillin	500 mg	Bacterio-	1.7 mL	500 mg/2 mL	7 r
	1 g	static	3.4 mL	1,000 mg/4 mL	7 r
	2 g	water	6.8 mL	1,000 mg/4 mL	7 r
	10 g		43.0 mL	1,000 mg/5 mL	7 r

Methylprednisolone concentrations for syringes:

40 mg/mL:	30 mg=0.75 mL	20 mg=0.5 mL	10 mg=0.25 mL	48 hr r
125 mg/mL:	100 mg=1.6 mL	80 mg=1.3 mL	60 mg=0.96 mL	48 hr r

Gentamicin concentrations for syringes or minibags:

40 mg/mL vial:	10 mg=0.25 mL	50 mg=1.25 mL	90 mg=2.25 mL
	15 mg=0.375 mL	55 mg=1.375 mL	95 mg=2.375 mL
	20 mg=0.5 mL	60 mg=1.5 mL	100 mg=2.5 mL
	25 mg=0.625 mL	65 mg=1.625 mL	105 mg=2.625 mL
	30 mg=0.75 mL	70 mg=1.75 mL	110 mg=2.75 mL
	35 mg=0.875 mL	75 mg=1.875 mL	115 mg=2.875 mL
	45 mg=1.125 mL	85 mg=2.125 mL	125 mg=3.125 mL

*r = refrigerated.

Once parenteral medication charts have been obtained or prepared, someone should be responsible for maintaining and updating them. Charts and reminders found in a pharmacy parenteral area usually signify a well-organized practice with the least amount of errors.

Table 19-5A. Example of IV rate charts*

Dose in mg/hr	Aminophylline† 1 g/250 mL	1 g/500 mL	1 g/1,000 mL
20 mg/hr	6 mL/hr	11 mL/hr	21 mL/hr
25	7	14	26
30	9	16	31
35	10	19	36
40	12	22	42
45	13	24	47
50	15	27	52
55	16	30	57
60	17	32	62
65	19	35	68
70	20	38	73
75	22	41	78
80	23	43	83
85	25	46	88
90	26	49	94
95	28	51	99
100	29	54	104
105	30	57	109
110	32	59	114

Starting doses range from 2 to 7 mg/kg/hr.

*Final solution volume is considered to be the diluent volume plus approximately 40 mL of aminophylline.
†Charts use IV tubing that delivers 60 gtt(drops)/minute.

Heparin†

25,000 units/500 mL NSS‡ or 50,000 units/1,000 mL NSS‡ solution

Flow rate, mL/hour	Units/hour delivered
8	400
10	500
12	600
14	700
16	800
18	900
20	1,000
22	1,100
24	1,200
26	1,300
28	1,400
30	1,500
32	1,600
34	1,700
36	1,800
38	1,900
40	2,000

‡NSS = 0.9% sodium chloride.

Another important area where standardized charts are needed is on the patient units. These should include charts for determining intravenous infusion rates.[21] The first step in developing infusion rate charts is to collaborate with nurses and physicians, preferably through the pharmacy and therapeutics committee, to establish standard medication concentrations to be used in the hospital. Examples of medications that may require rate charts are heparin infusions of 50 units/mL and aminophylline infusions of 1,000 mg in 250, 500, or 1,000 mL of diluent as well as standard dilutions for intravenous cardiac medications (table 19-5A). When the standard dilutions are established, charts to determine infusion rates for different dosages can be compiled. This guarantees continuity throughout the hospital, decreases chances of medication administration errors, and enables physicians to order drug dosages in milligram or microgram per minute, per hour, or per kilogram without calculating dilution concentrations and reduces waste.

Personnel

The personnel who will be involved in an admixture program must be carefully trained. Depending on the type or types of systems used, the number of additional personnel required will be extremely important. Regulations within a particular State may also dictate who may prepare intravenous admixtures. Some States prohibit technicians from preparing IV medications; other States will allow this practice (under the "direct" supervision of a registered pharmacist), as long as an adequate check system is established.

The reason different types of admixture systems dictate personnel requirements will become readily apparent once available systems are reviewed. If manufacturer-prepared products are used, additional personnel may be minimized. Pharmacies that use bulk medication to prepare individualized doses will require an increase in personnel. The majority of hospital pharmacies use a combination of several different types of systems.

The proper training of personnel in aseptic technique and sterile product information is necessary. This may entail sending staff to training courses or to other institutions to learn how to prepare parenteral medications. Once a proper training program is established, it must be maintained to accommodate personnel turnover. Self-study programs may be used along with on-the-job training. The American Society of Hospital Pharmacists also has several videotapes that are available for training IV personnel in the proper methods of aseptic technique and chemotherapy preparation.

Storage Space

As mentioned earlier, space is another important component of an admixture program. Once again, space will depend on the type of system one chooses to use, because the amount of space required for stocking supplies varies. Computer systems have made it possible for pharmacy admixture programs to function without being in close proximity to the central pharmacy or the pharmacist who may be profiling the medication orders. In evaluating space requirements, this should be kept in mind. If space is available outside of the pharmacy, even on a different floor, this is where the intravenous admixture preparation area could be located.

One last consideration on space is the patient care area. As mentioned, expanded refrigeration may be needed depending on the types of IV systems used. Additional storage space for IV sets and other administration devices may be required. Plain IV solutions are often stored as floor stock in patient care areas. (See the chapters on facility design and computerization in pharmacy in this handbook for further information.)

Economic Considerations

The preparation area, personnel, and equipment of an admixture program could have a great financial impact on the hospital, or more specifically, on the pharmacy's budget. The cost will be greatest if pharmacy was not involved in parenteral preparation and if additional pharmacy personnel, space, and equipment are required, without a reduction in nursing personnel. In this instance, the rationale for pharmacy involvement, recommendations of hospital and State regulatory agencies, and the support of nursing administration will be needed.

The type or types of system(s) that are incorporated will determine the additional cost to the hospital.[22-28] Presented in table 19-6 are examples of low- and high-cost programs in relation to the components of the system.

Table 19-6. Relative costs for parenteral admixture systems

	Cost*	Personnel	Equipment	Prep area	Waste
Premixed	moderate	low	low	low	low
Compounded	low	high	high	high	high
Drug Diluent system†	moderate	low	moderate†	low	low‡

*Acquisition costs.
†Two components for inventory and storage will add a relatively higher cost.
‡Waste will depend on where activation of the components is performed.

In conjunction with table 19-6, the acquisition cost of the parenteral products must be taken into consideration. Depending on the private or group purchasing contracts a hospital establishes, the cost of one system compared to another may vary. This is extremely important when evaluating systems, even if an admixture system is in place or the expansion of a system is being completed. With the inception of multihospital purchasing groups, the cost of intravenous solutions and accessory supplies for medication administration has actually decreased since the late 1970's and early 1980's.

Waste is another important economic factor in any parenteral admixture system.[8,29-31] Waste in an IV admixture system refers to prepared IV solutions that are not used (i.e., IV orders may be changed or discontinued after the product has already been prepared). Manufacturers' attempts to deal with the problem of waste are the single most motivating factor in the proliferation of the multitude of different types of admixture systems that are available today.

The stability of an admixture compounded in the pharmacy is often much less than that of a comparable product available premixed from the manufacturer (e.g., gentamicin 80 mg in 50 mL of 5 percent dextrose in water). The manufacturer's premixed product has an extended expiration date because it was manufactured under sterile conditions that cannot be duplicated in the pharmacy. Therefore, the use of premixed drugs may be associated with less waste than a system in which the pharmacy compounds the admixtures. However, premixed products also tend to be more costly; the cost savings associated with decreased waste of premixed products must be weighed against their greater acquisition cost. The schedule by which the pharmacy delivers the IV admixtures to the patient care area is also important.

Parenteral products are usually prepared in either 12- or 24-hour batches. Changes in dosages or medications made after the products are prepared may entail significant waste. Some pharmacy departments prepare admixtures in 6- or 8-hour intervals in order to decrease waste, but this procedure may require additional personnel. Therefore, the cost of product waste must be balanced with labor costs. Table 19-7 summarizes the points to be remembered when starting or expanding an intravenous admixture system.

Table 19-7. Steps involved in starting or expanding an IV admixture program

1. Review State and hospital governing regulations.
2. Review current recommendations from agencies or organizations that have standards of practice.
3. Prepare and gain support for rationale in starting or expanding a program.
4. Obtain approval from hospital administration.
5. Evaluate space and equipment requirements for different types of systems. Rely on help from manufacturers of different systems in coordinating data. Visit other hospital pharmacies to view actual systems in use.
6. Assess personnel requirements. The financial impact and availability of additional personnel may necessitate compromise in choosing one type of system over another.
7. Experiment with different types of systems. Manufacturers will readily help with trial evaluations.
8. Maintain communication between pharmacy and nursing when evaluating systems. Different systems may be more suitable for particular nursing units. The final program may contain several types of admixture systems.
9. Prepare or update a thorough policy and procedure manual for the type of system(s) that will be used.

Admixture Systems

The combination of two or more parenteral products in one container results in what is known as an "intravenous admixture." However, pharmacy may choose an admixture system that requires little or no involvement in the actual "compounding" of dosage forms. Such a system would rely on the use of ready-to-administer premixed products available from manufacturers. These products will meet the clinical needs of the majority of patients. Patients with specific medical requirements (e.g., volume restrictions, diabetics who may require sodium chloride diluents rather than dextrose) can be accommodated with specially compounded solutions. Typically, pharmacy-controlled IV programs use both types of admixture systems.

Medications that are given via the parenteral route may be given via intermittent or continuous infusion or by rapid direct injection (also known as IV push or bolus). The type of drug (e.g., antibiotic versus electrolyte) as well as the condition of the patient will usually determine the method of administration. Methods of parenteral drug administration will be discussed below along with the different types of admixture programs that can be used with each.

SMALL-VOLUME INTRAVENOUS INFUSIONS

Manufacturer's Drug Packaging

Sterile dosage forms are prepackaged in single-dose or multidose vials, ampules, syringes, glass bottles, or polyvinyl chloride or polyolefin plastic containers. These products may also be classified according to their therapeutic use: intravenous or irrigating solutions, intramuscular, subcutaneous, intradermal, intrathecal, sterile ophthalmic solution, diagnostic agents, or allergenic extracts.

Different types of prepackaged parenterals used in intravenous admixture systems will be discussed briefly. (See the bibliography for further information.)

Glass Ampules

Ampules are made entirely of glass and can be used to package drugs that may not be chemically compatible with plastic containers or rubber closures. An ampule file was originally used to score the neck of the ampule to facilitate opening. Today, the neck of the ampule may be prescored or inscribed with a ceramic paint to make it easier to open.[1]

The major disadvantage of using ampules to prepare parenteral products is that they may become contaminated with glass fragments upon opening. The solution in the ampule must be drawn into a sterile syringe using a filter needle. The filter needle must then be removed and a new sterile needle attached to the syringe prior to use. The filter needle will remove any glass particles that may have fallen into the ampule.

Single-Dose Vials

Drugs packaged in single-dose vials may be in the lyophilized (powdered) form or may already be in solution. Single-dose vials may be composed of glass or plastic with rubber closures or a spike- or pin-top closure. Single-dose vials with a pin top can be easily inserted directly into the stopper of an IV diluent bottle (they cannot be used with plastic IV bags), thereby eliminating the need to draw up the contents of the vial.

Drug in Solution

Single-dose vials that contain drugs in solution usually contain no preservatives. The correct dose of drug can be withdrawn from the vial using a needle and syringe and can be added to an intravenous bag or bottle. After a single use, the vial is discarded.

Lyophilized or Powdered Drugs

Powdered or lyophilized drugs are prepared by a freeze-drying process in which water is sublimed from the product after it is frozen.[32] Lyophilization helps to increase the shelf-life of products that would otherwise be unstable if packaged as aqueous solutions. Lyophilized products must be reconstituted with an appropriate diluent prior to use. The reconstitution of lyophilized drugs may be batch processed to save time. After dissolution, reconstituted parenteral products may be used immediately, or they may be refrigerated or frozen for future use, depending on the stability of the product. A unique type of single-dose vial is the double-chambered vial, which contains the lyophilized drug in the bottom chamber and the diluent in the top chamber. A stopper between the two chambers keeps the diluent separate from the powder. When pressure is exerted on the first rubber stopper at the top of the vial, it causes the second rubber stopper to be dislodged and allows the diluent to mix with the drug.

Multiple-Dose Containers

Manufacturer bulk bottles or multidose vials are also available for preparing intravenous admixtures. There are two general categories of multiple dose containers as follows.

Drug in Solution

Like single-dose vials, multidose vials are also available with drug already in solution. The primary difference between the two is that multidose vials will usually contain a bacteriostatic agent such as alcohol or phenol. Resealable rubber closures allow the vials to be reused after they have been punctured with a needle. Aseptic handling of multidose vials is more critical than with single-use vials. The risk for microbial contamination increases with repeated withdrawals from the vial. The chance of particulate contamination may increase due to the likelihood of coring with repeated punctures.

Lyophilized or Powdered Drugs

Manufacturer "bulk" bottles containing multiple doses of drug are reconstituted with a specified amount of diluent. Care must be taken in adding diluents to the bulk bottle. If an incorrect amount of diluent is added to the bulk bottle, the entire bottle may need to be discarded. These bottles are reconstituted similarly to single-use IV piggyback bottles, except that several doses of antibiotic can be drawn into syringes to be used with automated or gravity-fed syringe devices. Doses of drug from bulk bottles can also be drawn and added to IV bags or bottles.

It is important to place an expiration date on the bulk vials, since the shelf-life of the product will decrease once it is reconstituted. Recommended expiration dates are provided by each manufacturer for its own products.

Prefilled Syringes

Some medications are available in prefilled syringes from manufacturers. These syringes have several advantages. They are more convenient to use than ampules or vials; they make highly concentrated solutions available (e.g., morphine [25 mg/mL] syringe for morphine drips); they require minimal manipulation by pharmacy personnel and, therefore, provide increased assurance of sterility; they can be used quickly and easily in emergency situations.

Although prefilled IV syringes have many advantages over ampules and vials, it is important to separate single IV push medications from syringes intended for preparing IV admixtures (e.g., lidocaine 2 g for preparing IV admixtures versus lidocaine 100 mg IV bolus). Syringes not intended to be given by direct IV push should not be stocked on nursing units. Cost may be another disadvantage to using prefilled syringes. Comparable quantities of the same drug in vials or ampules often cost more when purchased in prefilled syringes.

Premixed IV Bags and Bottles

Intravenous medications may be supplied by the manufacturer in premixed and frozen premixed containers. Some drugs are also available from the manufacturer, ready to dispense in vials to which a small amount of diluent is added (CRIS®), or in vials that are attached to the diluent solution (ADD-Vantage®). These two types of systems also help to reduce preparation time and waste.

Lyophilized or Powdered Single-Dose Containers

Single doses of lyophilized or powdered drugs are available packaged in the final administration container (e.g., IV bag or glass bottle). These products are easily prepared for administration by adding an appropriate amount of diluent (e.g., 50-100 mL) to each container. These intravenous admixtures may be batch processed and frozen for future use.

INTRAVENOUS ADMIXTURE SYSTEMS

Before 1970, intravenous medications given intermittently were administered by direct intravenous push or bolus, or diluted in a volumetric chamber-type intravenous set (e.g., Metriset®, Buretrol®, Soluset®), (figure 19-3) using the patient's primary IV solution.[33] Drug in solution is placed into a chamber located on the primary IV line. The primary IV fluid is used to deliver the drug to the patient. Although volumetric IV sets are still in use today, medications are more commonly administered using the IV admixture systems described below.

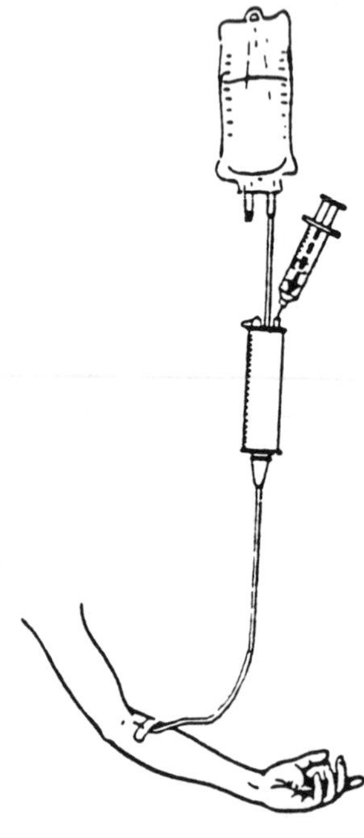

Figure 19-3. Volumetric chamber (i.e., Metriset®, Buretrol®, Soluset®) system. The IV additive is placed into the chamber attached to the primary large-volume IV tubing. Fluid from the primary IV delivers the drug to the patient.

Both glass and plastic IV containers are available today. Glass allows for quick and easy inspection of the container's contents for particulate matter. Plastic containers are translucent and require more careful inspection than glass. Plastic containers, on the other hand, are nonbreakable and allow for easy storage compared to glass.

Syringes

Syringes containing single or multiple doses of an individual drug may also be prepared by pharmacy. These syringes may be prepared by drawing the required amounts from single- or multiple-dose vials.

Bulk vials containing large quantities (e.g., 10-40 g) of drug are reconstituted with sterile water for injection or other diluent. Several doses can be drawn up from a single bulk vial. Single-dose vials, which may also require reconstitution, as well as ampules can be used to prepare syringes. The correct dose is drawn into a syringe (usually 5-60 mL), labeled, and delivered to the patient unit. Syringe pumps or gravity-fed syringe devices may be used to administer doses of drugs that are drawn up into syringes.

If syringes are used to deliver intermittent IV doses, a sufficient number of automated syringe pumps will need to be purchased by the hospital. The syringe pump can be set to deliver one dose of drug (e.g., chemotherapy) or several intermittent doses (e.g., antibiotics). If automated pumps (figure 19-4) are not available, the syringe can be placed in a plastic sleeve, and the dose delivered via a gravity-fed method (figure 19-5).

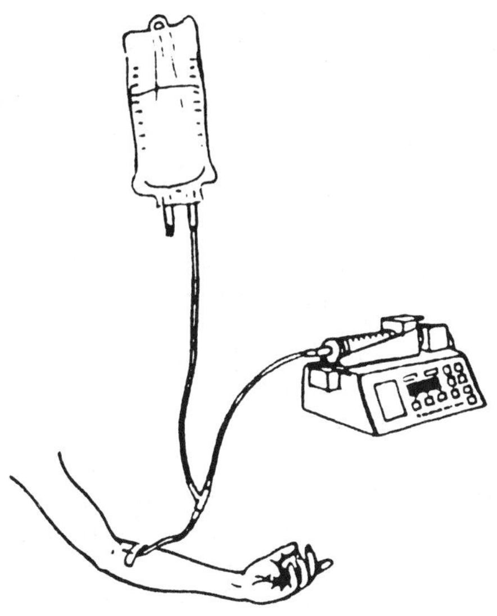

Figure 19-4. An automated syringe pump is shown here. The parenteral medication is drawn up into a syringe by pharmacy. Nursing attaches the syringe to the pump and activates the pump to deliver the dose(s) of medication.

Single-dose pumps require that a newly prepared syringe be placed onto the pump for each intermittent dose. Some multiple-dose pumps, on the other hand, can be programmed to deliver a 24-hour drug supply. The pump is activated daily by the nurse who initiates the first dose for the day. The pump will thereafter automatically deliver the correct dose at the appropriate interval.

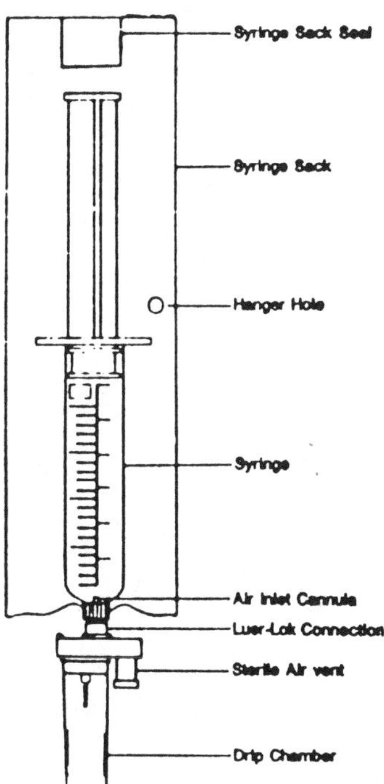

Figure 19-5. Gravity-fed syringe systems rather than automated syringe pumps may also be used to deliver intermittent IV infusions.

Some medications may need to be given by rapid intravenous injection (IV push) (figure 19-6). Syringes containing IV push medications will be prepared in a manner similar to syringes discussed above; however, an automated syringe pump or plastic sleeve will not be needed to administer the dose. The drug is delivered directly to the injection site (e.g., intravenous, intra-arterial, intracardiac) over a period of several seconds to minutes. Bolus doses of medication (e.g., aminophylline, lidocaine) may be given using a similar technique to rapidly increase serum concentrations and, therefore, achieve the therapeutic effect of a specific drug.

Small-Volume IV Systems

Intravenous admixture solutions may be administered by intermittent doses by means of a secondary or "piggyback" IV. A piggyback refers to a second intravenous solution, usually in a smaller volume of diluent than the primary IV. The piggyback is administered via a special connection (e.g., Y-site) on the IV tubing of the primary IV. The fluid level of the piggyback must be above that of the primary IV in order to flow properly (figure 19-7). The administration of a secondary IV (piggyback) through the same IV line as the primary IV eliminates the need for another injection or venipuncture site.

Premixed and Frozen Premixed Bags and Bottles

Premixed and premixed frozen intravenous preparations have helped to reduce pharmacy waste and labor costs. Manufacturer-premixed bags usually have a longer shelf-life than do specially compounded intravenous admixture solutions. Often, when a premixed IV drug is discontinued,

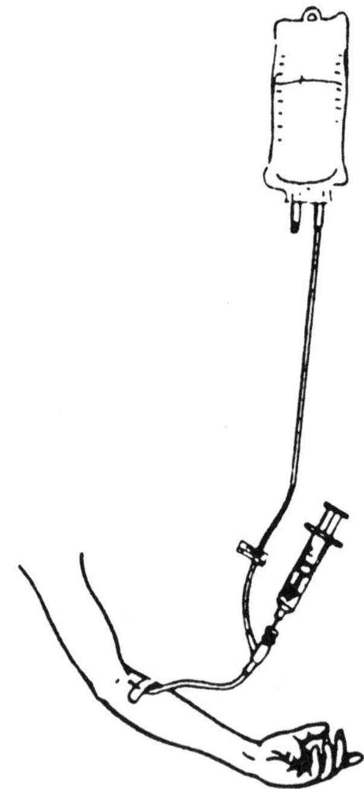

Figure 19-6. Intravenous medications may also be administered rapidly (IV push) through a special port in the primary IV tubing by first clamping off the primary IV before administering the IV push, or directly into a vein or heparin lock infusion port.

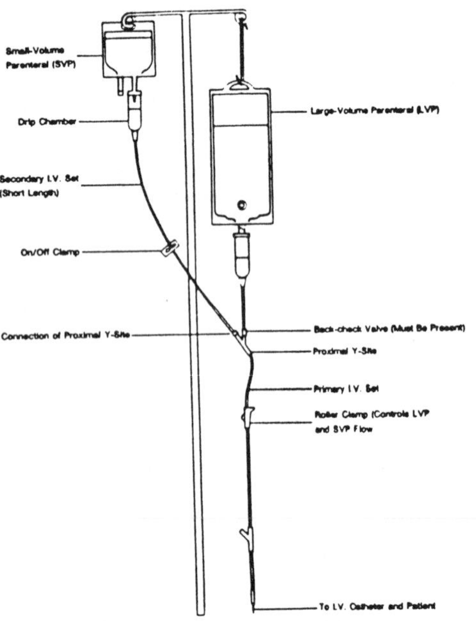

Figure 19-7. The bag/piggyback system is probably the most commonly used method of administering drugs such as antibiotics and H_2 antagonists. The bag can be attached to the primary IV tubing via a "Y-site," or may be directly administered to the patient through a heparin lock infusion port.

unused doses can be reused because of the extended expiration dating and increased assurance of sterility.

The major disadvantage of these products is their high acquisition cost compared to the same IV dose that is compounded manually. Premixed systems offer the least dosing flexibility and are available from limited sources; therefore, the likelihood of competitive bidding is reduced.

Premixed intravenous products prepared by the manufacturer contain both the diluent and drug already combined in a single unit-of-use IV bag or bottle. These premixed IV drugs are stored at room temperature and dispensed directly from the pharmacy without any product intervention. Each IV bag (e.g., piggyback) comes from the manufacturer in a plastic overwrap, which acts as a moisture barrier. Pharmacy only needs to remove the overwrap and attach a patient-specific label prior to dispensing. Premixed, frozen, intravenous piggybacks are also available from the manufacturer, but are delivered to the pharmacy frozen and need to be stored in a -20° C freezer. The frozen piggybacks are thawed prior to use. Frozen IV bags can be thawed by removing them from the freezer and placing them at room temperature for 1-2 hours or by placing them in a refrigerator for 8-16 hours. "Forced" thawing procedures using a microwave or warm-water baths are not recommended. Forced thawing methods may affect the stability of the drug or may compromise the bag seal. Once thawed, these IV bags should never be refrozen. After they are thawed, they are given an appropriate expiration date (per manufacturer recommendations), labeled, and dispensed to the patient unit.

Single-Dose Lyophilized or Powdered Drugs in Final IV Container

Some drugs (e.g., antibiotics) may be purchased as lyophilized powders in single-use/dose IV piggyback bags or bottles that are large enough to hold 50 or 100 mL of a compatible diluent. The original drug bottle or bag serves as the final IV container. Reconstitution of the piggybacks may be performed using automated devices designed to deliver the desired amount of diluent. Some of these devices are designed to reconstitute more than one piggyback simultaneously. Glass piggyback bottles and plastic IV bags may also be prepared in advance and frozen for future use. The IV bags require less storage space than the glass piggyback bottles. Dosing flexibility is limited with these single-use/dose containers. Only the volume of diluent or type of diluent (e.g., dextrose in water or sodium chloride) may be altered, but the dose itself cannot be changed. These bottles and IV bags are reconstituted with an appropriate amount of diluent by pharmacy and then dispensed to the patient care area. The original drug bag or bottle serves as the final IV container.

Compounded Intermittent IV Admixtures

Special orders for small-volume IV admixtures traditionally have been prepared by adding the drug (e.g., antibiotic or H_2-histamine antagonist) to a small plastic (polyvinyl chloride) IV bag or glass bottle containing 50-250 mL of 5 percent dextrose in water or 0.9 percent sodium chloride. This method of admixture preparation requires the most pharmacy labor, but also gives pharmacy more flexibility in preparing admixtures, since doses can easily be adjusted and diluents changed. Admixture drugs that are powdered or lyophilized will need to be reconstituted prior to addition to the IV bag or bottle. Medications that are already in solution will only have to be drawn into a syringe and injected into the bag or bottle. Some drugs may also be available in prefilled syringes, in which case pharmacy will only need to add the drug to the bag or bottle. This system also allows pharmacy to adjust the volume of each infusion for fluid-restricted patients by removing a portion of diluent before adding the drug. Sodium chloride diluents can also easily be used for diabetic patients, or dextrose solutions for cardiac patients, whenever indicated.

Special IV Admixture Systems

Controlled-Release Infusion System

This system uses drugs that are reconstituted in vials. Pharmacy will reconstitute each dose if it is in the powdered form. Then the vial of drug in solution is sent to the patient care area. A special IV tubing set containing a special adapter for the vial must be used with the primary intravenous solution. This adapter allows the nurse to attach the vial of drug in solution onto the primary IV tubing (figure 19-8). The adapter on the IV set is adjusted so that fluid from the primary IV runs into and out of the attached drug vial, delivering the drug to the patient. It should be noted that this system cannot be used with primary IV's that are running at less than 60 mL/hour.

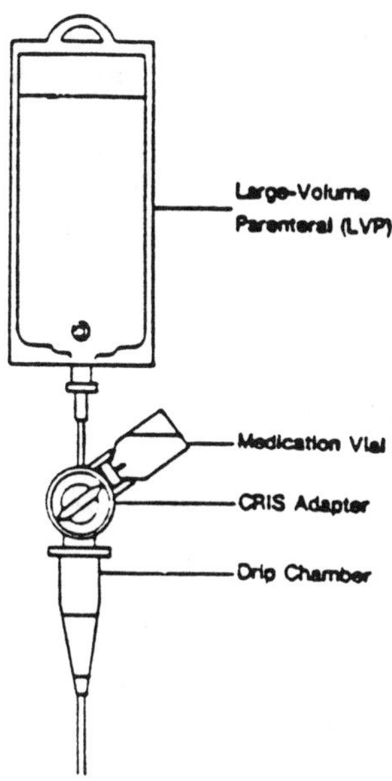

Figure 19-8. The controlled-release infusion system (CRIS™) requires a special primary IV set onto which a reconstituted vial of drug fits. The vial is spiked onto the set, and the CRIS™ adapter is turned so that fluid from the primary IV enters the spiked vial to deliver drug to the patient.

Specially Designed IV Bag With a Drug Vial Port

Minimal pharmacy labor is needed with this system, and drug waste may also be reduced. A specially designed vial, usually containing powdered drug, is attached to the top of an IV bag. This bag contains a port that will accommodate the drug vial (figure 19-9). Once the vial is attached to the bag by pharmacy, the bag is labeled and delivered to the patient unit. Prior to administration, the nurse activates the system by pulling on the vial stopper through the clear plastic bag. The drug in the vial falls into the diluent in the bag. The bag should be inverted to ensure adequate mixing of drug and diluent. Activation of the system may also occur in the pharmacy; the person activating the system should also check for any leakage at the vial/bag interface.[34] The expiration dating for this system is based on both the time of attachment of the drug vial to the IV bag and the time that the drug and diluent are mixed. Each drug has a specific manufacturer-recommended expiration date.

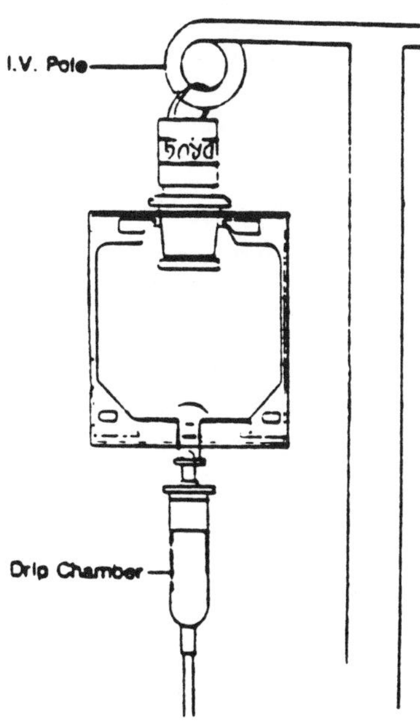

Figure 19-9. The ADD-Vantage™ system setup is shown here. Note the special port at the top of the bag, which holds the medication vial.

LARGE-VOLUME INTRAVENOUS INFUSIONS

Parenteral solutions that are administered continuously over 24 hours should also be included in the pharmacy's IV admixture program. These differ from intermittent infusions because they can be used to deliver large quantities of fluid to a patient. It is important that IV solutions that are administered intravenously are isosmotic (having an osmolality of approximately 300 mOsm). Parenteral solutions having higher osmolalities (i.e., TPN) will need to be given through a larger vein (i.e., superior vena cava) in order to avoid damage to peripheral veins. Continuous intravenous infusions may also be used to administer electrolytes, total parenteral nutrition solutions, and chemotherapy.

A common question from nursing regarding continuous IV infusions pertains to the overfill volumes in these solutions. Usually IV overfill volumes do not present a problem. However, a physician may request that a drug such as a chemotherapeutic agent be administered over a specific time interval. Nurses will need to know the total estimated volume of the parenteral product so that the IV rate (mL/hour) can be adjusted to deliver the drug over the desired time interval. The chart in table 19-8 gives approximate fill ranges for both small and large volume parenteral solutions.[35] Depending on the drug being administered, pharmacy may prepare IV solutions by adding the requested drug to the exact amount of diluent needed rather than using prefilled diluent bags or bottles.

Table 19-8. Approximate fill ranges for parenteral solutions[35]

Labeled volume (mL)	*Glass (mL)*	*Viaflex (mL)*
25	–	28 – 34
50	51 – 58	52 – 63
100	101 – 110	105 – 115
150	150 – 170	160 – 175
250	250 – 275	265 – 285
500	500 – 545	530 – 565
1,000	1,000 – 1,075	1,030 – 1,070
2,000	2,000 – 2,070	2,040 – 2,120
3,000	–	3,050 – 3,150

Although plastic IV bags are very popular, many institutions may use glass bottles. The openings of glass IV bottles are usually stoppered with a solid or vented rubber closure. Glass bottles are vacuum packaged; before use, the vacuum must be dissipated. When glass bottles are used, an internal air tube must be present or a vented set must be used to facilitate the flow of solution out of the bottle. The vented set or air inlet tube allows air to enter the bottle, which displaces the solution.

Premixed Large-Volume IV Solutions

Several continuous IV solutions are available commercially in large-volume (500-1,000 mL) flexible plastic (polyvinyl chloride) bags or semirigid plastic containers and glass bottles. Each IV bag is protected by an outer, tamper-resistant, moisture barrier plastic covering that is removed prior to use. The most popular solutions are 0.9 percent sodium chloride, 5 percent dextrose in water, and 5 percent dextrose in water with varying concentrations of sodium chloride (e.g., 0.9 percent, 0.45 percent, 0.3 percent, 0.2 percent). Different concentrations of dextrose (e.g., 10-50 percent) and sodium chloride (e.g., 0.2-3 percent) may also be purchased for compounding special IV solutions.

Plain IV solutions requiring no additives may be labeled and dispensed directly to the patient unit by pharmacy, or may be available as floor stock on each nursing unit, depending on established hospital policy.

Several large-volume parenteral products may be purchased premixed from the manufacturer (e.g., 5 percent dextrose in water and 0.45 percent sodium chloride with potassium 10, 20, 30 or 40 mEq/L). Premixed solutions containing magnesium, potassium, lidocaine, aminophylline, nitroglycerin, and dopamine are available. These premixed IV solutions require minimal pharmacy labor and help to reduce waste.

Compounded Large-Volume IV Solutions

Often, a specific concentration of a drug or electrolyte (e.g., potassium, magnesium) must be added to a dextrose and/or sodium chloride intravenous solution. It is the responsibility of the pharmacist to ensure that the IV preparation is stable, compatible, and safe. The pharmacist should also verify unusually high doses of drugs or electrolytes (e.g., potassium) with the ordering physician.

Advantages and Disadvantages of IV Admixture Systems

The type or types of IV admixture system(s) that are chosen by an institution should be determined by the items discussed in the section on Components of an IV Admixture Program. Every system will have advantages and disadvantages. As mentioned earlier, premixed products and frozen premixed products offer the least dosing flexibility, but they save pharmacy and nursing labor and also help to decrease waste. The special IV admixture systems discussed in this chapter also offer reduced labor and waste. These products, however, are available from limited sources; therefore, the competitive pricing potential is reduced.

The specially compounded bags are the most labor-intensive to prepare but often have the lowest acquisition cost. They do allow for more dosing options. Doses of medications can be easily changed prior to preparing these compounded bags or LVP's. Unfortunately, the expiration dating on compounded IV's is usually shorter than for the other systems. Unused doses that are wasted are usually greater with this system compared to the premixed, manufacturer's special systems.

Syringes that are used in place of small-volume intravenous bags or bottles may offer a cost advantage. Typically, syringes are less expensive and are relatively quick and easy to prepare. Disadvantages include the purchase of a sufficient number of automated syringe pumps or plastic hanging sleeves. Also, expiration dating for syringes may be less than for IV bags. As a result of the capitalizing of equipment expenditures and availability of prefilled syringes, these systems are gaining in popularity. The institution must carefully choose the IV system that will work best with the resources available to it.

Intravenous Infusion Control Devices

The purchase of electronic infusion devices used to administer intravenous infusions should be under the direction of one department or members of several departments (e.g., pharmacy, nursing, finance). Numerous types of infusion pumps are available on the market today. These pumps allow for multiple drug infusion programming, continuous and intermittent infusions, as well as ambulatory care therapy. The newest addition to the electronic infusion device market is an infusion pump that is programmed using a bar-coding system. A bar code is placed on the intravenous solution, which contains dose administration information. A special wand is passed over the bar code to transfer the coded information to the pump. Once the pump is programmed from the information on the bar code, it automatically sets itself to deliver the required amount of drug at the right time and rate.[36]

Guidelines should be established in the hospital's policies and procedures as to when an electronic infusion device is required for IV drug administration.[37,38] (Refer to reference 40 for an extensive discussion on infusion devices.)

The need or justification for infusion devices has been reported in the literature.[38-40] Often, infusion devices are needed to administer specific intravenous or enteral products. The use of infusion devices should be monitored by each institution to determine in which instances these pumps should be used.

Gravity-dependent administration systems may be used for administering some intravenous fluids. The IV flow rate in gravity-fed systems may be affected by several variables (e.g., viscosity, temperature, clot formation, patient's blood pressure). Since the therapeutic effect of many intravenous solutions is dependent upon accurate flow rates, electronic infusion devices should be used. Infusion controllers help to deliver a specific volume of IV solution mechanically or electronically, usually by counting drops. An infusion pump, on the other hand, uses a motorized pump to deliver a set volume measured in milliliters rather than drops. Critically ill patients will benefit from the use of electronic infusion devices.

Although pharmacy may have minimal input on the purchase and/or use of electronic infusion pumps, pharmacists are being consulted to assist with patient-controlled analgesia (PCA) pumps and programmable infusion pumps.

The PCA and programmable pumps allow the patient to be ambulatory while receiving intravenous medication. These devices can be used on the patient unit, but are designed for outpatient, home care use. Pharmacy may be involved with initiating a patient on one of these pumps while the patient is still hospitalized. Pharmacists play an important role in the use of these devices. Concentrations of medications to be used in these pumps must be calculated, and stability and compatibility information must be considered when these devices are used.

The cassettes or elastomeric reservoirs that contain the drug must be filled by pharmacy using the aseptic techniques discussed earlier in this chapter. To decrease the number of medication cassette or IV bag changes, a more concentrated solution may be prepared. Depending on how the medication will be administered—through peripheral or central access—drug osmolarity must be considered. It is important for the pharmacist to collaborate with the nurse, physician, and patient as to the proper use of these devices.

SPECIALIZED ADMIXTURES

The preparation of parenteral nutrition products, chemotherapeutic agents, intravenous and irrigation solutions, ophthalmics, and other medication may entail vastly different requirements for hospital pharmacy departments. Other chapters in this handbook that are devoted to these topics should be reviewed for a more complete discussion of these areas. Other references are listed in the bibliography at the end of this chapter. Presented below is a brief overview of two types of specialized admixtures.

Nutritional

Parenteral nutrition must be prepared in an aseptic environment using a laminar air-flow hood. Although amino acid solutions containing additives can be purchased, these solutions should be mixed with dextrose solutions, and often additional electrolytes are needed. Secondary intravenous transfer sets are used to mix the dextrose and amino acid components. These secondary sets have large-bore tubing to facilitate the transfer of solutions into a final container. Depending on the type of IV system that is used by the hospital, clamps and caps may also be needed to seal the final product.

Parenteral nutrition solutions, also referred to as total parenteral nutrition, require up to a dozen additives. Caution should be used in evaluating the compatibility of these additives (e.g., calcium, phosphorus). An array of mechanical devices is available to assist in the preparation of these products. Figure 19-10 shows one such product, which aids in adding electrolytes to parenteral nutrition solutions. This device can be reused and is helpful and cost effective when large quantities of solutions are prepared. It must be remembered that these aids are for use in a clean environment; therefore, thorough cleaning and disinfecting of these devices should be performed daily.

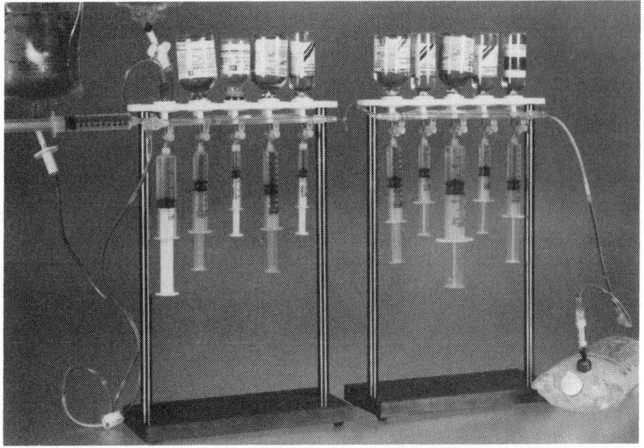

Figure 19-10. A mechanical admixture compounding device is shown here. This apparatus is convenient and easy to use for preparing admixtures that require several diluents.

A complete product check system is required with nutritional products. Most often, two pharmacists will check the calculations for addition of extra electrolyte quantities. When pharmacy technicians are preparing solutions, a pharmacist must check the ingredients before they are added to the final solution. Preprogrammed calculators or computer programs are available to assist in calculating the volume of ingredients for nutritional solutions. These are especially helpful in preparing neonatal and pediatric nutrition solutions that require very small volumes of additives.

Although not in the realm of this chapter, a nutritional support team with pharmacy representation can be extremely valuable in ensuring that proper solutions are ordered and waste is kept to a minimum.

Chemotherapy

Displayed in figure 19-2 is one of a number of vertical air-flow hoods available on the market. For the preparation of chemotherapy, a Class II, (Type A, B1, B2, or B3) vertical air-flow hood is recommended. It is preferable that the hood be vented to release exhaust to the outside atmosphere, but often this may be extremely costly or impossible because of the location of the hood. If a vertical hood is not available, a clean countertop or horizontal air-flow hood that is shut off may be used. These last two areas are not recommended, but may be used until a vertical air-flow hood is obtained. Table 19-9 lists components that should be used when preparing chemotherapy. Additional reference sources regarding this topic can be found at the conclusion of this chapter.

Table 19-9. Suggested equipment for chemotherapy preparation

- Vertical air-flow hood
- Eye-wash container
- Double latex gloves, respirators (not surgical masks), lint-free, low-permeability, long-sleeved, solid-front gown with tightly fitting cuffs, goggles, or safety glasses
- Separate biohazard disposal container
- Chemotherapy spill kit
- Aerosol protection devices (i.e., CytoGuard™)

The preparation and administration of parenteral products deserves serious attention by all health professionals involved with the process. A number of aspects deserve special attention including sterility, stability, incompatibility, solubility, proper labeling, and a thorough understanding of the administration systems involved. The patient must be the recipient of a quality product and must receive the attention required to administer and manage this important form of therapy. An admixture system is a dynamic, patient-oriented system that deserves continual evaluation. Such evaluation should lead to improvements in patient care, and the value to the hospital and patient of such a continually revised system cannot be overemphasized. As important changes occur in the compounding and administration of these products, pharmacy should respond by evaluating their place in the provision of quality care for the patients it serves. No IV admixture system should ever be considered perfect.

Note: The American Society of Hospital Pharmacists recently published draft guidelines on quality assurance for pharmacy-prepared sterile products (41). When these guidelines are finalized they will provide standards to assist in developing an intravenous admixture program.

REFERENCES

1. Turco S, King RE: *Sterile Dosage Forms, Their Preparation and Clinical Application.* Philadelphia, Lea & Febiger, 1987.
2. Akers MJ: Considerations in using the IV route for drug delivery. *Am J Hosp Pharm* 44:2528-2530, 1987.
3. National Coordinating Committee on Large Volume Parenterals: Recommendations to pharmacists for solving problems with large volume parenteral solution. *Am J Hosp Pharm* 33:231-236, 1976.
4. National Coordinating Committee on Large Volume Parenterals: Recommended methods for compounding intravenous admixtures in hospitals. *Am J Hosp Pharm* 32:261-270, 1975.
5. National Coordinating Committee on Large Volume Parenterals: System for the surveillance and reporting of problems with large volume parenteral solutions in hospitals. *Am J Hosp Pharm* 32:1251-1253, 1975.
6. National Coordinating Committee on Large Volume Parenterals: Recommendations for labeling of large volume parenterals. *Am J Hosp Pharm* 35:49-51, 1978.
7. National Coordinating Committee on Large Volume Parenterals: Recommended procedures for in-use testing of large volume parenterals suspected of contamination or of producing a reaction in a patient. *Am J Hosp Pharm* 35:678-682, 1978.
8. Mitchell SR: Monitoring waste in an intravenous admixture program. *Am J Hosp Pharm* 44:106-111, 1987.
9. Reilly KM: Problems in administration techniques and dose measurement that influence accuracy of IV drug delivery. *Am J Hosp Pharm* 44:2545-2550, 1987.
10. Pearlstein PH, Callison C, White M, et al: Errors in drug computations during newborn intensive care. *Am J Dis Child* 133:376-379, 1979.
11. Cohen MR, Davis NM: Assuring safe use of parenteral dosage forms in hospitals. *Hosp Pharm* 25:913-915, 1990.
12. Joint Commission on Accreditation of Hospitals: *Accreditation Manual for Hospitals.* Chicago, Joint Commission on Accreditation of Hospitals, 1990, pp 115-161.
13. American Society of Hospital Pharmacists: *Practice Standards of the American Society of Hospital Pharmacists 1989-90.* Bethesda, MD, American Society of Hospital Pharmacists, 1989.
14. Recommended standards of practice, policies and practices for intravenous therapy. National Coordinating Committee on Large Volume Parenterals. *Am J Hosp Pharm* 37:660-663, 1980.
15. Brzozowski DF, Lisitano RC, Patton JJ, et al: Pharmacists' opinions about and compliance with recommendations for intravenous admixture practices. *Am J Hosp Pharm* 44:2077-2084, 1987.
16. Ansel HC: The prescription. In *Remington's Pharmaceutical Sciences,* 16th ed. Easton, PA, Mack Publishing Co., 1980, p 1732.
17. Garner JS, Favero MS: CDC guidelines for the prevention and control of nosocomial infections. *Am J Infec Control* 14:110-129, 1986.
18. Gennaro AR: Analysis of medicinals. In *Remington's Pharmaceutical Sciences,* 17th ed. Easton, PA, Mack Publishing Co., 1985.
19. Clean room and work station requirements: Controlled environment (Fed. Std. No. 209B). Washington, DC, U.S. Government Printing Office, April 24, 1973.
20. Trissel LA: *Handbook of Injectable Drugs,* 5th ed. Bethesda, MD, American Society of Hospital Pharmacists, 1988.
21. Warren DW, Paladino JA, Adams-Warren CP, et al: Standardized charts to determine intravenous infusion rates. *Am J Hosp Pharm* 43:1914-1915, 1986.
22. Loeb AJ, Fishman DA, Koclis TR: Premixed intravenous admixtures: A critical challenge for hospital pharmacy. *Am J Hosp Pharm* 40:1041-1043, 1988.
23. Witte KW, Eck TA, Vogel DP: Decision analysis applied to the purchase of frozen premixed intravenous admixtures. *Am J Hosp Pharm* 42:835-839, 1985.
24. Kirschenbaun BE, Cacae L, Anderson RJ, et al: Personnel time and preparation costs for compounded versus premixed intravenous admixtures in three community hospitals. *Am J Hosp Pharm* 45:605-608, 1988.
25. Rapp RP: Hospital intravenous drug administration in the era of prospective payment. *Drug Intell Clin Pharm* 19:146-149, 1985.
26. Paxinos J, Hammel RJ, Fritz WL: Contamination rates and costs associated with the use of four intermittent intravenous infusion systems. *Am J Hosp Pharm* 36:1497-1503, 1979.
27. Smith TF, Kitrenos JG: Comparison of seven methods of preparing and administering cefazolin sodium small-volume injections. *Am J Hosp Pharm* 43:1930-1935, 1986.
28. Rapp RP: Considering product features and costs in selecting a system for intermittent IV drug delivery. *Am J Hosp Pharm* 44:2533-2538, 1987.
29. Vogel DP, Eck TA, Witte KW: Calculation of product waste in IV admixture programs. *Am J Hosp Pharm* 43:952-953, 1986.
30. Walter DJ: Documenting IV admixture product waste. *Am J Hosp Pharm* 43:1914-1915 (letter), 1986.

31. Salberg DJ, Newton RW, Leduc DT: Cost of wastage in a hospital intravenous program. *Hosp Formul* 19:375-378, 1984.
32. Osol A: *Remington's Pharmaceutical Sciences,* 16th ed. Easton, PA, Mack Publishing Co., 1980.
33. DeMonaco HJ: IV drug delivery: New technology for consideration. *J Intravenous Nurs* 11:316-320, 1988.
34. Foltyn Smith C, Amen RJ: Comparison of seven methods of preparing and administering small-volume injections. *Am J Hosp Pharm* 45:1896-1901, 1988.
35. Gabos C: Personal communication (letter) Baxter Healthcare Corporation, November 1989.
36. Anonymous: Abbott infuses IV business with growth. *Hospitals* (Jan 5):67, 1990.
37. Donnelly EB, Witte KW, LaPlume G: Interdisciplinary committee on infusion-control devices: Managing product use. *Am J Hosp Pharm* 45:589-594, 1988.
38. Alexander MR: IV infusion devices: Are they always justified? *Drug Intell Clin Pharm* 21:255-257, 1987.
39. Alexander MR, Kirking DM, Baron KA: Utilization of electronic infusion devices in a university hospital. *Drug Intell Clin Pharm* 21:630-633, 1987.
40. Kwan JW: High-technology IV infusion devices. *Am J Hosp Pharm* 46:320-335, 1989.
41. Draft guidelines on quality assurance for pharmacy-prepared sterile products. *Am J Hosp Pharm* 49:417, 1992.

ADDITIONAL READING

Quality Control

Akers M: *Parenteral Quality Control: Sterility, Pyrogen, Particulate Matter and Package Integrity Testing.* New York, Marcel Dekker, 1985.

Morris BG, Avis KE, Bowles GC, et al: Quality control plan for intravenous admixture programs. I: Visual inspection of solutions and environmental testing. *Am J Hosp Pharm* 37:189-195, 1980.

Morris BG, Avis KE, Bowles GC, et al: Quality control plan for intravenous admixture programs. II: Validation of operator technique. *Am J Hosp Pharm* 37:668-672, 1980.

National Coordinating Committee on Large Volume Parenterals: Recommended guidelines for quality assurance in hospital centralized intravenous admixture services. *Am J Hosp Pharm* 37:645-655, 1980.

Training

Hinshaw WR, Wilken LO Jr: Training personnel for intravenous admixture programs. *Am J Hosp Pharm* 29:1025, 1972.

Hunt ML: *Training Manual for Intravenous Admixture Personnel.* Chicago, Pluribus Press, 1989.

Hunt ML: Intravenous admixture training program for pharmacy personnel. *Am J Hosp Pharm* 31:467-471, 1974.

Latiolais CJ: Teamwork — the key to success in IV therapy. *Am J IV Therapy* 13, 1975.

Ray MD (ed): Training hospital pharmacy technicians. *Am J Hosp Pharm* 41:2595-2596, 1984.

Ross SR: Managing training programs for pharmacy employees. *Am J Hosp Pharm* 41:1173-1177, 1984.

Compatibility and Stability

Donn R: Intravenous admixture incompatibility program. *Bull Parenteral Drug Assoc* 24:98-103, 1970.

Fowler TJ: *Injectable Solutions and Additives: Compatibilities, Incompatibilities, Routes of Administration.* New York, Springer Publisher, 1971.

Ho NFH: Prediction of pharmaceutical stability of parenteral solution III. *Drug Intell Clin Pharm* 5:47-50, 1971.

Ho NFH, Goeman JA: Prediction of pharmaceutical stability of parenteral solution. *Drug Intell Clin Pharm* 4:69-72, 1970.

Kramer W, Inglott A, Cluxton R: Some physical and chemical incompatibilities of drugs for IV administration. *Drug Intell Clin Pharm* 5:211-228, 1971.

Parker EA: Parenteral incompatibilities. *Hosp Pharm* 4:14, 1969.

Sister Mary Edward: pH: An important factor in compatibility of additives in intravenous therapy. *Am J Hosp Pharm* 24:440, 1967.

Trissel LA: *Handbook of Injectable Drugs,* 5th ed. Bethesda, MD, American Society of Hospital Pharmacists, 1988.

Trissel LA: *Supplement to the Handbook of Injectable Drugs.* Bethesda, MD, American Society of Hospital Pharmacists, 1989.

Contamination

Akers MJ: Parenteral fundamental. Dynamics of microbial growth and death in parenteral products. *J Parenteral Drug Assoc* 33:372-388, 1979.

Davis NM, Turco S, Sivelly E: Particulate matter in IV infusion fluids. *Bull Parenteral Drug Assoc* 24:257, 1970.

Garvan JM, Gunner BW: Particulate contamination of intravenous infusion fluids. *Brit J Clin Prac* 25:119, 1971.

Hansen J, Helper C: Contamination of intravenous solutions of airborne microbes. *Am J Hosp Pharm* 30:326, 1973.

Lim JC: Technique for microbiological testing of in-use intravenous solutions and administration sets. *Am J Hosp Pharm* 36:1202-1204, 1979.

Maki D, Goldman D, Rhame R: Infection control in intravenous therapy. *Nursing Digest* 5, 1975.

Pappalardo G, Hirschi B, Pannatier A, et al: Comparative study between liquid and solid media for the detection of bacterial contamination in intravenous solution. *J Clin Pharm Ther* 13:411-416, 1988.

Turco SJ, Davis NM: Clinical significance of particulate matter: A review of the literature. *Hosp Pharm* 8:137, 1973.

Turco SJ, Davis NM: Glass particles in intravenous injections. *New Engl J Med* 287:1204, 1972.

Turco SJ, Davis NM: Particulate matter in intravenous infusion fluids — Phase 3. *Am J Hosp Pharm* 30:611, 1973.

Weil DC, Arrow PM: Safety of refrigerated storage of admixed parenteral fluids. *J Clin Microbiol* 26:1787-1790, 1988.

Cancer Chemotherapy

AMA Council report guidelines for handling parenteral antineoplastics. *JAMA* 253:1590-1592, 1985.

American Society of Hospital Pharmacists: Technical assistance bulletin on handling cytotoxic drugs and hazardous drugs. *Am J Hosp Pharm* 47:1033-49, 1990.

Clinical Oncological Society of Australia: Guidelines and recommendations for safe handling of antineoplastic agents. *Med J Aust* 1:426-428, 1983.

DeVita VT Jr, Hellman S, Rosenberg SA: *Cancer: Principles and Practice of Oncology,* Vol. I and II. Philadelphia, J.B. Lippincott, 1989.

Jones B, Frank R, Mass T, et al: Safe handling of chemotherapeutic agents: A report from the Mount Sinai Medical Center. *CA* (Sept/Oct):258-263, 1983.

Kuemmerle HP: *Antineoplastic Chemotherapy.* New York, Thieme Medical Publishers, 1984.

Kuemmerle HP: *Fundamentals of Clinical Chemotherapy,* Vol. I. New York, Thieme Medical Publishers, 1983.

Lokich J (ed): *Cancer Chemotherapy by Infusion.* Chicago, Pluribus Press, 1987.

National Study Commission on Cytotoxic Exposure: *Recommendations for Handling Cytotoxic Agents.* Boston, MA, Massachusetts College of Pharmacy and Allied Health Sciences.

OSHA work-practice guidelines for personnel dealing with cytotoxic (antineoplastic) drugs. *Am J Hosp Pharm* 43:1193-1204, 1986.

Recommendations for the safe handling of parenteral antineoplastic drugs. NIH Publication No.83-2621. Washington, DC, U.S. Government Printing Office.

Sather MR: *Cancer Chemotherapeutic Agents: Handbook of Clinical Data.* Boston, GK Hall, 1978.

Parenteral Nutrition

Dean RE: *Total Parenteral Nutrition: Standard Techniques.* Chicago, Pluribus Press, 1983.

Deitel M, Lloyd CS, Friedman KL, et al: Physical stability of a total nutrient admixture for total parenteral nutrition. *Can J Surg* 32:240-243, 1989.

Fong WL, Grimley GW: Peripheral intravenous infusion of amino acids. *Am J Hosp Pharm* 38:652-659, 1981.

Grant JP: *Handbook of Total Parenteral Nutrition.* Philadelphia, Saunders, 1979.

Hargus-Biehle K: *Guidelines for Developing a Home Parenteral Nutrition Program.* Memphis, American College of Apothecaries Research and Education Foundation, 1983.

King JC: *Guide to Parenteral Admixtures.* St. Louis, Cutter Laboratories, Pacemarq, Inc., 1973.

Rombeau JL, Caldwell MD: *Clinical Nutrition: Parenteral Nutrition,* Vol. 2. Philadelphia, Saunders, 1986.

General

Avallone HJ: Regulatory issues of parenteral equipment and systems. *J Parenteral Sci Technol* 42:89-93, 1988.

Balinsky W, Nesbitt S: Cost effectiveness of outpatient parenteral antibiotics: A review of the literature. *Am J Med* 87:301-305, 1989.

Barker KN (ed): *Recommendations of the National Coordinating Committee on Large Volume Parenterals for the Compounding and Administration of Intravenous Solutions.* Bethesda, MD, American Society of Hospital Pharmacists, 1981.

Caplik JF, Walters JK Jr: *Guidelines for the Preparation of Intravenous Admixture Solutions.* Cutter Medical, 1980.

Channell SR: *Manual of IV Therapy Procedures,* 2nd ed. Med Economics, 1985.

DeMuynck C, Remon JP, Colardyn F: Binding of drugs to end-line filters: A study of four commonly administered drugs in intensive care units. *J Clin Pharm Ther* 13:335-340, 1988.

Dubois M: Patient-controlled analgesia for acute pain. *Clin J Pain* 5(suppl 1):S8-S15, 1989.

Ensminger WD, Selam JL (eds): *Infusion Systems in Medicine.* Futura Publishing Co., 1987.

Ensminger WD, Selam JL: *Update in Drug Delivery Systems.* Futura Publishing Co., 1989.

Ford RD (ed): *Medication Administration and IV Therapy Manual.* Philadelphia, PA, Spring House Publishers, 1985.

Francke DE: *Handbook of IV Additive Reviews.* Reprinted by Drug Intelligence in Clinical Pharmacy, 1971.

Gahart BL: *Intravenous Medication: A Handbook for Nurses and Other Allied Health Personnel,* 4th ed. St. Louis, C.V. Mosby, 1988.

Hipwell CE, Mashford ML, Robertson MB: *Guide to Parenteral Administration of Drugs.* Boston, ADIS Health Science Press, 1984.

King JC, Macmillan MW: *Concise Guide to Parenteral Medications.* San Francisco, Pacemarq, Inc., 1989.

Knapp JZ, Kuschner HK, et al: Generalized methodology for evaluation of parenteral inspection procedures. *J Parenteral Drug Assoc* 34(1):14-61, 1980.

L'eff RD, Roberts RJ: *Practical Aspects of Intravenous Techniques for the Practicing Nurse, Pharmacist, Physician.* Bethesda, MD, American Society of Hospital Pharmacists, 1985.

L'eff RD, Stull JC: Accuracy, continuity and pattern of flow from five macrorate infusion pumps. *Am J Hosp Pharm* 45:361-365, 1988.

Morris ME (updated by Tierney M, Godbout L): *Intravenous Drug Therapy Manual,* 11th ed. Ottawa, Canada, Ottawa General Hospital, 1989.

National Coordinating Committee on Large Volume Parenterals. Recommendations to pharmacists for solving problems with large-volume parenterals — 1979. *Am J Hosp Pharm* 37:663-667, 1980.

New products and services in IV therapy. *J Intravenous Nurs* 11(2):139, 1988.

Piecoro JJ: Development of an institutional IV drug delivery policy. *Am J Hosp Pharm* 44:2557-2559, 1987.

Plumer AL: *Principles and Practice of Intravenous Therapy,* 4th ed. Boston, Little, Brown, 1987.

Primer: Current problems and innovations in intravenous drug delivery. *Am J Hosp Pharm* 44:2528-2557, 1987.

Pulliam CC, Upton JH: Pharmacy coordinated intravenous admixture and administration service. *Am J Hosp Pharm* 28:92, 1971.

Robinson ML: Hospitals poised to offer in-home IV therapy. *Hospitals* 63(14):16-20, 1989.

Sherrin TP, Miller WA, Latiolais CJ: Projecting staffing patterns from time study data in centralized intravenous admixture programs. *Am J Hosp Pharm* 29:1013, 1972.

Vogel DP, Eck TA, Witte KW: Calculation of product waste in IV admixture programs. *Am J Hosp Pharm* 43:952-953, 1986.

Wuest JR: Initiating an IV additive service 3. Development of policies and procedures. *Drug Intell Clin Pharm* 4:183-186, 1970.

Wuest JR: Initiating an IV additive service 4. Development of policies and procedures. *Drug Intell Clin Pharm* 4:279-282, 1970.

Wuest JR: Justifying an IV additive program. *Drug Intell Clin Pharm* 4:125-126, 1970.

Wuest JR: Staffing an IV additive service. *Drug Intell Clin Pharm* 4:153-154, 1970.

Zenk KE: Dosage calculations for drugs administered by infusion (letter). *Am J Hosp Pharm* 37:1304-1305, 1980.

CHAPTER 20

Adult Enteral and Parenteral Nutrition

KATHERINE TREXLER and JOHN MURRAY

BACKGROUND

Recognition of the need for nutritional intervention in the malnourished patient is not a new phenomenon. The advent of intravenous support occurred in the late 1960's when Dudrick et al.[1] described its use in beagle puppies. There then followed an explosive increase in its use and applications throughout the medical community, so that total parenteral nutrition (TPN) may now be considered as the standard of care for many conditions.[2] The state of the art has advanced significantly over the past 30 years so that adequate protein and calories can be provided to correct or to prevent nutritional deficiencies in most patients. Modern technology has produced a variety of access devices for both enteral and parenteral nutrition[3] as well as ancillary devices and nutrition formulas. Nevertheless, its use has not been without complications, some quite significant.[2]

As a result of some of the complications resulting from intravenous support and the recent recognition of the unique role of the gastrointestinal tract in the maintenance of immunofunction,[4] much attention has been given to the increased application of enteral feedings. Since the gut itself may serve as a barrier to infection and may also alter absorption of certain nutrients depending on the need for them, fewer complications may occur from this form of support. In addition, the enteral route is much less expensive than parenteral and is much more physiologic. Current development has now centered around identifying the patient who could benefit from nutrition support and enhancing his or her response.

As demands for cost-effectiveness in the health care setting become more rigorous,[5,6] carefully designed nutrition regimens play a major role in the overall therapeutic plan.[7,8] Formulas must be adjusted to provide individually prescribed total calories, protein, lipid, carbohydrate, electrolytes, and micronutrients for maintenance of good health and nutrition (table 20-1).

Team Function

To reduce the morbidity and mortality from nutrition support as well as to ensure its application in a safe and effective manner, the health care setting has recognized the necessity for a team approach.[9] The pharmacist has been involved in intravenous nutrition support services since their inception to supply safe and effective solutions.[10] The past decade has brought increased awareness and advances in the technology of nutrition support as well as new product development. Specialization of nutritional support has brought together physicians, nurses, pharmacists, and dietitians, each with their own responsibilities to provide parenteral and enteral nutrition.[11] The ideal nutrition support team (NST) has been conceptualized to include all these disciplines. However, few institutions have the luxury of starting with a full-time member from each. Usually teams start with one or two members and add others as the need arises.

General guidelines for roles and functions of various NST members exist but may vary depending upon the number and type of patients followed, whether the team is consultative or management oriented, and if a home nutrition support program is offered. The physician assumes the overall responsibility for the team and should be specifically trained in nutritional management.[12] The pharmacist's tasks include solution compounding, evaluation of drug-drug and drug-nutrient interactions, formula design, compatibilities, and metabolic monitoring.[13] Nutritional assessment, estimations of oral intake, enteral product evaluation and design, nutrient needs, and tube and transitional feedings are managed by the dietitian.[14] Nurses are responsible for catheter care, patient and staff education as well as metabolic monitoring.[15] Some teams have also incorporated a social worker to assist with emotional support and financing as well as a physical therapist for exercise programs.[16]

Benefits of an established NST include a decrease in septic, metabolic, and mechanical complications.[12,17] Documentation of quality assurance is necessary to ensure continued high standards of practice.[18] Discipline certification is also now becoming available and should be pursued by all practitioners.[19]

Consequences of Malnutrition

The alarming incidence of malnutrition in the hospitalized patient has been widely documented. Studies have shown that upon admission, approximately 20-50 percent of patients have some degree of impairment. Of increasing concern in American society is obesity, which also is detrimental to health. It is difficult to improve nutrition status while the patient is in the hospital without significant intervention, since meals are often withheld or interrupted for procedures or tests, and the hospital may be unable to provide the usual diet for a patient (e.g., ethnic). Medical treatment may also require a specialized diet that is unpalatable to the patient, such as low bacterial, low fat, or low sodium.

Starvation affects every organ, causing a decrease in organ mass and function (table 20-2). The consequences of malnutrition depend upon its degree, type, and duration as it interacts with the individual's clinical condition. The general lack of agreement on the accuracy and validity of physical and chemical assessment to identify or predict which patients have or will develop a deficiency or benefit from nutritional intervention further complicates decisions on nutrition support. Certainly malnutrition, whether primary or secondary to another disorder, is accompanied by a substantial risk for patient survival.

NUTRITIONAL ASSESSMENT

The roles of nutritional assessment are (1) to identify all patients who are malnourished regardless of age, body habitus, disease process, therapeutic regimen, or organ dysfunction; (2) to identify patients who would benefit from specialized nutritional feeding; and (3) to guide therapy and evaluate attainment of nutritional goals, whether the goal is to replete, maintain, or deplete body weight while maintaining or restoring lean body mass and function. The standard nutritional assessment includes multiple indices, such as diet history, physical exam, anthropometric measurements, visceral proteins, and immunological parameters, which reflect status of or changes in body mass.[20,21]

Diet History and Physical Exam

A detailed nutritional history can often be obtained from the patient or family member. The history includes weight changes (recent changes are more significant), previous intake, dental history, social history, presence of gastrointestinal disease, and history of stressful events such as surgery or trauma. Physical exam evaluates muscle wasting, mucosal changes, edema, and findings of deficiency syndromes.[20,21]

The nutritional history and physical exam are sometimes termed the "subjective global assessment" (SGA) (table 20-3). Some practitioners feel this inexpensive and easily performed method effectively accomplishes nutritional assessment goals and is helpful in identifying patients who will benefit from nutritional support.[22] It does not provide a record of body composition changes or assist in assessing nutritional changes.

Anthropometric Measurements

Anthropometric measurements attempt to separate body fat mass from fat-free mass to determine body composition. Variation from the normal population serves to stratify people into risk groups. Fat mass is evaluated by measuring skinfold thickness (usually triceps skinfold), which is proportional to subcutaneous fat.[23,24] Somatic muscle mass is determined by a calculation involving the midarm circumference and the triceps skinfold.[20,21] The measurements have several limitations as a result of wide variation in the general population, disproportionate fat distribution, change in total body water, subcutaneous emphysema, and measurement error.[23,25]

Table 20-1. Nutrient components contained in both parenteral and enteral nutrition

Nutrient	*Source*
Water	
Nitrogen	Eight essential amino acids, conditionally essential amino acids (e.g., histadine is essential in renal failure), plus various nonessential amino acids
Energy (carbohydrate and/or fat)	Multiple sources
Essential fatty acids	Linoleic acid, linolenic acid, arachidonic acid
Electrolytes	Salts Acetate Calcium Chloride Magnesium Phosphate Potassium Sodium Sulfate
Vitamins	Fat-soluble vitamins (A,D,E,K) Water-soluble vitamins Ascorbic acid (C) Biotin Cyanocobalamin (B12) Folic acid Nicotinic acid Pantothenic acid Pyridoxine (B6) Thiamine (B1) Riboflavin (B2)
Trace elements	Chromium Copper Iodine Iron Manganese Molybdenum Selenium Zinc

Table 20-2. Proposed relationship of lean body mass depletion and patient morbidty and mortality

Lean body mass depletion (%)	*Metabolic consequence*
10	Growth retardation (child), decreased muscle mass: skeletal, cardiac, smooth
15	Anemia, decreased visceral proteins
20	Impaired immune response, complement, antibodies, acute phase proteins
25	Impaired wound healing, response to trauma, impaired organ function, gut, liver, heart
28-30	Impaired adaptation, urinary tract infection, bed sores
>30	Nitrogen death

Reprinted with permission from Mirtallo JM, Ebbert ML: Enteral and parenteral nutrition. In Brown TR, Smith MC (eds): *Handbook of Institutional Pharmacy Practice.* Baltimore, Williams & Wilkins, 1986, pp 376-388.

Body weight is generally evaluated as percentage of ideal weight, usual weight, or weight change (table 20-4). Recent weight change is calculated as (change in weight/usual weight) x 100 percent.[20,21] Patient recall, commonly the source of usual weight, and fluctuating fluid status may make interpretation erroneous; nevertheless, weight change should be evaluated carefully, as significant weight loss is associated with a poor prognosis.[25-29]

Anthropometrics, although fraught with inaccuracies, somewhat address all three of the nutritional assessment questions. Weight loss, decreased subcutaneous fat, and decreased muscle mass together help identify malnourished patients, patients with little reserve, and those who may benefit from early nutritional therapy.[20,21] As a monitoring technique, anthropometrics are of little assistance short term, as they may only reflect fluid status changes.[30-32] However, repetitive measurements in the euvolemic patient with a single observer can give some valuable information for long-term therapy.[30,31,33]

Visceral Proteins

To evaluate visceral protein mass, the serum proteins albumin, transferrin, prealbumin (transthyretin), and somatomedin C may be measured (table 20-5).[21] Serum protein concentrations are assumed to reflect hepatic synthesis, which is directly related to substrate availability and/or visceral organ mass. Unfortunately, many other factors affect serum protein levels, including fluid status, liver function, renal function, acute stress, and colloid administration.[21,25,34] Albumin, with its long serum half-life (20 days) and large body pool (4-5 g/kg body weight), is a poor indicator of early protein malnutrition and only slowly recovers with refeeding.[21,25,35,36] If clinical status does not improve, it may never recover. However, it is a very good predictor of individual risk for morbidity and mortality and therefore helps identify those who may benefit from nutrition intervention.[20,21,32]

Transferrin, although not as sensitive as albumin, is useful in predicting risk.[20,21,32] Because of its shorter half-life (8-10 days) and smaller body pool (less than 100 mg/kg body weight), it is more sensitive to changes in nutritional status.[21,35,36] Prealbumin has an even shorter half-life (2 days) and smaller body pool (10 mg/kg body weight), making it more responsive to nutritional intake and therefore useful in assessing adequacy of nutritional support.[21,35,36] It is not useful in predicting nutritional risks.[32] Somatomedin C is being investigated to determine whether it offers any advantage over other serum proteins.[34]

Immune Competence

Depression of host immune response is associated with malnutrition, which may be reversed with nutritional repletion.[37] Immunocompetence is assessed by total lymphocyte count and delayed-type hypersensitivity skin reactions to a battery of skin test antigens. These tests, although affected by malnutrition, are also influenced by surgery, anesthesia, stress or injury, radiation therapy, chemotherapy, and steroids.[38] Unfortunately, the complexity of immune function prevents interpretation for any nutritional assessment goals.[25]

Table 20-3. Features of subjective global assessment (SGA)

Select appropriate category with a checkmark, or enter numerical value where indicated by "#."

A. History
1. Weight change
   Overall loss in past 6 months: amount = # ______kg
   % change from normal ______.
   Change in past 2 weeks: ________increase, ________no change, ________decrease.
2. Dietary intake change (relative to normal)
   ___No change,
   ___Change ___duration =#_____weeks.
   ___type:___suboptimal solid diet, ___full liquid ___hypocaloric liquids, ___starvation.
3. Gastrointestinal symptoms (that persisted for >2 weeks)
   ___none, ___nausea, ___vomiting, ___diarrhea, ___anorexia
4. Functional capacity
   ___No dysfunction (e.g., full capacity),
   ___Dysfunction ___duration =# ___weeks.
   ___type: ___working suboptimally ___ambulatory, ___bedridden.
5. Disease and its relation to nutritional requirements
   Primary diagnosis (specify)
   Metabolic demand (stress): ___no stress, ___low stress, ___moderate, ___high stress

B. Physical (for each trait specify: 0=normal, 1+ = mild, 2+ = moderate, 3+ = severe).
   #_____loss of subcutaneous fat (triceps, chest)
   #_____muscle wasting (quadriceps, deltoids)
   #_____ankle edema
   #_____sacral edema
   #_____ascites

C. SGA rating (select one)
   _______A = Well nourished
   _______B = Moderately (or suspected of being) malnourished
   _______C = Severely malnourished

Reprinted with permission from Detsky AS, Mclaughlin JR, Baker JP, et al: What is subjective global assessment of nutritional status? *J Parenter Enter Nutr* 11:8-13, 1987.

Table 20-4. Degree of protein calorie malnutrition

	Mild	*Moderate*	*Severe*
Percent ideal body weight	80-90%	70-80%	<70%
Percent usual weight	85-95%	75-84%	<75%
Recent weight change	1 week	1-2%	>2%
	1 month	5%	>5%
	3 months	7.5%	>7.5%
	6 months	10%	>10%

Reprinted with permission from Mirtallo JM, Ebbert ML: Enteral and parenteral nutrition. In Brown TR, Smith MC (eds): *Handbook of Institutional Pharmacy Practice.* Baltimore, Williams & Wilkins, 1986, pp 376-388.

Table 20-5. Visceral protein serum levels and nutritional status[21]

	Degree of deficiency			
Visceral protein	*Normal*	*Mild*	*Moderate*	*Severe*
Albumin g/dL	4-3.5	3.4-2.8	2.7-2.1	<2.1
Transferrin mg/dL	300-200	200-150	150-100	<100
Prealbumin mg/dL	29.6-15	15-10	10-5	<5

Function

Decreased oral intake and malnutrition correlate well with decreased muscle function. Provision of nutrition can improve muscle function in malnourished patients, but not to their previous well-nourished state.[25,39,40]

In the future, more functional measurements may be used to assess nutritional status or determine nutritional response.[41] The average length of time a person receives TPN at Duke University Medical Center is 17 days (national average, 11-29 days).[42] During this time, significant lean body mass accumulation does not occur and cannot be measured by current indices.[25,43] TPN has been shown to improve outcome in malnourished patients when given only 7-10 days preoperatively.[32,44] As body composition does not improve during this period, it is postulated that either a critically important small nitrogen pool is restored or conversion to an anabolic state protects against detrimental consequences. Although current indices cannot measure these changes, other functional assessments may further define this population.[41]

Other Measurements

Creatinine-height index, 3-methylhistidine excretion, bioelectric impedance, doubly labeled water, neutron-activation analysis, total body potassium, oxygen-18-labeled water, computerized tomography, and nuclear magnetic resonance have been used as other nutritional assessment tools.[21,25,45-55] These techniques offer little advantage over previously discussed measurements, require special equipment to perform, expose patients to radiation, and/or are too expensive to use routinely.

No single nutritional assessment tool provides all needed information. An objective, reproducible, responsive index to guide nutritional therapy is needed but currently is not available. By use of common techniques, patients have been separated into three categories. "Marasmus" is defined as a loss of somatic muscle and total body fat with normal visceral proteins. "Kwashiorkor" is defined as a loss of lean body mass occurring with low or poor-quality protein intake. "Marasmus-kwashiorkor" malnutrition is a combination of the previous types and is associated with the highest morbidity and mortality. These classifications are further divided into degrees of severity (i.e., mild, moderate, severe) and may occur in combination.[21]

INDICATIONS FOR NUTRITIONAL SUPPORT

When spontaneous oral nutrition is inadequate, another route of nutrition support must be considered. The published guidelines of the American Society of Parenteral and Enteral Nutrition (ASPEN) present clinical settings in which nutritional support should be included in care, in which it might be beneficial, and in which there is little benefit.[56,57] Enteral nutrition becomes the treatment of choice if the gastrointestinal (GI) tract is functional because of its economic, safety, and therapeutic advantages. The most important stimulus for growth and development of the intestinal mucosa is the presence of food within the bowel. The colonocyte is more dependent on luminal nutrition than the enterocyte.[58] Acute and chronic starvation may impair the barrier functions of the gut,[59] resulting in increased bacterial translocation in critically ill patients.[4] Long-term parenteral nutrition is unable to sustain the mucosa, and atrophy occurs. Lack of glutamine, ketones, short-chain fatty acids, and aspartate, major sources of fuel for the GI mucosa, in total parenteral nutrition may play a role in gut atrophy.[58,60,61,62]

Enteral nutrition is indicated when the patient is malnourished and unable to ingest adequate intake for at least 5 days (table 20-6).[56] Even the patient with a normal nutrition status does not benefit from starvation; therefore, if the intake is less than 50 percent of estimated requirement for the previous 7-10 days, consideration for placement of an enteral feeding tube must be given. If the patient is postoperative, careful evaluation must be made that bowel function has returned.

Table 20-6. Indications for enteral nutrition therapy

- Helpful
  - Severe dysphasia
    - Stroke, multiple sclerosis, head injuries, brain tumors, head and neck surgery, partial esophageal obstruction, esophageal fistula
  - Major burns
    - May stem hypermetabolic response[63]
  - Short gut syndrome (in conjunction with TPN)
    - 50%-90% resection
  - Low-output entercutaneous fistulae
    - Feed distally if in proximal gut
- Usually Helpful
  - Major trauma
  - Radiation therapy[64]
  - Mild chemotherapy
  - Liver failure
  - Severe renal dysfunction
- Limited or Undetermined Value
  - Intensive chemotherapy
  - Immediate postoperative or poststress period
  - Acute enteritis
  - <10% small bowel
- Not Useful or Contraindicated
  - Complete mechanical intestinal obstruction
  - Ileus
  - Severe diarrhea
  - High-output entercutaneous fistula
  - Severe acute pancreatitis
  - Shock
  - Aggressive nutrition support not desired by patient or legal guardian and such action being in accordance with hospital policy and existing law
  - Prognosis not warranting aggressive nutrition support

Adapted with permission from Guidelines for the use of enteral nutrition in the adult patient. *J Parenteral Enteral Nutr* 11:435-439, 1987.

If enteral support is unavailable or inadvisable, intravenous support may be instituted. Parenteral nutrition is generally not considered unless the anticipated duration would exceed 5 days. Increased levels of stress provide greater urgency to begin support. Further starvation may deplete the already minimal reserves, and the possibility of major organ dysfunction increases in patients with moderate to severe malnutrition. However, when gut function is difficult to assess, initiating both routes is advised to improve gut function, prevent inadequate nutrition intake, and speed the transition from parenteral. As soon as the enteral or oral route is well established, then IV support may be discontinued.

Parenteral nutrition is generally considered to be the standard of care in severe short bowel syndrome,[65] severe pancreatitis,[66] enterocutaneous fistulae,[67,68] diseases of the small intestine,[69,70] intractable vomiting, severe diarrhea,[71] and postoperative complications such as prolonged ileus (table 20-7). The identification of other patients who might benefit from intravenous nutrition support is more challenging.[57]

Table 20-7. Disease states benefiting from IV nutrition

Short bowel syndrome. If only 3-5 feet of small bowel remain, most patients cannot absorb adequate nutrients for survival immediately post-resection. With adequate support and time (6 months to 3 years), gut adaptation occurs, so many patients become independent of parenteral nutrition support. Provision of nutrients enterally is important in stimulating adaptation. If less than 3 feet remain, most patients will require life-long supplemental or total parenteral nutrition.[65]

Pancreatitis. Although nutritional support itself has little effect upon the course of the disease, it is generally able to maintain nutritional status. Total parenteral nutrition provides beneficial support during acute severe pancreatitis and optimizes the patient's condition if surgery is indicated. During mild pancreatitis or recovery from severe pancreatitis, jejunal enteral nutrition is preferable.[66]

Entercutaneous fistulae. Nutritional support and delay of surgical intervention can reduce the high morbidity and mortality of enterocutaneous fistulae. Many will close spontaneously; in others, nutritional status can be improved or maintained for subsequent surgical repair.[67,68]

Sepsis and burns. Aggressive and early nutritional support is essential to meet the accelerated metabolic rate. Some data suggest that early enteral support may reduce the hypermetabolic response. In burn patients, the use of enteral nutritional support avoids the high sepsis rate associated with central venous access.[63]

Inflammatory bowel disease. Nutritional support may be of some value in severe inflammatory bowel disease. Intractable Crohn's disease may remit when put at bowel rest with parenteral nutrition.[69] Closure of Crohn's-induced fistulae tends to occur only when the disease goes into remission. In less severe disease, reports of similar beneficial response have appeared with elemental diets.[70] Ulcerative colitis has not shown any abatement of the disease process during parenteral support, but nutritional deprivation is prevented. Variable results have been reported in radiation enteritis or the bowel effects of chemotherapy.[71]

Postoperative complications. Recovery of intestinal function after surgery may be delayed with ileus, retroperitoneal hematomas, intra-abdominal abscesses, bowel obstruction, and wound dehiscence. Profound malnutrition may result if nutrition support is not provided during this period of increased demands.

As no known medical condition improves with starvation, prevention of further decline in nutrition status should be a goal whenever possible. The ability to treat the underlying disease must also be considered during formulation of a therapeutic plan. A meta-analysis by Detsky et al.[72] has shown parenteral nutrition to be beneficial in the most severely malnourished patients in the perioperative setting, and a multicenter Veterans Administration (VA) trial on the effect of perioperative TPN on postoperative morbidity and mortality also demonstrated utility in the same population.[73] A second meta-analysis by Detsky and colleagues[74] on TPN in the cancer patient showed it to be of only limited value.

Urgent surgery should never be delayed for nutrition support (e.g., drainage of abscesses or exploration for small bowel obstruction). Nutritional support is of limited value in the immediate postoperative period; no impact on patient outcome has been observed, even though improved metabolic balance has been reported. Nutritional support is of no value when the prognosis does not warrant aggressive support or when risks of nutritional support exceed possible benefits.[57] The presence of profound shock, severe sepsis with hypotension, or multiple organ failure often makes nutrition support impossible, and attention should first be directed to correcting the underlying problem, then toward nutrition support. Provision of nutrition support to the terminally ill patient, especially in the situation where suffering will be prolonged and other therapy has been stopped, evokes very difficult ethical issues. Therefore, nutritional support should be withheld only after full discussion with the patient and appropriate family members, and in accordance with existing law.[57]

NUTRITIONAL REQUIREMENTS

Energy Requirements

Total energy expenditure is the summation of basal energy expenditure (BEE), activity energy expenditure, and stress-induced increases. As shown by Harris and Benedict,[75] the BEE can be estimated by measuring oxygen consumption (indirect calorimetry). They related this to body cell mass and produced the Harris-Benedict equations (table 20-8). There is a variability among individuals of about 5-10 percent from the mean population.[76]

Table 20-8. Harris-Benedict equation for basal energy expenditure (BEE in kcal)

Males: BEE = 66 + (13.7 x Wt) + (5 x Ht) – (6.8 x age)
Females: BEE = 665 + (9.6 x Wt) + (1.7 x Ht) – (4.7 x age)

Where: W = weight in kg
H = height in cm
A = age in years

Reprinted with permission from Long CL, Schaffel N, Greger JW, et al: Metabolic response to injury and illness: Estimation of energy and protein needs from indirect calorimetry and nitrogen balances. *J Parenter Enteral Nutr* 3:452-456, 1979.

The BEE as determined by the Harris-Benedict equation is multiplied by both an activity factor and an injury factor to give total energy expenditure. In ambulatory patients, physical activity may cause a 20-30 percent increase in energy expenditure. Patients confined to bed lack physical activity, and therefore have no appreciable rise in energy expenditure.[76] Traditionally, the injury factor, as given in figure 20-1, predicts the additional energy needs during stress. As these are predictive formulas, it is not uncommon to find energy expenditure underestimated or more commonly overestimated by as much as 30 percent.[77-80] These authors recommend conservative application of injury factors to the Harris-Benedict equation (table 20-9). The guidelines attempt to define nutritional goals based on the patient's body habitus using ideal body weight (IBW). The use of indirect calorimetry instead of predictive energy formulas to derive caloric needs is more accurate.[81]

Table 20-9. Nonprotein energy requirements of hospitalized patients*

Weight (% IBW)	Goal	Guidelines
<90-120	Maintenance	1.2-1.4 x BEE
>120	Depletion	< or = 1.0 x BEE

*If weight gain is desirable, an additional 500 kcal per day is added (3,500 kcal = 1 pound). During times of acute stress, overfeeding is not recommended.

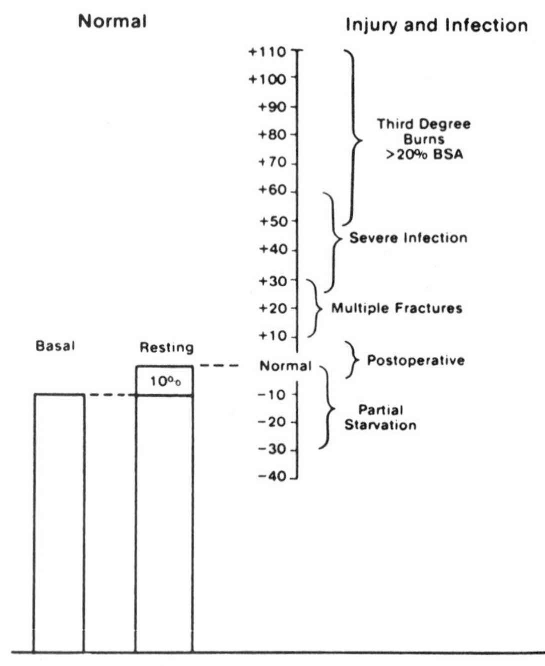

Figure 20-1. Resting energy expenditure

Reprinted with permission from Kinney JM (ed): *Assessment of Energy Metabolism in Health and Disease.* Columbus, OH, Ross Laboratories, 1980, pp 42-48.

Indirect Calorimetry

Humans are primarily aerobic organisms, and as such, oxygen consumption (VO_2) and carbon dioxide production (VCO_2) can be measured to estimate energy expenditure. This technique is termed "indirect calorimetry." Special metabolic carts for indirect calorimetry are available in the clinical setting to determine appropriate fuel requirements. Indirect calorimetry also measures the respiratory quotient (RQ), which is the ratio of carbon dioxide produced to oxygen consumed.[82] Use of each substrate produces its own RQ (table 20-10). RQ values greater than 1.0 are felt to represent net lipogenesis (production of fat).[83,84] RQ values less than 1.0 are associated with net lipolysis (fat oxidation).[84,85]

Influence of Calories and Protein on Body Composition

Lean body mass is affected by both nitrogen and energy intake. Nitrogen balance in depleted patients improves with increasing nitrogen or energy intake as long as neither is severely restricted (figures 20-2 and 20-3). On closer examination, it appears that generation of lean body mass (LBM) and/or fat can be controlled by the amount of protein and calories administered. Nitrogen balance improves as caloric intake increases. Once caloric intake exceeds 50-60 percent of energy expenditure, nitrogen accretion proceeds at a much slower rate and fat production increases. At this point, protein administration is the most important factor affecting nitrogen accretion. Since the aim is to preserve LBM, three nutritional goals can be defined depending on a patient's initial body habitus.[86] In marasmic patients (loss of fat and somatic protein), calories and protein can be provided for LBM as well as fat mass gain. If normal body weight is present but visceral protein stores depleted (i.e., kwashiorkor), the goal is LBM gain with fat mass maintenance. Finally, an obese patient may be best served by giving large doses of protein for LBM maintenance with low caloric intake for fat mass loss.[86,87] In nonstressed obese patients, this therapy is known as "protein-sparing modified fast."[88]

The relationship between calorie and protein needs can be expressed as calorie to nitrogen ratios given in table 20-11. The severity of illness and individual variation require modification of these recommendations to the individual patient (table 20-12).

Carbohydrates

Energy sources available for parenteral administration include carbohydrates and fat emulsions. Intravenous dextrose is the least expensive and most commonly used source of calories. It is available as d-glucose monohydrate, supplying 3.45 kcal/g. Concentrations of 10 percent or less are generally well tolerated by peripheral vein. Higher concentrations (up to 70 percent supplying 2.38 kcal/mL) are manufactured commercially but are hypertonic (up to 3,600 mOsm/L) and thus restricted to central venous administration. Dextrose is compatible with amino acid solutions, electrolytes, and fat emulsions within defined, stable ratios.[91]

Body carbohydrate stores are limited, with only 2,000-4,000 kcal stored as glycogen.[92] These stores are rapidly depleted during starvation or stress.[92] Glucose is produced via hepatic gluconeogenesis with a basal production rate of 2.5 mg/kg/min.[93] It is readily metabolized by all tissues in the body and is the main energy source for red cells, healing wounds, and, except in prolonged starvation, the central nervous system.[94-96] It stimulates insulin release, which in turn, promotes protein deposition in skeletal muscle.[92] It is required for lipid oxidation.[94,95] When infused with lipid, glucose is oxidized preferentially.[87,97] With infusion rates as low as 1.1 mg/kg/min, exogenous glucose depresses gluconeogenesis and prevents ketosis in nonstressed patients.[98] When it is given with amino acids at higher rates, positive nitrogen balance can be achieved.[76,94]

Table 20-10. Respiratory quotient values for metabolic fuels

Substrate	Reaction	Products	Kcal/LO_2	mL/min O_2 consumed / kcal of reactant	mL/min CO_2 produced / kcal of reactant	RQ CO_2 produced / O_2 consumed
Carbohydrate						
Glucose	Oxidation	CO_2+H_2O	5.01	200	200	1.00
Glucose	Lipogenesis	C_{54}LCT+CO_2+H_2O	18.22	4.5	61.7	13.71
Glucose	Lipogenesis	C_{55}LCT+CO_2+H_2O	13.95	7.4	63.9	8.67
Glucose	Lipogenesis	Palmitic acid +CO_2+H_2O	7.06	29.6	81.4	2.75
Fat						
C_{54}LCT	Oxidation	CO_2+H_2O	4.51	221	157	0.71
C_{55}LCT	Oxidation	CO_2+H_2O	4.48	223	157	0.705
MCT	Oxidation	CO_2+H_2O	4.705	213	154	0.725
Protein						
Amino acid	Oxidation	Urea+CO_2+H_2O	4.46	239	191	0.80
Amino acid	Lipogenesis	Tripalmitylglycerate +CO_2+H_2O	—	82.9	61.3	0.74
Other						
Glycerol	Oxidation	CO_2+H_2O	5.07	197	170	0.86

LCT=Long-chain triglycerides
MCT=Medium-chain triglycerides
Adapted with permission from Heymsfield SB, Erbland M, Caspar K, et al: Enteral nutritional support: Metabolic, cardiovascular, and pulmonary interrelations. *Clin Chest Med* 7:41-67, 1986.

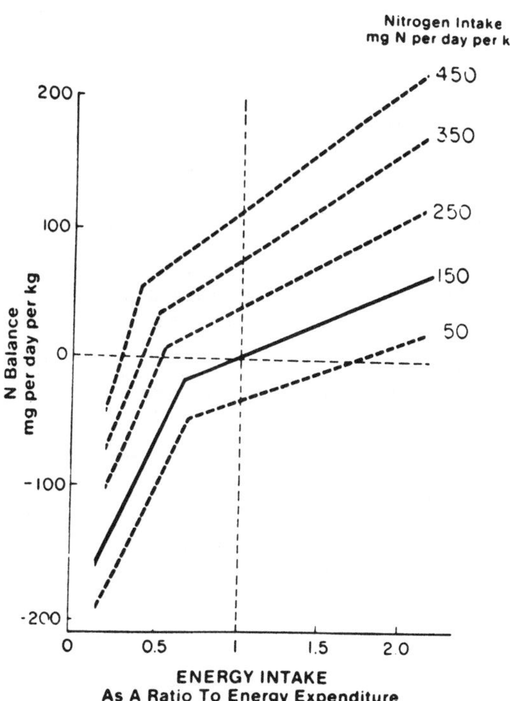

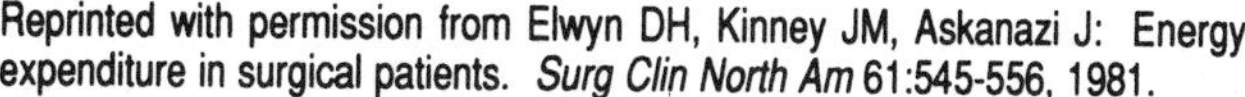

Figure 20-2. The relationship between energy and nitrogen intake and nitrogen balance in unstressed depleted patients

Reprinted with permission from Elwyn DH, Kinney JM, Askanazi J: Energy expenditure in surgical patients. *Surg Clin North Am* 61:545-556, 1981.

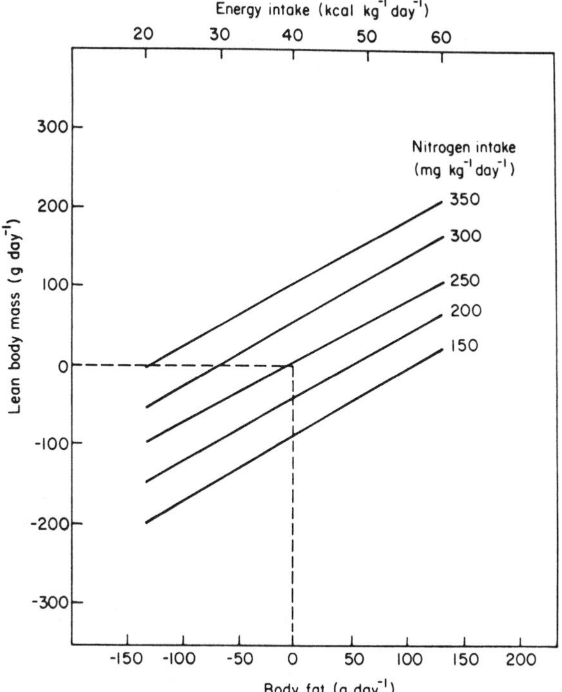

Figure 20-3. The relationship between energy and nitrogen intake and LBM and body fat production in mild to moderately stressed depleted surgery patients

Reprinted with permission from Hill GL, Church J: Energy and protein requirements of general surgical patients requiring intravenous nutrition. *Br J Surg* 71:1-9, 1984.

Table 20-11. Protein to calorie ratios

Stress level	Nonprotein calorie: Nitrogen ratio kcal:g N	Amino acids g/kg/day	Total nonprotein kcal
Nonstress starvation	150-200:1	0.8-1	25
Elective general surgery	100:1	1.5	25
Polytrauma	100:1	2	30
Sepsis/hypermetabolic state	90:1	2.5	35

Table 20-12. Examples of daily TNA/TPN formulas at full nutritional support*

Patients are 30-year-old euvolemic males with an ideal body weight of 70 kg and height of 180 cm with normal organ function in mild to moderate stress.

Solution	Weight		
	70 kg	50 kg	100 kg
Dextrose, g	500	360	315
Amino acids, g	105	100	115
Lipid, g	60	80	20
Fluid, mL	2,850	2,400	3,200
1,500 mL/m²			
Sodium, mEq	170	140	170
Potassium, mEq	100	85	85
Chloride, mEq	205	175	205
Acetate, mEq	20	20	20
Phosphorus, mmol	30	20	20
Magnesium, mEq	18	14	18
Sulfate, mEq	18	14	18
Calcium, mEq	15	12	15
Gluconate, mEq	15	12	15
Multivitamin	AMA/FDA	AMA/FDA	AMA/FDA
Vitamin K, mg	1	1	1
Zinc, mg	3	3	3
Copper, mg	1.2	1.2	1.2
Manganese, µg	300	300	300
Chromium, µg	12	12	12
Selenium, µg	40	40	40
Molybdenum, µg			
Additional vitamin C			
Additional zinc		as indicated	
Heparin			
Iron			
Regular insulin			

*TNA = total nutrient admixtures; AMA/FDA = American Medical Association and Food and Drug Administration recommended daily allowance for IV therapy.[89,90]

Optimal oxidation of glucose is achieved with infusion rates between 4 to 7 mg/kg/min, and administration above this may produce undesirable effects.[99] In the minimally to nonstressed patient, glucose administration above basal energy expenditure results in decreased lipolysis and increased lipogenesis with an RQ greater than 1.0. Energy expenditure, carbon dioxide production, and oxygen consumption are only slightly elevated.[83] With further stress, hepatic gluconeogenesis and overall glucose use increase, while optimal oxidation of exogenously administered glucose remains fixed.[92,99,100] Additional glucose infusion, especially beyond optimal oxidation rates at 4-5 mg/kg/min, causes slight suppression of lipolysis.[85,100] Net lipogenesis decreases, resulting in an RQ below 1.0.[101] Energy expenditure, carbon dioxide production, and oxygen consumption are significantly elevated.[102,103] Excess glucose has therefore been implicated in inducing respiratory failure and fatty liver without improving nutritional status.[101,103] This may be clinically significant in a few patients.

Hyperglycemia is a common occurrence when glucose is administered in injured patients. This not only predisposes patients to the risk of diabetic ketoacidosis and hyperosmolar hyperglycemic nonketotic coma but also may impair the immune response and prevent optimal glucose oxidation.[93] It is therefore necessary to administer exogenous insulin carefully to increase glucose clearance from the bloodstream and prevent hyperglycemia without inducing hypoglycemia. Judicious use of insulin has been recommended by different authors (table 20-13).[93,104] To prevent antibody formation, recombinant human insulin is used.

Table 20-13. Dosing of insulin in diabetics receiving TPN

I. Restrict initial dextrose content to 100-150 g.
II. Add about 50% of home daily insulin requirement to TPN as regular insulin
III. Take frequent measurements (at least q8h) of blood glucose and administer supplemental regular insulin as a subcutaneous dose according to the following scale:

Blood glucose (mg/dL)	IDDM† (insulin units)	NIDDM† (insulin units)	Stress diabetics (insulin units)
200-250	3	5	5
251-300	6	10	10
301-350	9	15	15
351-400	12	20	20

IV. Total the subcutaneously administered insulin given over a 24-hour period.
   A. If blood glucose levels have been <200 mg/dL with SQ administration, add two-thirds of the amount of subcutaneous insulin required to amount of insulin already in TPN.
   B. If blood glucose levels have been >200 mg/dL, add the total amount of subcutaneous insulin required.
V. The dextrose content may be slowly increased (100-150 g/day) to required needs by adjusting the TPN insulin to maintain the prior insulin-to-dextrose ratio, provided that at least 2 of the 3 blood glucose levels on the previous day have been <200 mg/dL.
VI. If the patient becomes hypoglycemic, treat appropriately (i.e., dextrose, d/c SQ insulin, change to TPN with less insulin and/or more dextrose). Many times reducing insulin by 30%-50% in next TPN bag is sufficient.

Adapted with permission from McMahon M, Manji N, Driscoll DF, et al: Parenteral nutrition in patients with diabetes mellitus: Theoretical and practical considerations. *J Parenter Enteral Nutr* 5:545-553, 1989.
†IDDM = insulin-dependent diabetes mellitus; NIDDM = non-insulin-dependent diabetes mellitus.

Alternative carbohydrate sources have been used to bypass the glucose intolerance of stress, reduce hyperosmolarity, prevent fluid and electrolyte abnormalities, or decrease the need for insulin; other sources include fructose, maltose, xylitol, and the polyols—sorbitol and glycerol.[94] Because of adverse effects, only glycerol is currently available.[105] It is marketed as ProcalAmine (Kendall McGaw, Irvine, CA) as a 3-percent glycerol and 3-percent amino acid solution for peripheral administration. Large fluid intakes are required with this product to meet total nutritional needs. In addition, glycerol administration does not stimulate insulin production, which is important in decreasing protein catabolism.[92]

Fat

Carbohydrate based TPN in the nonstressed patient causes decreased lypolysis and net lipogenesis.[97] Therefore, it is not surprising that numerous cases of essential fatty acid (EFA) deficiency have been reported when this single caloric source is used.[106,107] EFA (linoleic, arachidonic, and possibly linolenic) are needed for cellular integrity, pulmonary surfactant, immune competence, prostaglandin synthesis, normal platelet function, and central nervous system development. In order to prevent essential fatty acid deficiency (EFAD), 4 percent of total calories (100 g of intravenous fat per week) must be provided. To correct a known deficiency, 8-10 percent of total calories should be provided. Oral doses of safflower oil as low as 20 mL/day are reported to correct EFAD.[106]

Fat has become the second most commonly used fuel source. Current commercially available lipid emulsions (table 20-14) have proved beneficial in providing essential fatty acid and energy.[106] It is available as a 10-percent or 20-percent lipid emulsion providing 1.1 or 2 kcal/mL, respectively. Advantages over carbohydrate include low osmolarity (approximately 330 mOsm/L), making it more suitable for peripheral administration;[108] no effect on insulin needs or glucose management; decreased carbon dioxide production during oxidation; and another source of energy when carbohydrate infusion alone cannot meet requirements or is detrimental.[91] Fat does not decrease gluconeogenesis, but it does improve protein synthesis and appears to be as nitrogen-sparing as glucose.[109,110] The amount of fat that can be used safely and effectively is disputed.

Table 20-14. Commercial fat emulsion products[106]*

100% Soybean	*Manufacturer*	*50% Safflower 50% Soybean*
Liposyn III	Abbott	Liposyn II
Intralipid	Kabivitrum	
Nutrilipid	Kendall McGaw	
Soyacal	Alpha Therapeutic	
Travamulsion	Travenol	

*Products available in 10 and 20 percent concentrations. Products contain 1.2-percent egg phosphatides as emulsifying agents. Egg phosphatides vary in composition, perhaps making TNA compatibility different.[91]

Many adverse effects have been reported with lipid infusions (table 20-15). Before large doses of fat are advocated, the type, amount, rate of administration, and clinical setting must be considered.[91] All parenteral and most enteral products contain fat as long-chain fatty acids (LCFA). LCFA may be taken up by the reticuloendothelial system and inhibit clearance of bacteria from the bloodstream.[111,112] Currently available lipids probably should be limited to 30 percent of nonprotein calories, as this usually provides total caloric needs after optimal glucose administration and increased dosages may cause inhibition of the immune response.[113] Infusing lipids (see table 20-16) over 24 hours may improve oxidation and preserve immune function.[113] Increasing lipid administration to more than 30 percent of total calories in nonstressed individuals is usually well tolerated and may be beneficial in specific disease states such as cystic fibrosis or other severe pulmonary diseases.[101,103,114]

Table 20-15. Potential adverse reactions to IV fat emulsions[106]

Acute reactions	*Rapid infusion*	*Long-term effects*
Chest or back pain	Cyanosis	Eosinophilia
Chills	Headache	Fat overload syndrome
Febrile response	Nausea	Hepatomegaly
Pruritic urticaria	Oily taste in mouth	Jaundice due to cholestasis
Vomiting	Pain at injection site	Leukopenia
	Palpitations	Splenomegaly
	Tachypnea	Thrombocytopenia
	Wheezing	Transient liver function test elevations

Much exciting basic science and clinical research using alternative fat sources (e.g., medium-chain triglycerides, omega-3 fatty acids, short-chain fatty acids) is underway to overcome LCFA shortcomings and improve nutritional response.[62,115-117]

Table 20-16. Dosage of intravenous lipids[106]

SHOULD BE GIVEN OVER 4-24 hours*

	Adult	*Pediatric*
Test dose† for egg allergy (10% lipid)	1 mL/min over 15-30 min	0.1 mL/min over 15-30 min
Daily dose	0.5 g/kg/day increase 0.5 g/kg/day to max 2.5 g/kg/day	0.5 g/kg/day increase 0.5 g/kg/day to max 3-4 g/kg/day

*Because of bacterial growth potential, the Centers for Disease Control recommend maximum infusion times of 12 hours for lipid emulsions. When placed in TNA, increase hang times to 24 hours.[91]
†Patients who are allergic to eggs should not be exposed to the intravenous (IV) fat products, since egg phosphatides are used as the emulsifier. Test doses are usually not used with TNA administration.

Oxidation of lipid infusion is not measured in the clinical setting; however, monitoring serum triglyceride has been used to determine tolerance. Free fatty acid (FFA) measurements may be used as well but are not commonly available.[118] Serum triglyceride levels greater than 400 mg percent in the adult and greater than 250 mg percent in the pediatric patient may predispose patients to adverse effects (e.g., pancreatitis, kernicterus) and may indicate decreased oxidation.[106,119,120] (Institution values may vary.) If triglyceride levels are excessive and drawn appropriately, e.g., 6 hours after bolus infusion, the dose should be decreased and another level measured. Clearance of lipid may improve with continuous infusion;[113] however, continued poor clearance may require discontinuation of the lipid infusion. Lipid infusion can be resumed when clearance improves.

Serum lipemia does not correlate with FFA or triglyceride levels.[121] Although some advocate ignoring lipemic serum with normal triglycerides, a consistently lipemic serum is abnormal and may indicate accumulation of other metabolites.[122,123] For intravenous dosage recommendation, see table 20-16.

Protein

Protein administration is a very important factor determining preservation and production of lean body mass. Current commercial products (parenteral and enteral) provide protein of high biological value (high in essential amino acids).[124] Adaptation to low intakes of protein has been reported with minimum daily intakes of 0.3-0.4 g/kg/day.[94,125] Normal adults can maintain nitrogen equilibrium with the recommended daily allowance (RDA) of 0.8 g/kg/day. Hospitalized adult patients routinely require 1.0-1.5 g/kg/day, increasing to 2.0-2.5 g/kg/day with stress.[76,94] In assessing protein requirements, it is again important to determine nutritional goals based on a patient's nutritional and catabolic state (table 20-17).

Table 20-17. Protein requirements of hospitalized patients requiring TPN

Clinical state	Goal	Protein (g/kg/day)
Well nourished	Maintenance	0.8-1.5
Depleted	Repletion	1.5-2
Stressed	Support	2-2.5

Reprinted with permission from Dickerson RN: Energy and protein requirements of hospitalized patients receiving parenteral nutrition. *Hosp Pharm* 22:70-79, 1987.

The commercial protein source in parenteral nutrition is crystalline amino acids. Various formulas have been developed for use in peripheral, neonatal, renal, hepatic, stress, and volume-restricted patients. Standard formulas are comparable in amino acid profile and range in concentration from 3.5 percent to 15 percent, providing flexibility in nitrogen administration (table 20-18). Solutions are available with and without added electrolytes. On average, each gram of nitrogen is equivalent to 6.25 g amino acids; however, the products vary depending on the type of amino acids used.[124]

Table 20-18. Currently available standard amino acid products

Solution	Manufacturer
Aminosyn	Abbott
Travasol	Clintec Nutrition
Novamine	Clintec Nutrition
FreAmine III	Kendall McGaw

Reprinted with permission from Kastrup EK, Olin BR (eds): *Facts and Comparisons.* Philadelphia, J.B. Lippincott, 1990, pp 36b-37.

Patients in the acute-care setting are under great stress with accelerated gluconeogenesis. Prior recommendations for energy and protein may be inadequate to prevent net protein catabolism. Branched-chain amino acids (leuceine, isoleuceine, and valine) may serve as sources for gluconeogenesis and improve nitrogen balance in this population.[126] The effectiveness of this type of product (table 20-19) when administered for long periods of time has not been demonstrated and therefore is advocated only for brief periods early in the course of illness. Present clinical trials are inadequate to determine effect on morbidity and mortality.[127,128]

Table 20-19. Currently available parenteral nutrition products enriched for branched-chain amino acids (BCAA)

Amino acid product and concentration	Manufacturer	%BCAA
Branchamine 4% †	Clintec	100
Freamine 6.9% HBC	Kendall McGaw	45
Aminosyn-HBC 7%	Abbott	50

Reprinted with permission from Kastrup EK, Olin BR (eds): *Facts and Comparisons.* Philadelphia, J.B. Lippincott, 1990, p 37d.
†BCAA supplement. Must be added to standard product.

Micronutrients

The usual daily requirements for electrolytes, vitamins, and trace elements during parenteral and enteral nutritional support are listed in table 20-20. Rudman et al.[129] demonstrated in 1975 that anabolism could not occur without proper micro- and macronutrient administration. In addition, deficiencies and excesses of these nutrients may impair body homeostasis and lead to detrimental consequences. In considering micronutrient needs, careful thought must be given to disease state, organ function, loss of body fluids, present micronutrient level, nutritional status, macronutrient administration, route of administration, and drug and fluid administration. The management of fluid and electrolytes is beyond the scope of this chapter but can be explored elsewhere.[130-141]

Renal Disease

In hospitalized patients, renal insufficiency and renal failure are common occurrences. Whereas patients with acute renal failure have a high mortality rate, patients with chronic renal failure can survive for long periods of time. Renal failure is associated with decreased clearance of waste products, water, and electrolytes. To prevent toxicity, either intake must be modified or waste must be removed with dialysis.[142,143]

Minimum protein requirements of 0.3-0.4 g/kg/day must be given to maintain lean body mass in nonstressed patients, with stressed individuals requiring more.[94] Unfortunately, in renal failure, administration of large doses of protein causes the accumulation of urea and other waste products, which is associated with decreased platelet aggregation and mental status changes when blood urea nitrogen (BUN) levels are above 100 mg/dL.[143] In addition, high doses of protein may be associated with worsening renal failure.[144] Efforts to improve protein use and decrease urea production have used essential amino acids only or products high in branched-chain amino acids. Improved efficacy of these products has not been shown.[142]

Table 20-20. Daily adult electrolyte, trace element, and mineral and vitamin requirements

Nutrient	Parenteral	Enteral
Micronutrients		
Sodium	40-250 mEq	40-250 mEq
Potassium	30-200 mEq	30-200 mEq
Chloride	40-250 mEq	40-250 mEq
Acetate	10-80 mEq	10-80 mEq
Phosphorus	10-40 mmol	20-60 mmol
Calcium	4.5-20 mEq	400-1000 mg
Magnesium	2-45 mEq	4-27 mEq
Zinc	3-6 mg†	12-15 mg
Copper	1-1.5 mg	1.5-2 mg
Chromium	10-20 mcg‡	30-200 mcg
Manganese	150-800 mcg	2.2-2.5 mg
Molybdenum	100-150 mcg	150-500 mcg
Selenium	40-120 mcg	50-200 mcg
Iron	1-2 mg§	18-30 mg
Vitamins		
Multivitamin for IV¶	AMA/FDA	
enteral‖		RDA
Phytonadione (vit K)	1 mg	

Dosage needs to be adjusted to the individual, because the patient's clinical and nutritional status will affect dosage needs.
†Give additional zinc with GI losses. Add 4 mg/L for small bowel fluid lost; 6 mg/L of stool or ileostomy output.
‡Give 100-150 mcg chromium per day for 7-10 days for suspected cause of glucose intolerance unresponsive to insulin.
§Do not supplement unless documented iron deficiency.
¶The recommended daily allowance (RDA) for vitamins with the exception of vit K is provided in current intravenous preparations.
‖The amount of tube feeding required to provide the RDA varies with each product.

Prior to the initiation of dialysis, protein intake should be limited to prevent waste accumulation and further deterioration of renal function (0.6 g/kg/day).[144] In stressed individuals, this will be insufficient to prevent loss of lean body mass. The presence of dialysis and its route, frequency, and effectiveness may permit liberalization of protein intake as well as produce increased nitrogen losses. Amino acids are lost during dialysis in these ranges: hemodialysis, 2-9 g/day; peritoneal dialysis, 0.3-0.5 g/exchange; continuous arteriovenous hemofiltration, unknown but thought to be small.[143,144] Protein losses also occur during peritoneal dialysis in the range of 0.6 ± 0.5 g/hour of treatment, with increasing losses during episodes of peritonitis.[143] Recommendations for protein administration in patients on hemodialysis are 0.8-1.2 g/kg/day and for peritoneal dialysis, 1-1.5 g/kg/day, using standard amino acid products.[142] Nitrogen balance can be used to estimate needs, but losses from dialysis (i.e., urea, protein, amino acids) are not usually measured.[144] Severely restricting protein administration below recommendations may predispose patients to excessive waste of nitrogen and development of kwashiorkor.[143]

Estimated energy needs for patients with renal failure are similar to those for patients with normal renal function. As previously discussed, caloric intake above estimated needs may improve nitrogen balance but may also increase fat accumulation and carbon dioxide production. Without protein administration, provision of calories in excess of 300 kcal/day does not improve nitrogen balance.[76,125] In the delivery of nutritional support, the impact of dialysis on caloric intake must be considered, as peritoneal dialysis may deliver substantial carbohydrate calories. Insulin may be needed with the increased carbohydrate loading. Hemodialysis will remove glucose when a glucose-free bath is used. Hemofiltration may cause dehydration, requiring fluid replacement to maintain blood pressure. If dextrose solutions are used, caloric intake may be substantial (150 kcal/L of 5 percent dextrose).[143]

Type IV hypertriglyceridemia is common in renal failure. When lipids are administered, weekly monitoring of serum triglyceride level may prevent hyperlipidemia.[144]

Water and electrolyte excretion are usually impaired in renal failure; therefore, concentrated nutrient solutions and judicious use of electrolytes are important.[145,146] Vitamins and trace elements should be administered in doses consistent with the RDA and AMA recommendations. In patients with chronic renal failure, both deficiencies of and accumulation of micronutrients are reported.[144]

Hepatic Disease

The liver plays an integral role in production, elimination, and orchestration of body metabolism. In the failing liver, delivery of protein, energy, fluid, and micronutrients is very challenging and requires an individualized approach to medical and nutritional therapy.[144,147]

Provision of adequate protein in the presence of liver failure may cause elevated levels of ammonia, abnormal amino acid profile (decreased branched-chain amino acids and elevated aromatic amino acids), and hepatic encephalopathy. Protein administration should start at 0.5-0.75 g/kg/day and advance by 0.25 g/kg/day until requirements are met or intolerance occurs. Hepatamine (Kendall McGaw, Irvine, CA) and specialized enteral products with increased BCAA and decreased aromatic amino acids (AAA) are used when conventional amino acid products are not tolerated and serum amino acid profiles are abnormal. Limited clinical trials have demonstrated some improvement in encephalopathy as well as mortality, while others have not. Because of the additional cost, careful patient selection should be employed in using these products.[144,147]

Energy requirements are as discussed previously. Modification of glucose, insulin, and lipid dosing to prevent intolerance is usually necessary. Fluid and electrolyte administration is usually characterized as concentrated solutions with sodium restriction, and supernormal doses of potassium, phosphorus, magnesium, and chloride. Concurrent drug administration (i.e., antacids, furosemide, spironolactone, lactulose, etc.) may alter electrolyte requirements. Trace elements and vitamins are given to meet the RDA and AMA recommendations. Therapeutic supplements of zinc, folic acid, thiamine, pyridoxine, riboflavin, pantothenic acid, vitamin B12, and fat-soluble vitamins may be needed. Restriction of copper in patients with biliary obstruction should be considered.[144,147]

INTRAVENOUS ACCESS

Peripheral Nutrition

Parenteral nutrition may be administered via the peripheral or the central route. Peripheral nutrition has generally been reserved for individuals with good venous access who are expected to require intravenous support for only a limited amount of time, generally less than 2 weeks, and who are not malnourished or stressed.[148] Care must be taken to avoid hypertonic fluids, and osmolarity should not exceed 600-900 mOsm.[149,150] The approximate osmolarity of peripheral nutrition solutions can be computed by using the alligation medial method described in *Remington's Pharmaceutical Sciences*.[151] Lipid emulsions prove to be a beneficial source of nonprotein calories because they are isotonic. Amino acid concentrations are usually restricted to not more than 5 percent with dextrose at 12 percent. Volumes of infusion range from 2 to 4 L daily for full support. The addition of 1,000 U of heparin and 5 mg of hydrocortisone per liter may decrease the risk of phlebitis.[150]

Central Nutrition

Central venous access is the preferred route for total parenteral nutrition. Provision of nutrition support for extended periods of time requires administration into large veins with high blood flow, such as the superior vena cava, inferior vena cava, right atrium, or arteriovenous fistulae, because of the hyperosmolar nature of the fluid. The most commonly used cannulation site is the superior vena cava, using the infraclavicular approach to the subclavian vein. The catheter may be inserted percutaneously in the hospital room or may be a permanently implanted right atrial catheter placed in the operating room. Advantages of central access include patient comfort, as sites do not interfere with clothing; avoidance of phlebitis; and ability to establish long-term access. Greater flexibility of solution formulation is also possible, as osmolarity is not restricted.[152]

The demand for intravenous access has prompted development of several different types of central catheters. Percutaneous central lines are generally considered to be temporary. Right atrial catheters, however, are considered permanent lines and are tunneled to minimize bacterial tracking from the skin into the vein and to stabilize the line. They may even be placed subcutaneously as an implantable port. All central lines are now available as single as well as multiple lumen to facilitate simultaneous delivery of nutrition support, blood products, and drugs as well as blood sampling.[152]

Complications

Insertion complications are rare if catheters are placed by experienced physicians and a strict protocol for aseptic line care is consistently followed. Reported catheter complications include pneumo-, hemo-, and hydrothorax, subclavian artery puncture, uncontrolled bleeding at the puncture site, malposition of the catheter tip, local hematoma, brachial plexus and thoracic duct injury, air embolism, hemo- and hydromediastinum, subclavian vein thrombosis, embolism of catheter tip, infection, and catheter occlusion secondary to kinking. Confirmation of proper catheter placement by chest x ray is mandatory prior to initiation of parenteral nutrition.[152]

Although malposition is the most common complication of subclavian venous access, pneumothorax is the most common major one. The patient at greatest risk is thin, because the vein is close to the cupula of the lung with little intervening fat. Pneumothorax may be recognized by aspiration of air rather than blood via the catheter and complaint of sharp chest pain. If the patient is asymptomatic, withdraw and recannulate; if symptomatic, a chest x ray must be obtained immediately.

Central venous catheter-induced thrombosis has been reported to occur in 5-20 percent of patients, but may be higher, since it is often asymptomatic. Signs include swelling of involved arm, neck, and face or embolic showers. Upper extremity venography may be used for confirmation of thrombosis. The preferred form of therapy is prompt removal of the catheter and anticoagulation with heparin followed by warfarin therapy.[153] In highly selected cases, thrombolytic therapy has been employed.[154-157] Preventive measures include avoiding dehydration to improve venous return and cardiac output, use of small amounts of heparin in the parenteral fluid, and use of newer catheters made of less thrombogenic materials.[153,156,157]

Bacterial contamination of the catheter is a serious complication. Subclavian venous catheter sepsis rates for single-lumen catheters are generally 2-3 percent, with triple-lumen catheters higher at 6-7 percent.[158] *Staphylococcus aureus*, staph epidermis, entercocci, and fungus (especially *Candida*) have been particularly associated with catheter-related sepsis. Catheter sepsis may develop by many pathways, including introduction of microbes along the subcutaneous tract from the puncture site (the most common route), within the catheter itself, or hematogenous "seeding" from a remote site (urinary tract, lungs, wounds).[104,159,160] Rarely, the parenteral solution itself may be the source of infection, since microbial growth can occur in all types of intravenous nutrition products. The catheter should be removed if it is identified as the source of sepsis. Using appropriate techniques for catheter insertion and care, avoiding catheter violation, following strict aseptic technique during manufacture and compounding, and maintaining dedicated access for nutrition fluids alone may greatly reduce septic complications.[161]

IMPLEMENTING NUTRITIONAL SUPPORT

Metabolic and Electrolyte Complications

Abnormalities in serum electrolytes and metabolism are found frequently in patients receiving nutritional support.[135,140-141,162-164] Although all are certainly not attributable to the nutritional support, careful adjustment in the formula may ameliorate or even correct the problem. A list of the more common clinical findings is found in table 20-21, along with therapeutic recommendations.

Monitoring

A thorough assessment of fluid and electrolyte status, organ function, nutrition needs, and treatment goals must be made prior to the initiation of nutrition support. Routine monitoring must evaluate complications of therapy, changes in patient condition, and achievement of therapeutic endpoints. A suggested protocol is found in table 20-22. Blood and urine glucose must be measured regularly to avoid an osmotic diuresis and the potential for nonketotic hyperglycemic coma.

Nitrogen Balance

Nitrogen balance is the "gold standard" for assessing adequacy of nutrition support. For each gram of nitrogen lost or gained, 30 grams of lean body mass is lost or gained.[165] As protein is synthesized and catabolized, the net change can be determined by measuring nitrogen input and output (figure 20-4). In a healthy adult, nitrogen balance fluctuates, but net balance is zero. Malnourished people under nonstressful conditions, childhood growth, and pregnancy are situations in which a positive nitrogen balance of 4-6 g/day is attainable with provision of proper substrates.[76] The level of nitrogen loss may categorize degree of stress, as shown in figure 20-5. Provision of calories and/or protein will blunt catabolism, augment synthesis, and therefore decrease net nitrogen loss. In mild to moderate stress, zero or positive nitrogen balance may be attained with appropriate nutritional support depending on the current nutritional status.[76] In severe stress (where nitrogen balance is negative 15 g or more), it is unusual to attain even zero nitrogen balance, but nutritional support can significantly diminish net loss.[166]

Nitrogen loss is usually underestimated as a result of inadequate collection from all sites of loss. Most clinicians use urine urea nitrogen (UUN) and add a small correction factor for other nitrogen losses in the urine, skin, hair, and stool (figure 20-4).[167] This practice may not always be accurate, as stool, skin, and nonurea urine losses (e.g., ammonia, uric acid, and creatine) are quite variable. Often it is unknown if severely depleted patients are capable of generating positive nitrogen balance. Administration of excess nitrogen, except in certain disease states, is not harmful when monitored carefully. The aim is to make nitrogen balance positive 4-6 g/day in mildly to moderately stressed patients. This is intended to equate into 120-180 g lean body mass per day (1-2 lb per week). In severely stressed individuals (figure 20-5) receiving high protein intakes (2-2.5 g protein/kg), a nitrogen balance of 0-2 g/day is more realistic. In depleted nonstressed patients, if nitrogen balance is positive by a large amount (i.e., greater than 8 g) and protein and calorie administration is reasonable, it is unnecessary to adjust the regimen.

Nitrogen balance is not used routinely because collection is difficult. If a patient's response to nutritional therapy is not easy to evaluate (e.g., visceral proteins decline or do not improve, wounds do not heal, or anthropometric measurements decrease), a nitrogen balance study should be done. If the patient's response is negative, protein and/or calories may need to be increased. After a nutritional regimen change, 2 days should be allowed to attain new steady-state.[109,165] A 24-hour or more period of collection is usually more accurate.

Nutritional support is limited in its ability to improve nitrogen balance, especially in the severely stressed patient. Physical exercise has long been known to increase net protein synthesis and improve muscle function.[168-171] Unfortunately, in the critically ill, physical exercise is limited. Although it is very expensive, growth hormone

Table 20-21. Electrolyte and metabolic abnormalites during nutritonal support

Electrolyte	*Metabolic abnormality*	*Etiologies*	*Therapy*
Sodium	Hyponatremia	Fluid excess Na depletion	Fluid restriction Na replacement
	Hypernatremia	Osmotic diuresis Volume depletion Na excess	Free water administration No restriction
Potassium	Hypokalemia	K depletion Alkalosis Excess losses Drug therapy Refeeding	K replacement Mg replacement Replace losses Correct alkalosis
	Hyperkalemia	K excess Acidosis Renal failure	K restriction Correct acidosis
Calcium	Hypocalcemia	Blood transfusion Hyperphosphatemia Various diseases Hypoalbuminemia	Ca replacement Adjust value for low albumin
	Hypercalcemia	Various diseases Vitamin D excess Immobility	Restrict vitamin D Saline IV plus diuretics Drug therapy Ambulation
Magnesium	Hypomagnesemia	GI losses Drug therapy Refeeding	Mg replacement
	Hypermagnesemia	Renal failure Antacids	Mg restriction Switch antacid to nonmagnesium
Phosphate	Hypophosphatemia	Inadequate intake Antacids Alkalosis Alcohol ingestion Diabetic ketoacidosis Refeeding	Phosphate replacement Switch antacid to nonphosphate-binding
	Hyperphosphatemia	Renal failure Excess intake	Phosphate restriction
Disorder			
Metabolic acidosis	Hyperchloremia	Excess Cl Diarrhea Dehydration Renal insuffiency Hyperventilation	Bicarbonate or acetate replacement Decrease chloride load in TPN Volume replete
	Decreased bicarbonate	Diarrhea Renal insufficency Excess acid Hyperventilation	Bicarbonate or acetate replacement Decrease chloride load in TPN
Metabolic alkalosis	Hypochloremia	Vomiting NG suction Hypoventilation Excess acetate Loop diuretics	Give KCl of HCl Reduce TPN acetate H_2 blockers Acetazolamide
	Increased bicarbonate	Excess acetate Hypoventilation Vomiting NG suction	Give KCl or HCl Reduce TPN acetate H_2 blockers Acetazolamide
Glucose			
	Hyperglycemia	Stress Excess gluose Diabetes Infection Steroids Drugs	Control underlying disease Increase insulin Decrease glucose Use infusion pump
	Hypoglycemia	Excess insulin Too rapid TPN taper	Limit exogenous insulin Slower TPN taper Push D50W
Hepatic enzyme elevation		Excess caloric administration	Reduce calories Replace some glucose with fat Cycle feedings

Table 20-22. Protocol for patient monitoring

Daily	2-3 times/week	Weekly
Vital signs (temperature, pulse respirations, blood pressure)	Serum	Liver function tests
Continuous input and output	Hemoglobin	Albumin
Weight	Hematocrit	Total protein
Serum electrolytes	WBC	Transferrin
Sodium	Calcium	Prealbumin
Potassium	Phosphorus	Triglyceride
Chloride	Magnesium	Clotting studies
Bicarbonate		Zinc
BUN	Change when stabilized	Nitrogen balance
Glucose		
Urine (q6h)	Change to q12h when stabilized	
Glucose		
Acetone		
Specific gravity		
Electrolytes	As needed	
Arterial		
Blood gas	As needed	
Ammonia		

Nitrogen balance(NB) = Nitrogen intake(NI) – Nitrogen output(NO)

NI = Protein intake (g) / 6.25
(most commercial protein provides 1 g nitrogen per 6.25 g protein)*

NO = 24-hr UUN (g) + 2 g (nonurea urine losses)†
+ 2 g (insensible loss in skin, hair, stool)
+ body urea‡ + N dialysate

*Commercial proteins may have different nitrogen contents.[124]
†Total urinary nitrogen losses may be determined using Kjeldahl technique or new automated chemiluminescence system (Antek Instruments, Inc., Houston, TX).
‡Necessary if a significant change in BUN (i.e., ≥5 mg/dL).

Adapted with permission from Blumendrantz MJ, Kopple JD, Gutman RA, et al: Methods for assessing nutritional status of patients with renal failure. *Am J Clin Nutr* 33:1567-1585, 1980.

Figure 20-4. Formula for nitrogen balance

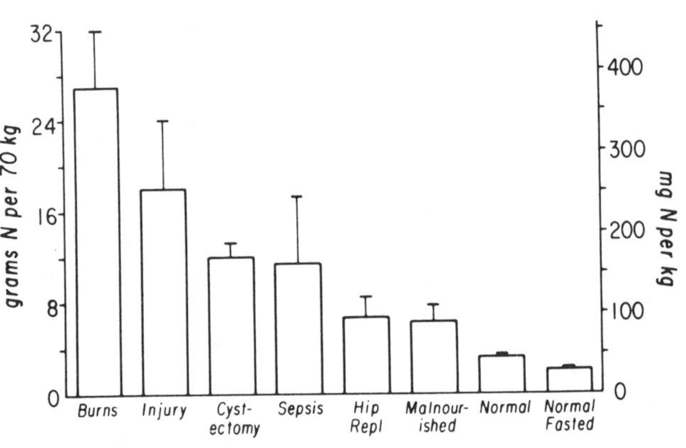

Figure 20-5. Nitrogen loss stratified by metabolic stress

Reprinted with permission from Elwyn DH: Protein metabolism and requirements in the critically ill patient. *Crit Care Clin* 3:57-69, 1987.

promotes anabolism and improves nitrogen balance when given in conjunction with nutritional support.[172,173] Further investigation is needed before therapeutic use is advocated.

DELIVERY OF PARENTERAL NUTRITION

Solution Preparation

Two types of parenteral nutrition solutions are commonly employed in the hospital setting. Total parenteral nutrition, or TPN, refers to hypertonic dextrose and amino acid mixtures with intravenous fat emulsion provided piggyback via the TPN line or through a peripheral vein. Total nutrient admixtures, or TNA (also "3-in-1"), have gained popularity over recent years and provide dextrose, amino acids, and fat in a single large-volume container. Depending upon the osmolarity of the final product, each may be administered via a central or peripheral line.

All types of solutions used in providing parenteral nutrition must be prepared in a laminar flow hood using strict aseptic technique.[174,175] Quality assurance procedures are needed to ensure a sterile final product. The hospital pharmacist involved in the IV compounding area should be knowledgeable in solution formulations as well as compatibility, sterility, and stability.[176,177] Automatic compounders using stock solutions offer much flexibility in preparing individual patient formulas. The final solution is measured by weight, with a tare balance, as amounts of the various components are calculated using their specific gravity. The use of the automatic compounder has enhanced the ability to provide patient-specific volumes as well as nutritional components that may be very beneficial to many different populations (e.g., renal failure may need concentrated; fistula patients may need diluted).

TPN solutions (dextrose-amino acid mixtures) with electrolytes are stable for 30 days, but may be at greater risk for microbial growth.[178,179] They may be prepared in bulk, by using commercial kits, or from products with standard electrolyte profiles. Industry has put considerable effort into providing adaptable products. Some institutions prefer individually formulated products. Volumes range from 750 mL to 4 L daily, depending upon the fluid tolerance and requirement of the patient.

Total nutrient admixtures require that the amino acid product be mixed with the lipid emulsion prior to the addition of dextrose, because the protein serves as a buffer between the alkaline IV fat and the acidic IV dextrose. A new automatic compounder, however, has been marketed that provides simultaneous delivery of amino acids, dextrose, and lipids. Stability was similar to the sequentially compounded formula after a 3-day storage period.[180]

Advantages of 3-in-1 admixtures are better tolerance of fat, no second infusion pump or piggybacking via the central or a peripheral line, and less nursing time. The Centers for Disease Control recommends lipid hang times of 12 hours when piggybacking lipids because of potential bacterial growth, but increases hang times to 24 hours when total nutrient admixtures are used because of decreased rate of bacterial growth.[181,182] Disadvantages include less stability, opacity with difficulty in making visual inspection, less electrolyte compatibility as a result of higher pH, inability to use a 0.22-μ filter, and potential catheter clogging. Since these 3-in-1 solutions are inherently unstable, they should not be stored for longer than 8 days. Ideally, these products should be used shortly after preparation, because the risk of aggregation of lipid particles increases with length of exposure. Total nutrient admixtures require the use of nonphthalate infusion bags and sets, as IV fat emulsion has the propensity to leach phthalates from phthalate-plasticized polyvinyl chloride (PVC).[91,183,184]

Inorganic phosphorus and calcium are incompatible in solution, forming insoluble CaPO4 precipitates. The presence of amino acids in the formula serves as a buffer and allows addition of both compounds to the solution in limited amounts, depending upon the type and amount of amino acid present, temperature, pH, and order of mixing.[91,184-186] Vitamins degrade significantly over 24-48 hours, so it is preferable to add these just prior to administration.[187]

Although the high osmolarity and low pH of TPN and TNA solutions provide a hostile environment for microbes, parenteral nutrition solutions support both bacterial and fungal growth. The most commonly isolated species include *Staphylococcus*, *Streptococcus*, and *Candida*.[161,188-190] Products may become contaminated during commercial manufacture, hospital compounding, or delivery. Methods of prevention of infusate-related contamination include adequate manufacturer quality assurance procedures, refrigeration, aseptic compounding, prompt use of fluids, and procedures to eliminate product-in-use violations.[161] Most hospitals have established 24-hour expiration times for these fluids to miminize infusate-related sepsis.[175]

Parenteral nutrition fluids may also be used as vehicles for drug delivery.[191] Advantages include diminished fluid loads, pump delivery for continuous infusion, decreased need for additional IV access, and less nursing time. Drugs that are commonly added to the nutrition solution include albumin,[192] heparin,[157] H_2 receptor antagonists,[193-195] and insulin.[196,197] Albumin can be added in any amount in nutrition solutions without lipid. If lipid is added, the albumin dose should be limited to 25 g/day to prevent emulsion instability. In addition, inline filters less than 1.2 μ will not allow albumin to flow through. Heparin is commonly added in low doses (1-3 μ/mL) to decrease the risk of fibrin sheath formation and subclavian vein thrombosis.[157] Recent evidence showing risk for heparin-induced thrombocytopenia has decreased this practice.[198] Higher doses of heparin for anticoagulation may be added to the formula but should be reserved for patients on stabilized regimens. Presently available H_2 receptor antagonists have been shown to be compatible for at least 24 hours. They are especially useful in this population to prevent metabolic alkalosis and stress ulceration and decrease fluid losses. Insulin is generally added to the nutrition solution as required for control of elevated blood sugars, as discussed earlier. Insulin has been shown to bind to the IV bag and tubing, depending on the type of solution, tubing, bag, and dose of insulin. Generally, this binding does not affect a patient's glucose control, because the insulin dose is titrated to the amount of glucose administered.[196,197] Insulin is also subject to removal by small micron filters.

Other drugs, such as hydrochloric acid,[91,199] aminophylline,[191] dopamine,[200] 5-fluorouracil,[200] some antibiotics,[200] morphine,[200] and steroids,[200] may be added to nutrition solutions under special circumstances. Restrictions on their use include incompatibility with certain components of the nutrition solutions and inability to adjust drug infusion rates.

Piggybacking medications via the TPN line should be avoided except when other access is unavailable, and then only when compatibility of the solutions is known. Possible alternatives to piggybacking medications with the TPN are using cyclic TPN to allow infusion of the medication while the TPN is off (i.e., amphotericin)[201] or connecting a compatible solution via Y-connector at the catheter hub under sterile conditions to use the same IV access without compromising sterility or infusion rate flexibility.

Administration

Intravenous pumps are used for delivery of parenteral nutrition to guarantee uniform rates of flow. Most patients receive a single 24-hour supply in a container ranging from 1 to 4 L, often with pump-specific tubing attached. An inline 0.22-μ filter may be used for bacteria, particulate matter, and air bubble removal. IV fat emulsions have particle sizes too large for this size filter, so that only a 1.2-μ filter may be used on lipids and 3-in-1 formulas. This larger size does not remove bacteria but may eliminate fungus.[91]

Peripheral nutrition generally is initiated at the desired rate, as caloric needs are less. Central support is usually begun at a lower rate and advanced as tolerated, or alternatively, started with partial rather than full calories. This practice helps to reduce some of the fluid and electrolyte shifts that occur with feeding. When central support is discontinued, the formula is generally tapered to half rate for at least 2 hours (preferably longer) to avoid hypoglycemia.[201,202]

Ambulatory patients, either in the hospital or at home, enjoy cyclic feedings, because this permits periods of freedom from the pump. Activity level, hygiene, and psyche may improve when patients are not attached to an infusion pump 24 hours daily. Cyclic delivery has also been advocated to prevent EFAD- and TPN-induced liver disease as well as improve hepatic function and nitrogen balance.[170,203] Improvement in nitrogen balance may depend on the level of stress.[204] The formula is delivered overnight, usually for 10-14 hours, and may require a taper on as well as a taper off.[205]

ENTERAL NUTRITION

Sites and Tubes

For short-term enteral feeding access, tubes may be passed from the nose to the stomach or small intestine. Nasogastric feedings generally employ a large-bore (16-18 gauge) tube, and feedings are usually given by bolus. Nasoduodenal or nasojejunal tubes are small-bore urethane or silicone tubes passed transpylorically, usually under fluoroscopy.[206] Feedings are usually continuous or cyclic as the small intestine is sensitive to both volume and osmolarity.

Long-term access may be accomplished by a gastrostomy placed surgically, endoscopically,[207] or radiologically into the stomach. This route offers the advantages of being physiologic and tolerant to large osmotic loads and bolus feedings. Disadvantages include increased risk of aspiration[208] and inability to use with delayed gastric emptying.

A feeding jejunostomy offers access to the jejunum by surgical,[209] endoscopic, or radiologic placement of either a feeding tube or a needle catheter. This system has a decreased risk of aspiration and can be used with gastric emptying problems, but it has the disadvantages of requiring a pump for administration and inability to use for bolus feeding.

Administration

The most common methods of enteral formula administration are intermittent bolus, intermittent gravity drip, and continuous and cyclic continuous/drip feedings. The type and placement of the enteral access are the primary determinants for the best method.[82,210] Bolus feeding is used for patients who have intact stomachs with gastrostomy, esophagostomy, pharyngostomy, or nasogastric tubes. Enteral infusion sets or syringes are used to deliver 250-400 mL boluses several times a day. Advantages are that they require little equipment, are more physiologic, and are less time-consuming, although the patient is at increased risk for aspiration.

Intermittent gravity feeding uses a formula container to deliver 200-400 mL over 20 to 60 minutes several times daily. An infusion pump is optional. Although aspiration remains a risk, gastrointestinal intolerance is minimized. Continuous delivery of enteral formula may improve GI tolerance further but requires increased equipment, nursing time, and expense and decreases the patient's mobility. Cycling the feeding to night time permits greater freedom to ambulate during the day. Most tube feedings are initiated as a continuous dilute formula, increasing rate and then concentration as tolerated until full support is achieved.

Formula Selection

The major components of enteral feedings are fat, protein, and carbohydrate. Each component may be present in the feeding as an elemental, partially digested, or intact source. Less digestive capability is required for the simpler forms, but osmolarity increases and palatability decreases. Supplements are tube-feeding products that may be administered orally as well as enterally, because they are palatable. These products are generally high in fat content and are flavored.

Specialty products are usually much more expensive. There has recently been extensive development of disease-specific enteral products for pulmonary, diabetic, hepatic, renal, stress, malabsorptive, and hypoalbuminemic disorders. In addition, fiber is also included in some formulas. Careful evaluation of the amount and function of small bowel must be made for proper formula selection. In response to the large number of enteral products commercially available, most institutions have developed enteral formularies.

Carbohydrates may be present as glucose or galactose, partially digested sugars such as sucrose and lactose, or intact sources such as starches, syrups, or glucose polymers. Carbohydrates provide 4 kcal/g and are usually the major source of calories in most enteral products. Lactose is generally not present because of the high incidence of lactase deficiency in the adult population. Disaccharides are the most palatable and require minimal digestion. Oligosaccharides require more digestion but reduce osmolarity. Most carbohydrates are present in a more complex form, as the simple sugars alone present a high osmotic load. Carbohydrates are converted to glucose and transported via the portal vein directly to the liver, which allows for first-pass metabolism and may prevent the hyperglycemia seen with parenteral glucose infusion.

Fat may come from natural or synthetic sources. Standard formulas have butterfat (from milk), lecithin, or vegetable oils (sunflower, safflower, corn, soy) as intact fat sources. Fat sources in partially digested products include medium-chain triglycerides (MCT), monoglycerides, and diglycerides. Fat is generally present in only small amounts in elemental products. MCT provides 8 kcal/g; other fats give 9 kcal/g. MCT oils do not require pancreatic enzymes for digestion; vegetable oils are more palatable and less expensive.

Protein can be administered in different forms according to digestive capacity and metabolic state and provides 4 kcal/g. Intact protein requires normal digestion; partially hydrolyzed smaller fragments such as oliopeptides, dipeptides, and tripeptides may be better tolerated in certain circumstances such as hypoalbuminemia and short bowel syndrome. Absorption of protein occurs by more than one mechanism, with simple amino acids requiring a sodium-dependent pump, which is slower and more readily saturated than specific carrier proteins for di-, tri-, and oligopeptides in the small bowel wall. Simple amino acid products are also unpalatable and thus are restricted to the tube feeding. Protein intake is dependent on the formula concentration and volume provided. Protein requirements can be met by adjusting the volume, selecting formulas with a different protein density, or adding protein or nonprotein modules to a standard formula.[210-212]

The quantity of calories needed to meet 100-percent RDA for minerals and vitamins varies from 1,060 to 3,000 mL. Electrolyte content also differs with each formula. The free water content ranges from approximately 80 percent in 1 kcal/mL formulas to 70 percent in the more concentrated ones. Each patient must be carefully evaluated to ensure that proper fluid volume is provided with the feeding. Formulas must be compared on a per calorie basis to ensure full nutrition support for a given electrolyte content. Some disease-specific formulas lack minerals, vitamins, and electrolytes and require supplementation.

Complications

Four types of complications can occur with tube feedings: metabolic, gastrointestinal, mechanical, and aspiration. One recent study found that 30-40 percent of patients on tube feedings have at least one metabolic complication;[162] another found that 52 percent of tube-fed patients required fluid or electrolyte modification.[213] Metabolic complications, both excesses and deficiencies, can occur with all nutrients,[214] so that judicious monitoring is necessary.

The most common complications with enteral feeding are gastrointestinal (table 20-23). Administration of medications via the feeding tube is also known to increase diarrhea.

Table 20-23. Gastrointestinal complications

Symptom	Solution
Diarrhea	
Lactose intolerance	Lactose-free formula
Fat malabsorption	Low-fat formula
	Pancreatic enzymes
	MCT formula
Hyperosmolar formula	Isotonic formula
	Dilute formula
Cold feeding	Warm to room temperature
Hypoalbuminemia	IV albumin
	Peptide formula
Bacterial contamination	Commercial formulas
	Change equipment q24h
	Hang time of 8 hr
	Sanitary technique
Rapid infusion rate	Decrease rate
	Concentrate formula
	Continuous versus bolus
Lack of bulk	Fiber formula
	Psyllium
Nausea	
Offensive smell	Polymeric formula
	Flavoring packets
Rapid infusion rate	Continuous feeding
	Bolus feedings <350 mL
	Decrease rate
High gastric residuals	Low-fat formula
	Isotonic formula
	Intestinal feeding
Constipation	
Lack of bulk	Fiber formula
	Add prune juice to feeding
	Increase free water

A clogged feeding tube is the most common mechanical problem.[214] Tubes frequently can be unclogged by dissolving pancreatic enzymes in sodium bicarbonate and irrigating.[215] Clogged tubes can be prevented by not administering crushed medications via the tube and flushing the tube well both before and after each use.[216]

Aspiration can occur whenever a tube feeding is given. The risk can be minimized by keeping the patient at a 30° angle while feeding; use of a low-fat formula; continuous rather than bolus feeding; drug therapy to promote gastric emptying; checking gastric residuals before each bolus feeding and withholding the feeding if the residuals are greater than 150 mL; checking gastric residuals during intestinal feeding, if possible, discarding gastric residuals greater than 150 mL, reinstilling remaining residuals, and continuing with the feeding;[214] intestinal feeding; and inflation of a tracheostomy cuff when available.

Tube feedings frequently do not provide adequate nutrition support as a result of inadequate delivery. Delays in refilling the containers, withholding feeding prior to procedures, delays in resumption, and poor tolerance to tube feedings in general all contribute to this problem. Preventive measures include ordering the infusion rate higher than predicted to allow for delays and educating health care providers on the importance of delivering the necessary amount of tube feeding each day.[217]

Nutrition Support in the Home

Delivery of both intravenous and enteral nutrition support outside the hospital setting is rapidly expanding.[218,219] The ability to provide home therapy is life-sustaining to those with short gut syndrome, among other conditions, and has enabled patients to resume a normal lifestyle. This therapy is also cost-effective. The advent of diagnosis-related groups (DRG's) and lack of adequate reimbursement for many hospitalized patients have accelerated interest in providing home nutritional care to other types of patients.[5,6] Clearcut benefits as well as a low incidence of complications should be primary goals of therapy. Pharmacists' involvement in attaining the JCAHO *Standards for Accreditation of Home Care* is considerable, involving compounding, delivery, and monitoring of all drug therapy.[220]

REFERENCES

1. Dudrick SJ, Wilmore DW, Vars HM, et al: Long term total parenteral nutrition with growth, development and positive nitrogen balance. *Surgery* 64:134-142, 1968.
2. Sitzmann JV, Pitt HA: The Patient Care Committee of the American Gastroenterological Association: Statement on guidelines for total parenteral nutrition. *Dig Dis Sci* 34:489-496, 1989.
3. Konstantinides NN: Parenteral access devices and enteral feeding tubes. *Nutr Supp Serv* 8(April):12-13, 1988.
4. Deitch EA, Winterton J, Ma L, et al: The gut as a portal entry for bacteremia: Role of protein malnutrition. *Ann Surg* 205:681-690, 1987.
5. Steinberg EP, Anderson GF: Implications of Medicare's prospective payment system for specialized nutrition services. *Nutr Clin Prac* 1:12-28, 1986.
6. Regenstein M: Reimbursement for nutrition support. *Nutr Clin Prac* 4:194-202, 1989.
7. ASPEN: Standards for nutrition support. *Nutr Clin Prac* 3:28-31, 1988.
8. ASPEN: Standards for nutrition support. Hospitalized pediatric patients. *Nutr Clin Prac* 4:33-37, 1989.
9. Ailor EJ, Shane R: Documentary benefits of a nutrition support team: A key to justification under DRGs. In *Topics in Clinical Nutrition*. Rockville, MD, ASPEN Publications, 1986, pp 8-13.
10. Skoutakis VA, Martinez DR, Miller WA, et al: Team approach to total parenteral nutrition. *Am J Hosp Pharm* 32:693-697, 1975.
11. Blackburn GL, Bothe AJ, Laheg MA: Organization and administration of a nutrition support service. *Surg Clin North Am* 61:709-720, 1981.
12. Hamaoui E: Assessing the nutrition support team. *J Parenter Enteral Nutr* 11:412-421, 1987.
13. ASPEN: Nutritional support pharmacist. *Nutr Clin Prac* 2:166-169, 1987.
14. ASPEN: Standards of practice. Nutritional support dietitian. *Nutr Clin Prac* 1:216-220, 1986.
15. ASPEN: Standards of practice. Nutrition support nurse. *Nutr Clin Prac* 3:78-80, 1988.
16. Hamaoui E, Rombeau JL: The nutrition support team. In Rombeau JL, Caldwell MD (eds): *Clinical Nutrition, Vol. 2. Parenteral Nutrition*. Philadelphia, WB Saunders, 1986, pp 237-256.
17. Dalton MJ, Schepers G, Gee JP, et al: Consultative total parenteral nutrition teams: The effect on the incidence of total parenteral nutrition-related complications. *J Parenter Enteral Nutr* 8:146-152, 1984.
18. Owens JP, Geibig CB, Mirtallo JM: Concurrent quality assurance for a nutrition-support service. *Am J Hosp Pharm* 46:2469-2476, 1989.
19. Task Force on Specialty Recognition and Certification of Nutritional Support Pharmacists. Executive summary of petition requesting recognition of nutrition support pharmacy as a specialty. *Am J Hosp Pharm* 45:162-170, 1988.

20. Grant JP: Nutritional assessment in clinical practice. *Nutr Clin Prac* 1:3-11, 1986.
21. Grant JP, Custer PB, Thurlow J: Current techniques of nutritional assessment. *Surg Clin North Am* 61:437-463, 1981.
22. Detsky AS, McLaughlin JR, Baker JP et al: What is subjective global assessment of nutritional status? *J Parenter Enteral Nutr* 11:8-13, 1987.
23. Bishop CW, Bowen PE, Ritchey SJ: Norms for nutritional assessment of American adults by upper arm anthropometry. *Am J Clin Nutr* 34:2530-2539, 1981.
24. Durnin JV, Womersley J: Body fat assessed from total body density and its estimation from skinfold thickness; measurements of 481 men and women aged from 16 to 72 years. *Br J Nutr* 32:77-97, 1974.
25. Jeejeebhoy KN, Baker JP, Wolman SL, et al: Critical evaluation of the role of clinical assessment and body composition studies in patients with malnutrition and after total parenteral nutrition. *Am J Clin Nutr* 5(supp):1117-1127, 1982.
26. Morgan DB, Hill GI, Burkinshaw L: The assessment of weight loss from a single measurement of body weight: The problems and limitations. *Am J Clin Nutr* 33:2101-2105, 1980.
27. Seltzer MH, Slocum BA, Cataldi-Belcher EL, et al: Important nutritional assessment: Absolute weight loss and surgical mortality. *J Parenter Enteral Nutr* 6:218-221, 1982.
28. Studley HO: Percentage of weight loss. A basic indicator of surgical risk in patients with chronic peptic ulcer. *JAMA* 106:458-460, 1936.
29. Ryan JA Jr, Taft DA: Preoperative nutritional assessment does not predict morbidity and mortality in abdominal operations. *Surg Forum* 31:96-98, 1980.
30. Collins JP, McCarthy ID, Hill GL: Assessment of protein nutrition in surgical patients—the value of anthropometrics. *Am J Nutr* 32:1527-1530, 1979.
31. Forse RA, Shizgal HM: The assessment of malnutrition. *Surgery* 88:17-24, 1980.
32. Buzby GP, Mullen JL, Matthews DC, et al: Prognostic nutritional index in gastrointestinal surgery. *Am J Surg* 139:160-167, 1980.
33. Edwards DAW, Hammond WH, Healey MJR, et al: Design and accuracy of calipers for measuring subcutaneous tissue thickness. *Br J Nutr* 9:133-143, 1955.
34. Mattox TW, Brown RO, Boucher BA, et al: Use of fibronectin and somatomedin-C as markers of enteral nutrition support in traumatized patients using a modified amino acid formula. *J Parenter Enteral Nutr* 12:592-596, 1988.
35. Church JM, Hill GL: Assessing the efficacy of intravenous nutrition in general surgical patients: Dynamic nutritional assessment with plasma proteins. *J Parenter Enteral Nutr* 11:135-139, 1987.
36. Ingenbleck Y, Schrieck HG, Nayer PB, et al: Albumin, transferrin and the thyroxine-binding prealbumin/retinol-binding protein (TBPA-RBP) complex in assessment of malnutrition. *Clin Chim Acta* 63:61-67, 1975.
37. McAkins JL, Pietsch JB, Bubenick O, et al: Delayed hypersensitivity: Indicator of acquired failure of host defenses in sepsis and trauma. *Ann Surg* 186:241-250, 1977.
38. McLoughlin GA, Wu AV, Saporoschetz I, et al: Correlation between anergy and circulating immunosuppressive factor following major surgical trauma. *Ann Surg* 190:297-304, 1979.
39. Keys A, Broseck J, Henschel L: *The Biology of Human Starvation.* Minneapolis, University of Minnesota Press, 1950.
40. Webb AE, Newman LA, Taylor M, et al: Hand-grip dynamometry as a predictor of postoperative complications: Reappraisal using age standardized grip strengths. *J Parenter Enteral Nutr* 13:30-33, 1989.
41. Jacobs DO, Mullen JL: Current status of total parenteral nutrition. In Sabiston DC Jr (ed): *Textbook of Surgery.* Philadelphia, WB Saunders, 1989, pp 39-52.
42. Nichols LE: Nutritional support services survey 1987, part III: Parenteral nutrition; clinical monitoring and assessment. *Nutr Supp Serv* 8(Aug):12-16, 1988.
43. Almond DJ, King RFGJ, Burkinshaw L, et al: Influence of energy source upon body composition in patients receiving intravenous nutrition. *J Parenter Enteral Nutr* 13:471-477, 1989.
44. Detsky AS, Baker JP, O'Rourke K, et al: Predicting nutrition-associated complications for patients undergoing gastrointestinal surgery. *J Parenter Enteral Nutr* 11:440-446, 1987.
45. Sinning WE, Lohman TG, Wilmore JA, et al: Comparison of anthropometry with bioelectric resistance measurements. *Med Sci Sports Exerc* 19:S39(abstract), 1987.
46. Jackson AS, Polluck ML, Graves JE, et al: Reliability and validity of bioelectric impedance in determining body composition. *J Appl Physiol* 64:529-534, 1988.
47. Schoeller DA, Taylor PB: Precision of the doubly labeled water method using the two-point calculation. *Hum Nutr Clin Nutr* 41C:215-223, 1987.
48. Lifson N, McClintock R: Theory of use of the turnover rates of body water for measuring energy and material balance. *J Theor Biol* 12:46-74, 1966.
49. Schoeller DA, Leitch CA, Brown C: Doubly labeled water method: In vivo oxygen and hydrogen isotope fractionation. *Am J Physiol* 250:R823-R830, 1986.
50. Biggin HC, Chen NS, Ettinger KV, et al: Measurement of whole body nitrogen by neutron activation analysis. *Nature* (New Biol) 236:187-190, 1972.
51. McNeill KG, Mernagh JR, Jeejeebhoy KN, et al: In vivo measurements of body protein based on the determination of nitrogen by prompt gamma analysis. *Am J Clin Nutr* 32:1955-1961, 1979.
52. Forbes GM, Hursh JM: Age and sex trends in lean body mass calculated from 40K measurements. *Ann NY Acad Sci* 110:255-263, 1963.
53. Enzi G, Gasparo M, Biondetti PR, et al: Subcutaneous and visceral fat distribution according to sex, age, and overweight, evaluated by computed tomography. *Am J Clin Nutr* 44:739-746, 1986.
54. Abrams HL, Cook PH, Berne AS, et al: Magnetic resonance imaging: Consensus conference. *JAMA* 259:2132-2138, 1988.
55. Mallard JR: Nuclear magnetic resonance imaging in medicine: Medical and biological applications and problems. *Proc R Soc Lond* 226:391-419, 1986.
56. ASPEN Board of Directors: Guidelines for the use of enteral nutrition in the adult patient. *J Parenter Enteral Nutr* 11:435-439, 1987.
57. ASPEN: Guidelines for use of total parenteral nutrition in the hospitalized patient. *J Parenter Enteral Nutr* 10:441-445, 1986.
58. Sakata T, von Engelhardt W: Stimulatory effect of short chain fatty acids on the epithelial cell proliferation in rat large intestine. *Comp Biochem Physiol* 74a:459-463, 1983.
59. Clarke RM: The time-course of changes in mucosal architecture and epithelial cell production and cell shedding in the small intestine of rat fed after fasting. *J Anat* 120:321-326, 1975.
60. Souba WW, Scott TE, Wilmore DW: Intestinal consumption of intravenously administered fuels. *J Parenter Enteral Nutr* 9:18-22, 1985.
61. Trocki O, Heyd TJ, Robb EC, et al: Carnitine supplementation vs. medium chain triglyceride in postburn nutritional support. *Burns* 14:379-387, 1988.
62. Koruda MJ, Rolandelli RH, Bliss DZ, et al: Parenteral nutrition supplemented with short-chain fatty acids: Effect on the small bowel mucosa in normal rats. *Am J Clin Nutr* 51:685-689, 1990.
63. Mochizuki H, Trocki O, Dominioni L, et al: Mechanism of prevention of postburn hypermetabolism and catabolism by early enteral feeding. *Ann Surg* 200:297-310, 1984.
64. McArdle AH, Wittnich C, Freeman CR, et al: Elemental diet as prophylaxis against radiation injury: Histological and ultrastructural studies. *Arch Surg* 120:1026-1032, 1985.
65. Gouttebel MC, Saint-Aubert B, Astre C, et al: Total parenteral nutrition needs in different types of short bowel syndrome. *Dig Dis Sci* 31:718-728, 1986.
66. Grant JP, James S, Grabowski V, et al: Total parenteral nutrition in pancreatic disease. *Ann Surg* 200:627-631, 1984.

67. Soeters PB, Ebeid AM, Fischer JE: Review of 404 patients with gastrointestinal fistulas. Impact of parenteral nutrition. *Ann Surg* 190:189-202, 1979.
68. Dombrowski SR, Mirtallo JM: Drug therapy and nutritional management of patients with gastrointestinal fistulas. *Clin Pharm* 3:264-272, 1984.
69. Ostro MJ, Greenberg GR, Jeejeebhoy KN: Total parenteral nutrition and complete bowel rest in the management of Crohn's disease. *J Parenter Enteral Nutr* 9:280-287, 1985.
70. Lochs H, Marosi L, Ferenci P, et al: Has total bowel rest a beneficial effect in the treatment of Crohn's disease? *Clin Nutr* 2:61-64, 1983.
71. Dickinson RJ, Ashton MG, Axon AT, et al: Controlled trial of intravenous hyperalimentation and total bowel rest as an adjunct to the routine therapy of acute colitis. *Gastroenterology* 79:1199-1204, 1980.
72. Detsky AS, Baker JP, O'Rourke K, et al: Perioperative parenteral nutrition: A meta-analysis. *Ann Intern Med* 107:195-203, 1987.
73. Buzby GP, Williford WO, Peterson OL, et al: A randomized clinical trial of total parenteral nutrition in malnourished surgical patients: The rationale and impact of previous clinical trials and pilot study on protocol design. *Am J Clin Nutr* 47:366-381, 1988.
74. McGeer AJ, Detsky AS, O'Rourke K, American College of Physicians: Parenteral nutrition in patients receiving cancer chemotherapy. *Ann Int Med* 110:734-736, 1989.
75. Harris JA, Benedict FG: *Biometric Studies of Basal Metabolism in Man.* Washington, DC, Carnegie Institute of Washington, publication No. 279, 1919.
76. Elwyn DH, Kinney JM, Askanazi J: Energy expenditure in surgical patients. *Surg Clin North Am* 61:545-556, 1981.
77. Feurer ID, Crosby LO, Mullen JL: Measured and predicted resting energy expenditure in clinically stable patients. *Clin Nutr* 3:27-34, 1984.
78. Foster GD, Knox LS, Mullen JL: Measured vs estimated TPN requirements. *J Parenter Enteral Nutr* 9:113(abstract), 1985.
79. Quebbeman EJ, Ausman RK, Schneider TC: A re-evaluation of energy expenditure during parenteral nutrition. *Ann Surg* 195:282-286, 1982.
80. Weissman C, Kemper M, Askanazi J, et al: Resting metabolic rate of the critically ill patient: Measured versus predicted. *Anesthesiology* 64:673-679, 1986.
81. Dickerson RN: Energy and protein requirements of hospitalized patients receiving parenteral nutrition. *Hosp Pharm* 22:70-79, 1987.
82. Heymsfield SB, Erbland M, Casper K, et al: Enteral nutritional support: Metabolic, cardiovascular, and pulmonary interactions. *Clin Chest Med* 7:41-67, 1986.
83. MacFie J, Holmfield JHM, King RFG, et al: Effect of the energy source on changes in energy expenditure and respiratory quotients during total parenteral nutrition. *J Parenter Enteral Nutr* 7:1-5, 1983.
84. Silberman H, Silberman AW: Parenteral nutrition: Biochemistry and respiratory gas exchange. *J Parenter Enteral Nutr* 10:151-154, 1986.
85. Carpentier YA, Askanazi J, Elwyn DH, et al: Effects of hypercaloric glucose infusion on lipid metabolism in injury and sepsis. *J Trauma* 19:649-654, 1979.
86. Dickerson RN, Rosato EF, Mullen JL: Net protein anabolism with hypocaloric parenteral nutrition in obese stressed patients. *Am J Clin Nutr* 44:747-755, 1986.
87. Goodenough RD, Wolfe RR: Effect of total parenteral nutrition on free fatty acid metabolism in burned patients. *J Parenter Enteral Nutr* 8:357-360, 1984.
88. Bistrian BR: Clinical use of a protein-sparing modified fast. *JAMA* 240:2299-2302, 1987.
89. Nutrition Advisory Group, AMA-Department of Foods and Nutrition: Multivitamin preparations for parenteral use. *J Parenter Enteral Nutr* 3:258-262, 1979.
90. Shils ME, Baker H, Frank O: Blood vitamin levels of long-term adult home total parenteral nutrition patients: The efficacy of the AMA-FDA parenteral multivitamin formulation. *J Parenter Enteral Nutr* 9:179-188, 1985.
91. Driscoll DF: Clinical issues regarding the use of total nutrient admixtures. *Drug Intell Clin Pharm* 24:296-303, 1990.
92. Wolfe BM, Chock E: Energy sources, stores, and hormonal controls. *Surg Clin North Am* 61:509-518, 1981.
93. McMahon M, Nasrullah M, Driscoll DF, et al: Parenteral nutrition in patients with diabetes mellitus: Theoretical and practical considerations. *J Parenter Enteral Nutr* 13:545-553, 1989.
94. Hill GI, Church J: Energy and protein requirements of general surgical patients requiring intravenous nutrition. *Br J Surg* 71:1-9, 1984.
95. Shreeve WW: *Physiological Chemistry of Carbohydrates in Mammals.* Philadelphia, WB Saunders, 1974.
96. Brennan MF, Horowitz GP: Total parenteral nutrition in surgical patients. *Adv Surg* 17:1-36, 1984.
97. Nordenstrom J, Carpentier YA, Askanazi J, et al: Metabolic utilization of intravenous fat emulsion during total parenteral nutrition. *Ann Surg* 196:221-231, 1982.
98. Crowe PJ, Dennison A, Royle GJ: The effect of pre-operative glucose loading on postoperative nitrogen metabolism. *Br J Surg* 71:635-637, 1984.
99. Wolfe R, O'Donnell T, Stone M, et al: Investigation of factors determining the optimal glucose infusion rate in total parenteral nutrition. *Metabolism* 29:892-900, 1980.
100. Burke SJF, Wolfe RR, Mullany CJ, et al: Glucose requirements following burn injury: Parameters of optimal glucose infusion and possible hepatic and respiratory abnormalities following excessive glucose intake. *Ann Surg* 190:274-285, 1979.
101. Askanazi J, Carpentier YA, Elwyn DH, et al: Influence of total parenteral nutrition on fuel utilization in injury and infection. *Ann Surg* 191:40-46, 1980.
102. Mann S, Westesnkow DR, Houtchens BA: Measured and predicted calorie expenditure in the acutely ill. *Crit Care Med* 13:173-177, 1985.
103. Herve P, Simmonneau G, Girard P, et al: Hypercapnic acidosis induced by nutrition in mechanically ventilated patients: Glucose vs fat. *Crit Care Med* 13:537-540, 1985.
104. Grant JP: *Handbook of Total Parenteral Nutrition.* Philadelphia, WB Saunders, 1980.
105. Freeman JB, Fairfull-Smith R, Rodman GH, et al: Safety and efficacy of a new peripheral intravenously administered amino acid solution containing glycerol and electrolytes. *Surg Gynecol Obstet* 156:625-631, 1983.
106. Roesner M, Grant JP: Intravenous lipid emulsions. *Nutr Clin Prac* 2:96-107, 1987.
107. Riela MD, Broviac JW, Wells M, et al: Essential fatty acid deficiency in human adults during total parenteral nutrition. *Ann Intern Med* 83:786-789, 1975.
108. Fujiwara T, Kawarasaki H, Fonkalsrud EW: Reduction of post infusion venous endothelial injury with Intralipid. *Surg Gynecol Obstet* 158:57-65, 1984.
109. Jeejeebhoy KN, Anderson GH, Nakhooda AF, et al: Metabolic studies in total parenteral nutrition in man. *J Clin Invest* 57:125-136, 1975.
110. Munro HN: General aspects of the regulation of protein metabolism by diet and by hormones. In Munro HN, Allison JB (eds): *Mammalian Protein Metabolism. Vol. 1.* New York, Academic Press, pp 381-481, 1969.
111. Hamawy KJ, Moldawer LL, Georgiett M, et al: The effect of lipid emulsions on reticuloendothelial systems function in the injured animal. *J Parenter Enteral Nutr* 13:614-619, 1985.
112. Seidner DL, Mascioli EA, Istfan NW, et al: Effects of long-chain triglyceride emulsions on reticuloendothelial system function in humans. *J Parenter Enteral Nutr* 13:614-619, 1989.
113. Abbott WC, Grakauskas AM, Bistrian BR, et al: Metabolic and respiratory effects of continuous and discontinuous lipid infusions. *Arch Surg* 119:1367-1371, 1984.
114. Skeie B, Askanazi J, Rothkopf M, et al: The beneficial effects of fat on ventilation and pulmonary function. *Nutrition* 3:149-154, 1987.
115. Trocki O, Heyd TJ, Waymack JP, et al: Effects of fish oil on postburn metabolism and immunity. *J Parenter Enteral Nutr* 11:521-527, 1987.

116. Sakata T, Yajima T: Influence of short-chain fatty acids on the epithelial cell division of the digestive tract. *Q J Exp Physiol* 69:639-648, 1984.
117. Mascioli EA, Babayan VK, Bistrian BR, et al: Novel triglycerides for special medical purposes. *J Parenter Enteral Nutr* 12(supp):127-132, 1988.
118. Untraucht S: Alterations of serum lipoproteins resulting from total parenteral nutrition with Intralipid. *Biochem Biophys Acta* 711:176-192, 1982.
119. Andrew G, Chan G, Schiff D: Lipid metabolism in the neonate. II. The effect of Intralipid on bilirubin binding in vitro and in vivo. *J Pediatr* 88:279-284, 1976.
120. Silberman H, Dixon NP, Eisenberg D: The safety and efficacy of a lipid-based system of parenteral nutrition in acute pancreatitis. *Am J Gastroenterol* 77:494-497, 1982.
121. Schreiner RL, Glick MR, Nordschow CD, et al: An evaluation of methods to monitor infants receiving intravenous lipids. *J Pediatr* 94:197-200, 1979.
122. Griffin E, Brechenridge WC, Kuksis A, et al: Appearance and characterization of lipoprotein X during continuous Intralipid infusions in the neonate. *J Clin Invest* 64:1703-1712, 1979.
123. Patsch JR, Soutar AK, Morrisett JD, et al: Lipoprotein-X: A substrate for lecithin: cholesterol acyltransferase. *Eur J Clin Invest* 7:213-217, 1977.
124. Miller SJ: The nitrogen balance revisited. *Hosp Phar* 25:61-70, 1990.
125. Gamble JL: Physiological information from studies on the life-raft ration. *Harvey Lect* 42:247-273, 1946-1947.
126. Cerra FB, Upson D, Angelico R: Branched chains support postoperative protein synthesis. *Surgery* 92:192-199, 1982.
127. Oki JC, Cuddy PG: Branched-chain amino acid support of stressed patients. *Drug Intell Clin Pharm* 23:399-408, 1989.
128. Brennan MF, Cerra FB, Daly JM, et al: Report of a workshop: Branched-chain amino acids in stress and injury. *J Parenter Enteral Nutr* 10:446-452, 1986.
129. Rudman D, Millikan WT, Richardson TJ, et al: Elemental balances during intravenous hyperalimentation of underweight adult subjects. *J Clin Invest* 55:94-104, 1975.
130. Zalman SA, Wasserstein A, Goldfarb S: Disorders of calcium and magnesium homeostasis. *Am J Med* 72:473-488, 1982.
131. Hyneck ML: Simple acid-base disorders. *Am J Hosp Pharm* 42:1992-2004, 1985.
132. Rose BD: New approach to disturbances in the plasma sodium concentration. *Am J Med* 81:1033-1040, 1986.
133. Klotz R: Do the crystalline amino acid formulas impact acid-base balance in the patient on parenteral nutrition? *Hosp Pharm* 23:78-82, 1988.
134. Kunau RT, Stein JH: Disorders of hypo- and hyperkalemia. *Clin Nephrol* 7:173-190, 1977.
135. Husami T, Abumrad NN: Adverse metabolic consequences of nutrition support: Micronutrients. *Surg Clin North Am* 66:1049-1069, 1985.
136. Baumgartner TG: *Clinical Guide to Parenteral Micronutrition*. 1st ed. Melrose Park, IL, Educational Publications, 1984.
137. Guidelines for essential trace element preparations for parenteral use. *JAMA* 241:2051-2054, 1979.
138. Narins RG, Jones ER, Stom ML, et al: Diagnostic strategies in disorders of fluid, electrolyte and acid-base homeostasis. *Am J Med* 72:496-520, 1982.
139. Stoff JS: Phosphate homeostasis and hypophosphatemia. *Am J Med* 72:489-495, 1982.
140. Thompson J, Hodges R: Preventing hypophosphatemia during total parenteral nutrition. *J Parenter Enteral Nutr* 8:137-139, 1984.
141. Niemiec PN, Vanderveen TW: Pharmacotherapeutic considerations during nutrition support. In Brown TR, Smith MC (eds): *Handbook of Institutional Pharmacy Practice*. Baltimore, Williams & Wilkins, 1986, pp 238-288.
142. Mirtallo JM, Kudsk KA, Ebbert ML: Nutritional support of patients with renal disease. *Clin Pharm* 3:253-263, 1984.
143. Feinstein EI: Nutrition in acute renal failure. In Rombeau JL, Caldwell MD (eds): *Parenteral Nutrition*. Philadelphia, WB Saunders, 1986, pp 586-601.
144. Brown RO: Nutritional considerations in major organ failure. In DiPiro JT, Talbert RL, Hayes PE, et al (eds): *Pharmacotherapy*. New York, Elsevier, 1989, pp 1638-1654.
145. Broyles JE, Brown RO, Vehe KL, et al: Fluid balance in fluid-restricted patients receiving 10% amino acids or 15% amino acids as part of parenteral nutrition. *Hosp Pharm* 24:995-998, 1989.
146. Simmons RS, Berdine GG, Seidenfeld JJ, et al: Fluid balance and the adult respiratory distress syndrome. *Am Rev Respir Dis* 135:924-929, 1987.
147. Barber JR, Teasley KM: Nutritional support of patients with severe hepatic failure. *Clin Pharm* 3:245-252, 1984.
148. Watters JM, Freeman JB: Parenteral nutrition by peripheral vein. *Surg Clin North Am* 61:593-604, 1981.
149. Gazitua R, Wilson K, Bistrian BR, et al: Factors determining peripheral vein tolerance to amino acid infusions. *Arch Surg* 114:897-900, 1979.
150. Isaacs J, Millikan W, Stackhouse J, et al: Parenteral nutrition of adults with a 900 milliosmolar solution via peripheral vein. *Am J Clin Nutr* 30:552-559, 1977.
151. Siegel FP: Tonicity, osmoticity, osmolality, and osmolarity. In Gennaro AR (ed): *Remington's Pharmaceutical Sciences*. Philadelphia, Mack Publishing Company, 1985, pp 1455-1472.
152. Grant JP: Catheter access. In Rombeau JL, Caldwell MD (eds): *Clinical Nutrition, vol 2. Parenteral Nutrition*. Philadelphia, WB Saunders, 1986, pp 306-315.
153. Forlaw L, Torosian MH: Central venous catheter care. In Rombeau JL, Caldwell MD (eds): *Clinical Nutrition, vol. 2. Parenteral Nutrition*. Philadelphia, WB Saunders, 1986, pp 316-330.
154. Rubenstein M, Creger WP: Successful streptokinase therapy for catheter-induced subclavian vein thrombosis. *Arch Intern Med* 140:1370-1371, 1980.
155. Stewart A, Mayre EE: Rapid resolution of subclavian vein thrombosis by tissue plasminogen activator (letter). *Lancet* 1:890, 1988.
156. Fabri PJ, Mirtallo JM, Ebhert ML, et al: Clinical effect of nonthrombotic parenteral nutrition catheters. *J Parenter Enteral Nutr* 8:705-707, 1984.
157. Fabri PJ, Mirtallo JM, Ruberg RL, et al: Incidence and prevention of thrombosis of the subclavian vein during total parenteral nutrition. *Surg Gynecol Obstet* 155:238-240, 1982.
158. Pemberton L, Lyman B, Lander V, et al: Sepsis from triple- vs. single-lumen catheters during total parenteral nutrition in surgical or critically ill patients. *Arch Surg* 121:591-594, 1986.
159. Benotti PN, Bistrian BR: Practical aspects and complications of total parenteral nutrition. *Crit Care Clin* 3:115-131, 1987.
160. Press OW, Ramsey PG, Larson EB, et al: Hickman catheter infections in patients with malignancies. *Medicine* 63:189-200, 1984.
161. Williams WW: Infection control during parenteral nutrition therapy. *J Parenter Enteral Nutr* 9:735-746, 1985.
162. Vanlandingham S, Simpson S, Daniel P, et al: Metabolic abnormalities in patients supported with enteral tube feeding. *J Parenter Enteral Nutr* 5:322-324, 1981.
163. Weinsier RL, Bacon J, Butterworth CE: Central venous alimentation: A prospective study of the frequency of metabolic abnormalities among medical and surgical patients. *J Parenter Enteral Nutr* 6:421-425, 1982.
164. Giner M, Curtas S: Adverse metabolic consequences of nutrition support: Macronutrients. *Surg Clin North Am* 66:1025-1047, 1986.
165. Elwyn DH: Protein metabolism and requirements in the critically ill patient. *Crit Care Clin* 3:57-69, 1987.
166. Shaw JHF, Wolfe RR: Influence of stress, depletion and/or malignant disease on the responsiveness of surgical patients to TPN. *Am J Clin Nutr* 48:144-177, 1988.
167. Spruill WJ, Wade WE, Beckett BE, et al: Determination of urinary urea nitrogen concentrations with modified blood urea nitrogen procedures. *Clin Pharm* 9:371-373, 1990.

168. Shangraw RE, Stuart CA, Prince MJ, et al: Insulin responsiveness of protein metabolism in vivo following bedrest in humans. *Am J Physiol* 255:E548-E558, 1988.
169. Herber FF, Scheidegger JR, Grunig BE, et al: Evidence that prednisone-induced myopathy is reversed by physical training. *J Clin Endocrinol Metab* 61:83-88, 1985.
170. Dietrick JE, Whedon GD, Shorr E: Effects of immobilization upon various metabolic and physiologic functions of normal men. *Am J Med* 4:3-36, 1948.
171. Sale DG, MacDougall JD, Alway SE, et al: Voluntary strength and muscle characteristics in untrained men and women and male body builders. *J Appl Physiol* 62:1786-1793, 1987.
172. Jiang Z, He G, Zhang S, et al: Low-dose growth hormone and hypocaloric nutrition attenuate the protein-catabolic response after major operation. *Ann Surg* 210:513-525, 1989.
173. Ziegler TR, Young LS, Manson JM, et al: Metabolic effects of recombinant human growth hormone in patients receiving parenteral nutrition. *Ann Surg* 208:6-16, 1988.
174. National Coordinating Committee on Large Volume Parenterals: Recommended methods for compounding intravenous admixtures in hospitals. *Am J Hosp Pharm* 32:261-270, 1975.
175. National Coordinating Committee on Large Volume Parenterals: Recommended guidelines for quality assurance in hospital centralized intravenous admixture services. *Am J Hosp Pharm* 37:645-655, 660-663, 665-667, 1980.
176. Stolar MH: Assuring the quality of intravenous admixture programs. *Am J Hosp Pharm* 36:605-608, 1979.
177. Levchuk JW, Nolly RJ, Lander N: Method of testing the sterility of total nutrient admixtures. *Am J Hosp Pharm* 45:1311-1121, 1988.
178. Parr MD, Bertch KE, Rapp RP: Amino acid stability in total parenteral nutrient solutions. *Am J Hosp Pharm* 42:2688-2691, 1985.
179. Kaminski MV, Harris DF, Collin CF, et al: Electrolyte compatibility in a synthetic amino acid hyperalimentation solution. *Am J Hosp Pharm* 31:244-246, 1974.
180. Tripp MG. Automatic 3-in-1 admixture compounding: A comparative study of simultaneous versus sequential pumping of core substrates on admixture stability. *Hosp Pharm* 25:1090-1096, 1990.
181. Simmons BP, Hooten TM, Wong ES, et al: Guidelines for the prevention of intravascular infections. Centers for Disease Control: Guidelines and control of nosocomial infections. *National Intravenous Therapy Association* 5:40-46, 1982.
182. Brown DH, Simkover RA: Maximum hang times for i.v. fat emulsions. *Am J Hosp Pharm* 44:282,284, 1987.
183. Driscoll DF, Baptista RJ, Bistrian BR, et al: Practical considerations regarding the use of total nutrient admixtures. *Am J Hosp Pharm* 10:650-658, 1986.
184. Brown R, Querica RA, Sigman R: Total nutrient admixture: A review. *J Parenter Enteral Nutr* 10:650-658, 1986.
185. Niemiec PW Jr, Vanderveen TW: Compatibility considerations in parenteral nutrient solutions. *Am J Hosp Pharm* 41:893-911, 1984.
186. Eggert LD, Rusho WJ, MacKay MW, et al: Calcium and phosphorus compatibility in parenteral nutrition solutions for neonates. *Am J Hosp Pharm* 39:49-53, 1982.
187. Das Gupta V, Allwood MC, Louie N: Stability of vitamins in total parenteral nutrition. *Am J Hosp Pharm* 43:2132, 2138, 2143, 1986.
188. Goldman DA, Martin WT, Worthington JW: Growth of bacteria and fungi in total parenteral nutrition solutions. *Am J Surg* 126:314-318, 1973.
189. Rowe CE, Fukuyama TT, Martinoff JT: Growth of microorganisms in total nutrient admixtures. *Drug Intell Clin Pharm* 21:633-638, 1987.
190. Vasilkis A, Apelgren KN: Answering the fat emulsion contamination question: Three in one admixture vs. conventional total parenteral nutrition in a clinical setting. *J Parenter Enteral Nutr* 12:356-359, 1988.
191. Baptista RJ: Medications compatible with hyperalimentation solutions. *Nutr Supp Serv* 3(May):18-20, 1983.
192. Mirtallo JM, Schneider PJ, Ruberg RL: Albumin in TPN solutions: Potential savings from a prospective review. *J Parenter Enteral Nutr* 4:300-302, 1980.
193. Tsallas G, Allen LC: Stability of cimetidine hydrochloride in parenteral nutrition solutions. *Am J Hosp Pharm* 39:484-488, 1982.
194. Bullock L, Fitzgerald JF, Click MR, et al: Stability of famotidine 20 and 40 mg/L and amino acids in total parenteral nutrient solutions. *Am J Hosp Pharm* 46:2321-2325, 1989.
195. Williams MF, Hak LJ, Dukes G: In vitro evaluation of the stability of ranitidine hydrochloride in total parenteral nutrient mixtures. *Am J Hosp Pharm* 47:1574-1579, 1990.
196. Marcuard SP, Dunham B, Hobbs A, et al: Availability of insulin from total parenteral nutrition solutions. *J Parenter Enteral Nutr* 14:262-264, 1990.
197. Seres DS: Insulin adsorption to parenteral infusion systems: Case report and review of the literature. *Nutr Clin Prac* 5:111-117, 1990.
198. Laster J, Cikrit D, Walker N, et al: The heparin-induced thrombocytopenia syndrome: An update. *Surgery* 102:763-770, 1987.
199. Mirtallo JM, Rogers KR, Johnson JA, et al: Stability of amino acids and availability of acids in total parenteral nutrition solutions containing hydrochloric acid. *Am J Hosp Pharm* 38:1729-1731, 1981.
200. Trissel LA: *Handbook on Injectable Drugs*, 5th ed. Washington, DC, American Society of Hospital Pharmacists, 1988.
201. Dickerson RN: Question: How fast can I taper TPN in a hospitalized patient? *Hosp Pharm* 20:620-621, 1985.
202. Wagman LD, Miller KB, Thomas RB, et al: The effect of acute discontinuation of total parenteral nutrition. *Ann Surg* 204:524-529, 1986.
203. Matuchansky C, Morichau-Beauchant M, Druart F, et al: Cyclic (nocturnal) total parenteral nutrition in hospitalized adult patients with severe digestive diseases. *Gastroenterology* 81:433-437, 1981.
204. Messing B, Pontal PJ, Bernier JJ: Metabolic study during cyclic total parenteral nutrition in adult patients with and without corticosteroid-induced hypercatabolism: Comparison with standard total parenteral nutrition. *J Parenter Enteral Nutr* 7:21-25, 1983.
205. McClary B, Rosen GH: Cyclic total parenteral nutrition. *Nutr Clin Prac* 5:163-165, 1990.
206. Grant JP, Curtas MS, Kelvin FM: Fluoroscopic placement of nasojejunal feeding tubes with immediate feeding using a nonelemental diet. *J Parenter Enteral Nutr* 7:299-303, 1983.
207. Namel JJ: Percutaneous endoscopic gastrostomies. A review. *Nutr Clin Prac* 2:65-75, 1987.
208. Kiver KF, Hays DP, Fortin DF, et al: Pre- and post-pyloric enteral feeding: Analysis of safety and complications. *J Parenter Enteral Nutr* 6:588(abstract), 1982.
209. Ryan JA, Page C: Intrajejunal feeding: Development and current status. *J Parenter Enteral Nutr* 8:187-198, 1984.
210. Chernoff R: Enteral feedings. *Am J Hosp Pharm* 37:65-74, 1980.
211. Heymsfield SB, Bethel RA, Ansley JD, et al: Enteral hyperalimentation: An alternative to central venous hyperalimentation. *Ann Int Med* 90:63-71, 1979.
212. Silk DBA: Diet formulation and choice of enteral diet. *Gut* 27(Suppl):40-46, 1986.
213. Cataldi-Betcher EL, Seltzer MH, Slocum BA, et al: Complications occurring during enteral nutrition support: A prospective study. *J Parenter Enteral Nutr* 7:546-552, 1983.
214. Hayes-Johnson V: Tube feeding complications: Causes, prevention, and therapy. *Nutr Supp Serv* 6(Mar):17-18, 1986.
215. Marcuard SP, Stegall KL, Trogdon S: Clearing obstructed feeding tubes. *J Parenter Enteral Nutr* 13:81-83, 1989.
216. Schwartz DB: Enteral therapy. In Lang CE (ed): *Nutritional Support in Critical Care*. Rockville, MD, ASPEN Publications, 1987, pp 99-111.
217. Abernathy GB, Heizer WD, Holcombe BJ, et al: Efficacy of tube feeding in supplying energy requirements of hospitalized patients. *J Parenter Enteral Nutr* 13:387-391, 1989.
218. Lees CD, Steiger E, Hooely RA, et al: Home parenteral nutrition. *Surg Clin North Am* 61:621-633, 1981.

219. Davey-McCrae JA, Hall NH: Current practices for home enteral nutrition. *J Am Diet Assoc* 89:233-240, 1989.
220. Joint Commission on Accreditation of Healthcare Organizations: *Accreditation Manual for Home Care*. Oakbrook Terrace, IL, JCAHO, 1991.

CHAPTER 21

Repackaging Pharmaceuticals in Institutional Practice

LAWRENCE J. PESKO

INTRODUCTION

Historically, institutionally based pharmacists have been responsible for repackaging pharmaceuticals for patient use. If we were to trace our roots back in time to early institutional practice, we would find that the packaging process was the end result of the culmination of the formulation and preparation process for oral and injectable medications. As pharmaceutical manufacturers began to prepare, package, and distribute commonly prescribed medications, the role of the institutional practitioner changed from formulator and packager to repackager of commercially prepared medications. In this context, the pharmacist would repackage bulk containers of medication into patient-specific containers of medication. The amount of medication that was repackaged into the patient container was generally predicated on the course of therapy or the average length of stay in the hospital for the patient. This type of packaging (from bulk containers into patient-specific containers called "unit-of-use packaging") marked the very beginnings of the unit dose concept and the idea of providing patient-specific medications as opposed to a general stock of medications on the nursing unit. Unit of use packaging was characterized by a package, either a vial, envelope, or plastic bag, containing several doses of medication (all the same type). The only thing that the container lacked was a prescription label with the patient's name on it. This label was affixed to the package prior to dispensing and contained the patient's name and often the directions for administration of the medication. Unit of use packaging, sometimes referred to as "prepackaging," was a suitable concept for inpatient or outpatient dispensing. An advantage to this type of dispensing process was that it allowed the pharmacist to prepare medications for administration prior to their anticipated request. This allowed the pharmacist to better plan and control important things like providing a double-check of the medications being administered by the nurse as opposed to the nurse selecting the medication from a generalized stock, reducing the overall cost of stocking medication on each nursing unit, and controlling pharmacy staffing requirements.[1-8]

The unit dose system of dispensing medication in organized health care settings has been the driving force behind repackaging programs as we know them today. Unit dose distribution is the standard by which all other distribution systems are measured.

As the benefits of unit of use packaging became publicized, further modifications took place in the dispensing processes that now have become known as the unit dose concept. In the unit dose system, single-unit packages are prepared containing a single and separate dosage form.[9] Examples of single-unit packages would include one tablet or one capsule, one teaspoonful (5 mL) of an oral liquid, one 50-mg (2-mL) syringe, or 2 g of a topical ointment. The important thing to remember about single-unit packages is that they contain only one distinct dosage form.

A third type of package is the "unit" or "single-dose package." This package is often confused with the single-unit package. The important difference between these two different packaging systems is that the single-dose package always contains the dose of the drug for a given patient. Therefore, a single-dose package may contain two tablets or two capsules in one package or container for a given patient if the dose calls for two tablets or two capsules. Single-unit packages will contain only one tablet or one capsule. Figure 21-1 shows the three different types of packaging systems that are used in institutional practice. A complete glossary of terms can be found at the end of this chapter.

The availability of single-unit and single-dose packaging of pharmaceuticals by the manufacturer of the product has reduced the need for the institutional practitioner to be involved in repackaging. However, not all medications are available in single-unit or single-dose packages. This is especially true for oral liquid medications and for parenteral medications, which often require reconstitution and dilution prior to administration.

In addition, new developments in automated packaging machines and in packaging materials, coupled with financial incentives gained through in-house packaging programs versus purchase of the drug already packaged by the manufacturer, have given greater importance to establishing institutional repackaging programs.

EXTEMPORANEOUS VERSUS BATCH REPACKAGING

One of the major advantages credited to unit dose drug distribution systems is that they decrease the total cost of

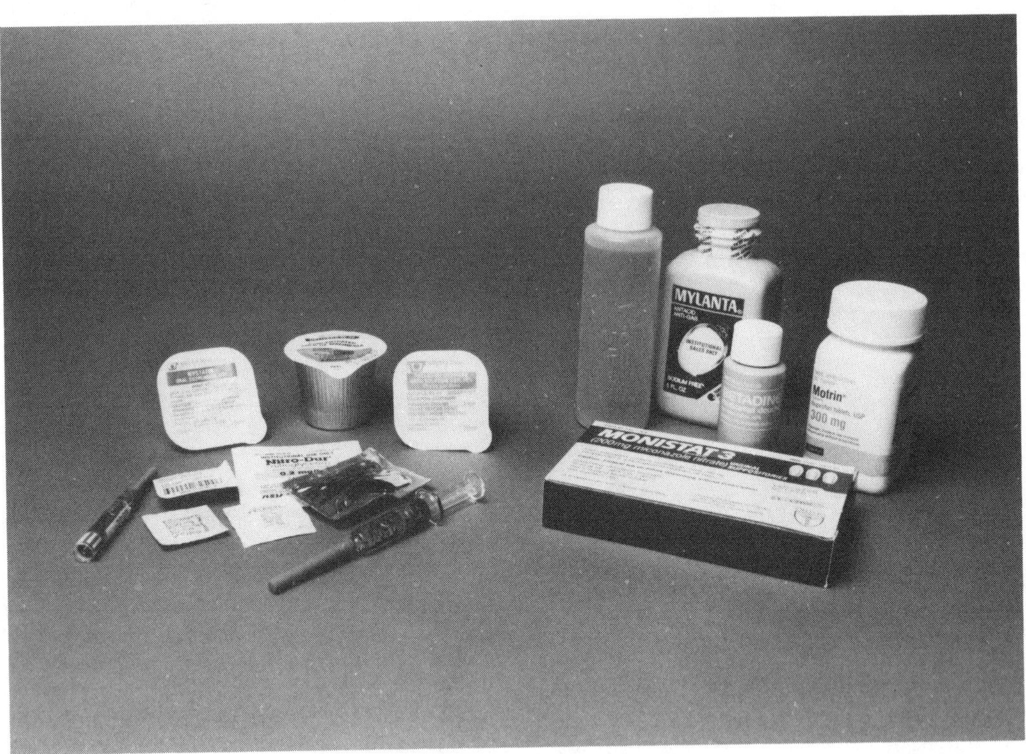

Figure 21-1. Examples of packages used in institutional practice

medication-related activities. This is achieved in part through greater control by the pharmacist over pharmacy workload patterns and staff scheduling. Repackaging medications in advance of when they are needed allows the pharmacist to take advantage of periods of reduced staff activity to lessen the demands of peak activity. In short, the pharmacist is able to stock up on repackaged medications to supply peak demand periods. This is the basic premise behind batch packaging versus extemporaneous packaging.

"Extemporaneous repackaging" is the process of repackaging medications on a day-to-day basis that will be used over a short period of time. Medications that are of a specific dosage and in a specific dosage form are prepared in limited quantities by a specific operator. These medications generally represent drugs that have limited or unknown stability in the package, or dosages of medications that are infrequently prescribed. Generally, the number of doses that are repackaged reflect the number of doses that will be consumed prior to the expiration date of the repackaged drug.

"Batch repackaging" can be defined as the repackaging of a specific dosage and dosage form of medication at a given time, by an assigned operator, in sufficient quantity to last a predetermined amount of time. Batch preparation lends itself to medications that are stable over an extended period of time in the package material and medications that are prescribed frequently in the institution. In addition, medications that meet these criteria and offer a financial incentive over the manufacturer's product may become candidates for batch repackaging from bulk supplies.

Batch repackaging offers several advantages over extemporaneous repackaging. Medications that are repackaged in batches lend themselves to production-controlled processes. Therefore, the incorporation of good manufacturing practices and end product testing are more likely to be achieved in batch repackaging programs than in extemporaneous repackaging programs.

Batch repackaging requires greater control methods than does extemporaneous repackaging because of the greater number of packages produced and the likelihood of affecting larger numbers of patients adversely. Finally, batch repackaging generally produces a final package that is less costly than the extemporaneously repackaged counterpart.

GENERAL REPACKAGING GUIDELINES AND GOOD MANUFACTURING PRACTICES

The American Society of Hospital Pharmacists' (ASHP) technical assistance bulletin on single-unit and unit dose packages of drugs states that drug packages must fulfill four basic functions: (1) protect their contents from deleterious environmental effects (e.g., photodecomposition); (2) protect their contents from deterioration resulting from handling (e.g., breakage and contamination); (3) identify their contents completely and precisely; and (4) permit their contents to be used quickly, easily, and safely.[10]

These guidelines have as their basis the *Good Manufacturing Practices for Finished Pharmaceuticals* (GMP) established by the U.S. Food and Drug Administration (FDA) in 1963. The *United States Pharmacopeia XXII* (USP)[11] states that "while these regulations are directed primarily to the drug manufacturers, the principles embodied therein may be helpful to those engaged in the practice of pharmacy..." The USP further states that, "Good manufacturing practices were established to describe the methods to be used in, and the facilities or controls to be used for, the manufacture, processing, packaging, or holding of a drug to assure that such drug meets the requirements of the act as to safety, and has the identity and strength and meets the quality and purity characteristics that it purports or is reputed to possess."

The *United States Pharmacopeia* lists several key areas that define GMP's and the requirements needed to meet these key areas. The key areas are (1) organization and personnel; (2) facilities; (3) equipment; (4) control of components and drug product containers and closures; (5) production and process controls; (6) packaging and labeling controls; (7) holding and distribution; (8) laboratory controls; and (9) records and reports.[12]

Organization and Personnel

There shall be a quality control unit that shall have the responsibility and authority to approve or reject all components, containers and closures, packaging materials and labels....

In the community hospital setting, this could range from a pharmacist checking a single product to a pharmacist dedicated completely to quality control.

Each person engaged in the manufacture, processing, packaging, or holding of a drug product shall have education, training, and experience to enable the person to perform the assigned functions.

This requirement could be applied to an in-house training program conducted by professional staff or through a certified community college training program or a certificate program of a professional organization (such as the ASHP Technician Training Program).

Personnel engaged in the manufacture, processing, or packaging shall wear clean clothing appropriate for the duties they perform. Protective apparel, such as head, face, hand, and arm coverings, shall be worn as necessary to protect drug products from contamination.

Personnel shall practice good sanitation and health habits. Any person shown at any time to have an apparent illness or open lesions that may adversely affect safety or quality of the drug product shall be excluded from direct contact with components, drug product containers, closures, and drug products until the condition is corrected or determined not to jeopardize the product.

These guidelines may apply to packaging sterile as well as nonsterile products. Certainly protective garments such as hair netting should be worn during packaging of oral liquids and solids. More extensive garments may be required in the preparation of sterile products. This could include hair netting, surgical masks, nonshedding particle over garments, and surgical gloves.

Commonsense dictates that employees with communicable illnesses and open wounds should not come into contact with products that may be ingested, injected, or applied topically. At a minimum, precautions should be taken to provide an environment that is at least as clean as a food preparation area for repackaging orally administered medications. Repackaging of sterile products will demand more stringent requirements.

Facilities

Any building or buildings used in the manufacture, processing, packaging, or holding of a drug product shall be of suitable size, construction, and location to facilitate cleaning, maintenance, and proper operations. Any such building shall have adequate space for the orderly placement of equipment and materials to prevent mixups between different components and to prevent contamination.

Although most hospitals do not perform enough repackaging to justify a separate facility, some of the basic constructs do hold true even in a small pharmacy. Basically, a separate area should be designated for repackaging drugs. The area should be clean and well lighted, with adequate ventilation and temperature controls. The repackaging area should be out of the mainstream of activity to limit traffic and to minimize disruption of personnel. The facility requirements are different for sterile product repackaging compared to nonsterile repackaging. These differences will be further explained in the subsection on sterile product repackaging.

The packaging area should be constructed of materials that allow for proper cleaning and disinfection of work surfaces. Trash and waste materials should be separated from the repackaging process. Food and beverages should not be allowed in the repackaging area.

The repackaging area should be large enough to eliminate the possibility of cross-contamination of products (repackaging products in the wrong containers, mislabeling, and, in the case of sterile products, microbial and particulate contamination, or any form of putting something in the package that was not intended to be placed in it). Cross-contamination resulting from drug product residue on equipment and work surfaces must be avoided.

Equipment

Equipment used in the manufacture, processing, packaging, or holding of a drug product shall be of appropriate design, adequate size, and location suitable to facilitate operations for its intended use and for cleaning and maintenance.

Equipment shall be constructed so that the surfaces that contact components or drug products shall not be reactive, additive, or absorptive so as to alter the safety, identity, strength, quality, or purity of the drug product beyond the official or other established requirements.

Any substance required for operation, such as lubricants or coolants, shall not come into contact with components or drug products so as to alter the drug product beyond the official or other established requirements.

Equipment must be cleaned, maintained, and sanitized at appropriate intervals to prevent malfunctions or contaminations.

Written procedures shall be established and followed for the cleaning and maintenance of equipment.

Records shall be kept of maintenance, cleaning, sanitizing, and inspection.

Automatic, mechanical, or electronic equipment or other types of equipment, including computers, or related systems that will be used in the drug preparation process, must be routinely calibrated, inspected, or checked according to a written program designed to assure proper performance.

Good manufacturing practices related to use of equipment in the repackaging of pharmaceuticals in hospitals can relate to those practices employed in industry. It is common for hospitals to use various strip packaging machines for single-unit packaging of oral solid medication. Hospitals may also use various liquid pumping devices for delivering oral liquid medications into glass and plastic vials. Different types of closure systems are available; some are automated for capping vials of oral liquids. Sterile product repackaging necessitates the use of laminar air-flow hoods, which should meet or exceed these same standards.

Pharmacists who are responsible for the selection of repackaging equipment must understand the GMP principles that are used to ensure the proper use of that equipment. Equipment that is reliable, safe, and has been proven to provide the type of package expected should be the guiding concern in the selection of such equipment. Equipment that is intended to be reused for other products must be able to be cleaned and disinfected or sanitized prior to the next production run to prevent cross-contamination of product.

Pharmacists who are responsible for selecting equipment must make certain that the products that they intend to repackage with the equipment are compatible with the equipment. This becomes especially important in selecting pumping devices that may come in contact with a variety of chemical solvent systems. In addition, the selection of cleaning solutions and disinfectants and sanitizers must be considered in selecting equipment.

Pharmacists are responsible for ensuring that automated equipment and computer-driven equipment has programs available for testing reliability and calibration of instrumentation.

Control of Components and Drug Product Containers and Closures

Components and drug product containers and closures shall at all times be handled and stored in a manner to prevent contamination. Bagged or boxed components of drug product containers, or closures, shall be stored off the floor and suitably spaced to permit cleaning and inspection.

Most hospital pharmacies are able to meet this requirement without any trouble, since they generally store all drugs and associated materials off the floor.

Drug product containers and closures shall not be reactive, additive, or absorptive so as to alter the safety, identity, strength, quality, or purity of the drug beyond the official or established requirements.

Packaging materials must not only protect the product from the outside, they must be nonreactive with the product placed within them. An excellent example of this problem would be using a plastic container to repackage an oral liquid that uses an organic solvent system. Chances are that the organic solvent system would interact with the container to leach materials out of the container into the solution, form new products from reactions with the container, or have components absorb or adsorb onto the container from the solution.

Container closure systems shall provide adequate protection against foreseeable external factors in storage and use that can cause deterioration or contamination of the drug product.

Most drugs deteriorate as a result of being exposed to oxygen and moisture. Therefore, repackaging materials that can minimize moisture permeation and eliminate other harmful external environmental factors are generally regarded as materials of choice. It is important to note here that it is not only the components that must adhere to these requirements, but the finished package. We discuss specific requirements of repackaging materials and closure systems later in this chapter, when we discuss oral solid repackaging systems.

Production and Process Controls

There shall be written procedures for production and process control designed to assure that the drug products have the identity, strength, quality, and purity that they purport or are represented to possess. Any deviation from the written procedures shall be recorded and justified.

Most hospital pharmacies satisfy this requirement by developing repackaging control cards. These cards outline the products, components, and procedures that are to be followed in repackaging a given drug dosage and dosage form. The procedures should be specific to that product and no other product. It is also generally accepted that a repackaging card is established for each dosage of a given product. If a pharmacy were to repackage dexamethasone tablets in several different strengths, then a card would be needed for each strength. Examples of production control procedures will be presented later in this chapter when we cover policies and procedures.

Actual yields and percentages of theoretical yield shall be determined at the conclusion of each appropriate phase of manufacturing the drug product. Such calculations shall be performed by one person and independently verified by a second person.

Usually, a technician will calculate the theoretical yield of the repackaging of a bulk container of drug, which is then verified by the pharmacist who checks the final product. The pharmacist is generally checking to see how close the actual yield is to the theoretical yield. This is a very important step in verifying the content of the product being repackaged.

Packaging and Labeling Control

There shall be written procedures describing in sufficient detail the receipt, identification, storage, handling, sampling, examination and/or testing of labeling and packaging materials.

Most hospitals do not buy preprinted labels. Most labels that are used for repackaged medications are generated by the hospital pharmacy by typewriters or word processing equipment. Many automated packaging machines have label-printing capabilities built into the equipment. An important point that is highlighted in this requirement is the examination of packaging materials. A visual examination of glass vials for cracks and the inspection of paper-foil laminates for proper adhesiveness are important parameters that the hospital pharmacist can check in a repackaging program.

Labels and other labeling materials for each different drug product, strength, dosage form, or quantity of contents shall be stored separately with suitable identification. Obsolete and outdated labels, labeling, and other packaging materials shall be destroyed.

Most hospital pharmacy packaging programs require labels to be prepared separately from the actual packaging process. Automated packaging machines have the capacity to prepare labels as part of the repackaging process; therefore, this is an extremely important recommendation. Misbranding of repackaged products can occur if different lots of labels are not kept separate from each other. Additional labels should never be prepared. Only the number of labels needed to address the theoretical yield should be prepared. Extra labels must be discarded to prevent misbranding of other products. Labeling is one of the most common areas of error in the repackaging process.

Packaged and labeled products shall be examined during finishing operations to provide assurance that the containers and packages in the lot have the same label.

This process is always completed as a final check by the hospital pharmacist.

To assure that a drug product meets applicable standards of identity, strength, quality and purity at the time of use, it shall bear an expiration date determined by appropriate stability testing. Expiration dates shall be related to any storage conditions stated on the labeling.

Most hospital pharmacies do not routinely conduct stability studies on repackaged medications. Many pharmacies do not have the resources or the expertise to conduct such studies. The FDA has made provisional expiration dating for drugs whose stability is unknown. These guidelines are discussed later in this chapter.

Holding and Distribution

Written procedures describing the warehousing of drug products shall be established and followed. They shall include: quarantine of drug products before release by the quality control unit; storage of drug products under appropriate conditions of temperature, humidity, and light so that the identity, strength, quality, and purity of the drug products are not affected.

This requirement is generally met by the conditions that prevail in most hospital pharmacies. Pharmacists should have in writing the conditions under which drugs will be stored. If conditions differ for repackaged medications, those conditions should be noted in writing. This could be in the form of a policy and procedure.

A system of quarantine should be developed for medications that are repackaged in remote areas of the pharmacy or on off shifts and cannot be checked immediately. This type of system might require affixing a quarantine sticker to the finished product prior to its final check and release.

Laboratory Controls

For each batch of drug product, there shall be appropriate laboratory determination of satisfactory conformance to final specifications for the drug product, including the identity and strength of each active ingredient, prior to release.

There shall be appropriate laboratory testing, as necessary, of each batch of drug product required to be free of objectionable microorganisms.

There shall be a written testing program designed to assess the stability characteristics of drug products. The results of such stability testing shall be used in determining appropriate storage conditions and expiration dates.

Most of these conditions are never met in the hospital pharmacy. There are provisions for assigning short expiration dating to products of unknown stability. Some hospital pharmacies that repackage sterile products do engage in some limited sterility testing programs. However, these programs are not intended to provide statistical significance to their results. The tests are intended as a gross review of sterility.

Records and Reports

Records shall be maintained for all components, drug product containers, closures, and labeling for at least 1 year after the expiration date.

A written record of major equipment cleaning, maintenance and use shall be included in individual equipment logs.

Batch production and control records shall be prepared for each batch of drug product produced and shall include complete information relating to the production and control of each batch. These records shall include:

(a) Dates of production,
(b) Identification of each component used in the manufacturing process,
(c) Identification of equipment used,
(d) Weights and measures of the components used,
(e) In-process and laboratory controls,
(f) Statement of actual yield,
(g) Complete labeling control records including samples of the labels,
(h) Description of the drug product containers and closures, and
(i) Identification of the persons performing each step of the process.

Most pharmacists would agree that keeping accurate records of the repackaging process is extremely important for several reasons. First, records may be needed to determine the components that make up the final product in the event that a recall of one or more of the components occurs. A second reason to keep complete and accurate records of the repackaging process is to provide an in-process accountability and a final product accountability system. Records of repackaging serve as an important component of the quality control process. Often errors may be detected by comparing lot numbers of individual components and the log sheet of the components used. Weights and measures become important pieces of information if actual yield does not closely approximate theoretical yield. Finally, records and reports are important from a historical perspective to determine if the institution's repackaging program is efficient. Examination of packaging and waste records can assist the pharmacist in adjusting the quantity produced. This review identifies drugs that can be repackaged in batches and those that should be repackaged extemporaneously.

Good manufacturing practices should form the foundation of a repackaging program. Although not always directly applicable to the institutional pharmacist, good manufacturing practices do support many of the specific guidelines that have been established for institutionally based repackaging programs. Pharmacists wishing to modify existing repackaging programs should keep in mind the tenets of good manufacturing practices.

SPECIFIC GUIDELINES FOR REPACKAGING PROGRAMS

As mentioned earlier, the ASHP technical assistance bulletin on single-unit and unit dose packages of drugs states that drug packages must fulfill four basic functions: (1) protect their contents from deleterious environmental effects, (2) protect their contents from deterioration resulting from handling, (3) identify their contents completely and precisely, (4) permit their contents to be used quickly, easily, and safely.[10]

Repackaging Materials

Repackaging materials and the package itself must possess the physical characteristics to protect the drug from deleterious external elements such as light, heat, moisture, air, and, in the case of sterile products, microbial contaminants. The material must not deteriorate during the shelf-life of the drug. Packages should be lightweight and made of materials that do not interact with the dosage form. In this context, repackaging materials should not absorb, adsorb, or chemically interact with the drug. Materials that are recyclable or biodegradable are preferred over those that are not.

Packages should be constructed so that they do not deteriorate with normal handling. They should be easy to open and use, and their use should not require any additional training or experience. Packages should allow for inspection of their contents by the person administering the medication, unless the pharmaceutical properties of the drug prevent its exposure to light.

The *United States Pharmacopeia XXII* defines containers and closures based upon the degree of protection of the contents.[13] These are defined as follows:

> Light-resistant containers protect the drug from the effects of incident light by virtue of the specific properties of the material of which it is composed, including any coating applied to it. If protection from light is required, a clear and colorless or a translucent container may be made light-resistant by means of an opaque enclosure.
>
> Well-closed containers protect the contents from extraneous solids and from loss of the drug under ordinary or customary conditions of handling, shipment, storage, and distribution.
>
> Tight containers protect their contents from contamination by extraneous liquids, solids, or vapors, from loss of the drug, and from effervescence, deliquescence, or evaporation under ordinary or customary conditions of handling, shipment, storage, and distribution.
>
> Hermetic containers are impervious to air or any other gas under ordinary or customary conditions of handling, shipment, storage, and distribution.

The *USP XXII* also establishes guidelines for assigning expiration dates for oral solids and liquids that are repackaged based on the moisture permeability of the final package. Therefore, the type of repackaging materials and the closure system chosen for a given dosage form can affect the expiration date of the final product.[14]

> An official dosage form is required to bear on its label an expiration date assigned for the particular formulation and package of the article. This date limits the time during which the product may be dispensed or used. Because the expiration date stated on the manufacturer's or distributor's package has been determined for the drug in that particular package and may not be applicable to the product where it has been repackaged in a different container, repackaged drugs dispensed pursuant to a prescription are exempt from this label requirement. It is necessary, therefore, that other precautions be taken by the dispenser to preserve the strength, quality and purity of drugs that are repackaged for ultimate distribution or sale to patients.
>
> The following guidelines and requirements are applicable where official dosage forms are repackaged into single-unit or unit-dose containers or mnemonic packs for dispensing pursuant to prescription.
>
> Labeling—It is the responsibility of the dispenser, taking into account the nature of the drug repackaged, the characteristics of the containers, and the storage conditions to which the article may be subjected, to determine a suitable beyond-use date to be placed on the label.

The USP clearly points out that it is the responsibility of the pharmacist to know the type and quality of the packaging materials and the associated closure systems employed in developing the final package. The USP further states:

> Such a date is not later than the expiration date of the original package. In the absence of stability data to the contrary, such date should not exceed (1) 25% of the remaining time between the date of repackaging and the expiration date on the original manufacturer's bulk container, or (2) a six month period from the date the drug is repackaged, whichever is earlier.

The monograph for meeting the criteria for a single-unit container for capsules and tablets states: "To permit an informed judgment regarding the suitability of the packaging for a particular type of product, the following procedure and classification scheme are provided for evaluating the moisture-permeation characteristics of single-unit and unit dose containers." A complete description of the moisture permeation test is provided in the quality control section of this chapter.

The classification scheme derived from this test procedure designates the package types as class A, least amount of moisture permeation; class B, more moisture permeation; class C, more moisture than class B; and class D, highest amount of moisture permeation.

Manufacturers of repackaging materials and repackaging equipment describe their products based on the type of package that is achievable—class A, B, C, or D—with class A being the best and class D the worst. It is generally regarded that class A or class B packages are needed to extend the stability of a repackaged product beyond the few days following repackaging.

The package types most often found in institutional practice include those used for oral solids, oral liquids, injectables, respiratory medications, and topical medications.

Oral Solids

Oral solids may be packaged in blister packages or in pouch packages. *Blister packages* are composed of an opaque and nonreflective backing that is usually used for printing or labeling. The backing should be easily peelable from the blister portion of the package, and, is generally composed of paper or a foil/paper laminate. Backing that is made entirely of paper may vary in thicknesses from light (about the thickness of construction paper) to heavy (about the thickness of light cardboard).

The blister portion is composed of a dome or bubble of transparent material that is flat bottomed. The transparent material is a plastic. The plastic may be either high-density or low-density polyethylene or a combination of polyethylene densities and polypropylenes. Polyvinyl chloride (PVC) has also been used as a blister package plastic.

Blister packages are more rigid than the pouch package and therefore may protect the contents of the container better. However, blister packages do not lend themselves to automated repackaging systems found in institutional practice. Automated blister packaging is generally confined to the pharmaceutical industry. However, blister packages are used for manually operated repackaging programs in institutional practice.

Pouch packages have one or both sides composed of an opaque, nonreflective surface intended for printing. This surface is generally composed of a paper/foil laminate. The opposing side of the pouch can be made of the same paper/foil laminate, a paper/foil/polyethylene laminate, or a transparent polyethylene-coated cellophane.

The pouch package is probably the most popular repackage used mainly for batch repackaging. The pouch package lends itself to relatively inexpensive automated machinery applications in institutional practice. Figure 21-2 shows examples of blister and pouch packaging.

Oral Liquids

Oral liquids are always repackaged into rigid or semirigid containers. The most popular containers include vials, cups, and oral syringes.

Glass or plastic vials are the most frequently used containers for oral liquids. They are composed of the glass or plastic reservoir and a closure system that is generally a rubber stopper or a screw cap made of plastic or metal. The screw cap is generally lined with a paper/vinyl inner cap. The rubber stopper is frequently made of butyl rubber with an aluminum or plastic overseal to hold the stopper in place.

Some plastic and glass vials use a paper lined aluminum foil cap as a closure system. The paper/aluminum foil cap is affixed to the vial by crimping the top over a lip in the vial. Wheaton Laboratories provide both glass and plastic vials and closure systems. (A complete listing of manufacturers can be found at the end of this chapter in Appendix 21-A.)

BAXA Corporation manufactures a plastic oral liquid vial with a unique closure system that employs a plastic ball that fits into a small filling hole in the bottom of the vial. The ball provides a friction fit to prevent the escape of liquid from the container. The top of the vial has a paper/foil laminate pulloff tab that allows for labeling or just serves as a tear-off seal.

Oral syringes are similar to injectable syringes except that they are not sterile and will not accept a needle. They are specifically designed not to accept a needle to prevent accidental injection into the patient. Oral syringes are composed of either a glass barrel and a plastic/rubber plunger or a plastic barrel and a plastic plunger.

Plastic cups are infrequently used to repackage liquid medications. They are mentioned here because they are the only liquid containers that lend themselves to automated filling, sealing, and labeling machinery. Machinery may be used for filling and sealing vials and syringes, but these are considered manual, not automated, processes.

Glass containers are the reservoir most commonly used in repackaging, usually in the form of glass vials; however, glass syringes are also used for oral liquids. Glass is frequently chosen for the following four factors:

1. *Inertness.* Although the alkalinity of glass can sometimes present problems with solutions that are pH sensitive, glass in comparison to other packaging materials is relatively inert and free from incompatibilities. Although there are four different types of glass, type I and type II glass are the types generally used for repackaging.[15]
2. *Visibility.* The clarity of glass allows for product recognition. Amber-colored glass is generally used for repackaging, which prevents recognition of solutions based on color; however, volume can be seen.
3. *Stability.* Glass does not deteriorate under general handling and storage conditions encountered in institutional practice. Glass is also considered environmentally safe.
4. *FDA acceptance.* Glass containers are generally the containers against which all other containers are judged.[16]

Plastics began to be used for repackaging pharmaceuticals in the 1980's. The use of plastics was slow at first because of the many potential and actual problems associated with these materials. Autian[17-19] has divided these problems into five broad categories: (1) permeation, (2) leaching, (3) sorption, (4) chemical reaction, and (5) alteration or stability of the material.

It is important to point out that many of these problems can be avoided by knowing the composition of the plastic and the chemical and physical properties of the liquid being repackaged. Examples of oral liquid packages are shown in figure 21-3.

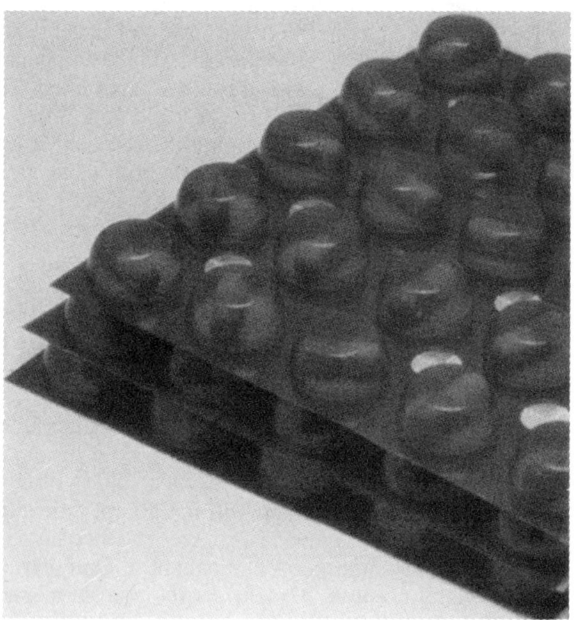

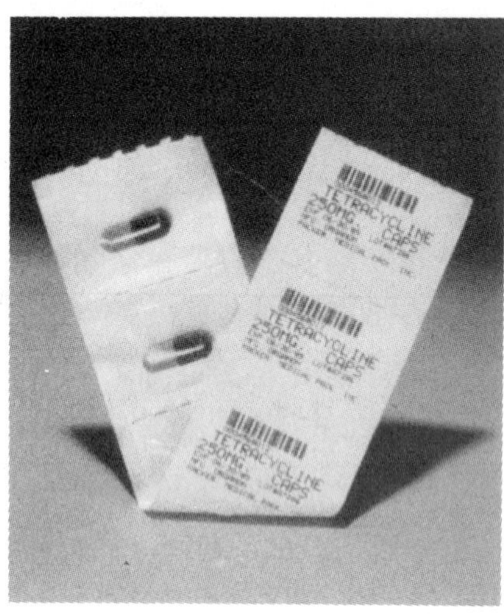

Figure 21-2. Types of oral solid packaging. Two of the general types of oral solid packaging are represented by the pouch package on the right and the blister package on the left.

Injectables

Repackaging of injectable medications requires sterile, pyrogen-free containers. Glass syringes, glass, empty evacuated vials, and plastic syringes are the containers used for repackaging sterile injectables. Intravenous admixture systems are discussed in chapter 19 of this handbook; therefore, this discussion of injectable repackaging materials is limited to syringes and vials.

Glass syringes are composed of type I glass and have a rubber/plastic plunger. The tip, which accepts the needle, is ground glass to allow a friction fit of the needle hub. Glass syringes are available in 1 mL, 3 mL, 5 mL, and 10 mL sizes from Becton-Dickenson.

Plastic syringes are available in clear plastic and amber plastic from several manufacturers. These syringes range in size from 0.5 mL to 60 mL.

A third type of syringe is a combination of glass/plastic and rubber. Smith and Nephew manufactures a syringe that has a detached plunger. It allows for a different method of filling, which is discussed later in this chapter.

Empty sterile glass vials are available as type I glass in 2 mL, 5 mL, 10 mL, and 30 mL sizes. Most of these vials have grey butyl rubber stoppers with aluminum overseals as their closure system, are terminally steam sterilized (sterilized after they have been assembled), and contain few drops of residual water. Figure 21-4 shows examples of the various containers used to repackage injectable medications.

Respiratory Medications

Some pharmacists repackage medications that are intended to be used in respiratory treatments. These medications are generally injected into devices that aerosolize the liquid for delivery to the lungs. Respiratory medications that require repackaging have packaging requirements similar to those of injectable medications. The container should be sterile and free from pyrogens. If a syringe is employed to contain the respiratory medication, it should not accept a needle in order to prevent the possibility of injecting the medication into the patient. This is the same premise used in developing oral syringes, which do not accept a needle. Respiratory syringes are available from Smith and Nephew in clear and amber glass in 3 mL and 5 mL sizes.

Topical Medications

Topical medications that are in ointment or cream vehicles can be repackaged into glass or plastic jars. Topical creams and gels that are intended for administration into the vagina may be repackaged into vaginal syringes specifically designed for this purpose and are available in a 5 mL size from BAXA Corporation. These syringes can be purchased with a tube adapter to fit almost any size tube of ointment or cream.

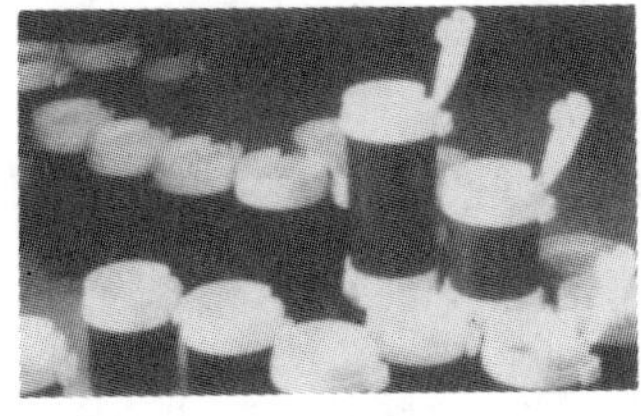

A

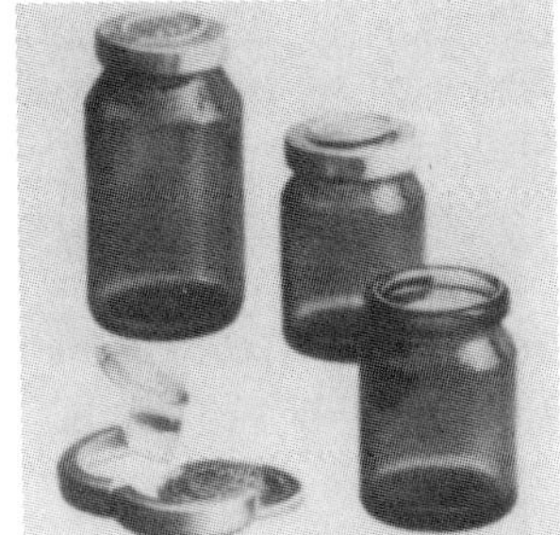

B

D

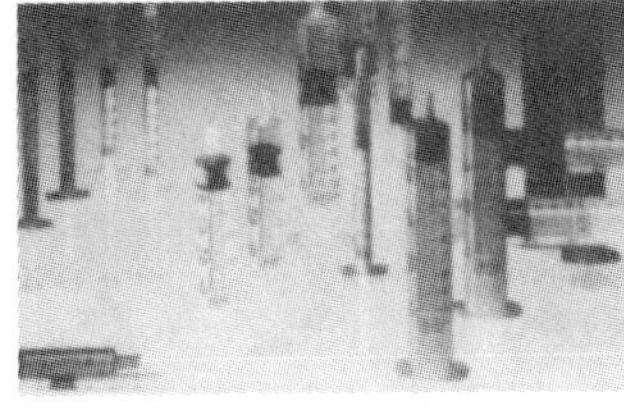

C

Figure 21-3. Some examples of oral liquid packages are represented by: (A) Flip-top plastic vials, (B) Wheaton glass vials with crimp-on lids, (C) Plastic oral syringes, and (D) Baxa Exacta-Med system vials.

Repackaging Equipment and Filling Devices

The two most important components in ensuring a quality package are the packaging materials and the closure system. The pharmacist who is engaged in repackaging must strive to make the final package as nearly perfect as possible. If the highest quality materials available are used for the package without proper equipment to ensure a quality seal, the final product will not satisfy GMP's. Conversely, with use of the best equipment available and poor materials, the final package will fail.

Most of the repackaging equipment that is available to the institutional practitioner can be categorized as manual, semiautomated, or fully automated. We explore these systems as they pertain to repackaging of oral solids, oral liquids, and injectables. One point to keep in mind is that the more manual the system, the more variability is introduced in the package quality and the lesser chance the product has of attaining a class A or class B rating.

Oral Solids

Oral solids are the most commonly repackaged medication. A greater number of repackaging systems are available for repackaging oral solids than for any of the other

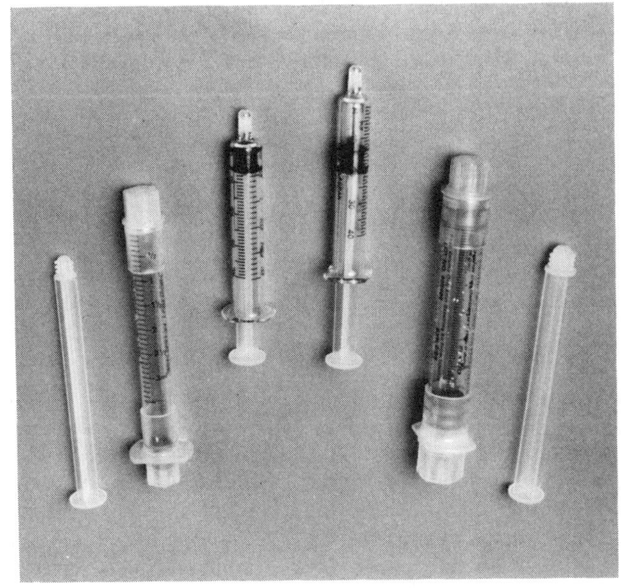

Figure 21-4. These are some examples of glass and plastic syringes that are available for packaging injectable medications.

dosage form. The reason for the variety of oral solid repackaging systems is that the majority of doses dispensed in institutions are oral solids, and oral solids do not present the contamination and cleaning problems posed by liquids and injectables.

Manually operated oral solid repackaging systems use either a pouch package or a blister package. Each of these two systems can be further subdivided into pouch packages that use heat sealing or adhesive sealing, and blister packages that use heat sealing or adhesive sealing. As a rule, adhesive systems produce class B, C, or D packages; heat sealing systems generally produce class A, B, C, or D packages.

Manual pouch repackaging systems use a thin mill plastic bag (usually polyvinyl chloride), which is clear or made of light-resistant materials. The tablet or capsule is dropped into the bag, and the bag opening is sealed with an adhesive. This system provides a class D package. Manual pouch systems can also use a heat sealer in the form of a hot knife blade to seal the end of the plastic bag. This provides a better seal; however, the package usually remains a class D package (mainly because of the packaging material). A label is typed on regular label stock and affixed to the bag. This system is generally reserved for extemporaneous packaging.

Manual blister repackaging systems use a plastic blister package that is made of a clear polyvinyl chloride or a polyvinyl chloride/low-density polyethylene plastic laminate. The blisters or bubbles come in various sizes, depending on the type (tablet or capsule) or size (large or small) of the product being repackaged. The blisters can be filled on a tabletop or placed in specially designed holders to cradle the package. Once the blisters are filled with the drug, a backing made of paper, foil/paper, or vinyl/foil/paper is attached to the blister by removing a protective covering on adhesive strip and applying pressure to the blister and the backing material. Blister packages that are to be heat sealed use a similar system to the adhesive system; however, the backing and blister are heated in what best can be described as a waffle-making iron. The heat seal press places heat and pressure on the backing material, while the blisters remain protected by the well-like device they sit in.

The adhesive blister package can create a class B, C, or D package. The heat seal blister system can create a class A, B, C, or D package. An example of a blister packaging system is shown in figure 21-5.

Automated oral solid repackaging systems have been available to the institutional practitioner since the 1960's. Today's machines represent the latest technological advancements in computerized labeling, hot stamp printing, and mechanical simplicity.

Automated oral solid repackaging systems, sometimes called "unit dose strip packaging machines," operate in basically the same fashion. They all produce a pouch package that is made up of two polyethylene/foil/paper laminates or a polyethylene/foil/paper laminate and a polyethylene/cellulose laminate. Tablets or capsules are manually fed into a wheel that drops the dose into a pouch that is formed by two heated wheels, and the product is sealed. Individual packages are separated by a serrated knife blade, which perforates the strip of pouches as they pass out of the machine. The polyethylene/foil/paper is imprinted with the required information by means of a stencil/ink system (wet or hot stamp) or a computer-generated printing system that is tied into the packaging machine. The printing process occurs before the dose is dropped into the pouch.

Automated repackaging machines can package from 60 to 120 doses of a single drug per minute. A device can be attached to the top of the automated strip packaging machine to eliminate the need for an operator to feed tablets and capsules into the wheel. The device is called a Robotic Solid Oral Unit Dose Feeder and is made by Econodose, Inc. (see figure 21-6).

One automated strip packaging system does not really fit the mold of the other automated systems discussed, Baxter's ATC 212 system. The ATC 212 system is a totally automated, microprocessor-based system used to manage and dispense and package patient oral solid drug orders processed through the pharmacy. It consists of two parts: the ATC machine itself and the computer that drives the machine.

The upper portion of the ATC machine has the capacity to bulk store and individually package up to 212 different tablets and capsules (see figure 21-7).

Each storage canister is specifically calibrated to the unique dimensions of the particular drug product it dispenses. Because the working mechanisms of each of the canisters are tailored specifically to the product it handles, inadvertent breakage and filling incorrect quantities of tablets or capsules is prevented.

The lower portion of the ATC machine contains the machinery where each drug item is individually strip packaged and labeled. The ATC 212 system produces sealed, completely labeled, unit dose packages in a continuous strip that can be sorted by medication or by administration time. Label information may be tailored to meet specific needs of each institution.

The ATC 212 system can be operated in two basic modes: stand-alone and mainframe. In the stand-alone mode, the ATC 212 is driven by a personal computer. If the pharmacy has access to a mainframe computer, the ATC 212 system can be operated by interfacing the patient medication information from the mainframe system through the personal computer.

The ATC 212 system packages 25 doses per minute (which is slower than other packaging machines). However, it can package up to 212 different drugs without requiring special setup and cleanup operations, whereas the other automated devices can package only one drug at a time.

Oral Liquid Medications

Oral liquid repackaging systems can be divided into two categories, manual and automated. Some semiautomated systems are basically manual systems that have some automated fluid delivery system associated with the filling process.

Manual repackaging systems for oral liquids can be divided into those that use a glass or plastic vial as the reservoir for the liquid medication and those that use a glass or plastic syringe. Manual repackaging systems that require vials have three different closure systems: screw cap vials, vials that have permanently affixed tops and small fill holes for medication, and vials that require the addition of a cap that must be crimped. An operator uses syringes, burettes, pipettes, and graduates to measure and administer the liquid into the vial.

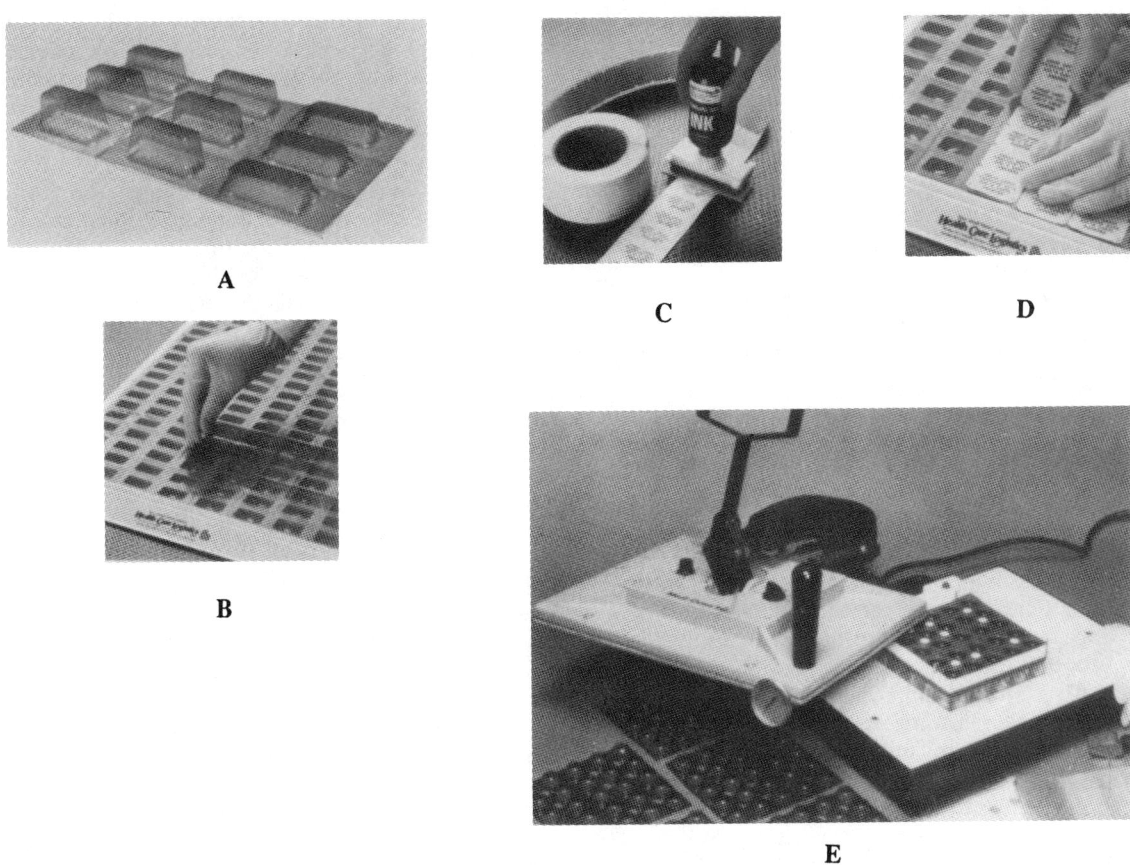

Figure 21-5. Here are two examples of blister packaging systems. An example of a pressure-sensitive blister system is shown in A-D: (A) Examples of blister package, (B) Medication being placed into blister package wells, (C) Backing of the blister package being imprinted with label, (D) Pressure-sensitive backing being applied to the blister package. A heat and pressure system is shown in E.

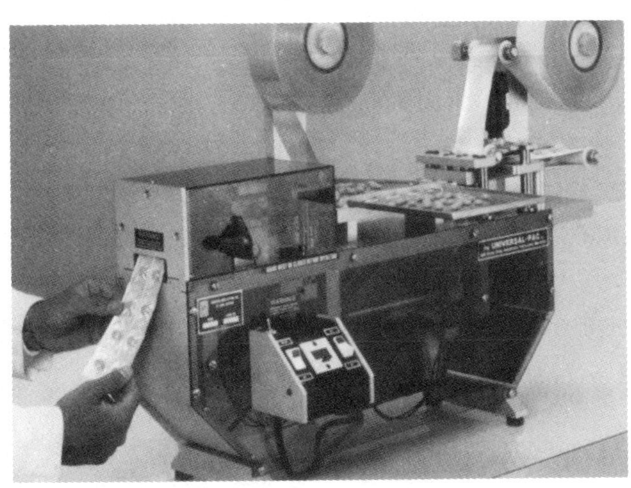

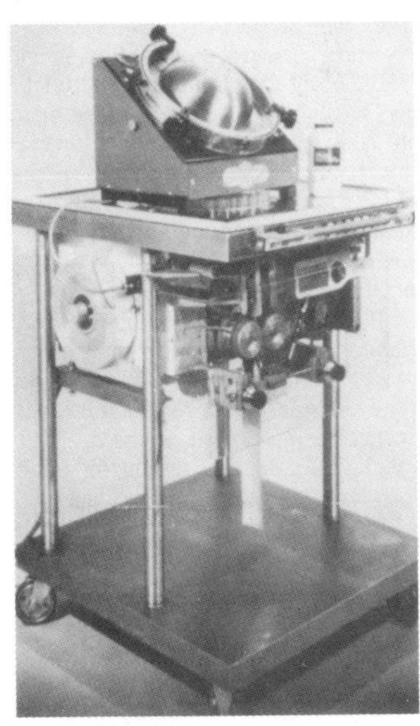

Figure 21-6. On the left is a picture of a strip-packaging machine used to package oral solid dosage forms. On the right is a picture of a strip-packaging machine with a robotic head that automatically feeds tablets and capsules to the packaging machine.

Manual systems for oral liquids that have syringes as their final container may employ one of two methods of repackaging. The first method relies on the operator transferring the liquid to a suitable vessel (such as a beaker) and withdrawing the liquid into the syringe. An ordinary syringe can be used for this process if the number of dosage units is relatively small. However, many pharmacists choose to use a Cornwall syringe (often referred to as a "magic syringe") to speed the filling process. The Cornwall syringe method also offers greater reliability in fill volumes, since the syringe is preset with the appropriate volume to dispense.

There are also preset and precalibrated systems that use a burette instead of a syringe. These systems have been popular in laboratory applications in which liquid chemicals are repeatedly added to reaction vessels. One dispensing burette is specifically designed to dispense liquid medications. The system is called the Versa-fil 120 and is made by Wheaton Laboratories (see figure 21-8).

In the second method, the operator attaches a specially designed cap to the bulk bottle that allows a syringe to be introduced into the bottle; the contents are then withdrawn via the syringe by inverting the bottle (see figure 21-9).

Semiautomated systems are manual systems that use some piece of automated equipment as part of the filling or sealing process. Semiautomated systems generally offer greater consistency and reliability in the final product by ensuring an accurate fill volume and, in some cases, a better closure seal (in the case of crimped vials).

Like manual systems, semiautomated systems can be grouped into systems that use a vial as the drug reservoir and those that use a syringe as the final container. Because the semiautomated filling machines (pumps) can be used with either container, we will consider the differences in these systems based on the type of pump used. Pumps can be subdivided into syringe pumps and peristaltic pumps.

Syringe pumps get their name not from filling syringes but from using a syringe as a measuring and filling chamber prior to expelling the liquid into the final container (either a syringe or a vial). Syringe pumps operate on the same principle as do Cornwall syringes. However, syringe pumps use a mechanical process for drawing back and pushing forward on the plunger. The volume to be dispensed into the container is preset based upon the draw-back setting and the type of syringe selected for the machine. Burron Medical manufactures a syringe pump fluid dispensing system called the Multi-Ad pump (see figure 21-10).

Peristaltic pumps get their name from the form of pumping action that they employ in delivering fluid. These pumps use peristaltic action, which is created by a series of roller wheels being pulled across a length of tubing. As each wheel passes over the tubing, the tubing is crimped and a small volume of fluid is forced along its pathway down the tubing (see figure 21-11). Peristaltic pumps offer several advantages over syringe pumps. These advantages include a faster rate of delivery for larger volumes (10 mL and above) and the ability to deliver fairly viscous liquids.

One of the major problems encountered with peristaltic pumps is calibration. If a large number of units are to be produced, the pump will probably require frequent recalibration. Syringe pumps do not experience this problem to the same extent as peristaltic pumps. In addition, syringe pumps are more accurate and reliable for delivering fluid volumes of less than 10 mL.

As with most mechanical devices, these pumps come with several convenience factors. Most of the pumps display the volume of fluid being dispensed and the number of dispensing cycles (number of units filled), fill cycle times can be set automatically with rest periods established between each fill, and alarms are available to alert the operator to an empty container. Pumps also are furnished with foot pedal actuators that allow the operator to control the delivery/rest cycle of the fill.

Two *fully automated* liquid repackaging machines are available to institutional pharmacists (see figure 21-12). Both machines use similar principles in filling, sealing, and labeling the medication. They use plastic cups as the fluid reservoir, and the sealing system is a polyvinyl/foil/paper overseal. The overseal acts as the label stock, and the labeling is directly printed on the seal as the machine fills and seals the product in much the same way as the automated oral solid packaging machines. The systems employ a peristaltic pump that pumps liquid from a fluid reservoir into each cup as the cups pass by the filling orifice. A predetermined amount of fluid is dispensed into each container. The overseal is attached using heat and pressure until a strong bond is made between the cup and the polyvinyl/foil/paper seal. The individual finished packages are separated when the machine cuts the overseal paper between cups. Both machines are equipped with a variety of sensors that detect and signal problems associated with the fill cups, sealing foil, printing tape, and general machine failures. These machines are capable of producing 20-32 units per minute. Their application is packaging liquids with volumes of 15 mL, 30 mL, or 45 mL. The final package produced by these machines can attain a class A rating.

Injectables

The institutional pharmacist does not have available a fully automated system for repackaging injectable medications. Injectable medications must be packaged manually or with a semiautomated process similar to those processes used to repackage oral liquid medications.

The manual system currently employed for filling injectable medications into syringes uses a sterile Cornwall-like syringe in a metal pipetting holder and an automatic double valve to form the basis of this pressure-fill system (see figure 21-13). Drugs from ampules or vials are individually filtered and pooled under aseptic conditions in sterile, empty evacuated containers. The container storing the injection to be packaged is connected to the inlet port of the automatic valve by sterile tubing. A sterile disposable stopcock is affixed to the male Luer port of the automatic valve to convert it, at right angles, to the necessary female Luer filling port. The filling syringe is calibrated to the desired delivery volume, plus any additional volume that may be necessary to overfill the administration syringe (repackaged product). Sterile disposable syringes are placed on the stopcock port and filled. The filled syringe is then removed from the filling port, and a sterile disposable tip is affixed to the hub.[20]

Semiautomated systems use a similar approach to the manual system. The only difference is that pumps are used in place of the Cornwall syringe. This is very similar to the progression seen in oral liquid repackaging. In fact, the same pumps used to repackage oral liquid medications are used to repackage injectables. The only difference is in the

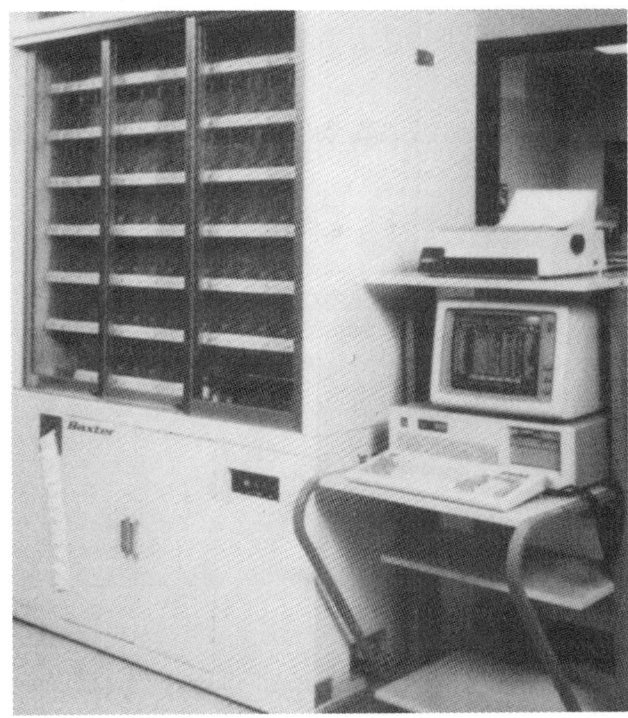

Figure 21-7. An example of Baxters' ATC 212 machine. Notice the drug storage canisters on the top of the machine. The strip packaging comes out of the bottom of the machine.

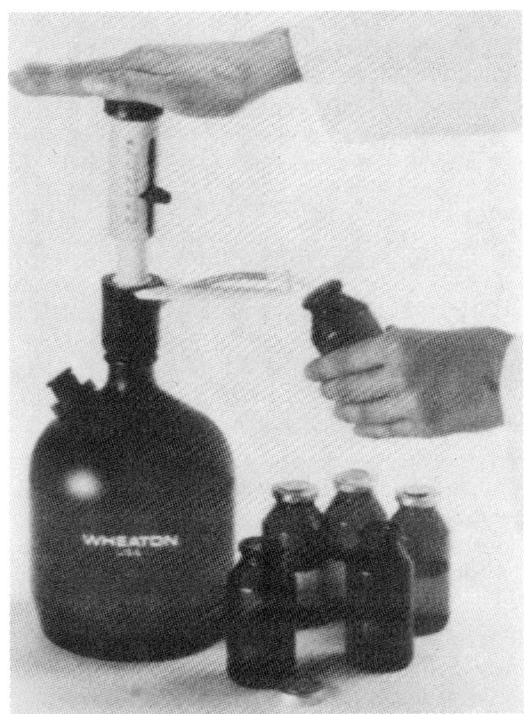

Figure 21-8. A Wheaton pipetting system for filling oral liquids into glass vials. A Wheaton vial is featured in this example.

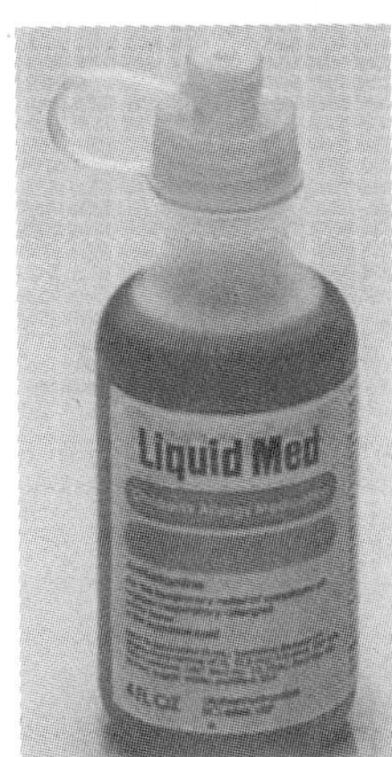

Figure 21-9. This is a bottle of medication which has been fitted with a Baxa special cap. The cap will flip open to accept an oral syringe. The oral syringe is filled by inverting the bottle and withdrawing the contents into the syringe.

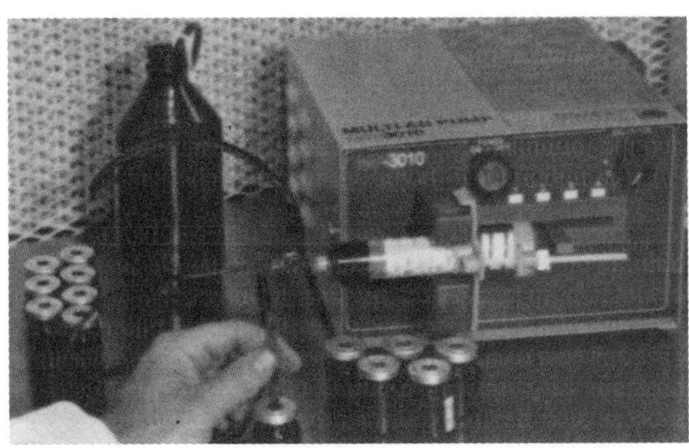

Figure 21-10. This is an example of Burron's Multi-AD syringe pump. Here the pump is shown delivering an oral liquid into a presealed Wheaton glass vial.

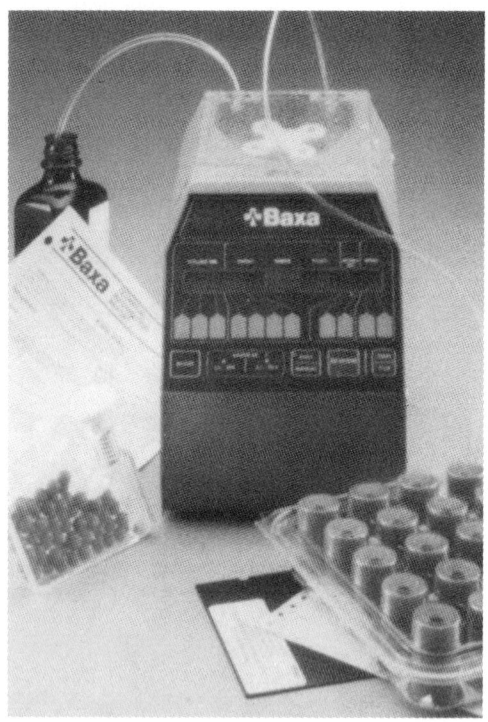

Figure 21-11. This is an example of a peristaltic pump. Notice the pumping chamber on the top of the pump is equipped with four roller heads. This pump is delivering an oral liquid into Baxa Exacta-Med containers.

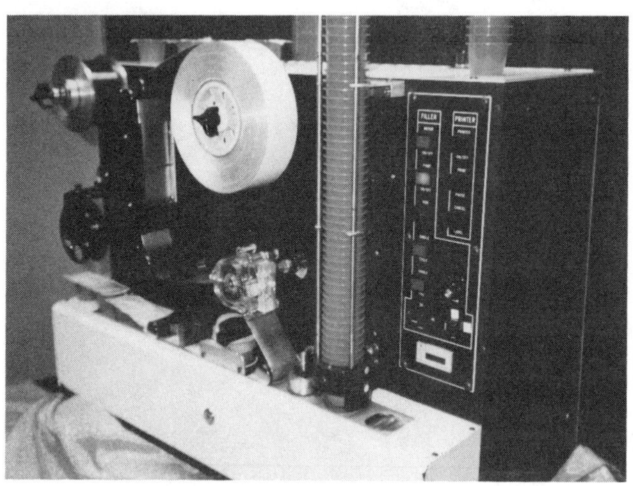

Figure 21-12. This is a Medical Packaging's automated liquid packaging machine. Notice the plastic fill cups that are in the front of the machine. The large roll of foil/paper is used to seal the top of the cup once medication has been pumped into it.

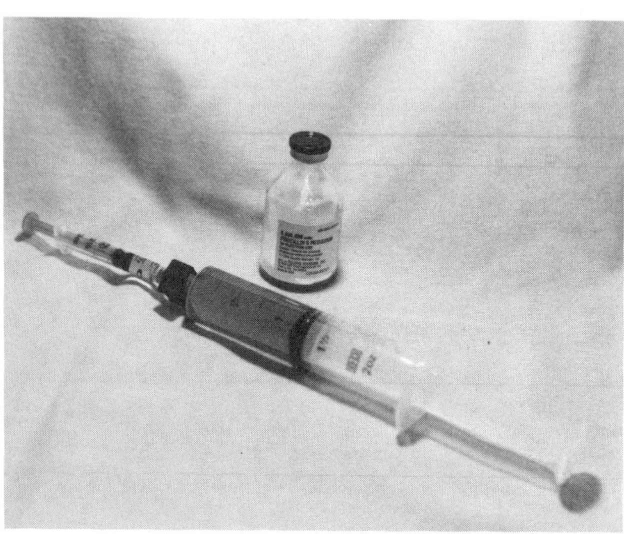

Figure 21-13. This is a front fill manual method for filling syringes.

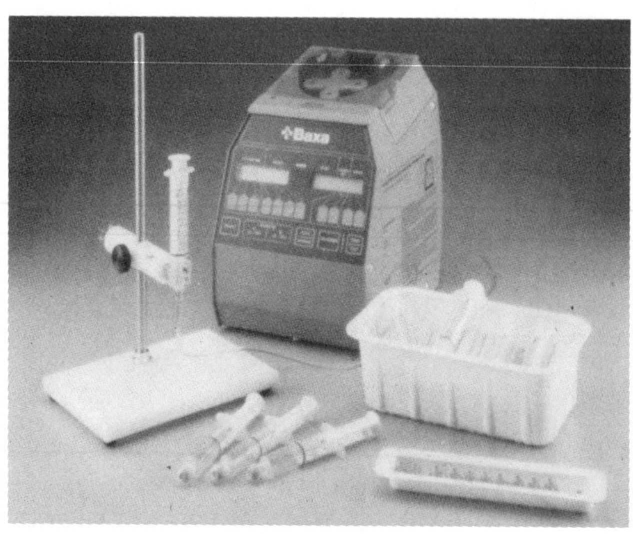

Figure 21-14. This is an example of a sterile filling system that is using a peristaltic pump to fill the syringe. The same peristaltic pump can be used to fill oral liquids. The tubing that is being used to fill these syringes must be sterile.

type of tubing that is used with the pump. Injectable drugs require sterile tubing, whereas oral liquid repackaging requires nonsterile tubing. (Figure 21-14 shows an example of a sterile syringe filling operation.)

Labels and Labeling Systems

Considerable technical advances have occurred in the area of labeling since the first edition of this handbook was published, in part as a result of the technical achievements that have been realized by applying computers to institutional practice. In particular, the personal computer has greatly improved the quality and efficiency of the label production process.

Before we discuss some of the technical achievements in label production, we need to review the labeling requirements for repackaged medications. Current Federal labeling requirements must be adhered to, with reference to the ASHP technical assistance bulletin on single unit and unit dose packages of drugs.[10] (See chapter 9, Appendix 9-B, which contains the text of this ASHP technical bulletin.)

The technical bulletin states that the control number or the lot number should appear on the package. The lot number is the number assigned by the repackager to the dosage form being repackaged. The lot number is often generated from the date the product is repackaged, and an additional number or letter is added to designate the order in which the dosage form was repackaged that day. An example of this type of assignment system is as follows:

Lot Number: A123091

This product was the first product that was repackaged on December 30, 1991. Another example would be as follows:

Lot Number: A913012

This product was made on the same day as the above date, but the date is displayed backwards.

It is important to point out that the lot numbering system should be simple to use. The more complicated the system, the greater the likelihood for errors to occur in assigning the lot number and in interpreting the lot number.

Technical Achievements

As mentioned earlier, the widespread use and availability of personal computers has dramatically changed the way labels are prepared. In the past, typewriters, memory card typewriters, paper stencils, adjustable printing plates, and preprinted labels obtained from specialty houses or commercial printers were the tools by which labels were obtained for repackaged products. Today, most of that has changed. Preprinted labels may have some benefit in certain applications; however, the majority of labels are customized and are printed by computer using a variety of programs and printers.

Record Keeping

Maintaining accurate and complete records of the repackaging process is a necessity mandated through standards of practice and governmental regulation. A good record-keeping system can facilitate the maximal use of technical support personnel in a repackaging operation by providing a focal point for a quality assurance program. Accurate records can assist the manager in inventory management and in monitoring the efficiency of the repackaging process.[21,22]

Record-keeping systems characterized by index cards, notebooks, and various filing systems are fast becoming a thing of the past. Like labeling systems, record-keeping systems are now becoming computerized. Computer programs provide easier and often quicker access to information. Computer record-keeping programs provide more flexibility in the quantity and type of information that can be gathered to form production reports.

The types of records that should be kept for a repackaging program include formulation records, prepackaging records, and daily repackaging logs.

Formulation Record

This file serves to provide pertinent information to the repackaging technician about container type, labeling information, stability, processing equipment, and hazardous materials information on a drug-by-drug basis. An example of the type of information contained in this file system for cloxacillin sodium would be:

Drug: Cloxacillin Sodium
Strength: 250 mg
Dosage Form: Capsule
Packaging Material: Poly/Foil to poly/foil
Equipment: MPL strip packager
Precautions: This is an antibiotic. The operator should use gloves and mask during production. Expiration Dating: Use FDA Guidelines

A Sample Label:

Cloxacillin Sodium
250 mg
Lot number:
Expiration date:

Prepackaging Record

This record is also filed on a drug-specific basis. The file should contain the following information:

- Name of the drug
- Strength
- Date the repackaging occurred
- Original manufacturer's data:
  - Manufacturer's name
  - Lot number
  - Expiration date
- Repackager's data:
  - Lot number assigned
  - Expiration date assigned
  - Quantity repackaged
- Signature:
  - Person packaging
  - Person checking

This record is drug specific to allow several batches to be entered into this record. Therefore, this particular record would contain information on all the repackaging runs of a given drug (see figure 21-15).

It is important to point out that the repackaging record and the formulation record can be combined into one record for a given drug.

Daily Repackaging Log

This record serves to list on a daily basis all repackaging activity. The log is used to track production records for a given shift or person and should contain the following information:

Drug/strength/form repackaged
Lot number assigned
Quantity packaged
Extemporaneous or batch
Person repackaging

This record is not a necessity, but many pharmacies find it helpful in tracking daily activities. It can serve an important function as a lot number assignment recording form, if the lot number is determined by the date and order in which the product was repackaged.

Quality Control and End Product Testing

A well-defined quality control and end product testing program is essential to ensure the continuous production of high-quality repackaged medications. Since many products and several technicians and pharmacists may be involved in repackaging medications, strict adherence to the principles of good manufacturing practices is essential to a program of quality control.

The control of quality takes on a bimodal function in the repackaging process. These controls include in-process controls and end product testing.

In process controls include written procedures, formal training of the operators of the system, maintenance of equipment, evaluation of the dosage form prior to packaging, and checkpoints during the process.[23]

Written Procedures

Written procedures need to be developed for every aspect of the repackaging operation. Procedures should include general guidelines about cleanliness; labeling format; assignment of expiration dates; container size in relation to the size or volume of the drug being repackaged; operational procedures for the setup, operation, and cleanup of equipment; the type and detail of records; and quality assurance and testing procedures.

Changes to procedures must be communicated in writing, and the procedure should be revised and the date of revision noted in the procedure book. All procedures should be reviewed annually to ensure that they reflect current practice.

Training Programs

One of the more important and most often neglected aspects of a quality control program is a formal training program. A formal training program is important in ensuring that every employee associated with the repackaging program is provided the same information, in the same manner, with the same degree of importance. Formal training programs lend themselves to promoting consistency and standardization. A training program can pay for itself by avoiding the loss of medication, supplies, and personnel time associated with the improper repackaging of a product. Training programs can also help to lengthen the useful life of equipment by demonstrating proper operating procedures, proper cleaning and maintenance, and the proper way to adjust and repair improperly working machinery.

There are so few training programs established in institutional practice because they tend to be resource intensive. However, teaching aids such as programmed texts and video presentations can help to minimize resource expenditures in this area of quality control.

Maintenance of Equipment

Most equipment that is used in the repackaging process requires some form of maintenance. Maintenance can be part of the daily operation of the equipment, or it can be a scheduled maintenance. Unfortunately, most pharmacies do not perform regularly scheduled maintenance on their equipment, and a few do not even perform preventive maintenance.

The proper maintenance of equipment is important from two perspectives. First, regularly scheduled preventive maintenance can extend the life of equipment. The extension of the equipment's life expectancy can lead to decreased overhead in the repackaging operation. Second, preventive maintenance will translate into less frequent downtimes resulting from equipment failure. Maintenance of equipment will also ensure that it is operating to the specifications of the manufacturer and that the quality of the package is as good today as when the equipment was first purchased.

Checkpoints

"Checkpoints" refer to those steps in the repackaging process that are crucial to ensuring a high-quality package. It is important to double-check each anticipated step to ensure a successful outcome. Examples of checkpoints include:

1. Double-checking the product to be packaged to ensure that it is the drug and dosage form that are supposed to be repackaged. It is also important to ensure that the starting product is within date.
2. Double-check the fill volumes to ensure that the amount of liquid delivered is proper for the dose and the container selected.
3. Double-check any calculations that may be needed to reconstitute a product to arrive at a given dosage.
4. Double-check the information that is on a label stencil or on a computer screen to ensure that the label is complete and accurate (e.g., spelling).

End product testing is the type of quality control that most industries practice. End product testing requires sampling the final product and determining if it meets all the standards that it met before being subjected to the repackaging process. Examples of end product testing include sterility testing of a sterile product or testing the moisture permeability of a package for a solid or liquid oral dosage. Content uniformity and potency can be tested by a number of applicable chemical analyses.

KETTERING MEDICAL CENTER
Department of Pharmaceutical
Packaging Division

REPACKAGING WORKSHEET

Name of Product__________
Dosage Form__________
Dosage Strength
or Concentration__________
Amount/Packaged Unit__________
Container Type and Size__________
Drug Code Number__________

Auxiliary Label __________

Special Considerations (Storage, Stability, Packaging Materials, Delivery Volume, etc.)
____
____
____

Item No.	Date	Manufacturer's			Pharmacy Exp. Date	Units Pkg'd	Pharmacy Control No.	Pkg'd By:	Approved By:			Date Released
		Name	Lot No.	Exp. Date					Drug	Quan.	Label	
1												
2												
3												
4												
5												
6												
7												
8												
9												
10												
11												
12												

Label Format:

Label Samples
Reverse Side

Figure 21-15. This is an example of a repackaging control record.

Testing for Sterility

Sterility testing can be conducted in the institutional setting by obtaining one of several kits that are on the market for this purpose. The kits provide a nondestructive method for testing the solution in question by filtering the solution through a 0.22-μ filter (which catches the bacteria). The filter is then submersed in a nutrient broth that will promote the growth of aerobic organisms. The broth is incubated and observed daily for evidence of microbial growth (as shown by turbidity). If the solution does turn turbid, it is generally sent to the microbiology department for analysis. Through identification of the organism, the source of contamination may be determined. For example, if the organism turned out to be *Staphylococcus epidermis*, it is likely that the contamination was through contact with skin.

This type of random sterility testing will not detect low-level or incidental contamination in batch production programs. However, it will give an indication if gross contamination is occurring in the production process.

Testing for Moisture Permeation

Testing for moisture permeation can be conducted fairly easily; however, few pharmacists ever perform this end product test. The test for moisture permeation can be conducted on packages intended for oral solid and oral liquid medications.

The *USP XXII* test for moisture permeation is as follows:[24]

> Dry 10 suitable desiccant tablets* at 110° C for 1 hour prior to use. Use pellets weighing approximately 400 mg each and having a diameter of approximately 8 mm.
>
> *Method I — for pouch and blister packages*
>
> Seal not less than 10 unit dose containers with 1 pellet in each, and seal 10 additional, empty unit dose containers to provide controls, using finger cots or padded forceps to handle the sealed containers. Number the containers, and record the individual weights† to the nearest mg. Weigh the controls as a unit and divide the total weight by the number of controls to obtain the average control weight. Store the containers at 75 ± 3% relative humidity and at a temperature of 20 ± 2° C (a saturated system of 35 g of sodium chloride with each 100 mL of water placed in the bottom of a desiccator maintains the specified humidity). After a 24-hour interval or a multiple thereof, remove the containers from the chamber and allow them to equilibrate for 15 to 60 minutes in the weighing area. Again record the weight of the individual containers and the combined controls in the same manner. Return the containers to the humidity chamber. Calculate the rate of moisture permeation, in mg per day, of each container by the formula:
>
> $$(1/N)[(W_f - W_i)-(C_f - C_i)]$$
>
> in which N is the number of days expired in the test period; $(W_f - W_i)$ is the difference, in mg, between the final and initial weights of each test container; and $(C_f - C_i)$ is the average of the difference, in mg, between the final and initial weights of the controls, the data being calculated to two significant figures.†
>
> *Suitable moisture-indicating desiccant pellets are available commercially from sources such as Medical Packaging, Inc., 11-10 Ilene Court, Belle Mead, NJ 08502.
>
> †Accurate comparisons of class A containers may require test periods in excess of 28 days if weights are performed on a class A prescription balance.
>
> *Results*
>
> The individual unit dose containers are designated class A if not more than 1 of 10 containers tested exceeds 0.5 mg per day in moisture permeation rate and none exceeds 1 mg per day; they are designated class B if not more than 1 of 10 containers tested exceeds 5 mg per day and none exceeds 10 mg per day; they are designated class C if not more than 1 of 10 containers tested exceeds 20 mg per day and none exceeds 40 mg per day; and they are designated class D if the containers tested meet none of the moisture permeation rate requirements.*
>
> *With the use of the desiccant described herein, suitable test intervals for the final weighing, W_f, are: 24 hours for class D; 48 hours for class C; 7 days for class B; and not less than 28 days for class A.

CONCLUSION

Historically, institutionally based pharmacists have been responsible for repackaging pharmaceuticals for patient use. The unit dose system of drug distribution in the institutional setting has continued to demand that medications be provided in a ready to use package. Until manufacturers of drugs can provide all their products in unit-of-use form, the institutionally based pharmacist will continue to be responsible for repackaging medications.

Pharmacists who are engaged in repackaging medications must adhere to the basic principles of good manufacturing practices. Pharmacists can ensure that high-quality repackages are produced by taking advantage of the technology that is available today. This technology includes the application of computers, equipment, and end product testing programs geared to the institutional practitioner. No effort should be spared to ensure that the repackaged medication is of the highest quality attainable.

GLOSSARY OF TERMS

Batch repackaging — a process by which many containers of medication are prepared. The amount of medication packaged in this process is contingent on the use rate for the medication and the expiration date that must be assigned to the final package.

Blister package — a semirigid package that is generally reserved for oral solid medications. The package is composed of two parts: a backing, which is usually made up of a paper/foil material, and a front or facing material, which is a plastic with a small blister or bubble in it that holds the medication. The blister portion of the package can be either clear or amber.

Extemporaneous packaging — the planning process involved in the repackaging of medications. Extemporaneously repackaged medications are packaged as needed, not in advance of the prescription.

Good manufacturing practices (GMP) — guidelines that have been established by the U.S. Food and Drug Administration in 1963 to represent standards of operation in manufacturing practice. They are the standards by which the pharmaceutical industry's manufacturing practices are gauged.

Pouch package — a flexible package that is composed of two parts. The package is generally made of a paper/foil laminate that is joined to another paper/foil laminate or to a clear cellophane-like material to form a small pouch.

Prepackaging — the process of packaging a drug before it is needed. Prepackaging is repackaging in advance or in anticipation of a medication order.

Repackaging — the process of taking a medication from one container and placing it into another container. Generally the original container is the manufacturer's container.

Single-dose package — a package that contains one dose of the medication. This type of package could contain two tablets or two capsules of medication if that was the dose ordered.

Single-unit package — a single unit of medication. Examples would include one tablet, one syringe, one ampule, one teaspoonful, or 1 g.

Strip package — the type of oral solid package that is formed by most automated oral solid repackaging machines. The package is so named because it comes off the machine in one continuous strip that has perforations between the doses. Individual doses are removed by tearing the perforation.

Unit of use packaging — a drug package that contains the amount of medication necessary for the period of treatment. This type of package generally applies to patient-specific containers that often contain several doses of the medication.

REFERENCES

1. Siater WE, Hripko K: The unit dose system in a private hospital. Part two: Evaluation. *Am J Hosp Pharm* 25:641-648, 1968.
2. Smith WE, Mackewicz DW: An economic analysis of the PACE pharmacy service. *Am J Hosp Pharm* 27:123-126, 1970.
3. Hynniman CE, Hyde GC, Parker PF: How costly is medication safety. *JAHA* 45:73-78, 1971.
4. Schnell BR, Hammel RW: A comparison of unit-dose costs under various hospital drug distribution systems. *Can J Hosp Pharm* 24:122-127, 1971.
5. Rase BE: A cost study of single unit medication packaging. *Am J Hosp Pharm* 25:434-436, 1968.
6. Beste DF: An integrated pharmacist-nurse approach to the unit-dose concept. *Am J Hosp Pharm* 25:397-407, 1968.
7. Gibson CA: Unit dose: Increased cost or savings. *Can J Hosp Pharm* 24:222-223, 1971.
8. Oglivie RI, Reudy J: Adverse drug reactions during hospitalization. *Can Med Assoc J* 97:1450-1457, 1967.
9. Beckerman JH: The logistics of a drug distribution system: Packaging, labeling and storage. *Am J Hosp Pharm* 24:63-65, 1967.
10. American Society of Hospital Pharmacists. ASHP technical assistance bulletin on single unit and unit dose packages of drugs. *Am J Hosp Pharm* 46:806, 1989.
11. U.S. Pharmacopeial Convention: *US Pharmacopeia-National Formulary, USP XXII-NF XVII*, 1990 ed. Rockville, MD, U.S. Pharmacopeial Convention, 1990, p 1671.
12. U.S. Pharmacopeial Convention: *US Pharmacopeia-National Formulary, USP XXII-NF XVII*, 1990 ed. Rockville, MD, U.S. Pharmacopeial Convention, 1990, pp 1673-1675.
13. U.S. Pharmacopeial Convention: *US Pharmacopeia-National Formulary, USP XXII-NF XVII*, 1990 ed. Rockville, MD, U.S. Pharmacopeial Convention, 1990, p 8.
14. U.S. Pharmacopeial Convention: *US Pharmacopeia-National Formulary, USP XXII-NF XVII*, 1990 ed. Rockville, MD, U.S. Pharmacopeial Convention, 1990, p 1574.
15. U.S. Pharmacopeial Convention: *US Pharmacopeia-National Formulary, USP XXII-NF XVII*, 1990 ed. Rockville, MD, U.S. Pharmacopeial Convention, 1990, p 1570.
16. Proceedings of seminar on drug stability as effected by environment and containers. Washington, DC, Food and Drug Administration, 1967.
17. Autian J: Drug packaging in plastics, Part I. *Drug Cos Ind* 102:47, 1968.
18. Autian J: Drug packaging in plastics, Part II. *Drug Cos Ind* 102:54, 1968.
19. Autian J: Drug packaging in plastics, Part III. *Drug Cos Ind* 102:79, 1968.
20. Stach PE: Method for the aseptic filling of unit dose syringes. *Am J Hosp Pharm* 31:762, 1974.
21. Proksch RA: Compounding and repackaging—a need for complete records. *Hosp Pharm* 15:344-355, 1980.
22. Henry B, Auberman J: Unit dose prepackaging: A guide for development of policies and procedures. *Hosp Pharm* 15:357-363, 1980.
23. Patel JA, Curtis EG, Phillips GL: Quality control guidelines for single unit packaging of parenterals in the hospital pharmacy. *Am J Hosp Pharm* 29:947-951, 1972.
24. U.S. Pharmacopeial Convention: *US Pharmacopeia-National Formulary, USP XXII-NF XVII*, 1990 ed. Rockville, MD, U.S. Pharmacopeial Convention, 1990, pp 1575-1576.

ADDITIONAL READING

Beck AV: Hospital unit-dose packaging. *Hosp Topics* 46:49-54, 1968.

Benya TJ: Records—a control device in production. *Am J Hosp Pharm* 23:385, 1966.

Feldman MJ, Sourney PF, Kaul AF: Determining the date of manufacture of drug products for lot numbers. *Am J Hosp Pharm* 36:1545, 1979.

Gupta VD, Stewart KR, Gupta A: Stability of oral solid drugs after repackaging in single-unit containers. *Am J Hosp Pharm* 37:165-169, 1980.

Kenna FR: Strip packaged medications. *Hosp Topics* 44:104, 1966.

Mandl FL, Greenburg RB: Legal implications of preparing and dispensing drugs under conditions not in a product's official labeling. *Am J Hosp Pharm* 33:814, 1976.

Miller RW: Pharmaceutical manufacturers and unit dose packaging. *Am J Hosp Pharm* 24:76, 1967.

Nold EG: Stability of drugs repackaged into unit dose containers. *Am J Hosp Pharm* 34:1294, 1977.

Reamer JT, Grady LT: Moisture permeation of newer unit dose repackaging materials. *Am J Hosp Pharm* 35:787-793, 1978.

Reamer JT, Grady LT, Shangraw RF, et al: Moisture permeation of typical unit dose repackaging materials. *Am J Hosp Pharm* 34:35-42, 1977.

Ritter FT: Panel discussions: Unit dose dispensing—container manufacturers' viewpoint of unit dose packaging. *Bull Parent Drug Assoc* 22:175, 1968.

Sacharow S: A guide to unit-dose packaging. *Drug Cos Ind* 103:90-161, 1968.

Stolar MH: Expiration dates of repackaged drug products. *Am J Hosp Pharm* 36:170, 1979.

Varsano J: Pharmaceuticals in plastic packaging. Part I. *Drug Cos Ind* 104:72, 1969.

Varsano J: Pharmaceuticals in plastic packaging. Part II. *Drug Cos Ind* 104:88, 1969.

Varsano J: Pharmaceuticals in plastic packaging. Part III. *Drug Cos Ind* 104:98, 1969.

Appendix 21-A

MANUFACTURERS OF PACKAGING EQUIPMENT AND SUPPLIES

Containers and closures

Abbott Laboratories
Hospital Products Division
1 Abbott Park Road
Abbott Park, IL 60064
(empty vials)

BAXA Corporation
13760 East Arapahoe Road
Englewood, CO 80112
(containers, closures, and filling systems)

Becton-Dickenson and Company
1 Becton Drive
Franklin Lakes, NJ 07417
(syringes and syringe tips)

Burron Medical, B. Braun of America
824 12th Avenue
Bethlehem, PA 18018
(containers and filling systems)

Lyphomed Inc
Division of Fujisawa, USA, Inc.
Parkway North Center/3 Parkway North
Deerfield, IL 60015
(empty vials)

Medi-Dose/EPS Inc.
1671 Loretta Avenue
Feasterville, PA 19053
(containers and closures)

Sherwood Medical
1831 Olive Street
St. Louis, MO 63103
(syringes and closures)

Smith and Nephew
1845 Tonne Road
Elk Grove Village, IL 60007
(containers)

3-M Company
3M Center
220-8W
St. Paul, MN 55144
(tamper-evident closures and seals)

West Company
1041 West Bridge Street
Phoenixville, PA 19460
(containers and all closure components)

Wheaton Laboratories
1501 North Tenth Street
Millville, NJ 08332
(containers and equipment)

Automated Packaging Equipment

Baxter Healthcare Corporation
1 Baxter Parkway
Deerfield, IL 60015
(ATC machine)

Econodose, Inc.
1236 Watson Ave.
Ypsilanti, MI 48917

Euclid Spiral Paper Tube Corporation
339 Mill Street, P.O. Box 458
Apple Creek, OH 44606
(equipment and supplies)

Medical Packaging Inc.
11-10 Ilene Court
Belle Mead, NJ 08502
(equipment and supplies)

Odessa Packaging
202 North Bassett Street
P.O. Box 487
Clayton, DE 19938
(equipment and supplies)

CHAPTER 22

Extemporaneous Formulations and Quality Assurance

ALBERT J. SZKUTNIK

As pharmacy has evolved, much emphasis has been placed on clinical services in institutional practice, overshadowing the importance of extemporaneous compounding. Although most products purchased by pharmacists are prefabricated by pharmaceutical manufacturers, there remains a need for some basic compounding. Unfortunately, extemporaneous compounding is often not available in hospitals to the extent the physicians would prefer.

A review of the literature reveals that many articles written by researchers have included formulations that can be useful but are not commercially available. Physicians have found it difficult to obtain products when compounding is required. Various reasons have been given and include limited manpower and lack of stability data.

In the hospital, extemporaneous formulations can satisfy three categories of need: (1) compounding of products individually, (2) enhancement and support of clinical services and investigational protocols, and (3) limited bulk compounding. A successful program of extemporaneous formulations must involve a committed pharmacy practitioner and a supportive medical staff. An important factor is the recognition by the director of the pharmacy department that compounding remains an important service of institutional pharmacy practice.

Pride in producing an elegant product possessing necessary stability and bioavailability is of prime importance; efficacy is best judged by the patient and the clinician. Extemporaneous compounding expertise comes from knowledge and experience. There are daily challenges to one's ability in a large institution, and a competent and reliable compounding capability is one of the attributes of a truly superior pharmacy service.

Preparations compounded include oral and external solutions, syrups, elixirs, oral suspensions, ointments, creams, lotions, suppositories, capsules, powders, and dental and ophthalmic formulations. Extemporaneous compounding by a number of individuals of the same product may produce variations in the product if an established procedure is not followed.

Collection, retrieval and maintenance of data for future use are essential. A 3" x 5" rotary file card can supply enough information to support a written log of most formulations. These index cards or a notebook can be used, but a notebook tends to be cumbersome if the files continue to expand. Data are provided for each new compounded product outlining the formulation, procedure, storage instructions, expiration date, any peculiarities encountered, and observations noted during the preparation of the prescription. Pharmacists should never trust their memory. Standardization of formulas reduces the potential for error related to calculations on the part of the physician and the pharmacist. The same information can be computerized using a data base program. Unfortunately all personnel may not be computer literate, and accessing data from a file may take more time than retrieving information from a rotary file.

All compounding cards should be filed alphabetically by generic name of the active ingredient. If the preparation has more than one active ingredient, several cards of the same formulation may be needed as a cross-reference system. Patient profile cards may also be referenced alphabetically by last name. An example of a compounding card can be seen in figure 22-1.

Spironolactone Suspension 2 mg/cc(1)

Spironolactone Tablets 100 mg		#6
Cologel[R]		100 mL
Cherry Syrup	q.s.	300 mL

Grind tablets to a fine powder with mortar and pestle. Add a small amount of distilled water to form uniform thick paste. Add Cologel[R] in portions and triturate well. Add cherry syrup by geometric dilution while triturating and a sufficient quantity of syrup to make the total volume 300 mL.

Note: Use manufacturer's tablets as specified in the formulation. Using another manufacturer's tablets can result in unpredictable stability and bioavailability. The appearance of the product may change, such as the viscosity and color, causing visual concern by the patient about the potency of the product.

Expiration time: 60 days

SHAKE WELL KEEP IN REFRIGERATOR

Figure 22-1. Example of a compounding card

The importance of a file card for each preparation cannot be overemphasized. Calculation errors are an everyday concern. Two pharmacists should scrutinize any preparation for errors in calculations before a file card is made. The compounding pharmacist should always check that the calculations are correct before dispensing.

To continue with the example, the following information should be entered on the back of the prescription:

Spironolactone tablets 100 mg #6
Mfr:
Lot # 3456
Exp:
Cologel[R] 100 mL
Mfr:
Lot # 3G45A
Exp:
Cherry Syrup q.s. 300 mL
Mfr:
Lot # 900606M05
Exp:

Placing the above information in mixing sequence along with the pharmacist's initials can aid in tracking any error that may occur and prevent future occurrences.

The following information should be entered on a patient record card:

Carlson, Debbie Ward 51 Weight 10 kg
Phone number: 576-2400

Spironolactone Suspension 2 mg/cc

Spironolactone tablets 100 mg		#6
Cologel[R]		100 mL
Cherry Syrup	q.s. (as much as needed)	300 mL

Sig: 4 cc (8 mg) t.i.d. (3 times/day)

Expiration time: 60 days
SHAKE WELL KEEP IN REFRIGERATOR

(Reverse side of card)

Date Dispensed - 300 mL AJS
Date Dispensed - 300 mL AJS
Sig: 5 cc (10 mg) t.i.d. (signifies change in directions at the above date)

Extemporaneous and the occasional bulk-compounded preparation should be entered into a daily tracking log of manufactured products. The log (figure 22-2) should provide the following information: (1) institution's lot number of the compounded product, (2) name of the product, (3) quantity produced, (4) destination (patient's name, ward, clinic), (5) extemporaneous or bulk compounded, (6) preparer's initial, and (7) initials of the person double-checking the preparation.

One example of an institutional lot number for extemporaneous and bulk-compounded pharmaceuticals is 911001M03. In this example, the 91 refers to the year; 11, to the month; 01, the day of month; M, manufactured (compounded) product; and 03, third preparation prepared that day. If a "P" is substituted for the letter "M," it would mean the item was prepacked. Unit dose would use the letter "U." Each pharmacy element can have a letter designation of its own. The lot number at a glance will tell where the product originated. Each element of the pharmacy that has a letter designation must also have a daily log as described above. Reconstituted preparations and half-tablets for unit dose should also be recorded in the log. If an error occurs, the pharmacy can retrace its steps and determine how to avoid the same error in the future.

Extemporaneous compounded prescriptions should be kept in a separate file for easy retrieval. Outpatients should be urged to phone the pharmacy at least 2 days in advance of a refill. This provides the compounding pharmacist with a reasonable period of time to prepare the compounded prescription while meeting other obligations of a more immediate nature.

SYRUPS AND SUSPENSIONS

Pediatric and geriatric patients, patients with swallowing difficulties, and nasogastric intubated patients may require liquid dosage forms of commonly prescribed medications. The pharmacist may be called upon to prepare medications in oral liquid formulations if no commercially available preparation is obtainable. A limiting factor in compounding oral liquids is the lack of stability and bioavailability studies of preparations compounded from capsules and tablets into syrups and suspensions. Oral liquid formulations with documented stability and bioavailability can be compounded with assurance that the product will maintain the labeled potency until the expiration date. Two sources of information on compounding oral liquids are the American Society of Hospital Pharmacists[1] (ASHP) *Handbook on Extemporaneous Compounding*, and Rappaport's,[2] *Extemporaneous Dosage Preparations for Pediatrics*.

Oral suspensions are an important dosage form for the dispersion of soluble and insoluble powders.[3-5] The concentration of a suspending agent such as a liquid methylcellulose concentrate may have to be adjusted according to the tablets and capsules used. Refrigeration of compounded preparations that use methycellulose tends to increase the viscosity. If the viscosity is too pronounced, the patient may not be able to shake the bottle to pour its contents or disperse the solids, which may settle. Proper homogeneity must be maintained to dispense a uniform dose of medication after the product is shaken.[6]

Green, blue, or violet tablets, when compounded with colored syrups, often result in a product with an unacceptable appearance. Alternate strengths of tablets may be used to circumvent the color problem. The most visually pleasing suspensions are prepared from orange, red, yellow, peach, and pink solid dosage forms. The pharmacist must also be aware of the possibility of tartrazine being a color component of some solid dosage forms, which may cause an allergy problem in some patients.

When preparing the suspension, the pharmacist should add a small amount of distilled water to the finely ground powder of the solid dosage form in a mortar, then triturate until a smooth, thick paste results. Particles floating in the suspension reduce the acceptability of appearance and raise questions as to the uniformity of a individually dispensed dose. The liquid methylcellulose is then added in small amounts to the paste until all the methylcellulose is incorporated. The use of a commercially available liquid methylcellulose concentrate facilitates incorporation and saves time. Add portions of the vehicle, while triturating, to the desired volume.

Adequate preservation of the formulation may require more than one preservative. There is no single preservative that fulfills the requirements of all preparations. Published

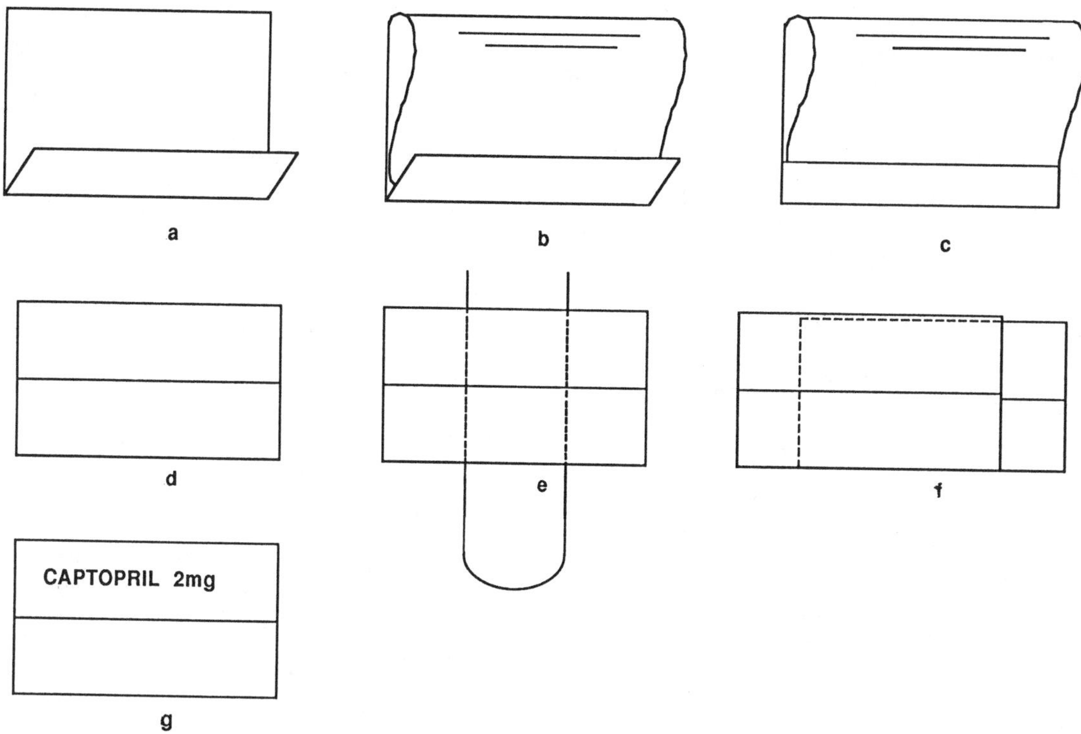

Figure 22-2. Folding a powder paper

literature and microbial studies at the institution can serve as sources of information as to the selection of the proper preservative. Preservatives listed in table 22-1 are sufficiently soluble in aqueous formulations and have demonstrated properties that are antibacterial and antifungal. A ratio of 10 to 1, methyl and propylparahydroxybenzoic acid, respectively, attributed to the solubility of each, potentiates the effect of each to achieve the desired antimicrobial result.[7]

Table 22-1. Pharmaceutically useful preservatives

Preservative	*Concentration*
Alkyl esters of parahydroxybenzoic acid	0.001-0.2
Benzoic acid and its salts	0.1-0.3
Sorbic acid and its salts	0.05-0.2

Adapted and reprinted with permission from Boylan JC: *Liquids. The Theory and Practice of Industrial Pharmacy,* 2nd ed. London, Henry Kimpton Publishers, 1976.

Syrups having approximately 85 percent (w/v) sucrose retard microbial growth by exhibiting an ex-osmotic effect on micro-organisms. Other agents such as glycerin, polyethylene glycol, propylene glycol, and sorbitol in sufficient quantities in syrups containing less than 85 percent (w/v) sucrose will have a similar ex-osmotic effect.[7]

It is possible to calculate the amount of alcohol used for its preservative action in syrups whose sugar content is less than 85 percent (w/v). Grote and Walker[8] used the principle of "free water." Eighty-five percent (w/v) sucrose, which is equal to 65 percent (w/w), will preserve itself as simple syrup. The following concentrations will preserve a specified amount of a liquid preparation: 1 mL glycerin preserves 2 mL of preparation: 1 g solids preserves 1 mL of preparation; 1 g sugar preserves 1.18 mL of preparation.

The amount of preserved solution is subtracted from the total volume of preparation, leaving "free water," which must be preserved. Alcohol is added to the "free water" so that the concentration is 18 percent. In the *U.S. Pharmacopeia* (USP) *XII* edition, syrups presented with low alcoholic content, when recalculated for sucrose, glycerin, and solid content, were shown to have an alcohol content based on "free water" above the 15 to 18 percent required for preservability.

Five to ten percent alcohol or an adequate amount of preservative should be added so that a dilution of the syrup does not support microbial growth. Surface evaporation and condensation of the solvent in a closed environment can cause surface dilution, resulting in a medium susceptible to microbial contamination. Ethanol vaporizers, because they have greater vapor pressure than water at the surface of the liquid, minimize the possibility of microbial growth because of surface dilution.[7] Ethanol also serves as a solvent for alcohol-soluble ingredients.

Because of the high concentration of sucrose, syrups generally have fewer solvent capabilities for salts than water. In preparing syrups having water-soluble salts, it is necessary to dissolve the salts in a minimal amount of distilled water before mixing with a syrup base.

The interaction between Tween 80 and methyl and propyl paraben produces a surfactant-preservative complex with the resulting loss of antibacterial activity.[7] This points to the need to investigate the combination of commonly used preservatives and pharmaceutical adjuvants.

Diluting the syrup makes it more prone to microbial growth if a preservative is not added. The patient should be advised to store the syrup in the refrigerator and discard the syrup after the expiration date.

If other sources or grades of flavorings are used, the amount needed must be adjusted. Do not overflavor. Experimentation in combining two or more flavors to enhance disguise of taste of medication(s) may bring worthwhile dividends in patient acceptance (table 22-2).

Table 22-2. Flavors for syrups and suspensions

Taste sensation	*Recommended flavor*
Salty	Butterscotch, maple, apricot, peach, vanilla, wintergreen mint
Bitter	Wild cherry, walnut, chocolate, mint combinations, passion fruit, mint spice, anise
Sweet	Fruit and berry, vanilla
Sour	Citrus flavors, licorice, root beer, raspberry

Adapted and reprinted from Boylan JC: *Liquids. The Theory and Practice of Industrial Pharmacy*, 2nd ed. London, Henry Kimpton Publishers, 1976.

Pediatric departments tend to prefer syrups and suspensions that are devoid of preservatives and colors. Many of the pediatric liquid preparations are prepared from medications meant for adults but are used for infrequent pediatric disease states. Pharmacists prefer to refrigerate these products to optimize stability and preservability.[9]

Informed decisions as to how to proceed in compounding a liquid dosage form will necessitate more detailed information from the manufacturer before the preparation is prepared from a solid dosage form. Some manufacturers will either suggest a formulation with stability data or refer to an article published in the literature. A few manufacturers are less cooperative.

Physicians must be informed about the limitations of the stability of a preparation as well as the need for clinical observation of the patient when formulations with perceived limited stability are compounded. Cooperation of the physician is essential in gathering information about the clinical success (bioavailability) of the preparation. Stability studies of the preparations at the institution should be carried out but may be beyond the capabilities of some institutions.

POWDERS

Powders are an alternative for drugs that cannot be compounded into liquid form. Powders eliminate many of the incompatibilities and instabilities associated with drugs in liquid form.

Powders are suited for children who have difficulty in swallowing capsules and tablets. This dosage form has its share of problems, such as administering bitter substances, protecting deliquescent and efflorescent medications from moisture, and protecting from exposure to light. Lactose is often used to make suitable dilutions of the medication. Each powder is individually weighed to ensure uniform dosage.

If food does not interfere with drug bioavailability, honey, jam, preserves, or flavored syrup mixed with the powder can mask the unpleasant taste of the preparation. Since these preparations have a high sugar content, diabetics will have to use artificially sweetened beverages, where appropriate, to mask the taste. Powders should not be mixed with milk or formula because of the possibility of children developing a dislike for milk or formula.

Powders having stable characteristics can be dispensed in ziplock bags with the air expelled and a silica gel desiccant enclosed. Parents must be told the bags are not child-proof containers and must be secured. Drugs formulated into powder papers that may deteriorate when exposed to environmental factors are best dispensed in wide-mouth, light-resistant, tight containers with a desiccant inside. The outside of the container should contain a label notifying the patient "DESICCANT INSIDE. DO NOT REMOVE. KEEPS CONTENTS DRY. DO NOT EAT."

Each powder paper must be individually labeled with the name of the drug and its strength. If a drug with various strengths is made for members of a family, it is necessary to label and package each prescription individually. The contents should be indicated on self-sticking colored labels so that each family member gets his or her individually colored label on the powder paper. Different colors reinforce the existence of varying potencies and prevent mixing of the powders among individuals.

The procedure of folding powders as is conventionally taught leaves something to be desired. If the powder is accidentally dropped by the patient, the contents are partially or totally lost. Figure 22-2 shows a progression of steps that are used in producing a powder that is totally enclosed but readily accessible to the patient when a dose is required. A standard 3 1/2" x 4 1/2" powder paper can comfortably hold up to 750 mg of powder that is the consistency of lactose. A spatula blade 1 3/4" wide by 10" long whose handle is weighed down by a heavy object(s), such as a book, extending 6 inches over the counter can act as a fine bending tool. A device made of thin metal with the dimensions above can be used.

In section 2a of figure 22-2, the bottom of the paper is folded 1/4." A number of powder papers (5-6 at one time) can be folded and placed in neat rows, closely aligned, as is convenient for the pharmacist, ready to accept the weighed out powder at their center. The upper edge of the paper is folded forward over the powder into the crease previously folded (section 2b). The 1/4" fold is folded over (section 2c). The lower edge of the paper is folded over away from the individual until it divides the paper at its center with the right side 1/16" higher than the center line and the left side 1/16" lower than the center line (section 2d). The paper is held as it was folded and centered over the blade of the spatula (section 2e). Each flap is bent over the sides and under the spatula (section 2f). The powder is flipped over, and the right narrower side of the paper is bent into the pocket formed in the wider left side (section 2g). There is no need to crease the sides of the powder paper. Repetition and attention to neatness are essential in producing powders that are uniform in size. With experience, productivity increases.

Individual powders as folded can be dispensed in any suitable container without the annoying prospect of the powder being lost from its powder paper containment. Each powder is labeled with the contents on a self-sticking label affixed to the top front portion of the powder paper (section 2h).

OPHTHALMICS

In preparing ophthalmic solutions, proper consideration must be given to buffering, isotonicity, preservation, sterility, viscosity, and packaging. Most compounded ophthalmic solutions are dilutions of concentrations of commercially prepared preparations or formulations that appear in the literature and are not available. Ophthalmic ointments and suspensions are rarely compounded. When the concentration of drug is less than 2.5 to 3 percent, generally the drug can be dissolved in an isotonic vehicle without causing undue eye discomfort.[10]

Packaging material, pH, and buffering contribute to the stability of the preparation. Packaging material should not interfere with the efficacy or stability of the preparation. Ophthalmic solutions are packaged in either sterile glass or plastic (polypropylene) containers that provide for dosing the preparation in drops. Plastic ophthalmic containers can be sterilized by gas sterilization and glass containers by steam sterilization in the institution's sterilization service.

USP/National Formulary (NF) *XXI/XVI*[11] lists an isotonic phosphate buffer solution with a pH range of 5.9 to 8.0. The buffer is composed of two solutions that can be mixed in varying amounts to produce a variety of pH's. Solution 1 is composed of monobasic sodium phosphate, anhydrous 8 g, sterile water q.s. to 1,000 mL; solution 2 is composed of dibasic sodium phosphate, anhydrous 9.47 g, sterile water q.s. to 1,000 mL. Table 22-3 specifies the amount of each solution required when mixed to give the pH shown.

Table 22-3. Isotonic phosphate buffer vehicle for ophthalmic preparations

Monobasic sodium phosphate solution, mL	Dibasic sodium phosphate solution, mL	Resulting buffer solution, pH	Sodium chloride required for isotonicity, g/100 mL
90	10	5.9	0.52
80	20	6.2	0.51
70	30	6.5	0.50
60	40	6.6	0.49
50	50	6.8	0.48
40	60	7.0	0.46
30	70	7.2	0.45
20	80	7.4	0.44
10	90	7.7	0.43
5	95	8.0	0.42

Reprinted with permission from the *USP/NF XXI/XVI.* Rockville, MD, U.S. Pharmacopeial Convention, 1984, p 1338.

Table 22-4 lists drugs usually encountered when compounding ophthalmic prescriptions.

The right column shows the resulting volume when 1 g of drug is dissolved in sterile water and a sufficient quantity of sterile water is added up to the specified volume of isotonic solution. Solutions containing less than 1 g of drug can be calculated by direct proportion. To minimize the discomfort of hypertonicity caused by dissolution of the drug in the isotonic phosphate buffer solution, the *USP/NF* suggests dissolving the drug first in sterile water to make an isotonic solution. Then, add isotonic phosphate buffer solution containing sufficient preservative to bring the solution to the calculated volume. Limited stability has been shown when salts of pilocarpine, eucatropine, scopolamine, and homatropine are added to isotonic phosphate buffer solution.[11]

Table 22-4. Isotonic solution that can be prepared from 1 g of drug and sterile water

Drug (1.0 g)	Volume of isotonic solution (mL)
Atropine sulfate	14.3
Benoxinate hydrochloride	20.0
Boric acid	55.7
Butacaine sulfate	22.3
Chloramphenicol sodium succinate	15.7
Chlorobutanol (hydrous)	26.7
Cocaine hydrochloride	17.7
Colisatimethate sodium	16.7
Dibucaine hydrochloride	14.3
Ephedrine hydrochloride	33.3
Ephedrine sulfate	25.7
Epinephrine bitartrate	20.0
Epinephrine hydrochloride	32.3
Eucatropine hydrochloride	20.0
Fluorescein sodium	34.3
Homatropine hydrobromide	19.0
Homatropine methylbromide	21.0
Neomycin sulfate	12.3
Penicillin G potassium	20.0
Phenacaine hydrochloride	22.3
Phenylephrine hydrochloride	35.7
Phenylethyl alcohol	27.7
Physostigmine salicylate	17.7
Physostigmine sulfate	14.3
Pilocarpine hydrochloride	26.7
Pilocarpine nitrate	25.7
Piperocaine hydrochloride	23.3
Polymyxin B sulfate	10.0
Procaine hydrochloride	23.3
Proparacaine hydrochloride	16.7
Scopolamine hydrobromide	13.3
Silver nitrate	36.7
Sodium bicarbonate	72.3
Sodium biphosphate	44.3
Sodium borate	46.7
Sodium phosphate (dibasic, heptahydrate)	32.3
Streptomycin sulfate	7.7
Sulfacetamide sodium	25.7
Sulfadiazine sodium	26.7
Sulfamerazine sodium	25.7
Sulfathiazole sodium	24.3
Tetracaine hydrochloride	20.0
Tetracycline hydrochloride	15.7
Zinc sulfate	16.7

Reprinted with permission from *USP/NF XXI/XVI.* Rockville, MD, U.S. Pharmacopeial Convention, 1984, p 1339.

Table 22-5 lists preservatives commonly used in ophthalmic solutions. Benzalkonium chloride is incompatible with anionic drugs and nonionic surfactants in elevated concentrations. Phenylmercuric acetate or nitrate should replace benzalkonium chloride when nitrates or salicylates are present. A precipitate may occur when phenylmercuric acetate is added to some solutions containing chlorides. Solutions containing chlorobutanol should be buffered from pH 5.0 to 5.5. Unbuffered neutral or alkaline solutions containing chlorobutanol are susceptible to decomposition at room temperature. The amount of preservative added should be effective in the formulation and packaging used.[11]

Table 22-5. Preservatives used in ophthalmic solutions

Frequently used preservatives	*Concentration*
Benzalkonium chloride	0.01% (1:10,000)
Phenylmercuric nitrate	0.002% (1:50,000)
Phenylmercuric acetate	0.002% (1:50,000)
Chlorobutanol	0.5%
Phenylethyl alcohol	0.5%

Increasing the viscosity of the ophthalmic solution prolongs the contact of the medication with the tissue of the eye. The *USP/NF XXI/XVI*[11] states that a pharmaceutical grade of methylcellulose (e.g., 1 percent if the viscosity is 25 cP, or 0.25 percent if 4,000 cP) or other suitable thickening agent such as hydroxypropyl methylcellulose or polyvinyl alcohol is occasionally added. Ophthalmic solutions whose viscosity has been increased must be free from visible particulate matter.

Ophthalmic solutions can be made sterile by passing the solution in a syringe through a 0.22-μ filter into a sterile ophthalmic container. The *USP/NF* considers this method the "preferred method." Sterilization using an autoclave is another preferred method if the preparation is not detrimentally affected.[11] Filtering solutions through a 0.22-μ membrane filter clarifies and removes bacteria and fungal contamination. All work that uses aseptic technique should be conducted in a laminar flow hood, which minimizes the possibility of airborne particles and microbial contamination.

SUPPOSITORIES

Suppositories are usually prescribed for their local or systemic effect. The most commonly used routes of administration for suppositories are rectal and vaginal. Rectal suppositories are an alternative route for systemic absorption of medication for patients who cannot tolerate oral dosage forms. Medication(s) should be in a readily absorbable form and in close contact with rectal mucosa.

Urethral suppositories are rarely compounded. Urethral molds can be fashioned by wrapping foil around a small-diameter glass rod or glass tubing which is then withdrawn, leaving a cavity for the melted base. The amount of base to be poured is calculated by trial and error.

USP/NF XXI/XVI[11] lists the following suppository bases: cocoa butter, glycerinated gelatin, hydrogenated vegetable oils, mixtures of polyethylene glycol of various molecular weights, and fatty esters of polyethylene glycol.

The release of the active ingredient(s) is dependent upon the suppository base and physical form of the drug. The range of doses administered via the rectal route usually is from one-half to two or more times the oral route except for potent medications. Specifications for suppository bases can be found in the text, *The Theory and Practice of Industrial Pharmacy.*[12]

In compounding a prescription, if no base is indicated, cocoa butter (theobroma oil) is usually the base of choice and most widely used. Cocoa butter has several disadvantages: it can melt in warm weather and become rancid; it softens or liquefies when drugs (e.g., chloral hydrate, phenol, and volatile oils) are added; priming of the mold is necessary to release the suppositories; and overheating can cause a lowering of its melting point. The amount of cocoa butter displaced by a drug can be ascertained by the replacement factor[12-14] or by the following method:

1. Cocoa butter, because of its low-volume contraction, will stick to the surface of the mold. Coat the mold with tincture of green soap or mineral oil in order for the suppositories to be released.
2. Melt the base and pour into a mold to make three suppositories and chill. Remove and obtain an average weight of a suppository. Retain this information in a file for future use.
3. Mix active ingredient(s) with less than the total amount of base required for three suppositories. Pour the melted mixture into the mold. Add sufficient melted base to make three suppositories and chill. Remove and obtain an average weight of a suppository.
4. Subtract the weight of the medication from the weight of the suppository with the active ingredient. This will determine the amount of base displaced by the medication when compared to the weight of suppository made from the base in step 2.

One of many alternative suppository bases is Witepsol®, which contains glycerol esters of mixtures of saturated vegetable fatty acids in which lauric acid predominates. It is offered in a wide variety of series to fit a number of suppository formulations.

The Witepsol S series is well suited for production of vaginal suppositories. The series S58 contains a protective agent, which reduces irritation as a result of the added drug. It also contains a small amount of a nonionic emulsifier, which increases the dispersion of the active ingredient and acts to moisten the mucosa. It has a low melting point and meets the requirements for producing vaginal suppositories. Suppositories can be stored at room temperature.

In calculating the amount of ingredients necessary for preparing suppositories, allowance should be made for losses in the process of mixing and pouring suppositories. It is advisable to calculate for one or two extra suppositories, depending upon the quantity needed. When controlled substances are incorporated into a base, any excess should be disposed of according to the prevailing State and Federal laws.

As with any suppository base, the bioavailability of the drug is dependent upon the characteristics of the medication and the formulation of the base. Clinical assessment will be needed to determine efficacy.

CAPSULES

Capsules have an advantage over tablets because they can be made extemporaneously in the pharmacy without need for sophisticated equipment. The process of filling capsules is convenient and relatively simple.

Some patients find it easier to swallow capsules than tablets. The advantage of capsules is that medication having an unpleasant taste or odor can be masked within a gelatin coat, which disintegrates within minutes upon entering the stomach. Capsules used in extemporaneous formulations are of the hard gelatin type, ranging in sizes from Number 5 (smallest) to Number 000 (largest). Gelatin capsules come in clear as well as a large range of solid colors. The capsules generally available to pharmacists are clear gelatin. The manufacturers of capsules will usually provide a guide on the side of the box the capsules come in as to the weight of powder each size capsule will hold. Dosage and formulation can be individualized by the physician to fit the therapeutic need of the patient.

Since small children have difficulty in swallowing solid dosage forms, capsules (as a source of premeasured dose, not a solid dosage form) are an alternative to powders for pediatric doses. If food-drug interactions and bioavailability are of no concern, the contents of capsules can be sprinkled or mixed with honey, jam, or apple sauce to disguise the taste immediately prior to ingestion. As with powders, the pharmacist must be aware of the diabetic patient where sugar-containing foods may be contraindicated.

Experience has shown that individuals who have difficulty in swallowing prefer the smallest capsule available to contain the quantity of powder required. If the capsule required is relatively large, the dose can be divided into two smaller capsules as one dose.

The usual method of preparing the powder prior to filling capsules is to reduce the particle size of the active ingredient(s) to a fine, uniform powder with mortar and pestle, whether in solid dosage form (tablet or contents of capsule) or commercially available raw material. Lactose is the preferred diluent in preparing the powder for the filling of capsules because of its compressibility. A drop of pure food coloring is added to the powder to ensure uniform distribution of the drug before the diluent is added by geometric dilution. Accurate, uniform distribution is important when small quantities of potent drugs are triturated with the diluent. No coloring is necessary if the active ingredient is present in a color tablet.

Before the capsules are filled, the hands should be washed thoroughly with a germicidal soap, such as chlorhexidine gluconate, to remove bacteria and dirt. Plastic or latex gloves or finger cots should be worn to prevent accumulation of perspiration on the fingers being transferred to the surface of the capsules. The powder is placed in the center of a paper and compressed lightly when half of the paper is folded over. The height of the compressed powder should be 1/3 the height of the body of the capsule. This height is important in preventing the soiling of the fingers, and ultimately the capsules, with the powder. The capsule body is separated from the cap and inverted open end down in the compressed powder, using the same compression pressure for each capsule. The cap is positioned on the body, and the capsule is tapped cap down on the working surface so that the powder is evenly distributed in the capsule. The balance is tared with an empty capsule. The empty capsule is removed and the filled capsule is weighed. If the weight of the capsule is over the calculated weight, some of the powder is removed from the capsule; if the weight of the capsule is under, powder is added to the cap of the capsule until the proper weight is reached. Each capsule must be weighed separately to ensure uniformity of dosage from capsule to capsule. Attention to precise mixing and weighing of the capsules is critical when potent drugs are needed for milligram or fractional milligram doses.

As a result of small losses of powder during the filling of capsules, it is advisable to calculate for a few more doses so that the quantity of capsules required is met. The remaining portion of unused powder is discarded. If controlled substances are involved the excess powder is disposed of according to State and Federal laws. The size of the capsule is annotated on the prescription for future reference in the event the prescription is refilled. Some pharmacists use the symbol of a triangle with the capsule size inserted, e.g., △. Accumulation of powder can be removed from the surface of capsules by shaking with granular sugar and then wiping with a towel or tissue.

States may require an expiration date on dispensed medications. The stability of the preparation will dictate the length of the expiration date. Some expiration dates may be derived empirically.

LIMITED BULK COMPOUNDING

As the need for extemporaneous compounding expands, a suitable alternative to increase productivity must be taken into account. Preparing syrups and suspensions in bulk from capsules and tablets is not always feasible. Inadequate formulations, lack of long-term stabilities, and infrequent use all contribute to the unsuitability of bulk compounding of these preparations. Pharmacists may also discover that it may not be in their best interest to prepare stock syrups and suspensions because of the variety of concentrations that may be encountered in individual patients. The preferred method would be to formulate the preparations at the time the patient submits the prescription.

The dermatology service, more than any other service, usually requires the greatest variety and percentage of extemporaneously compounded prescriptions. Limited bulk compounding of external preparations can have many advantages: patient waiting time is reduced to dispensing a prepackaged product in a relatively short period of time; standardizing formulations and eliminating variations in products save the hospital in material and personnel costs; and producing small to moderate quantities of preparations that normally would be extemporaneously compounded affords time for development of additional preparations.

Some institutions publish a dermatology formulary listing all commercial and in-house products prepared by the pharmacy. This facilitates standardization of demand for compounded prescriptions. The dermatology formulary also simplifies the prescribing of standard formulas favored by the dermatologists and is valuable to the education of residents in prescription writing. Revision of the formulary occurs once a year.

Formulas that serve as guides to development of creams, lotions, gels, and ointments can be located in the literature or obtained from companies supplying raw materials to the cosmetic and pharmaceutical industry. Scientific literature and trade journals are another source. (See Appendixes 22-A, 22-B, and 22-C.

Factors such as stability, appearance, feel, and release characteristics of drugs from the formulated base must be derived through experimentation. Introduction of recently developed safe materials opens new approaches to solving old problems.

Some areas that can benefit from limited bulk compounding are obstetrics and gynecology (progesterone suppositories, Prostin E2 gel, specialty creams and ointments), dentistry (dental therapeutic emollients, gargles, diagnostic agents), pediatrics (specialty creams and ointments), and surgery. Limited bulk compounding of preparations normally produced on an individual basis increases productivity.

Investigational protocols using single- and double-blind studies for clinical trials will need compounded dosage forms and placebos. The pharmacist who has been trained in designing protocols can assist the investigator in the pharmaceutical requirements.[15] A pharmacist experienced in compounding can be extremely useful by aiding the investigator to optimize the formulation considered. The incorporation of pharmaceuticals and placebos into capsule, liquid, and semisolid forms (creams, ointments) is within the capability of most institutions. Large quantities of capsules for protocols can be produced by using semiautomated machinery with a capacity of 1,500-3,000 capsules per hour.

Asking what must be accomplished and how it is to be conceived is of primary importance in formulation and procedure. Variations of the formula should be monitored so that no more than one variable is adjusted to accurately evaluate the effects of the change.

To ensure quality, a set of control procedures with predetermined parameters for uniformity are established that provide a standard to validate the output and performance during the compounding process. Defective products cannot be compensated because of the weakness in the formulation or compounding process. Compounded preparations are evaluated on an ongoing basis as part of the stability process.

Expiration dates are based on trial studies, expiration dates of ingredients, and information from the literature and trade journals. Some expiration dates must be derived empirically.

The type of testing will depend upon the range of options on hand. High-performance liquid chromatography, gas chromatography, or other sophisticated equipment can be used. Methods used should conform to the standards of the recognized Pharmacopeias. Periodic organoleptic inspection methods can be used on a retained sample to spot early signs of instability or microbial contamination.

REFERENCES

1. American Society of Hospital Pharmacists: *Handbook of Extemporaneous Compounding*. ASHP Special Interest Group on Pediatric Pharmacy Practice, 1987.
2. Rappaport PL: Extemporaneous dosage preparations for pediatrics. *U.S. Pharmacist* (March):H1-H12, 1984.
3. Scheer AJ: Practical guidelines for suspension formulation. *Drug Cos Ind* 128(4):40, 1981.
4. Scheer AJ: Practical guidelines for suspension formulation. Drug *Cos Ind* 128(5):39, 1981.
5. Scheer AJ: Practical guidelines for suspension formulation. *Drug Cos Ind* 128(6):52, 1981.
6. Kennon L, Storz G: *Pharmaceutical Suspensions: The Theory and Practice of Industrial Pharmacy*, 2nd ed. London, Henry Kimpton Publishers, 1976, pp 162-183.
7. Boylan JC: *Liquids: The Theory and Practice of Industrial Pharmacy*, 2nd ed. London, Henry Kimpton Publishers, 1976, pp 541-566.
8. Grote JW, Walker P: Studies in the preservation of liquid pharmaceutical preparations. *J Am Pharm Assoc* 35:182-187, 1946.
9. Tucker L: Pediatric suspensions—a crying need. *Am Pharm* NS19(11):21-22, 1979.
10. Mullins JD: Ophthalmic preparations. In *Remington's Pharmaceutical Sciences*, 17th ed. Easton, PA, Mack Publishing Co., pp 1553-1566.
11. USP/NF XXI/XVI: *Pharmaceutical Dosage Forms*. Rockville, MD, U.S. Pharmacopeial Convention, pp 1333-1342.
12. Anschel J, Lieberman HA: *Suppositories: The Theory and Practice of Industrial Pharmacy*, 2nd ed. London, Henry Kimpton Publishers, 1976, pp 245-269.
13. Zopf LC, Baug SM: Medicated Applications. In *Remington's Pharmaceutical Sciences*, 14th ed. Easton, PA, Mack Publishing Co., p. 1621.
14. Buchi J: *Pharm Acta Helv*, 20:403, 1949.
15. Gallelli JF, Hiranaka PK, Grimes GJ: Investigational drugs in the hospital. In *Handbook of Institutional Pharmacy Practice*, Thomas R. Brown and Mickey C. Smith, eds. 2nd ed. Baltimore, Williams & Wilkins, pp 471-506.

Appendix 22-A.

PERIODICALS

All subscriptions are free to qualified subscribers.

Pharmaceutical Technology
Aster Publishing Corp.
P.O. Box 10955
Eugene, OR 97440-2955

Pharmaceutical Manufacturing
2416 Wilshire Boulevard
Santa Monica, CA 90403

American Laboratory
P.O. Box 4048
Woburn, MA 01888-9918

LC.GC
Aster Publishing Corp.
P.O. Box 10955
Eugene, OR 97440-9843

Appendix 22-B.

BOOKS AND JOURNALS

The Theory and Practice of Industrial Pharmacy, 2nd ed.
Philadelphia, PA, Lea & Febiger, 1970

Remington's Pharmaceutical Sciences.
Easton, PA, Mack Publishing Co.

USP/NF (National Formulary).
United States Pharmacopeial Convention, Inc.
12601 Twinbrook Parkway
Rockville, MD 20952

Drug and Cosmetic Industry
P.O. Box 6150
Duluth, MN 55806

Manufacturing Chemist
Morgan-Grampian pic
Royal Sovereign House
40 Beresford Street
London SE 18 68Q
United Kingdom

Appendix 22-C.

SOURCES OF MATERIALS AND EQUIPMENT

Croda Inc.
183 Madison Avenue
New York, NY 10016
(supplier of raw materials to cosmetic and pharmaceutical companies; source of formulations, information, and samples; samples of materials can be used to produce experimental formulations)

Huls America Inc.
80 Centennial Ave
P.O. Box 456
Piscataway, NJ 08854
(supplier of raw materials to cosmetic and pharmaceutical companies; source of formulations, information, and samples; supplies a series of suppository bases under the name Witepsol®)

Ruger Chemical Co., Inc.
P.O. Box 806
Hillside, NJ 07205
(supplies bulk chemicals in quantities that most institutions use)

Erweka Instrument Corp.
56 Quirk Rd.
Milford, CT 06460
(supplies various sizes and shapes of precision suppository molds ranging from a capacity of 6 to 500 suppositories)

Wheaton
1000 N. 10th St.
Millville, NJ 08332
(source of polypropylene ophthalmic containers)

Scientific Instruments & Technology Corp.
P.O. Box 6906
Piscataway, NJ 08854
(source of capsule filling machinery)

CHAPTER 23

Investigational Drugs in the Hospital

CLARENCE L. FORTNER

Investigational drugs are agents that are being considered for commercial marketing, but have not yet been approved by the Food and Drug Administration (FDA) for use in humans.

Practical information on the proper administrative management and handling of investigational agents is still sparse, even though the regulations governing investigational agents were initiated in 1938.[1] In 1962, the Kefauver-Harris Drug Amendments to the U.S. Federal Food, Drug, and Cosmetic Act expanded clinical investigational drug studies that came under Federal regulation to require the collection of data on both safety and efficacy of a drug.[2]

PRECLINICAL STUDIES

Before an investigational agent can be administered to humans, the preclinical toxicology, pharmacology, and pharmacokinetics of the drug must be evaluated. Additionally, a source for the bulk drug and a preliminary formulation must be determined. This information will determine if the new agent is suitable for testing in humans. A flowchart for development of an antineoplastic drug is outlined in figure 23-1. Other kinds of experimental agents development would follow a similar procedure.

Preclinical Trials
- I. Acquisition of new agent
- II. Screening for activity
- III. Formulation and production of new agent
- IV. Toxicology

Clinical Trials
- I. Phase I
  - A. Maximally tolerable dose (MTD)
  - B. Pharmacology
  - C. Therapeutic effect
- II. Phase II
  - A. Determine if drug is effective
  - B. Dose/Response relationship
  - C. Toxicity
- III. Phase III
  - A. Compare new therapy to existing standard therapy, similar to way it would be on the market
  - B. Determine the optimum dose and schedule
  - C. Toxicity

FDA Approval for Commercial Use

Figure 23-1. Outline of antineoplastic drug development process

Potential new drugs are obtained from many different sources. They frequently are discovered at academic institutions, pharmaceutical industry, and various research-oriented centers. Preclinical investigators may voluntarily submit potential compounds for activity screening from any of these organizations. Other potential sources of new drugs are analogs, which are structural modifications of an active drug, developed in an attempt to improve the pharmacological and/or the physical properties of the parent compound.

Preclinical studies with an agent begin with the process of identifying and eliminating duplicate compounds. The remaining compounds are subjected to further structural and activity analyses to reveal novel compounds not previously tested. Further studies are conducted on the remaining compounds based on previously tested compounds. Some pharmaceutical companies use in vivo prescreening tests for the compounds that still appear promising. With some cancer agents, for example, the drug screen for antitumor activity is a single murine lymphocytic leukemia, P388. In the past, the National Cancer Institute (NCI) has used this in vivo screen, but in recent years it has changed to a disease-oriented screening procedure. This NCI process uses human tumor cell lines based on an in vitro screening program. This screening system can accommodate up to 10,000 to 20,000 agents each year in 60 different human tumor cell lines. It is expected that this process will be a more accurate method to identify activity as well as accelerate the screening process. Human tumor cell lines may identify a new generation of drugs with clinical potential against human tumors. Drugs showing activity will most likely be subjected to additional screening for activity such as schedule dependency studies. Knowing whether a drug's activity is schedule dependent assists in developing a rational pharmacological plan for the ultimate use of the drug in humans. The next steps in the drug development process are to scale up the production for the bulk drug and to formulate the initial dosage form that will be used in preclinical toxicology studies and early clinical trials.

FOOD AND DRUG ADMINISTRATION REGULATIONS

Before starting clinical trials with a new drug, the sponsor of the new agent must submit a notice of Claimed Investigational Exemption for an Investigation Drug (FDA

1571 form) to the FDA.[3] This commonly is called an "Investigational New Drug (IND) Application." The IND includes information on the chemistry as well as the preclinical data and any previous clinical results in addition to a proposed clinical protocol. The sponsor must wait 30 days before initiating clinical trials. This allows the FDA time to review the IND.

Investigators wishing to conduct clinical trials with this new agent are required to complete and submit a signed Statement of Investigator (FDA 1572 form) to the sponsor, e.g., pharmaceutical manufacturer, National Cancer Institute, or the FDA if the investigator is to be the sponsor.[4] The completed FDA 1572 form provides the sponsor with information about the investigator's qualifications. This information includes the investigator's name and address, education, training, and experience. Additionally, information is provided about the research facility, institutional review board (IRB), clinical laboratories used, other investigators involved, and protocol identification and procedures. The investigator's legal responsibilities are also listed on this form. Finally, the investigator must sign and date this form, indicating willingness to follow FDA regulations.

When clinical trials commence, they involve three progressive study phases. Each phase uses a protocol(s) that will be described in detail. However, the sponsor must have an approved protocol for the clinical trial before it can begin.

PROTOCOL

A protocol is a plan that outlines the objectives of a clinical research trial. A protocol must be prepared and then approved by both the investigator's local IRB and the sponsor of the investigational agent before a patient can be entered into the clinical trial. The protocol should have clear and attainable scientific goals that can be completed in a reasonable period. If the protocol is overly complicated or complex, it will be doomed to failure. The protocol should be a complete document similar to that outlined in figure 23-2, which details the procedures that investigators will follow to conduct the study and collect data.

1. Title page
2. Table of contents
3. Introduction and scientific background
4. Objective(s) of the clinical trial
5. Pharmaceutical information
6. Patient eligibility criteria
7. Procedure of patient entry on study
8. Treatment plan
9. Criteria for response assessment
10. Procedure in event of responses, no response, and toxicity
11. Dose modification for toxicity
12. Off-study criteria
13. Statistical considerations
14. References
15. Records to be kept
16. Copy of a model informed consent

Figure 23-2. Basic elements of a research protocol

The protocol document itself should begin with a title page. It should contain not only the title of the protocol but the names, addresses, and telephone numbers of the investigators, co-investigators, and the involved institutions. A table of contents should follow the title page. The scientific portion of the protocol should begin with the preclinical and any clinical data available, explaining the rationale for the new clinical trial. The aims described in the protocol are based on these scientific data.

The pharmaceutical section should contain, at a minimum, the mechanism of action, chemistry, pharmacokinetic data, and toxicities of the drug. The pharmaceutical data must include the formulation available, its storage, preparation, stability, safe handling procedures, and supplier.

The next section of the protocol should include the criteria for patient eligibility and the procedure for patient entry into the clinical trial. The treatment plan should be complete, and described in a step-by-step fashion. It should include the dose to be administered and schedule, the laboratory data to be collected, the patient requirements, the duration of therapy, treatment evaluation(s), and post-treatment evaluation(s). The protocol must contain criteria to measure patient response to treatment. These criteria must include objective parameters and procedures to test both positive and negative responses. Toxicity criteria and reporting methods should be outlined. If toxic effects require dosage reduction, these modifications should be specifically delineated in the protocol. Any dosage changes for a patient must be clearly documented and taken into consideration in the final analysis of the trial.

The statistical methods used for the interim and final analyses should be clearly outlined. This should include the number of patients to be studied and the duration of the treatment. The protocol should include examples of all clinical, research, and regulatory forms for recording data during the study. The protocol should include a copy of a model informed consent for this clinical trial. The protocol may contain additional information, depending on the nature of the trial. Finally, the protocol should contain a procedure to be followed to discontinue patient treatment for scientific, toxicity, ethical, or personal reasons, should they arise.

INSTITUTIONAL REVIEW BOARD

Human research can yield great benefit in developing new approaches to treating disease. However, research on humans has caused some safety and ethical concerns, which were first noted in the Nuremberg War Crimes Trials. The Nuremberg Code of 1947 set standards for judging scientists who conducted biomedical studies on concentration camp prisoners during World War II. This code has been modified many times. In 1971, the Food and Drug Administration issued regulations governing the institutional review board. In 1981, revised regulations governing the composition, operation, and responsibilities of IRB's were published.[5] IRB approval is required for the use of all investigational agents and devices used in clinical trials using FDA-regulated products.

The IRB has the responsibility to review ongoing research to ensure that the rights and welfare of patients involved in clinical trials are protected. No patient can start on a research protocol before the protocol, including the informed consent form, is approved by the IRB.

The IRB shall consist of at least five members, with differing backgrounds, who understand the regional and cultural population differences, and are sensitive to community attitudes. The board should consist of both men and women. The membership should not be made up of only one profession, and one member must be a nonscientist, e.g., lawyer, clergyman, or teacher. One member must not be associated with the institution, and the lay member must be present for all votes. The board may have individuals with expertise in specific areas to aid in the review of special situations. No one participating in the clinical trial may be involved in the board's decision. A majority vote is required for approval. An institution may override the IRB approval of a study; however, it may not approve a protocol disapproved by the board.

The FDA regulations require the IRB to develop and follow written procedures and continually review the study as it progresses. These should include review of research at intervals appropriate to the degree of risk but not less than once per year. They should also include a determination as to which projects need verification from sources other than the investigator. They should ascertain that no material change in the research has occurred since the IRB approval. The IRB has the responsibility of reviewing, changing, and approving or disapproving the informed consent document to be used in the clinical trial.

The Department of Health and Human Services Office of Protection From Research Risk, as well as the FDA, has regulations governing the IRB process. This office organizationally is located in the Office of the Director of the National Institutes of Health. Its function includes the negotiation of assurances of compliance with regulations for protection of human subjects and guidance of ethical concerns involving human subjects in clinical trials.

INFORMED CONSENT

An informed consent is required in clinical trials that are federally regulated or funded.[6] The informed consent provides information about the treatment and/or the drug that the patient is considering, written in easy to understand language. This document explains the objectives of the clinical trial, including the potential benefits and risks associated with it, as well as alternative treatments available. The patient must read the document and be encouraged to ask questions. Additionally, the investigator or a designee should orally explain the information to the patient. The informed consent process is a continuing process for the life of the clinical trial. Therefore, the patient should continue to ask questions and get additional information as the clinical trial proceeds. The patient should be informed about new therapies or risks associated with the therapy as they become available. There are required elements of an informed consent that must be used for federally funded or regulated studies (see figure 23-3).

The informed consent document approval is the responsibility of the local IRB. The investigator must obtain a written informed consent from the patient or the patient's authorized representative before an investigational drug can be administered. Only in extreme emergency circumstances can a patient be administered a test agent without informed consent.

CLINICAL TRIALS

Clinical trials involve systematic research in humans to test a new treatment based on preclinical studies, when the therapeutic benefits and risks involved are not known. The primary goals of clinical trials are to determine safety, therapeutic activity and toxicity of the new agents or treatment method in humans. Clinical trials progress through three premarketing phases, each of which is designed to answer a particular scientific question.

The primary scientific objective in a phase I clinical trial is to determine a maximally tolerated dose. However, when dose-limiting toxicities, the reversibility of toxicities, and the therapeutic activity are observed, they should be recorded. Therapeutic activity is limited in this phase of a clinical trial. Phase I trials usually use healthy adult volunteers. However, in diseases such as cancer, known toxic drugs must be evaluated in patients with the specific disease; the patients used must have cancer. Patients selected to participate in these trials must not be undergoing any other treatment for their disease. They should have normal physiological parameters and a life expectancy of at least several months. Baseline clinical tests are conducted including a history and physical examination, a complete laboratory screening, electrocardiogram, chest x ray, etc. Significant abnormal findings might make the patient ineligible for the clinical trial. Phase I studies involve only a few patients. The initial starting dose administered in

A. Basic elements of informed consent
The following information shall be provided to each patient:
1. A statement that the study involves research.
An explanation of the purpose of the research.
The expected duration of the subject's participation.
A description of the procedures to be followed.
Identification of any experimental procedures.
2. A description of any reasonably foreseeable risks or discomforts.
3. A description of any benefits to the subject or to others that may be expected.
4. Disclosure of alternative procedures for treatment, if any, that would be advantageous to the patient.
5. A statement describing the extent to which confidentiality will be maintained and a statement that the Food and Drug Administration may inspect the records.
6. For research involving more than minimal risk, an explanation as to whether any compensation and/or medical treatment is available if injury occurs. An explanation of the medical treatments provided and where further information may be obtained.
7. An explanation of whom to contact for answers to pertinent questions about the research and research subject's rights and whom to contact in the event of a research-related injury.
8. A statement that participation is voluntary and refusal to participate will involve no penalty or loss of benefits.
A statement that the subject may discontinue participation at any time without penalty or loss of benefits otherwise entitled.

B. Additional elements of informed consent
When appropriate, one or more of the following elements of information shall also be provided:
1. Statement that treatment may involve unforeseeable risk for the patient (embryo or fetus, if the patient is or may become pregnant).
2. The investigator may terminate the patient's participation without regard to the patient's consent.
3. Additional costs may occur.
4. The consequences of the patient's decision to withdraw from the research.
5. The right of the patient to be informed of new findings.
6. The approximate number of patients involved in the study.

Figure 23-3. Elements of informed consent

Source: *Fed Reg* 46(17):8951-8952, 1981.

these trials is determined from the preclinical data. Separate phase I protocols are usually used to evaluate different dosage schedules. The dose in each trial is escalated in separate groups of patients using a mathematical method, such as the modified Fibonacci search scheme. The dose is increased to the point of toxicity, then it is reduced to a dose that can be safely administered. Once the highest safe dose has been determined, the new agent can be advanced to the second phase of the drug development process. The phase I trials are difficult, but are a most important step in determining if the drug is suitable to continue on in the development process. Clinical data, pharmacology, and the pharmacokinetic data obtained from the trial must be evaluated, which will yield information on the toxicities, dose, and schedule to be used in the phase II trials.

The goals of phase II clinical trials are to determine whether the new drug has clinical activity and to expand knowledge of the dose, schedule, and toxicity. Phase II trials frequently provide further nontherapeutic and toxicity data beyond those obtained in the phase I trials. The protocols for these clinical trials define more study parameters than a phase I protocol. Eligibility criteria for patients is strict. Baseline data such as cardiac function, hematologic, hepatic, renal parameters, and liver function are evaluated and recorded.

Phase II trials are conducted by investigators trained in a particular medical specialty related to the disease being investigated. However, the protocol should clearly describe the objectives and define the assessment criteria for the final analysis of the patient's response to the new drug. The number of patients entered into the protocol will vary depending on the clinical response experience on the initial cadre of patients enrolled. If none of the first 14 patients respond, then the agent has a greater than 95 percent chance of not being effective in the disease. Normally, the trial will be stopped at this point. If 1 or more of the first 14 patients responds, then the trial will expand to 30 or 40 patients. Drugs that show activity without significant or irreversible toxicity will advance to a phase III clinical trial.

Phase III clinical trials are designed to compare a new treatment to an existing standard treatment or a placebo. These trials involve a large number of randomly assigned patients from a few hundred to several thousand. Frequently, these trials involve more than one investigator per protocol and may involve several institutions. The National Cancer Institute and National Institute of Allergy and Infectious Diseases have established large, well-organized groups of investigators worldwide to assist in the accrual of patients with cancer and acquired immunodeficiency syndrome (AIDS) for their clinical trials.

The phase III data are evaluated to determine whether the clinical activity of the new agent has increased patient response and/or survival compared to the standard therapy. These trials may be blinded and randomized with a placebo or a standard therapy. During phase III clinical trials, the sponsor continues to collect toxicity data to evaluate the safety of the investigational agent when it is administered to a large number of patients. Additional information on the proper dose and schedule also may be obtained, especially when the disease has several different stages. Commonly, treatments may be more effective at different stages within the disease.

INVESTIGATIONAL AGENTS FOR NONRESEARCH USE

There are several procedures through which physicians may obtain investigational agents for treatment of individual patients outside of the clinical trial mechanism. These are usually promising new agents that may be helpful for desperately ill patients who have no other known therapy available to them.

The emergency use of an investigational drug or biological agent is defined as the use of an agent for an individual patient in an emergency circumstance in which the standard acceptable treatment is not available.[7] In this situation, there is inadequate time to obtain IRB approval. In addition, the patient does not meet the criteria of an existing clinical trial for the drug, or an approved protocol does not exist. However, if there is time, the physician should try to contact the sponsor of the drug for approval under its IND. Should the sponsor refuse to approve the use of the agent, the physician may contact the FDA for an individual IND. The use of an investigational agent in an emergency situation should be reported to the IRB within 5 working days.

Informed consent is required from the patient or his or her legal authorized representative. If the patient is not able to communicate and the legal representative is not available, the patient's physician and a physician not associated with the clinical investigation must certify in writing that an emergency situation exists. Any subsequent use of the agent does require IRB review in advance of administration.

Investigational drugs also may be available for treatment of individual patients in nonemergency situations. During the course of the development of a drug, evidence of therapeutic activity will frequently become apparent. With this apparent activity, the sponsor will occasionally make the agent available to physicians to treat their patients on a case-by-case basis outside of the clinical trial. An investigational agent made available in such situations is commonly referred to as a "compassionate IND." There is no regulation in the Code of Federal Regulations (C.F.R.) describing this mechanism. However, the National Cancer Institute has a similar mechanism referred to as a "special exception," which is described in its drug master file with the FDA. This mechanism provides drugs to desperately ill patients who are not eligible for a clinical trial, when clinical trials are not available, or when the patient refuses to participate in a clinical trial. The procedures used for a drug under the special exception mechanism are outlined in figure 23-4. Other sponsors may follow similar procedures if they obtain FDA approval and are willing to release the agent for use in this manner. IRB approval and patient informed consent are required when investigational drugs are obtained by the "special exception" mechanism.

Since 1976, the National Cancer Institute, with the approval of the FDA, has made certain investigational agents available to physicians for treatment under a mechanism referred to as "Group C." This mechanism is the forerunner of the FDA treatment IND or protocol process that began in 1987.[8] The treatment IND (Group C) is different from the "special exception (compassionate)" use mechanisms in that it has FDA preapproved protocols using the drug in a specific treatment and disease. Treatment IND's permit the sponsor to distribute investigational drugs to physicians for

Drug Management and Authorization Section, IDB, CTEP
Division of Cancer Treatment, NCI, NIH
Executive Plaza North, Room 707-A
9000 Rockville Pike
Bethesda, Maryland 20892

NATIONAL CANCER INSTITUTE PROCEDURE FOR MANAGEMENT OF INVESTIGATIONAL DRUGS ACQUIRED FOR COMPASSIONATE TREATMENT OF INDIVIDUAL PATIENTS

Food and Drug Administration (FDA) regulations and National Cancer Institute (NCI) policy require the following steps to be completed as indicated:

1) Statement of Investigator (FDA 1572): Since you are not registered as an investigator, it is required that you complete and sign the enclosed FDA 1572 form and return it to the above address within 10 working days in order to receive additional drug.

2) Protocol: A brief protocol must be submitted for each patient which describes the treatment plan, toxicity, efficacy, and monitoring procedures. For your convenience we have designed a standard protocol form which is included and must be completed. The original and three copies must be returned to the above address within 10 working days.

3) Institutional Review Board Approval: You must obtain Institutional Review Board approval prior to treatment of the patient and retain documentation of this approval in the patient's medical record.

4) Informed Consent: You must write an informed consent which must be signed by the patient and retained in the patient's medical record. The consent should include a reasonable statement about the side effects of the drug. The informed consent must address each of the eight elements required under FDA regulations, as detailed on the accompanying sheet.

5) Final Patient Report: Upon completion of therapy, you must provide NCI a report of the treatment experience, which describes toxicity and efficacy. We have enclosed the form(s) be used. Please return this form(s) to the Drug Management and Authorization Section at the above address.

6) Adverse Drug Reactions: Report by phone [(301) 496-7957)] to the Investigational Drug Branch within 24 hours all life-threatening and lethal (grade 4 and 5) unknown adverse drug reactions. A written report must follow in 10 working days. Report in writing within 10 working days all grade 4 and 5 known reactions (except grade 4 myelosuppression) and grade 2 and 3 unknown reactions. Grade 1-3 known reactions should be reported as part of the progress summary. Toxicity rating scale and adverse drug reaction reporting forms are enclosed. All reports should be mailed to:

Investigational Drug Branch
P.O. Box 30012
Bethesda, Maryland 20824

7) Investigational Drug Accountability: The enclosed drug accountability record must be maintained and retained in your records. These records may be inspected upon request by an authorized representative of the FDA, the NCI, or the drug company.

8) Failure to submit items 1, 2, and 6 in a timely manner will prevent any further drug shipments and may result in recall of drug.

9) Drug Reorders: Additional drug may be requested by completing a Clinical Drug Request Form. You may only order more drug for the patient specifically named on this protocol. The patient's first name and initial of last name should be indicated on the Clinical Drug Request. A blank request form is enclosed in each drug shipment. Telephone orders will not be accepted.

SE-N Revised 11/89

Figure 23-4. NCI procedure for managing special exception/compassionate use

treatment of individual patients provided that the following criteria are met:

1. The patient must have either a serious or immediately life-threatening disease.
2. No satisfactory alternative therapy is available.
3. The drug currently must be in a controlled clinical trial.
4. The sponsor is pursuing marketing approval with due diligence.

The National Cancer Institute continues to use the Group C mechanism rather than the treatment IND mechanism. There are small differences between the two mechanisms. The primary difference is that the Health Care Financing Administration of the Department of Health and Human Services will pay for care with Group C drugs. To obtain treatment IND drugs, the physician should contact the pharmaceutical company directly. To get a Group C drug, the physician should telephone the NCI, Drug Management and Authorization Section, at (301) 496-5725. The NCI procedure for management of investigational drugs for Group C use is outlined in figure 23-5 and Group C drugs available from the NCI are listed in figure 23-6.

The use of drugs in the treatment IND or Group C mechanism requires informed consent; however, the FDA may waive the IRB requirement, usually after a central IRB has approved the protocol. The local IRB still has the right to either review the protocol or accept the FDA waiver.

USE OF INVESTIGATIONAL DRUGS IN THE LABORATORY

Investigators may request that the pharmacy provide a study drug from a clinical protocol for an experiment in a laboratory research animal or in vitro test.[9] Clinical supplies reserved for clinical trials should not be used. Investigational agents for laboratory use should be requested directly from the sponsor. The pharmacy may assist the investigator in obtaining the agent, but it should not provide an investigational agent designated for a clinical trial. Many sponsors will require that these requests be submitted in writing with details of the intended use, quantity of drugs needed, and duration of the study. The labeling on these agents will contain its own caution. For drugs, the caution will read: "CAUTION: Contains a new drug for investigational use only in laboratory research animals or for test in vitro. Not for use in humans." For biological agents, the legend will read: "CAUTION: Contains a biological product for investigational in vitro diagnostic test only."

The investigator receiving the agent must assure the sponsor that the drug will not be used in humans. The investigator must return all unused product to the sponsor. The sponsor may authorize in writing alternative methods of disposal of unused supplies of the agent. This alternative method must ensure that humans will not be directly or indirectly exposed to the agent.

INVESTIGATIONAL USE OF COMMERCIAL DRUGS

Physicians may use a commercial drug for a nonapproved indication for treatment of their patients. However, they have a responsibility to be well informed about the drug's use in this indication, as do others directly involved in the dispensing and administering of the agent. In addition, they should use the drug based on firm scientific information and good medical evidence and maintain good medical records of use and results of treatment. The physician under these circumstances may alter the dose, schedule, or route of administration. These changes can be very helpful to the patient and may be appropriate for his or her medical treatment. Frequently, manufacturers delay obtaining FDA approval for a new indication until after the new and effective therapies are established in the literature. Physicians who decide to employ a drug for a nonapproved use should be aware of their State's practice codes and any potential liabilities.

When a commercial drug is used in an investigational clinical trial for unapproved use, additional regulations should apply. With an intent to get information about safety or efficacy for a new indication, an IND submission is generally required. Even when an IND submission is not required, it may be in the best interest of the investigator and the sponsor to submit one, especially if the data will be used to obtain FDA approval of the drug for this new indication. When a drug is used in a clinical trial without an IND submission, the institutional review board may still choose to monitor the trial.

PHARMACY-BASED INVESTIGATIONAL DRUG SERVICE

The pharmacy department should be responsible for the management of investigational drugs. The Joint Commission on Accreditation of Healthcare Organizations (JCAHO) states that drug management within the hospital should be under the supervision of the pharmacy department.[10] This should include proper storage, distribution, and control of investigational drugs. Also, the American Society of Hospital Pharmacists (ASHP) has published guidelines for the use of investigational drugs in institutions.[11] These guidelines include recommendations for the basic principles in handling investigational drugs and guidelines for the organized health care setting, for the pharmacists, and for the pharmaceutical industry to consider.

To abide by the standards of practice of the JCAHO and ASHP, the pharmacy should be responsible for obtaining, storing, preparing, distributing, and recording information for all investigational drugs used within the hospital. These goals must begin with the pharmacist having a good professional relationship, especially with the investigator, and to some degree with the person or organization, e.g., the pharmaceutical company, National Institutes of Health, etc., that took the responsibility to initiate the clinical trial; this entity is also known as the sponsor. The pharmacist should have access to the clinical protocol and any known drug information, including all pharmaceutical data, safe handling procedures, record-keeping requirements, and methods to properly administer the investigational agent to the patient. This information should be in the protocol; if it is not, the pharmacist may obtain it from the sponsor. The standards of practice for managing investigational drugs are similar for investigators in private practice and for investigators in large research hospitals.

Clinical trials involve many professionals and supportive hospital personnel as well as patients and their families.

Drug Management and Authorization Section
Investigational Drug Branch
CTEP, DCT, NCI, NIH
Executive Plaza North, Room 707-A
Bethesda, Maryland 20892
(301) 496-5725

NATIONAL CANCER INSTITUTE PROCEDURES FOR MANAGEMENT OF INVESTIGATIONAL DRUGS ACQUIRED FOR GROUP C/TREATMENT PROTOCOL USE IN INDIVIDUAL PATIENTS

Food and Drug Administration (FDA) regulations and National Cancer Institute (NCI) policy require the following steps to be completed as indicated:

1. Statement of Investigator (FDA 1572): Since you are not registered as an investigator, it is required that you complete and sign the enclosed FDA 1572 form and return it within 10 working days to the above address in order to receive additional drug.

2. Institutional Review Board Approval: The NCI has obtained an exemption from the FDA eliminating the requirement for IRB approval. However, you should check with your IRB to determine whether its local policy requires approval.

3. Informed Consent: You must obtain written informed consent which must be signed by the patient and retained in the patient's medical record. For your convenience, a model informed consent document is included in the enclosed protocol.

4. Adverse Drug Reactions: All life-threatening and lethal (grade 4 and 5) unknown (not listed in the protocol as known toxicities) adverse drug reactions must be reported by phone [(30l) 496-7957] to the Investigational Drug Branch within 24 hours. A written report must follow within 10 working days. All grade 4 and 5 known reactions (except grade 4 myelosuppression) and grade 2 and 3 unknown reactions must be reported in writing within 10 working days. Common toxicity criteria and adverse drug reaction reporting forms are in the protocol appendices. All reports should be mailed to:

   Investigational Drug Branch
   P.O. Box 30012
   Bethesda, Maryland 20824

5. Investigational Drug Accountability: Investigational drug accountability records (enclosed) must be maintained and retained in your files. These documents may be inspected upon request by an authorized representative of the FDA and the NCI.

6. Quality Assurance: All patient records are subject to review for quality assurance as described in the protocol under, "Patient Records and Quality Assurance".

7. Failure to comply with item 1, and 6 in a timely manner may prevent any further drug shipments and may result in recall of drug.

8. Drug Reorders: Additional drug may be requested by completing a Clinical Drug Request Form. You may only reorder drug for a patient previously registered on this protocol. The patient's first name and initial of last name must be indicated on the clinical Drug Request Form. A blank request form is enclosed in each drug shipment for use with reorders. Telephone orders will not be accepted.

GC-N Revised 11/89

Figure 23-5. NCI procedure for managing group C drugs

National Cancer Institute
Division of Cancer Treatment, CTEP
Investigational Drug Branch
Drug Management and Authorization Section
(301) 496-5725

Policy For Group C Drug Distribution

Group C agents are investigational drugs provided by the National Cancer Institute to properly trained physicians for the treatment of individual patients who meet the eligibility criteria. Agents within this category have been approved by the Food and Drug Administration for the treatment of the specific cancer identified in the guideline protocol.

I. **Group C drugs are provided for the treatment of patients as indicated below:**

Drug	Approved Group C Use
a) Amsacrine*	Refractory Adult Acute Myelogenous Leukemia (AML) Single agent use only
b) Azacytidine*	Refractory Acute Myelogenous Leukemia (AML) Single agent use only
c) Erwinia Asparaginase*	Acute Lymphoblastic Leukemia (ALL), for patients allergic to E. Coli L-Asparaginase
d) Fludarabine Phosphate	Refractory Chronic Lymphocytic Leukemia
e) Hexamethylmelamine*	Refractory Ovarian Carcinoma, Single agent use only
f) Pentostatin*	Hairy Cell Leukemia, in patients refractory to or intolerant of Alpha-Interferon
g) Teniposide*	First Relapse or Refractory Acute Lymphocytic Leukemia (ALL) Combination therapy with cytarabine

* The FDA has granted a waiver from local IRB Approval. See paragraph 5 on the next page.

II. **Group C Drugs Available only at Approved Cancer Centers**

Interleukin-2 (Alone or in conjunction with Lymphokine Activated Killer Cells)	Metastatic or Unresectable Renal Cell Carcinoma or Unresectable Malignant Melanoma

Figure 23-6. Group C drugs available from NCI

The pharmacist definitely has a collaborative role in the clinical trial involving investigational drugs.

OBTAINING INVESTIGATIONAL DRUGS

The pharmacy may obtain investigational drugs for the investigator's clinical trials or for individual patients being treated with investigational drugs outside the clinical trial. Under either circumstance, the investigational agents remain the property of the sponsor, even while they are in the possession of the pharmacy or the investigator.

Sponsors may provide various quantities of investigational drugs to investigators at the beginning of the trial. Sponsors may estimate the amount of drug that will be required to complete the protocol, and then ship that amount to the investigator initially. The pharmacist should determine the space requirements and any special storage requirements such as additional refrigerator or freezer space prior to receiving the drugs. In contrast, sponsors such as the National Cancer Institute provide no more than an 8-week supply of drug at any one time. Unlike other sponsors, however, NCI provides a special drug request form to investigators to order investigational drugs as needed. In addition, study drugs may be obtained electronically from the NCI by using the pharmacy's personal computer and modem. This method reduces the time to receive the drugs from the NCI from 14-21 days to 4-7 days.

Investigational drugs may be ordered and shipped directly to the pharmacy if approved by the sponsor and the investigator. The National Cancer Institute strongly suggests that investigators designate the pharmacy department to order, store, prepare, dispense, and account for investigational drugs. When the pharmacy is responsible for the investigational drug management of the patient, investigator and sponsor will be better served. The drugs will be prepared and dispensed by the pharmacist in a standard method in accordance with each protocol. The security and control of the investigational drugs will be maintained similarly to the other drugs in the hospital.

When investigational drugs are obtained from sponsors for the treatment of a patient outside a clinical trial, it is even more important that these drugs be managed by the pharmacy department. This further complicates the distribution and accountability systems by increasing the number of physicians requesting these agents; they frequently are not familiar with the FDA regulations and the sponsor policies governing investigational drugs. It should be remembered that the physician cannot take investigational drugs that are intended for clinical trials and use them for treatment purposes, except in emergency circumstances when the patient does not meet the criteria of the protocol and the sponsor or FDA cannot be reached. Similarly, drugs obtained for treatment (nonresearch) use cannot be used outside of the guidelines agreed to between the physician and sponsor. Policies and procedures established by the pharmacy for handling investigational drugs should provide methods to control drug activities while meeting the requirements of the institution, the sponsor, and the FDA.

ADVERSE DRUG REACTION REPORTING

The investigator must report to the sponsor adverse reactions caused by or suspected to be caused by the new agent. If the reaction was a lethal or a life-threatening toxicity, it must be reported within 24 hours and all others, within 10 days.

INVESTIGATIONAL DRUG ACCOUNTABILITY

The investigator ordering the investigational drugs has agreed by signing the Statement of Investigator, FDA form 1572, to maintain accountability records for the disposition of investigational drugs. This responsibility includes retaining packing slip, drug use records, drug transfer, and return records. All unused drug must be disposed of in a fashion consistent with the sponsor's policies, and documentation of disposition must be maintained by the investigator. In many institutions, the pharmacy department is responsible for these activities.

The sponsor of the investigational drug will usually provide a form(s) to account for the drug. This will vary from a list of requirements to that of a standard accountability form. The complexity of the sponsor's accountability procedures may relate to the number of investigational agents and the number of investigators used to conduct clinical trials. The National Cancer Institute requires that investigators use only their "Investigational Drug Accountability Record" form (figure 23-7).[12] One form is used for each investigational agent for a particular individual protocol. If more than one investigational agent is used in a protocol, a separate form must be used for each agent. Similarly, if the same drug is used in more than one protocol, then a separate form is used for each drug and protocol that is associated. Separate drug accountability records must be maintained for each strength or dosage form of a drug. This form has been designed to be used where the drug is stored and dispensed. Other drug transactions may be recorded on the form, e.g., receipts, transfers to other locations, unused drug disposition, broken vials, etc. In addition to the "Investigational Drug Accountability Record," the NCI system uses forms to return unused drugs entitled the "Return Drug List" form (figure 23-8) or the "Transfer Investigational Drugs Form" (figure 23-9). The first form allows for the return of the unneeded drug to the NCI repository. The second form permits the transfer of drugs from a terminated protocol to an active protocol within the same institution.

QUALITY ASSURANCE

The pharmacy department should be responsible for the quality assurance of investigational drug accountability records.[13] The records should be legible and complete, and periodic audits of records should include the following information:

1. A comparison of amount of drugs received to that drug dispensed and the current inventory.
2. The date and quantity dispensed, which should agree with the date the dose was ordered on the patient's chart.
3. Whether the order was written by an investigator participating in the protocol.
4. Whether the patient was properly registered on the protocol.
5. A comparison of the amount of drug on the phar-

Form approved:
OMB No. 0925-0240
Expires: 6/30/91

National Institutes of Health
National Cancer Institute

Investigational Drug Accountability Record

PAGE NO. ________

CONTROL RECORD ☐

SATELLITE RECORD ☐

Name of Institution

Protocol No. (NCI)

Drug Name, Dose Form and Strength

Protocol Title

Dispensing Area

Investigator

Line No.	Date	Patient's Initials	Patient's I.D. Number	Dose	Quantity Dispensed or Received	Balance Forward / Balance	Manufacturer and Lot No.	Recorder's Initials
1.								
2.								
3.								
4.								
5.								
6.								
7.								
8.								
9.								
10.								
11.								
12.								
13.								
14.								
15.								
16.								
17.								
18.								
19.								
20.								
21.								
22.								
23.								
24.								

NIH-2564
9-85

Figure 23-7. NCI's Investigational Drug Accountability Record Form

NOTE NEW RETURN ADDRESS

Properly complete all sections to receive credit for the return.

NATIONAL INSTITUTES OF HEALTH
NATIONAL CANCER INSTITUTE

RETURN DRUG LIST

Return only drugs supplied by the National Cancer Institute

The drugs listed below were ordered by:
(One investigator per form only)

Dr. ______________ No. ______________

Address:

FOR NCI USE ONLY

R.D. NUMBER

DATE RECEIVED

SIGNATURE OF AUTHORIZING OFFICAL

DATE OF AUTHORIZATION

	PROTOCOL OR IND NUMBER	NSC NUMBER	DRUG NAME	STRENGTH & DOSE FORM (Specify vials, capsules, tablets)	QUANTITY (Specify vials or bottles)	MANU-FACTURER	LOT NUMBER	DESCRIPTION	ACTION
A									
B									
C									
D									
E									
F									
G									
H									
I									
J									

INSTRUCTIONS

1. Remove attached sheets
2. Type all information—one item or protocol per line. Fill in all sections completely.
3. DO NOT cross the double line into shaded area marked FOR NCI USE ONLY.
4. Sign and date list.
5. Pack the drugs well to minimize breakage and leakage.
6. Enclose the completed list with the drugs and return to:

NCI Clinical Repository
ERC INTERNATIONAL
649 E/F Lofstrand Lane
Rockville, MD 20850

Signature:

Date:

Individual preparing this list
(if other than the investigator)

Title:

Telephone Number:

RETURN RECEIPT
To obtain a return receipt, fill in the appropriate mailing address in the space provided to the right.

1. Destroy
2. Return to stock
3. Return to Manufacturer
4. Quarantine
5. Quarantine-RFF
6. Return to sender

Figure 23-8. NCI's Return Drug List

Form approved:
OMB No. 0925-0240
Expires: 6/30/91

National Institutes of Health
National Cancer Institute

Transfer Investigational Drug Form
Investigational Drug Accountability

Investigator Transferring Drug: Dr. *	NCI Investigator No.	Date of Transfer

Name of Institution

Street	City	State	Zip Code

This form is to be used for intra-institutional transfer only for the following reasons. (Please check one of the boxes below.)

Completed Protocol ☐ Unused Drug Obtained for Special Exception Protocol ☐

The following drug(s) required for NCI approved protocol(s) are being transferred to NCI approved protocol(s) for

Investigator ______________________*. No. ______________.
Investigator Receiving Drug   NCI Investigator No.

Received on NCI Protocol No.**	Transferred to NCI Protocol No.	NSC Number	Drug Name	Strength & Formulation	Quantity	Manufacturer and Lot No.

Authorized Signature (Investigator or Designee)

Telephone Number

*Use One Form Per Set Of Investigators.
**No Additional Drug Will Be Supplied For This Protocol No.

All Requested Information MUST Be Supplied In Order For Form To Be Valid.

NIH-2564
1/89

Return Form To:

Drug Management and Authorization Section
Investigational Drug Branch
Cancer Therapy Evaluation Program
Division of Cancer Treatment, NCI, NIH
Executive Plaza North, Room 707A
Bethesda, MD 20892

Figure 23-9. NCI's Transfer Investigational Drug Form

macy shelf with the balance on the accountability records.

6. Whether all unused drug is transferred to an active protocol with sponsor approval or returned to the sponsor.

Using these or similar audit procedures will ensure that no investigational drug is misused, that FDA regulations and sponsor policies are satisfied, and that no discrepancies exist. Good records should reduce differences arising among the investigators, the sponsor, and the FDA.

Accountability records must be maintained by the investigator for 2 years after the investigation is discontinued for an indication or 2 years following the date that a New Drug Application is approved by the FDA for an indication being investigated.

SECURITY

The security of investigational drugs must be of concern to the investigator and the institution. Investigational drugs should be kept in a secure area, accessible only to authorized individuals. The pharmacy normally would have adequate security as it does for other noninvestigational drugs. However, this may require a separate locked area for investigational drugs, depending on the complexity and current security system in the pharmacy, to protect them from unauthorized personnel. Investigational agents subject to the Comprehensive Drug Abuse Prevention and Control Act of 1970 must have adequate precautions taken, including storage in a securely locked, substantially constructed cabinet or enclosure with limited access, to prevent theft or diversion into illegal channels.

SUMMARY

The pharmacy department should have a close collaboration with investigators and other individuals involved in all clinical drug trials within the institution. The obvious role of the pharmacist would be to obtain, store, prepare, dispense, and account for the disposition of all investigational agents. Details of these procedures should be a part of the department's policy and procedure manual. Pharmacists will ensure that these agents are being managed and controlled according to the procedures set forth by the investigator and sponsor. These control procedures will further ensure the investigator that expiration dates and adequate levels of drug supplies are being monitored on a scheduled basis. The centralized storage of investigational drugs ensures that all patient doses will be prepared in accordance with the procedures outlined in the protocol and dispensed properly for administration to the patient. When clinical trials require randomization and blinding, the pharmacist is in an excellent position to collaborate with the investigator, statistician, and sponsor. The pharmacist should play a major role in managing drug-related issues in the clinical trial. The pharmacist should be involved in the clinical monitoring as the clinical trial progresses and in the reporting of adverse drug reactions. Finally, the pharmacist should provide drug information to all individuals involved in the study and maintain dispensing information needed as the clinical trial progresses.

REFERENCES

1. 52 Stat 1040, 1938.
2. Kelsey FO: The Kefauver-Harris amendments and investigational drugs. *Am J Hosp Pharm* 20:515-517, 1963.
3. 21 C.F.R. 312.40, April 1, 1989.
4. 21 C.F.R. 312.53, April 1, 1989.
5. *Fed Reg* 46(17):8958-8980, 1981.
6. *Fed Reg* 46(17):8942-8952, 1981.
7. 21 C.F.R. 312.36, April 1, 1989.
8. 21 C.F.R. 312.34, April 1, 1989.
9. 21 C.F.R. 312.160, April 1, 1989.
10. Joint Commission on Accreditation of Healthcare Organizations: *Accreditation Manual for Hospitals*. Chicago, IL, JCAHO, 1989.
11. ASHP guidelines for the use of investigational drugs in organized health-care setting. *Am J Hosp Pharm* 48:315-391, 1991.
12. *Investigational Drug Accountability*. Bethesda, MD, National Cancer Institute, 1991, NIH No. 2564.
13. Tankanow RM, Savitsky ME, Volger BW, et al: Quality assurance program for a hospital investigational drug service. *Am J Hosp Pharm* 9:962-969,1989.

ADDITIONAL READING

Johnson J, Temple R: Food and Drug Administration requirements for approval of new anticancer drugs. *Cancer Treat Rep* 69:1155-1157, 1985.

Marsoni S, Wittes R: Clinical development of anticancer agents—National Cancer Institute perspective. *Cancer Treat Rep* 68:77-85, 1984.

Ryan ML, Colvin CL, Tankanow RM: Development and funding of a pharmacy-based investigational drug service. *Am J Hosp Pharm* 44:1069-1074, 1987.

Stolar M (ed): *Pharmacy-Coordinated Investigational Drug Service*. Bethesda, MD, American Society of Hospital Pharmacists, 1986.

Temple R: Government viewpoint of clinical trials. *Drug Information J* (Jan-Jun):40-47, 1982.

CHAPTER 24

Drug Use Evaluation

MARK W. TODD

There is no question that pharmacy practice in the 1990's will be exciting. Now, more than ever, the safe and effective use of drugs cannot only be talked about; these important aspects must be demonstrated. Advances in drug therapy and biotechnology are being implemented at a staggering pace. This trend will undoubtedly continue, and the profession of pharmacy must position itself in a leading role for ensuring appropriate use of these agents. For years we have been able to show that drugs are frequently used inappropriately.[1-4] Now we must change our emphasis and accept the challenge that we have presented ourselves. That is, we must demonstrate positive patient outcome by optimizing drug therapy.

Spiraling health care costs have raised serious questions about the quality of care or value these dollars buy. Health care expenditures (7 percent of which are drugs) have risen from 6 percent to 12 percent of the Nation's gross national product during the past 25 years.[5] This represents a rise of 5 percent to a projected 15 percent of the entire Federal budget between 1970 and the early 1990's. It is no wonder that insurance companies, the Federal Government, accreditation agencies, and most important, the patient, are now focusing on value for the health care dollar spent by seeking assurance of improved patient outcome. Drug use evaluation (DUE) will serve as an important tool for demonstrating that drugs are of value to patient care by ensuring they are used safely, effectively, and economically ("safe, effective, and economical" drug use henceforth will be referred to as "appropriate").

The practice of DUE has become an essential part of pharmacy practice and will continue to grow in importance throughout the 1990's. A well-planned and legitimate DUE program will not only help to position the practice of pharmacy as an essential component of patient care but will help to continue to reshape pharmacy practice from a product-oriented to a patient-oriented profession. This activity has become so important not only to pharmacy practice, but also to the practice of medicine within institutions, that the Joint Commission on Accreditation of Healthcare Organizations (JCAHO) now mandates this activity as an essential component of quality assurance.[6] The American Society of Hospital Pharmacists (ASHP) likewise describes DUE as an important component of pharmacy practice.[7] Ensuring that drugs are used appropriately has now evolved into a quality assurance activity directly tied to patient care and ultimately patient outcome. DUE may be one of the best opportunities pharmacy practice has been provided. Our profession cannot afford to miss this opportunity. There is no question that DUE can improve patient care, avoid unnecessary costs, and firmly establish pharmacy practice as a clinical profession.

This chapter discusses the evolution of DUE from the early days of antibiotic usage review. It also reviews the JCAHO standards and explores ways to establish a DUE program. Examples of the DUE process are presented as well as common pitfalls encountered in attempting to establish and manage a DUE program.

DUE DEFINED

A DUE program has been defined as a "structured ongoing organizationally authorized quality assurance process designed to ensure that drugs are used appropriately, safely, and effectively."[7] In our health care environment, economical use of drugs should also be given high priority and, therefore, become a component of this definition. Other terms frequently used in the past to describe DUE function have included "antibiotic use review" (AUR), "drug utilization review" (DUR), and "drug use review" (DUR). These terms are now obsolete and in many cases only described quantitative drug use. The above DUE program definition focuses on qualitative drug use, assimilating the best of AUR and DUR approaches.[8,9] The words "usage" and "use" are frequently used interchangeably. ASHP refers to DUE as drug "use" evaluation; the JCAHO uses the term drug "usage" evaluation. However, the meaning is the same.

THE EVOLUTION OF DUE

DUE has matured into a quality assurance activity now mandated by the JCAHO.[6] The purpose of this activity is to ensure appropriate drug therapy. In 1976, Brodie and Smith[10] published an important paper that defined the DUR process (as it was referred to then) as an ongoing and well-conceived program that reviews, analyzes, and interprets the patterns of drug use in an organized health care setting compared with objective criteria or standards. The following year, Brodie et al.[11] described an important five-principle model for performing DUE in a hospital, which serves as the blueprint today. In 1978, Stolar[12] helped to further conceptualize the DUR process. He stated that in order for a DUR program to ensure the quality of drug use, it must be continuous, authorized, and structured; must measure the use of drugs against predetermined criteria; and importantly, initiate changes in drug use that does not meet these criteria. This helped to distinguish the DUR study from the DUR program. Stolar stated that a DUR study can be quantitative or qualitative. Quantitative studies involve the collection, organization, and reporting of the amount of drug use. The quality of drug use cannot be determined conclusively from these types of data. Quantitative DUR studies may or may not be part of an ongoing activity and are usually a pharmacy function. Qualitative DUR studies, on the other hand, are multidisciplinary activities that evaluate the appropriateness of drug use based on predetermined criteria. They are usually one-time examinations of a specific drug or class of drugs or sometimes a specific disease. With use of criteria, the quality of drug use can be measured. A combination of both types of DUR studies may be used to determine patterns, amounts, and quality of drug use. As Stolar emphasized, individual DUR studies do not generally have any lasting impact, are not an integral component of patient care, and provide no followup to determine if corrective measures were successful (assuming problem areas were identified).

In contrast, the DUR program is ongoing and a part of patient care. The program is "the system by which quality drug use is defined, measured, and ultimately achieved."[12] DUR programs are qualitative studies *plus* corrective action (usually education), prescriber feedback, and reevaluation.

When developing standards for how drug use should be evaluated within the institution, the JCAHO relied heavily on the concepts just discussed.[13] Early in the 1980's, the JCAHO focused on AUR; DUE itself was not mentioned in these standards. Antibiotics had received considerable attention in the literature because of their high use, high cost, and subsequent reports of frequent inappropriate use. The JCAHO felt it necessary to build standards to help monitor and prevent this problem from recurring. From 1981 to 1983, the term "AUR" appeared in the standards several times as it pertained to the medical staff, inpatients, emergency department, ambulatory care, and infection control. The responsibility for performing AUR was that of the medical staff with the assistance of the department of pharmacy. In 1984 and 1985, the AUR requirements were expanded and more specifically stated that antibiotics must be reviewed everywhere within the institution and compared to objective written criteria for use. The standards went so far as to state that the medical staff must review the appropriateness, safety, and effectiveness of the prophylactic, empiric, and therapeutic use of all antibiotics in all patient care areas based on established criteria. In 1986, the standards were again revised. At this time, the emphasis on antibiotics was eliminated. Specifically, the standards stated that DUE be performed as a criteria-based, ongoing, planned, and systematic process for monitoring and evaluating the prophylactic, empiric, and therapeutic use of drugs to ensure that such uses are appropriate, safe, and effective.[6] These standards have not changed as of 1990.

JCAHO STANDARDS FOR DUE

The JCAHO standards for performing DUE can be found within the medical staff chapter of the 1990 *Accreditation Manual for Hospitals*[6] (see table 24-1). Although the JCAHO has developed a framework for DUE, this standard is still in its infancy. Because it has been available and in practice only since 1986, not only do practitioners have difficulty in implementing this type of program, JCAHO surveyors who apply these standards to individual institutions have difficulty with their interpretation. Therefore, inconsistencies in surveyors' interpretations and expectations are common.

The DUE function is the responsibility of the medical staff, to be performed with the cooperation of the department of pharmacy. It must be an ongoing, criteria-based, systematic process. Theoretically, all drugs, not just antibiotics, must be monitored for effectiveness, safety, and appropriateness. JCAHO standards indicate that certain drugs be monitored more frequently than others. These standards include those that are known to cause adverse effects or interact with other drugs in a manner that may be harmful, those that are more prone to cause problems in certain patient groups (such as the elderly or renally impaired), those that are most frequently prescribed, and those that are designated by quality assurance activities (e.g., hospital infection control program). It is interesting to note that there is no mention of costly drugs in these standards. The standards also require that at least quarterly reports of all the findings and actions taken as a result of a DUE program be documented and disseminated to the appropriate members of the medical staff and hospital quality assurance committee or personnel. This standard is so important that it is also emphasized that results of DUE activities should be considered in the medical staff's reappointment and privileges.

Every institutional pharmacist should read, study, and understand these standards. They are extremely important to pharmacy practice and should be viewed as an excellent opportunity to work closely with the medical staff in ensuring appropriate use of drugs.

DUE STUDY DESIGNS

The assessment of drug use can be performed through a retrospective, concurrent, or prospective study design. Each of these types has its advantages and disadvantages. A *retrospective review* is the simplest to implement and perform. Drug therapy that has already been administered to a patient is reviewed to determine if that therapy met the approved criteria. This type of review is used frequently in research and can provide an enormous amount of information over extended periods of time. Studies can be performed as time permits and generally require limited resources. The obvious disadvantage of retrospective review is that it will not have any immediate impact on patient care. Another serious disadvantage is the reliance of retrospective evaluation on written documentation in the patient's medical record. Documentation of this type can be absent, incomplete, or vague, leading the reviewer to subjective interpretation.

A *concurrent review* provides the opportunity for corrective actions to be taken while the patient is still in the institution. For example, a review process may be in place that scans all potential theophylline and cimetidine drug interactions. Although the patient may already have received this drug combination, a concurrent review would allow therapy in that patient to be altered if necessary. This method has the advantage of affecting patient care more

Table 24-1. The 1990 Joint Commission on Accreditation of Healthcare Organizations, Standards for Performing Drug Usage Evaluation

MS.6.1.3 Drug Usage Evaluation.

MS.6.1.3.1 Drug usage evaluation is performed by the medical staff as a criteria-based, ongoing, planned and systematic process for monitoring and evaluating the prophylactic, therapeutic, and empiric use of drugs to help assure that they are provided appropriately, safely, and effectively.

MS.6.1.3.1.1 This process includes the routine collection and assessment of information in order to identify opportunities to improve the use of drugs and to resolve problems in their use.

MS.6.1.3.2 There is ongoing monitoring and evaluation of selected drugs that are chosen for one or more of the following reasons:

MS.6.1.3.2.1 Based on clinical experience, it is known or suspected that the drug causes adverse reactions or interacts with another drug (or drugs) in a manner that presents a significant health risk;

MS.6.1.3.2.2 The drug is used in the treatment of reactions because of age, disability, or unique metabolic characteristics;

MS.6.1.3.2.3 The drug has been designated, through the hospital's infection control program or other quality assurance activities, for monitoring and evaluation; and/or

MS.6.1.3.2.4 The drug is one of the most frequently prescribed drugs.

MS.6.1.3.3 The process for monitoring and evaluating the use of drugs

MS.6.1.3.3.1 is performed by the medical staff in cooperation with, as required, the pharmaceutical department/service, the nursing department/service, management and administrative staff, and other departments/services and individuals;

MS.6.1.3.3.2 is based on the use of objective criteria that reflect current knowledge, clinical experience, and relevant literature; and

MS.6.1.3.3.3 may include the use of screening mechanisms to identify, for more intensive evaluation, problems in or opportunities to improve the use of a specific drug or category of drugs.

MS.6.1.3.4 Written reports of the findings, conclusions, recommendations, actions taken, and results of actions taken are maintained and reported at least quarterly through channels established by the medical staff.

MS.6.1.3.5 As appropriate, the results of drug usage evaluation are considered in the medical staff reappointment and privilege delineation processes, and in the conduct of quality assurance activities.

directly than retrospective review. However, the logistics of locating a problem and intervening quickly requires a more sophisticated process than that of the retrospective review. Physicians must be available for diplomatic and assertive pharmacist consultation for this process to be effective.

Performing a *prospective review* has the advantage of altering drug therapy before the patient receives it. A good example of a prospective review process would be a protocol or specific written criteria for use. This method serves as an excellent teaching opportunity for pharmacists, but can create confrontations with physicians if not done tactfully. A major disadvantage to prospective evaluation is that a very organized and well-defined approach to drug therapy surveillance is needed, compared with the retrospective or concurrent design. All pharmacists must be involved, and daily routines may be interrupted for the process to work. Immediate access to patient information is required, making the system more difficult to implement for centralized practitioners.

More DUE activities need to be prospective, or at least concurrent, in nature to effectively measure and improve quality of drug therapy and ultimately outcome in an individual patient. Inherently, the practice of pharmacy is a prospective review process. Medication orders are reviewed at the time they are received, and if a problem exists, the medication is not provided to the patient until problems with therapy have been discussed with the prescriber. Although this occurs every day, standards for clinical practice have not been developed; therefore, an objective measure of quality is lacking.

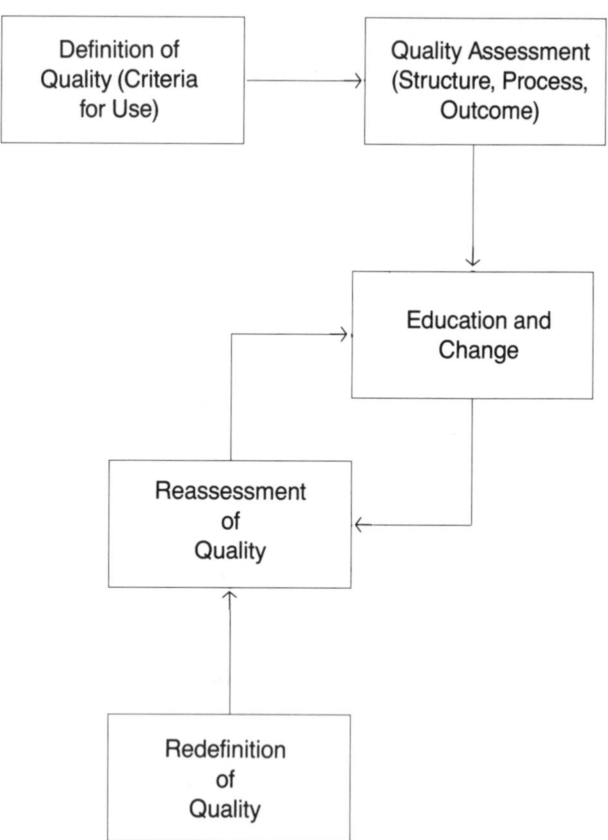

Figure 24-1. The quality assurance cycle

Source: Stolar MH: Conceptual framework for drug usage review, medical audit and other patient care review procedures. *Am J Hosp Pharm* 34:139-145, 1977.

PERFORMING DRUG USE EVALUATION

DUE can be easily visualized as a quality assurance activity as illustrated in figure 24-1. This framework should serve as the model for any DUE program. The process of establishing and maintaining a DUE program can be complex and frustrating. Although the development of the specific steps is somewhat arbitrary, the following "cookbook" approach should help to conceptualize and perform DUE as an effective quality assurance activity.

1. Assign responsibility.
2. Assess overall drug use patterns.
3. Identify specific drugs and drug classes to be monitored and evaluated.
4. Develop criteria for drug use.
5. Collect and organize data.
6. Evaluate drug use as compared with criteria.
7. Take actions to solve problem or improve drug use.
8. Assess the effectiveness of the actions taken and document improvement.
9. Communicate information to appropriate individuals and groups within the organization.

Assign Responsibility

The JCAHO DUE standards assign the responsibility for DUE to the medical staff. In most institutions, the pharmacy and therapeutics (P&T) committee would be the logical group to manage these activities. The P&T committee has the advantage of being a medical staff committee; pharmacy is well represented; it is in a direct reporting relationship with the executive committee of the medical staff; and its inherent responsibilities are to oversee all aspects of drug use within the institution. Some institutions may elect to establish a medical staff DUE committee (on which pharmacists should serve) or place responsibility of DUE with the quality assurance committee. Wherever the responsibility lies, it must be with a group that is well respected by the institution, has pharmacy representation, and has sufficient authority to give the program legitimacy. It should also be one with which the department of pharmacy can build and maintain excellent rapport.

Assess Drug Use Patterns

A logical place to start with the DUE process is to establish which drugs are the most commonly used within the institution. These patterns are generally recognized by members of the medical staff and pharmacy staff who have worked in an institution for several years and are based on the scope of the services provided by the institution. Although the JCAHO standards imply that many drugs or drug classes should be reviewed at all times for appropriateness, there simply are not enough resources to perform this activity. It is not necessary to constantly review drugs that are being used appropriately. A drug use report that quantifies drug use should serve as a starting point for individual DUE studies. This quantitative report should also identify which departments within the institution most frequently use specific medications. This could prove to be vital in performing individual DUE studies, because input would be sought from those departments for criteria development, and those departments might be targeted for educational activities and corrective actions. The ability to identify specific prescribers would also be valuable in helping educational activities to be better focused.

Identify Specific Drugs to Be Monitored and Evaluated

Establishing which drugs or classes of drugs to monitor within a DUE program should not be difficult. The JCAHO provides guidelines for which drugs should be considered for the review process. The standards basically mention three broad categories of drug use: (1) those that are used most frequently, (2) those that have the greatest relative risk to patients if used inappropriately, and (3) those that in the past have had problems associated with their use. Another possible mechanism for identifying drugs to evaluate would be for the individual medical departments within the institution to identify the drugs that they prescribe frequently, those that they perceive to have the least knowledge about, or those they feel may be the most hazardous to patients. Some of these drugs or classes of drugs may be similar among departments and can form the basis for initial evaluation. Another mechanism for ranking drugs for evaluation is development of a DUE matrix. Individual drugs or groups of drugs are listed on one axis of the matrix, and on the other, their characteristics (in this example, high volume, high risk, or problem prone). A drug that meets all three of these characteristics would have a total numerical value of 3. Similarly, a drug that is only high volume and not high risk or problem prone would be assigned a numerical value of 1. Therefore, those drugs or groups of drugs with the highest numerical value should be evaluated first. Any process that is used for identifying drugs for evaluation should be documented to meet JCAHO requirements for a systematic process.[14]

Develop Criteria for Use

Criteria are used to measure the quality of drug use. Criteria have been defined as "predetermined elements against which aspects of the quality of a medical service may be compared."[15] Well-written criteria often have several components or elements pertaining to drug therapy monitoring and other aspects of drug use for any given drug to help define whether or not that drug was used appropriately. Although there are no rules for writing criteria, they should be objective (explicit) rather than subjective (implicit). The objective criteria will help to ensure consistency when different individuals evaluate drug therapy. Subjective criteria allow for interpretation on the part of the reviewers and may lead to less meaningful results.

Developing criteria for use can be time consuming. Since it is essential that medical staff approval be obtained prior to performing the DUE study, the physician specialist should be consulted and be a part of criteria development. This is difficult to do in a busy institution where practitioners frequently do not have the time or the patience to sit down and construct these criteria. Therefore, a drug information service, through the direction of the P&T committee, could play a vital role in criteria development by conducting initial literature reviews, organizing a multidisciplinary approach, and serving as the catalyst for staff involvement. Of course, any member of the P&T committee or department could provide this important push. Many institutions are also creating pharmacy-based DUE specialist positions, which should prove important in organizing and managing the DUE program.

Criteria for use should reflect the standard of medical practice. They should be current, literature based, and reflective of the medical staff's experiences. Examples of items to include in criteria for use are appropriate indications, dose, potential drug interactions, important laboratory tests to monitor prior to and during drug therapy, complications, and specific patient care outcomes (see table 24-2). Another means of objectively measuring quality of drug therapy would be to develop criteria addressing whether the right dose of the right drug reached the right patient at the right time.[9]

One DUE program describes an effective method for developing criteria for use on an ongoing basis.[16] A P&T committee policy requires that criteria for use of a particular drug be submitted, along with the formulary addition request for that drug. This provides a mechanism for developing and approving criteria as drugs are added to the formulary and used in the institution. A flowchart depicting this process of adding drugs to the formulary and approval of criteria for use is shown in figure 24-2.

Developing criteria from scratch is not always necessary. ASHP has published an excellent resource containing numerous criteria sets.[17] The entire criteria set or portions can be used for evaluating drug therapy, but should be adapted to meet the needs of the individual institution. These criteria are well written, well referenced, and complete.

Another good source for criteria is the "Drug Utilization Review" newsletter published monthly by American Health Consultants, Inc. The newsletter frequently publishes criteria that have been developed by various individuals across the country.[18] An often overlooked resource is colleagues, many of whom are willing to share their criteria and DUE study results. This can be facilitated by subscribing to an individual institution's newsletter or using electronic bulletin boards. Whatever source is used to develop criteria for use, the two key points to remember are (1) the criteria must be written in an objective, not subjective, manner, and (2) the criteria must be approved by the medical staff in order to give the criteria authority.

Collect and Organize Data

Collecting data can be accomplished through either the retrospective, concurrent, or prospective review process discussed earlier. Drug therapy data are routinely available for review within institutions. For example, the medical record is the most common data source used for collecting information. Other types of data sources include nonformulary requests, special drug or drug class order forms, laboratory reports, medication administration records, adverse drug reaction reports, and even incident reports. Some data sources may need to be created as a part of an institution's DUE program. In some institutions, data

Table 24-2. Criteria for use of terfenadine

No.	Elements	Standard 100%	Standard 0%	No.	Exceptions	No.	Instructions – data retrieval
	Justification of use						
1	Patient with at least one of the following: (a) documented seasonal allergic or perennial rhinitis or conjunctivitis in adult intolerant of sedative effects of antihistamines (b) documented seasonal allergic or perennial rhinitis or conjunctivitis in child of >3 years old intolerant of sedative effects of antihistamines (c) documented histamine-mediated skin disorders unresponsive to standard therapy with cyproheptadine, dyphenhydramine, or hydroxyzine AND	X		1A	None	1	History and physical (H&P), physician orders, progress notes
2	Previous, documented unsuccessful trial with at least one of less sedating antihistamines (e.g., brompheniramine, chlorpheniramine, cyproheptadine, triprolidine)	X		2A	Occupation requiring alertness precludes potential for drowsiness	2 2A	H&P, physician orders, progress notes H&P, progress notes
	Critical (Process) Indicators						
3	Appropriate oral dosage prescribed: (a) adults: 120 mg/day as single dose or two divided doses (b) children: 3-5 years—15 mg BID 6-12 years—30 mg BID	X		3A	In obese (>120% ideal body weight) child 6-12 years, 60 mg orally BID prescribed	3 3A	H&P, physician orders, progress notes H&P, physician orders, nursing notes, progress notes
4	Use of other antihistamines discontinued at least 6 hr prior to terfenadine therapy	X		4A	If previous antihistamine is extended-release product, allow 12 hr	4,4A	H&P, physician orders, medication administration record (MAR), progress notes
5	Concurrent antihistamine therapy not present	X		5A	Concurrent antihistamine may be given instead of evening terfenadine dose in patient experiencing insomnia or nightmares with terfenadine therapy	5 5A	H&P, physician orders, MAR, progress notes H&P, physician orders, nursing notes, progress notes
	Complications				**Critical Preventative/ Responsive Management**		
6	Gastrointestinal effects: abdominal distress, nausea, vomiting, change in bowel habits, and/or increased appetite		X	6A 6B 6C	Identify other drug and nondrug causes Give terfenadine with meals and/or decrease terfenadine dosage If severe reaction, discontinue terfenadine or switch to alternative therapy	6,6A 6B,6C	Nursing notes, progress notes Physician orders, MAR, nursing notes, progress notes
7	Central nervous system effects: drowsiness, headache, fatigue, dizziness, depression, insomnia, tremor, confusion, and/or nightmares		X	7A 7B 7C	Identify other drug and nondrug causes If mild reaction, give terfenadine as single daily dose or decrease terfenadine dosage If severe reaction, discontinue terfenadine or switch to alternative therapy	7 7A 7B,7C	Nursing notes, progress notes Nursing notes, progress notes, physician orders Physician orders, MAR, nursing notes, progress notes

Table 24-2. Criteria for use of terfenadine (continued)

No.	Elements	Standard 100%	Standard 0%	No.	Exceptions	No.	Instructions – data retrieval
8	Anticholinergic effects: dry mouth, nose, and/or throat		X	8A	Identify other drug and nondrug causes	8	Nursing notes, progress notes
				8B	If mild reaction, administer sugarless hard candy or fluids	8A	Nursing notes, progress notes, physician orders
				8C	If severe reaction, discontinue terfenadine or switch to alternative therapy	8B,8C	Physician orders, MAR, nursing notes, progress notes
9	Cardiac effects: palpitations, tachycardia, and/or cardiac arrhythmia		X	9A	Identify other drug and nondrug causes	9	Nursing notes, progress notes
				9B	If mild reaction, decrease terfenadine dosage	9A	Nursing notes, progress notes, physician orders
				9C	If patient symptomatic, discontinue terfenadine or switch to alternative therapy; provide symptomatic care and supportive therapy	9B,9C	Physician orders, MAR, nursing notes, progress notes
10	Musculoskeletal symptoms		X	10A	Identify other drug and nondrug causes	10	Nursing notes, progress notes
				10B	If mild reaction, decrease terfenadine dosage	10A	Nursing notes, progress notes, physician orders
				10C	If severe reaction, discontinue terfenadine or switch to alternative therapy; provide symptomatic care and supportive therapy	10B,10C	Physician orders, MAR, nursing notes, progress notes
11	Hypersensitivity reaction: anaphylaxis (difficulty breathing, wheezing, laryngeal edema, flushing, or rapid pulse), rash, and/or urticaria		X	11A	Discontinue terfenadine or switch to alternative therapy	11	Nursing notes, progress notes
				11B	Provide supportive therapy, which may include steroids, epinephrine, and diphenhydramine	11A,11B	Physician orders, MAR, nursing notes, progress notes
	Outcome Measures						
12	Documented adequate relief of allergic symptoms	X		12A	Patient expired	12	Nursing notes, progress notes
				12B	Patient developed respiratory infection	12A-12C	Progress notes
				12C	No subsequent visit or communication with outpatient		

Source: *Criteria for Drug Use Evaluation*, vol.1, Bethesda, MD, ASHP, 1989, pp 3-5.

generated by pharmacists upon review of medication orders are used prospectively.[16] When necessary (based on criteria), pharmacists contact prescribers after the order is written but before the drug is administered. The pharmacists' recommendations are recorded on a checklist indicating discrepancies between a physician's order and approved criteria for use. The information generated on the drug therapy intervention documents is then entered into a data base manager program using a personal computer to organize and report the data.

Collection of the data would be impractical without the use of the computer. Over the past several years, several practical articles have been published that describe how computers facilitate collection and organization of DUE data. Some are described as mainframe systems within the institution,[19] and others use personal computers with common spreadsheet programs such as Lotus 1-2-3.[20,21] Computer programs have proven to be faster, more accurate, and more consistent than manual processing of data. Programs also allow the data to be sorted by drug, drug class, physician, indication, patient, service or any category the user wishes to evaluate. Performing DUE activities on a large scale without the use of computers would be difficult at best.

Evaluate Drug Use

Once the data are collected, they must be organized in ways that identify patterns of drug use within the institution. Some institutions find it useful to organize drug use data by the specific physician, service or department, and patient. This information allows for specific corrective action to be taken if needed (e.g., a letter from the P&T committee chair to an individual physician about inappropriate prescribing).

The data should be evaluated using a team approach by the individuals or committee responsible for the DUE program. Even though specific criteria for use may not have been met in certain situations, it may not necessarily mean that the use was inappropriate. The DUE committee or P&T committee may find that the violation of the criteria is minor and no corrective action should be recommended. In other cases, recommendations for corrective action must be formulated.

Take Actions to Solve Problems or Improve Drug Use

Implementing corrective action when inappropriate drug use is identified may be difficult. Departments of pharmacy can be placed in a precarious situation. It would not be advantageous for the medical staff to feel that the pharmacists serve as watchdogs or police in this process. Corrective action must come from the medical staff and not be perceived as coming strictly from the pharmacy.

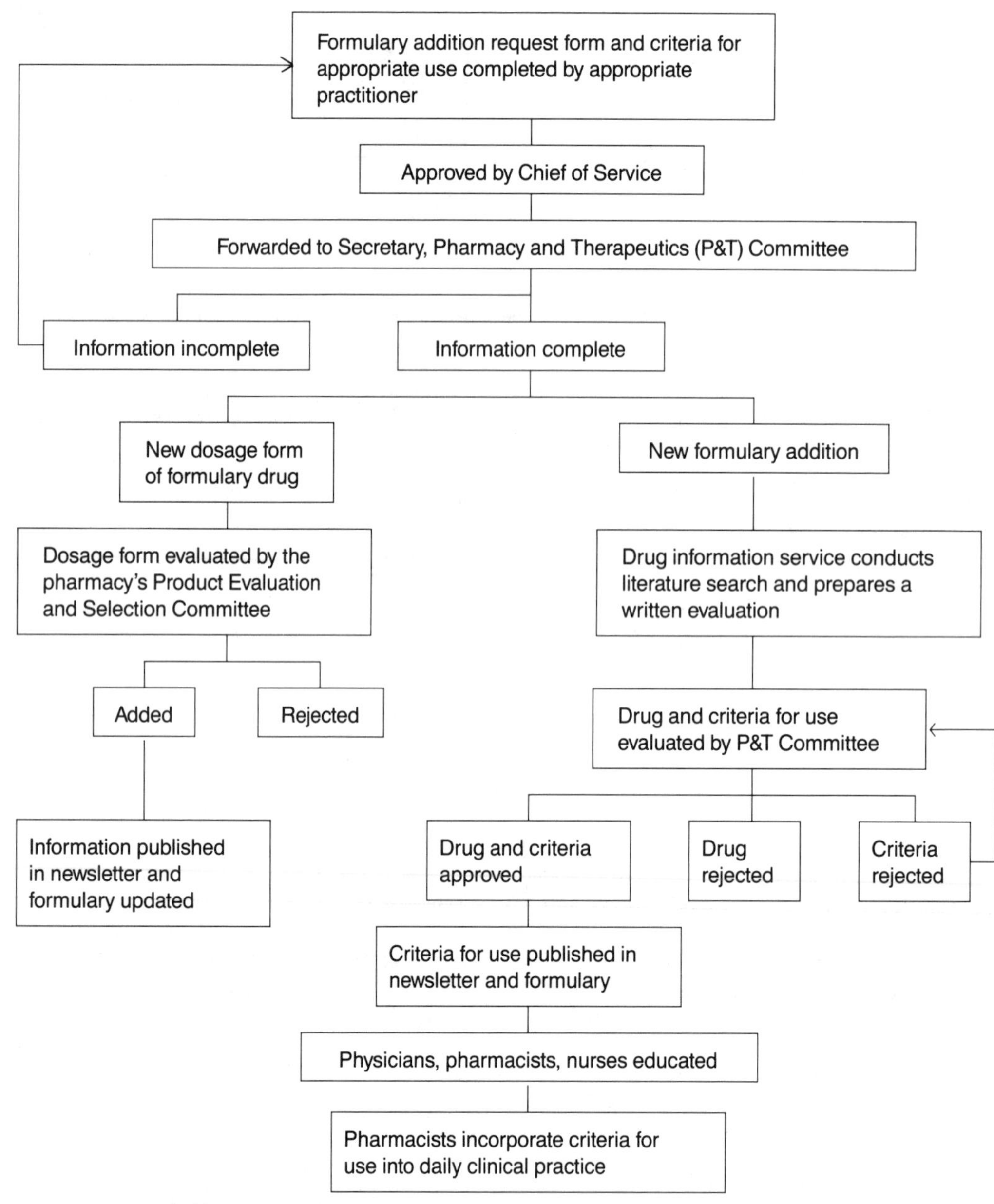

Figure 24-2. Flowchart describing a formulary addition policy and criteria for use approval

Source: Todd MW, Keith TD, Faith MT, Jr, et al: Development and implementation of a comprehensive, criteria-based drug-use review program. *Am J Hosp Pharm* 44:533, 1987.

Many different actions can be taken, depending on the situation and the magnitude of the problem. A simple mechanism for initiating corrective action is a letter from the chair of the P&T committee. The letter should be very specific, it should identify the specific cases or data for which the corrective measures are suggested, and clearly state the purpose of performing the DUE and why it is important to the institution and the medical staff. The letter should be specific as to the plan of corrective action, that is, who is to implement the change, what exactly is to be changed, and how it could be accomplished. In some institutions, the chair of each department involved in cases that fail to meet DUE criteria is asked to address the specific cases in his or her monthly departmental quality assurance activities. The P&T committee suggests in a letter that these particular cases be reviewed at the departmental meeting and that the department chair take any disciplinary or educational actions that may be necessary. An effective and usually preferable corrective action or measure is through education. Pharmacists can play a vital role in providing continuing education through seminars, newsletters, discussions at morning reports, formal presentations at grand rounds, and informal presentations on daily patient care rounds. The department of pharmacy may wish to target a specific drug, group of drugs, or specific physicians, departments, or services. Whatever mechanism is employed, it is important that it be used consistently and in a professional manner.

DUE programs provide an excellent opportunity to incorporate DUE activities and P&T committee policy into daily clinical pharmacy practice. For example, the practicing physician can use criteria for a particular drug approved by the P&T committee every day on rounds while reviewing patient drug orders or while having informal conversation with the physicians. DUE can, thereby, facilitate the evolution of pharmacy into a patient-oriented profession.

Assess the Actions Taken and Document Improvement

Once corrective actions have been taken to solve problems or improve drug use, a mechanism must be in place to assess whether or not the actions taken did indeed change therapy as intended. This would require a reevaluation of the drug or group of drugs previously reviewed, which is why it is so important to have a continuous, ongoing program that systematically assesses and reassesses appropriate use of drugs. An example of an ongoing type of evaluation would be a criteria-based target drug program. selected drugs can be evaluated on a quarterly basis. If no problems are detected with a particular drug, it is dropped from the review process and replaced by another target drug. Problem drugs remain on the target drug list until the problem is resolved. This system determines whether corrective actions are effective and might be used to identify whether individual physicians are involved. There are no guidelines as to how often a particular drug or class of drugs should be reviewed. Problem drugs might receive greater attention than others.

Communicate Relevant Information to Appropriate Individuals

Effective communication is essential for a successful DUE program. A clear plan must be in place that describes exactly who receives what type of information. All results of the DUE program should be communicated through channels established by institutional policy (e.g., P&T committee, quality management committee). It should be clearly defined who will be making recommendations for corrective actions and what type of feedback is expected. The JCAHO recommends that the medical staff's executive committee be provided with the conclusions, recommendations, and actions of DUE at least quarterly.[6] Results of DUE must also be considered in the medical staff reappointment and privilege delineation processes and in the conduct of quality assurance activities.[6] Although the exact role of the P&T committee in reappointment and privilege delineation is not known, it is clear that the results of DUE are important. In some programs, the burden of medical staff reappointment and privilege delineation rests with the department chair in keeping with medical staff bylaws. An example of a DUE study and the reporting of findings, actions, and results appears in table 24-3.

EXAMPLES OF DUE PROGRAMS

Even with the evolution of DUE into an essential quality assurance activity, very few DUE programs have been described in the literature. Only one report describing a comprehensive criteria-based program has been published during the last 5 years.[12] In this program, conducted at a university teaching facility, criteria for use are approved by the P&T committee at the time a drug is added to the formulary. These criteria are then incorporated into the daily practice responsibilities of all pharmacists. Pharmacists are responsible for contacting physicians when the criteria are not met and for recommending alternative therapy. The pharmacists document all actions taken and supply data for quarterly P&T committee reports. The pharmacists are also relied on extensively for education and problem solving. Figure 24-3 describes the pharmacists' practice responsibilities within this DUE program.

PITFALLS

Several pitfalls to be avoided in performing DUE activities are described below.

1. The most crippling is when the program has no authority. A DUE program working independent of the medical staff most likely will be ineffective. The medical staff must be involved in order for the program to have legitimacy.
2. A lack of organization can prove detrimental to the program. Without a clear definition of the roles of the individuals involved (who will develop criteria, who will communicate with other medical departments, who will collect data, who will evaluate the data), the program will flounder. Policies and procedures should be written so that the organizational process is clearly documented and there is no confusion as to who has what responsibility.

Table 24-3. Example of a completed DUE study emphasizing appropriate documentation

Drugs:	Cimetidine and Ranitidine
Aspect of care:	Use in ambulatory care
Indicator:	Duration and dosage of H_2 blocker as indicated in department protocol (clinical criteria accompanied this indicator)
Threshold/ (Performance):	95%/(29%)
Findings and action:	Monitoring and evaluation showed widespread inappropriate duration and dosage of these drugs. In addition, in 25% of cases, the drugs were not used for appropriate indications. To remedy this departmentwide problem, the director first shared these results of ongoing drug usage evaluation with staff. Subsequently, the chief of gastroenterology gave a presentation to the department, discussing the hazards of empiric therapy with H_2 receptor antagonists, potential drug interactions, and appropriate dosages and treatment durations with these agents.
Results:	During the next two months, in 75% of cases, dosage and duration were appropriate. In addition, in 90% of cases, the drugs were given for appropriate indications. Although these results still reached the thresholds for evaluation, the improvement was significant; the director continued to discuss use of these drugs with staff and expected that performance would continue to improve. Monitoring was continued to determine whether the improvement would occur or whether further action would be necessary.

Reprinted with permission from the Joint Commission on Accreditation of Healthcare Organizations: *Examples of Drug Usage Evaluation*, Chicago, JCAHO, 1989, p 57.

3. Operating the DUE program in a vacuum with poor communication will cause the program to fail. It is important that everyone involved understand the DUE process and its importance to the institution, the medical staff, and the department of pharmacy. A coordinator for DUE activities should be appointed and be responsible for all communications. Constant discussions involving DUE activities are important at the P&T committee level. A standing P&T committee agenda item that includes DUE can be a major impetus for constant education and discussion.
4. Poor documentation can ruin a DUE program. All DUE studies should be well documented, including the recommendations made, followup actions implemented, and evaluation of actions taken. Documentation should be readily retrievable.
5. Not involving all pharmacists in the DUE activity is a mistake. Successful programs have incorporated the criteria for use into daily pharmacy practice to ensure that P&T committee decisions are carried out on a consistent basis. The pharmacist is the logical and appropriate professional to conduct an initial evaluation of drug therapy within the DUE program structure.

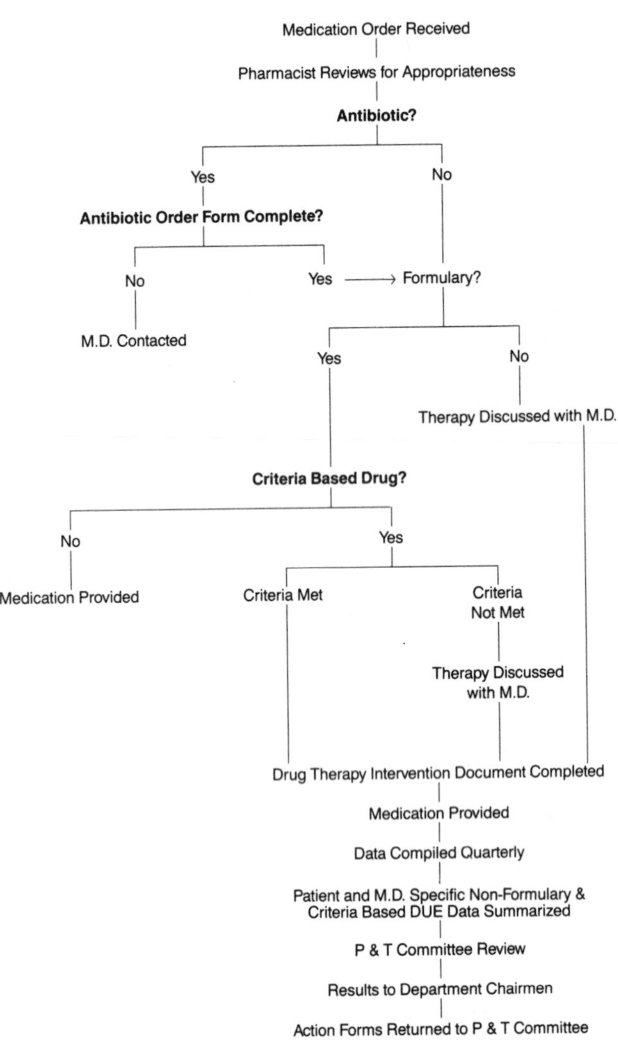

Figure 24-3. Example of pharmacists' practice responsibilities in an ongoing DUE program

CONCLUSION

DUE has evolved into an essential quality assurance activity and provides an innovative and challenging approach to clinical pharmacy practice. DUE is maturing from an isolated activity that is not a part of practice into an integral infrastructure for ensuring the appropriate use of drugs. The Federal Government, insurance companies, hospital administrators, and patients will continue to place enormous emphasis on DUE activities. Drugs must be used safely, effectively, and at the lowest possible cost. The profession of pharmacy must position itself as a leader in this arena. No one yet has the answers for establishing the ideal DUE program. Computer applications must be used. Innovative ways of relating quality drug use with patient outcome must be established. DUE is a dynamic process and an important tool for bringing pharmacists closer to a patient-oriented profession.

REFERENCES

1. Kunin CM, Tupasi T, Craig NA: Use of antibiotics. A brief exposition of the problem and some tentative solutions. *Ann Intern Med* 79:555-560, 1973.
2. Helling OK, Norwood GH, Donner JD: An assessment of prescribing using drug utilization review criteria. *Drug Intell Clin Pharm* 16:930-934, 1982.
3. Kelly WN, White JA, Miller DE: Drug usage review in a community hospital. *Am J Hosp Pharm* 32:1014-1017, 1975.
4. Ives TJ, Frey JJ, Furr SJ, et al: Effect of an educational intervention on oral cephalosporin use in primary care. *Arch Intern Med* 147:44-47, 1987.
5. Wagner L: State of the Union cost-control focus fails to satisfy industry. *Mod HealthC* (Feb 5):2, 1990.
6. Joint Commission on Accreditation of Healthcare Organizations: *Accreditation Manual for Hospitals, 1990*. Chicago, JCAHO, 1989.
7. ASHP guidelines on the pharmacist's role in drug use evaluation. *Am J Hosp Pharm* 45:385-386, 1988.
8. Myers CE: Keeping up-to-date with Joint Commission requirements: The case of drug-use evaluation. *Am J Hosp Pharm* 45:64, 1988.
9. Coe CP, Louviere ML: Preparing the pharmacy for a JCAH survey. Bethesda, MD, American Society of Hospital Pharmacists, 1986.
10. Brodie DC, Smith WE Jr: A conceptual model for drug utilization review. *Hospitals* 50:143-149, 1976.
11. Brodie DC, Smith WE Jr, Hlynka JN: Model for drug usage review in a hospital. *Am J Hosp Pharm* 34:251-254, 1977.
12. Stolar MH: Drug use review: Operational definitions. *Am J Hosp Pharm* 35:76-78, 1978.
13. Joint Commission on Accreditation of Hospitals: *Accreditation Manual for Hospitals*, 1980-1986 standards. Chicago, JCAH, 1980-86.
14. Joint Commission on Accreditation of Healthcare Organizations: Examples of Drug Usage Evaluation. Chicago, JCAHO, 1989.
15. Department of Health, Education, and Welfare. *PSRO Program Manual*. Washington, DC, Department of Health, Education, and Welfare, 1974.
16. Todd MW, Keith TD, Foster MT Jr: Development and implementation of a comprehensive, criteria-based drug-use review program. *Am J Hosp Pharm* 44:529-535, 1987.
17. American Society of Hospital Pharmacists: *Criteria for Drug Use Evaluation*, vol. 1. Bethesda, MD, ASHP, 1989.
18. Criteria swap. *Drug Utiliz Rev* 5:15-16, 1989.
19. Scarafile PA, Campbell BD, Kilroy JE, et al: Computer-assisted antibiotic review in a community hospital. *Am J Hosp Pharm* 42:313-315, 1985.
20. Stolar MH: Developing drug-use indicators with a computerized drug database and a personal computer software package. *Am J Hosp Pharm* 44:1075-1086, 1987.
21. Burnakis TG: Facilitating drug-use evaluation with spreadsheet software. *Am J Hosp Pharm* 46:84-88, 1989.

CHAPTER 25

Drug Therapy Monitoring

THOMAS D. KEITH and MALCOLM T. FOSTER, JR.

INTRODUCTION AND HISTORY

The essence of pharmaceutical care rests with drug therapy monitoring (DTM). The pharmaceutical literature from the past 15 years is rich with articles involving pharmacists' monitoring of adverse drug reactions,[1-9] therapeutic drug monitoring,[10-27] therapeutic selection and effectiveness,[28-39] and appropriateness and cost-effectiveness.[39-44] As momentum built for pharmacists involvement in DTM, the profession felt a clear need to direct these efforts in expanded patient care. That need was addressed in 1985 at the Hilton Head Island Invitational Conference entitled, "Directions for Clinical Practice in Pharmacy."[45] One of the more important results of the conference was the development of the fundamental purpose of the profession of pharmacy, i.e., "to serve society by ensuring the safe and appropriate use of drugs." Another important outcome of the conference was the recognition of the lack of an organized management approach to the provision of clinical pharmacy services, i.e., drug therapy monitoring.

These results later compelled the American Society of Hospital Pharmacists (ASHP), through its Council on Professional Affairs, to develop an ASHP statement on the "Pharmacist's Clinical Role in Organized Health Care Settings."[46] In that statement, ASHP stated "that pharmacists in organized health care settings bear a major responsibility for ensuring optimal clinical outcomes from all drug therapy." The statement further provides 15 examples of clinical services. The following three examples are particularly relevant to DTM:[46]

1. Drug therapy monitoring and communicating relevant findings and recommendations to other health care professionals who are also responsible for the patient's care. Drug therapy monitoring includes an assessment of:
   a. The therapeutic appropriateness of the patient's drug regimen.
   b. Therapeutic duplication in the patient's drug regimen.
   c. The appropriateness of the route and method of administration.
   d. The degree of patient compliance with the prescribed drug regimen.
   e. Drug-drug, drug-food, drug-laboratory, or drug-disease interactions.
   f. Clinical and pharmacokinetic laboratory data to evaluate the efficacy of drug therapy and to anticipate side effects, toxicity, or adverse effects.
   g. Physical signs and clinical symptom relevant to the patient's drug therapy.

   Findings from drug therapy monitoring activities enable pharmacists to make appropriate interventions to increase the effectiveness and minimize potential risks of drug therapy. Interpretation of such data may stimulate the formulation or revision of therapeutic plans in consultation with prescribers and other health care practitioners. Drug therapy monitoring should be conducted as an ongoing activity in all health care settings, although not every aspect of such monitoring may be needed for every patient.
2. Monitoring, detecting, documenting, reporting, and managing adverse drug reactions.
3. Participation in drug use evaluation and other quality assurance programs.

These examples offer a fundamental list of areas in which DTM can be initiated. It should be emphasized that the findings from DTM are of value only if they are communicated to the appropriate clinician(s) *and*, where problems are identified, alternatives are suggested. It may be necessary to provide documentation that links the patient illness, the drug therapy problem, and the suggested alternative. Face-to-face communication with clinicians may be more productive in ensuring change than a written note, and it may also provide the opportunity to establish a trusting relationship between pharmacist and physician.

In addition to communicating the findings from DTM, it is also important for the pharmacist to be reminded continually of several factors that may influence the outcome of DTM, such as drug cost, automation, new drug modalities, and new DTM standards.

With regard to standards, it should be noted that the Joint Commission on Accreditation of Healthcare Organizations (JCAHO) has provided impetus for DTM by the pharmacist through its "Agenda for Change Objectives."[47] JCAHO has changed its posture from simply monitoring antibiotic use retrospectively via drug use review to a proactive stance of requiring concurrent or prospective drug therapy monitoring of all drug use in the health care setting. This major change has presented the pharmacist with an enormous opportunity to expand the profession's role in DTM in a variety of settings.

The Basics

Is DTM a common service provided in most hospitals? In her 1990 national survey of hospital-based pharmaceutical services, Crawford[48] found that almost 80 percent of the hospitals responded that pharmacy staff members regularly provided drug therapy monitoring, which was defined as, at a minimum, (1) review of the patient's chart and (2) oral or written followup with the prescriber when indicated. About half of those who responded indicated that the interventions were being documented in the patient's medical record.

Is DTM so complex that most pharmacists are not sufficiently accomplished to participate? There is not an easy answer to this question, because there is probably not a single blueprint that will be universally acceptable. To begin, it must be clearly understood that physicians have the ultimate responsibility for outcomes related to their prescribing. Therefore, physician support for the monitoring process is important. Beyond physician support, the pharmacist must develop an organized approach to monitoring. This approach is usually one in which the mechanisms for monitoring have been tailored by each pharmacist to his or her skill level and meet service criteria by the pharmacy department. It is essential that pharmacists develop an appreciation and understanding of the general process that led the physician to diagnose and prescribe a particular drug or drugs.

A rather simple and yet reasonably well-organized approach is suggested as follows:

1. Identify the medication(s) that have been prescribed by the physician.
2. Work backwards and identify the problems or diagnoses that led the physician to prescribe the medication(s). This may require a review of nurses notes and/or a visit with the patient. Do not overlook the obvious such as laboratory evaluations, dietary intake, etc. It is also important (either at this point or later) to consider the cost of therapy relative to the problems and condition of the patient.
3. After carefully completing steps 1 and 2, outline a list of objective and subjective parameters to evaluate outcome. For example, if a patient was prescribed an antihypertensive, it is approriate to monitor blood pressure, patient somatic complaints, patient demeanor, etc., to determine if the therapy is effective in meeting the objectives.
4. Ensure that medication is being administered to the patient according to the instructions provided. Therefore, a review of medication administration records is required. It would not be prudent to conclude that therapy is ineffective only to find out that the medication is not being given to the patient.
5. If the desired therapeutic response does not occur or if adverse events occur with therapy, close the drug therapy process loop by communicating the findings to the physician. Keep in mind that DTM requires multidisciplinary collaboration and should be supported in the institution by the medical staff and the pharmacy and therapeutics (P&T) committee.
6. If the monitoring process discovers that the therapy did not achieve the desired result or produced an adverse event, use one or more alternatives for communication to the physician. This is vital to the success of the program, since successful alternatives are likely to enhance multidisciplinary respect.
7. View this process as a continuum that demands daily diligence. Over time, the clinical experience gained through such a monitoring program is extremely valuable.

Many patients may benefit from monitoring of therapeutic drug concentration once therapy is begun. Appropriate monitoring should result in maximizing the safety and efficacy of drug therapy. Additionally, such monitoring should ensure appropriate use of serum blood levels and reduce the use of these laboratory tests resulting from inappropriate timing.[49] Monitoring of therapeutic drug concentration has been established as an effective method of optimizing therapy with a number of drugs.[50] Table 25-1 provides a list of drugs (perhaps not exhaustive) for which evidence supports the value of monitoring.

Once the correct therapeutic drug level has been established, the patient should be monitored for the desired effect, adverse drug reactions (ADR's), signs of toxicity, and drug interactions. Effective DTM can result in decreased ADR's, decreased length of stay, and decreased cost.[51,52]

If drug therapy continues past the patient's stay in the hospital, patient compliance with drug therapy should be monitored. In some cases, hospital pharmacists have continued their DTM in the ambulatory setting.[53] Relevant findings and information resulting from DTM should continually feed back into the process to ensure optimal drug therapy.

Table 25-1. Therapeutic drug monitoring

Strong evidence supporting	*Evidence supporting*
Amikacin	Amitriptyline
Gentamicin	Carbamazepine
Methotrexate	Chlorpromazine
Phenobarbital	Desipramine
Phenytoin	Digoxin
Procainamide	Disopyramide
Quinidine	Ethosuximide
Theophylline	Imipramine
Tobramycin	Lidocaine
	Lithium
	Nortriptyline
	Primidone
	Salicylates
	Valproic acid
	Vancomycin

Reprinted with permission from McCoy HG, Cipolle RJ: Toward optimal drug therapy: Benefits of therapeutic drug monitoring. *Postgrad Med* 74(4):122, 1983.

COMPONENTS OF A DRUG THERAPY MONITORING PROGRAM DRUG USE POLICY

Historically, drug therapy monitoring programs have been developed solely by departments of pharmacy. These programs were managed by one or several pharmacists and had little to do with the major thrust of the department. They usually covered only a fraction of the patients in the hospital and had no formal authority or responsibility. In many cases, the major purpose of these programs was monitoring of therapeutic drug serum concentration.

Ideally, the development of a DTM program should begin with the drug therapy policy-making body within the institution, the P&T committee. Therapeutic policy, after appropriate consideration and input, should flow from the P&T committee to the department of pharmacy, and the pharmacy should serve as the implementation and clinical management arm. These policies should become the basis for the DTM program and should reach the level of the individual pharmacist in daily practice.

A comprehensive and aggressive DTM program must have the undivided support of the pharmacy management team. The fundamental philosophy of the department should nurture the basic precepts of total pharmaceutical care. To be effective in DTM, the entire department must see itself as that component of the institution that ensures appropriate use of drugs in a cost-effective manner. If it does, every function performed by the department will project an image of professional concern and caring. A DTM program must promote the safe, efficient delivery and administration of medications as well as their appropriate use.

DRUG INFORMATION

An effective drug information resource within a department of pharmacy is essential to an effective DTM program. This need not be a formal drug information center, since many hospitals are not yet capable of providing such a center. However, as the therapeutic role of the pharmacist continues to expand in the hospital, a department must create a source of unbiased therapeutic information and evaluation. This source, whether formal or informal, should become the drug therapy policy development and recommending mechanism within the department of pharmacy. This source should take an active role in directing the efforts of the P&T committee toward drug use policy development and appropriate use criteria for drugs that are meaningful and manageable. These policies and criteria should then be incorporated into the pharmacist's daily practice responsibilities. This drug information source should work cooperatively with all clinicians in the institution, especially the pharmacists who are involved in DTM. The drug information activities that are needed to support an effective DTM program include the following:

1. P&T committee management and support.
2. Development of appropriate use criteria for drugs.
3. Development of drug use policies.
4. Indepth review of new drugs requested for formulary addition.
5. Role as the management arm of the drug use evaluation program and adverse drug reaction reporting program.

EFFECTIVE CLINICAL MANAGEMENT

One of the greatest challenges to institutional pharmacy practice in this decade will be to develop effective clinical management skills. It is essential to have in place at least basic clinical management principles for a DTM program to function effectively. Basic principles of clinical management are listed in table 25-2.

Table 25-2. Basic principles of clinical management

1. To ensure accountability for the clinical responsibilities of their positions.
2. To ensure that all pharmacists understand their clinical responsibilities.
3. To ensure that job descriptions include clinical responsibilities.
4. To ensure that the mission statement of the department clearly indicates the clinical role of the pharmacist.
5. To ensure that policies and procedures are in place for clinical activities.
6. To ensure that there is an organized approach to clinical practice throughout the department.
7. To ensure that formal feedback mechanisms are developed to document drug therapy intervention.
8. To ensure that quality assurance standards are in place to measure the pharmacist's effectiveness in drug therapy intervention.

FACTORS THAT AFFECT DRUG THERAPY MONITORING ACTIVITIES

As the profession of pharmacy has progressed in its ability to provide more direct patient care services, several factors have had a positive impact both directly and indirectly in setting the stage for advances in the pharmacist's ability to provide DTM. These factors include pharmacy education, automation, new drugs, drug costs, and the changes in standards of care.

Pharmacy Education

We have witnessed a major change in pharmacy education over the past 15 years, and this change is continuing. Strong emphasis in college curricula is being placed on the pharmaceutical care that embraces the many facets of DTM. Recent pharmacy graduates are more confident in their ability to monitor therapy. This continuing influx of well-educated and well-trained patient care pharmacists into the institutional setting has provided departments of pharmacy with a major resource to meet the challenges placed before them.

Automation

The enormous strides that have been made in pharmacy computer systems have provided departments of pharmacy with increased ability to direct the knowledge base of pharmacy practice toward drug therapy monitoring activities. These systems also provide the practicing pharmacist with a wealth of data that can be applied to drug therapy monitoring. In many cases, computer systems are designed to include drug interaction screening, drug duplication, and serum level monitoring. Additionally, these systems provide drug use data which can be useful in identifying drugs that require intense monitoring. For example, increased use of a particular drug over time may indicate inappropriate use. Evaluation of such data may result in the development of specific criteria that the pharmacist can use to promote appropriate use. As the sophistication of these pharmacy computer systems increases, pharmacy practice will continue to move toward a therapeutic knowledge base, thereby improving the ability of the practicing pharmacist to monitor therapy effectively.

New Drugs

The discovery by the pharmaceutical industry and subsequent release of many new drug entities by the Food and Drug Administration (FDA) has presented the pharmacist with an opportunity to become more involved in drug therapy monitoring. Increasing emphasis on safety, efficacy, and the cost-effective use of these agents has encouraged the pharmacist to assume a more prominent role in drug therapy monitoring. As more and more drugs enter the market, greater emphasis is being placed on their appropriate use within the institution. Biotechnology is already providing a new challenge to practitioners that will grow in the future.

Drug Costs

The cost of drugs increased dramatically in the 1980's. The cost of prescription drugs has jumped 135 percent since 1980; inflation rose 53 percent.[54] This trend may continue in the 1990's. As more and more high-technology drugs are introduced, there will be increased scrutiny of their use in an effort to contain cost. Controlling drug cost in the institution in the past received little attention from hospital administrators, mainly because drugs represented only about 5 percent of the hospital's operating budget. However, as drug costs continued to soar and became a larger portion of the hospital budget and reimbursement to hospitals decreased, hospital administrators turned to departments of pharmacy for assistance in controlling and reducing these costs. Once again, the hospital pharmacist is in a unique position to balance therapy with cost.

Changes in Standards of Care

Over the past several years, the JCAHO has increased its emphasis on quality assurance and positive patient outcomes. This has spawned new standards[47] for drug use evaluation (DUE) for pharmacists and physicians. These new standards deal more with patient care aspects than with the technical aspects of pharmacy practice. Additionally, these quality assurance standards for drug use evaluation have presented an opportunity for pharmacists to incorporate them into their daily practice. Such activities emphasize the appropriate use of drugs within the institution where a structured drug therapy monitoring program is required.

The JCAHO has also begun to increase its emphasis on adverse drug reaction monitoring. This also has presented the pharmacist with an opportunity to incorporate ADR monitoring in daily activities. Although DUE and ADR monitoring are medical staff as well as pharmacy standards, the pharmacist plays a major role in the daily implementation and ongoing success of these proactive drug therapy monitoring activities.

These somewhat fragmented yet related factors have emerged and point to the need for a systematic, well-organized, structured drug therapy monitoring program that has major links with the medical and hospital staff and is managed by the department of pharmacy.

DRUG THERAPY MONITORING STANDARDS

Just as the JCAHO has developed standards for the monitoring and evaluation of health care quality, the profession of pharmacy should develop standards for monitoring drug therapy. These standards should reflect the necessary components of the drug therapy monitoring activity and ensure positive patient outcomes and results. Table 25-3 is offered as a beginning for such a task.

Table 25-3. Suggested standards for drug therapy monitoring

STANDARD I

The DTM activity should be managed by the department of pharmacy with appropriate medical staff support and guidance and be provided by qualified pharmacists capable of promoting the appropriate use of drugs in the institution.

STANDARD II

The drug therapy monitoring activity should gain its legitimacy from the therapeutic decision and policy development mechanism within the hospital and medical staff.

STANDARD III

The department of pharmacy must have the appropriate support activities to carry out the drug therapy monitoring activity.

STANDARD IV

Written policies and procedures should be in place to define specifically how the drug therapy monitoring activity is carried out and should address responsibility and accountability.

STANDARD V

Quality assurance mechanisms should reflect the impact of drug therapy monitoring activities on patient care. This information should be used by the therapeutic decision and policy development mechanism within the hospital.

SUMMARY

In summary, drug therapy monitoring activity promises to be one of the most challenging aspects of institutional pharmacy practice throughout the 1990's. As the profession of pharmacy continues to move toward a therapeutic information-based practice and as automation continues to progress in managing the technical aspects of pharmacy practice, drug therapy monitoring responsibilities will dominate the pharmacist's role in the organized health care setting. Outside factors, such as mounting economic pressures in health care, high-tech drug products, and increased emphasis on quality of care, will continue to create opportunities for pharmacists to become more involved in therapeutic policy development and management in the hospital. And last, pharmacy education will continue to provide clinically competent pharmacists to meet the demand of the health care industry.

REFERENCES

1. Bennett BS, Lipman AG: Comparative study of prospective surveillance and voluntary reporting in determining the incidence of adverse drug reactions. *Am J Hosp Pharm* 34:931-936, 1977.
2. Collins GE, Clay MM, Falletta JM: A prospective study of the epidemiology of adverse drug reactions in pediatric hematology and oncology patients. *Am J Hosp Pharm* 31:968-975, 1974.

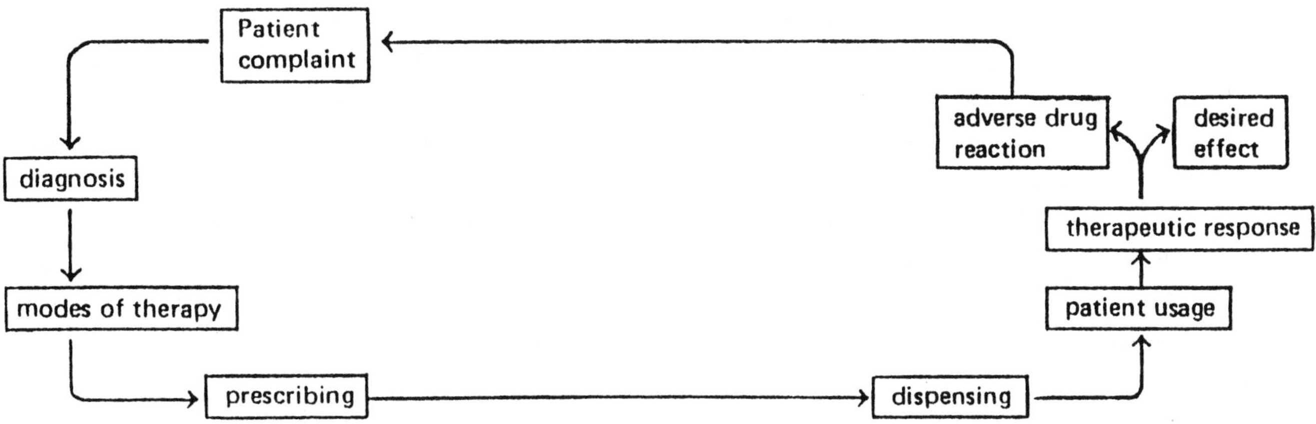

Figure 25-1. The drug therapy process. Adapted from B. Katcher: *Failures in drug therapy.* Continuing Education in Health Sciences, University of California at San Francisco, School of Pharmacy, 1972.

3. Dick ML, Winship HW III, Wood GC: A cost effectiveness comparison of a pharmacist using three methods for identifying possible drug related problems. *Drug Intell Clin Pharm* 9:257-262, 1975.
4. Greenlaw CW: Evaluation of a computerized drug interaction screening system. *Am J Hosp Pharm* 38:517-521, 1981.
5. Hassall TH, Daniels CE: Evaluation of three types of control chart methods in unit dose error monitoring. *Am J Hosp Pharm* 40:970-975, 1983.
6. Knapp DE, Knapp DA, Speedie MK, et al: Relationship of inappropriate drug prescribing to increased length of hospital stay. *Am J Hosp Pharm* 36:1334-1337, 1979.
7. Kwan TC, Washba WW, Wildeman RA: Drug interactions: A retrospective study of its epidemiology, clinical significance and influence upon hospitalization. *Can J Hosp Pharm* 32:12-16, 1979.
8. Levy M, Lipshitz M, Eliakim M: Hospital admissions due to adverse drug reactions. *Am J Med Sci* 277:49-56, 1979.
9. McKenney JM, Wasserman AJ: Effect of advanced pharmaceutical services on the incidence of adverse drug reactions. *Am J Hosp Pharm* 37:243-247, 1980.
10. Bollish SJ, Kelly WN, Miller DE, et al: Establishing an animoglycoside pharmacokinetic monitoring service in a community hospital. *Am J Hosp Pharm* 38:73-76, 1981.
11. Boatman JL, Wertheimer AI, Zaske D, et al: Individualizing gentamicin dosage regimens in burn patients with gram-negative septicemia: A cost-benefit analysis. *J Pharm Sci* 68:267-272, 1979.
12. Boatman JL, Zaske DE, Wertheimer AI, et al: Cost of individualizing aminoglycoside dosage regimens. *Am J Hosp Pharm* 36:368-370, 1979.
13. Dice JE, Burckart GJ, Woo JT, et al: Standardized versus pharmacist-monitored individualized parenteral nutrition in low birth-weight infants. *Am J Hosp Pharm* 38:1487-1489, 1981.
14. Gentry SM, Keith TD, McMillan DM, et al: Evaluation of the ordering of serum theophylline concentrations. *Am J Hosp Pharm* 38:1937-1939, 1981.
15. Greenlaw CW, Blough SS, Haugen RK: Aminoglycoside serum assays restricted through a pharmacy program. *Am J Hosp Pharm* 36:1080-1083, 1979.
16. Herfindal ET, Bernstein LR, Kishi DT: Effect of clinical pharmacy services on prescribing on an orthopedic unit. *Am J Hosp Pharm* 40:1945-1951, 1983.
17. Kelly WN, Gibson GA, Miller DE: Obtaining reimbursement for clinical pharmacokinetic monitoring. *Am J Hosp Pharm* 39:1662-1665, 1982.
18. Lawson LA, Blouin RA, Parker PF: Quality assurance for a clinical pharmacokinetic service. *Am J Hosp Pharm* 39:607-609, 1982.
19. Lehmann CR, Leonard RG: Effect of theophylline pharmacokinetic monitoring service on cost and quality of care. *Am J Hosp Pharm* 39:1656-1662, 1982.
20. Lewis KP, Cooper JW, McKercher PL: Pharmacist's effect on digoxin usage and toxicity. *Am J Hosp Pharm* 33:1272-1276, 1976.
21. Maddox RR, Vanderveen TW, Jones EM, et al: Collaborative clinical pharmacokinetic services. *Am J Hosp Pharm* 38:524-528, 1981.
22. Moore TD, Schneider PJ, Nold EG: Developing reimbursable clinical pharmacy programs: Pharmacokinetic dosing service. *Am J Hosp Pharm* 36:1523-1527, 1979.
23. Moore RA, Tonnies FE: Aminoglycoside dosing service provided by baccalaureate-level pharmacists. *Am J Hosp Pharm* 41:98-105, 1984.
24. Rich DS, Mahoney CD, Jeffrey LP, et al: Evaluation of a computerized digoxin pharmacokinetic consultation service. *Hosp Pharm* 16(1):23-27, 1981.
25. Rietscha WJ, Heissler JF, Paulson MF, et al: Collaborative clinical pharmacokinetics service in a community hospital. *Am J Hosp Pharm* 41:473-477, 1984.
26. Schloemer JH, Zagozen JJ: Cost analysis of an aminoglycoside pharmacokinetic dosing program. *Am J Hosp Pharm* 41:2347--2351, 1984.
27. Taylor JW, McLean AJ, Leonard RG, et al: Initial experience of clinical pharmacology and clinical pharmacy interactions in a clinical pharmacokinetics consultation service. *J Clin Pharm* (Jan):1-7, 1979.
28. Abramowitz PW, Ludwig DJ, Mansur JM, et al: Controlling moxalactam and cefotaxime use with a target drug program. *Hosp Pharm* 18:416-420, 1983.
29. Abramowitz PW, Nold EG, Hatfield SM: Use of clinical pharmacists to reduce cefamandole, cefoxitin, and ticarcillin costs. *Am J Hosp Pharm* 39:1176-1180, 1982.
30. Alexander MR, Ambre JJ, Liskow BI, et al: Therapeutic use of albumin. *JAMA* 241:2528-2529, 1979.

31. Barriere SL, Conte JE Jr: Aminoglycoside use monitored by clinical pharmaceutical services. *Am J Hosp Pharm* 36:1209-1211, 1979.
32. Britton HL, Schwinghammer TL, Romano MJ: Cost containment through restriction of cephalosporins. *Am J Hosp Pharm* 38:1897-1900, 1981.
33. Greenlaw CW: Antimicrobial drug use monitoring by a hospital pharmacy. *Am J Hosp Pharm* 34:835-838, 1977.
34. Maki DG, Schuna AA: A study of antimicrobial misuse in a university hospital. *Am J Med Sci* 275:271-282, 1978.
35. Moss J, Wyatt G, Christopherson D, et al: A prospective drug utilization review on the prescribing of oral and parenteral cephalosporins. *Hosp Form* (Dec):1589-1601, 1982.
36. Norris SM: Evaluation of gentamicin prescribing after drug use review. *Am J Hosp Pharm* 39:1529-1530, 1982.
37. Powell SH, Lantos RL: Concurrent pharmacist monitoring of gentamicin therapy. *Am J Hosp Pharm* 38:77-78, 1981.
38. Rihn TL, Debalko JN, Keys PW: Audit of lidocaine use. *Am J Hosp Pharm* 38:1017-1021, 1981.
39. Shapiro M, Townsend TR, Rosner B, et al: Use of antimicrobial drugs in general hospitals; patterns of prophylaxis. *N Engl J Med* 301:351-355, 1979.
40. Suzuki NT, Pelham ID: Cost benefit of pharmacist concurrent monitoring of cefazolin prescribing. *Am J Hosp Pharm* 40:1187-1191, 1983.
41. Seligman SJ: Reduction of antibiotic costs by restricting use of an oral cephalosporin. *Am J Med* 71:941-944, 1981.
42. Noel MW, Paxinos J: Cephalosporins: Use review and cost analysis. *Am J Hosp Pharm* 35:933-935, 1978.
43. Martucci HJ, Parry MF: Cephalosporin cost reduction. *Hosp Form* (Apr):396-403, 1981.
44. Todd MW, Keith TD, Foster NT: Development and implementation of a comprehensive, criteria-based drug-use review program. *Am J Hosp Pharm* 44:529-535, 1987.
45. Proceedings of invitational conference on "Directions for Clinical Practice in Pharmacy," *Am J Hosp Pharm* 42:1287-1342, 1985.
46. *Practice Standards of ASHP, 1988-89*. Bethesda, MD, American Society of Hospital Pharmacists, 1988, p 15.
47. Joint Commission on the Accreditation of Healthcare Organizations: *Accreditation Manual for Hospitals, 1990*. Chicago, JCAHO, 1989.
48. Crawford SY: ASHP national survey of hospital-based pharmaceutical services, 1990. *Am J Hosp Pharm* 47:2665-2695, 1990.
49. Taylor WJ, Robinson JD, Slaughter RL: Establishing a pharmacy-based therapeutic drug monitoring service. *Drug Intell Clin Pharm* (Nov):818-824, 1985.
50. McCoy HG, Cipolle RJ: Toward optimal drug therapy: Benefits of therapeutic drug monitoring. *Postgrad Med* 74(4):121-134, 1983.
51. Bollish SJ, Kely WN, Miller DE, et al: Establishing an aminoglycoside pharmacokinetic monitoring service in a community hospital. *Am J Hosp Pharm* 38:73-76, 1981.
52. McKenney JM, Wasserman AJ: Effect of advanced pharmaceutical services on the incidence of adverse drug reactions. *Am J Hosp Pharm* 36:1691-1697, 1979.
53. Conte RR, Kehoe WA, Nielson N, et al: Nine-year experience with a pharmacist-managed anticoagulation clinic. *Am J Hosp Pharm* 43:2460-2464, 1986.
54. Gorman C: The price isn't right. *Time* 135:56-58, 1990.

CHAPTER 26

Adverse Drug Reactions

KAREN E. KOCH

INTRODUCTION

Adverse drug reactions (ADR's) are the cause of significant morbidity and mortality. Consequently, ADR's are viewed as the unavoidable price we pay in exchange for the benefits of modern drug therapy. It is estimated, however, that at least half of all ADR's are avoidable.[1-4] This presents a tremendous challenge to all health care providers to improve health care by providing the benefits of modern drug therapy while reducing the risks.

Pharmacists are in an excellent position to meet this challenge because of their indepth knowledge of pharmacology and their roles in selecting, dispensing, and monitoring drug therapy. The objectives of many current clinical pharmacy activities should be to prevent ADR's as much as they are to maximize drug therapy.[2]

DESCRIPTION OF AN ADR

The term "adverse drug reaction" is frequently interchanged with "adverse drug event" or "untoward drug experience" or "drug misadventure" and is often thought of as the serious extension of a "side effect" of drug therapy. The World Health Organization (WHO) and the Food and Drug Administration (FDA) have both developed useful definitions of ADR's. The FDA defines an "adverse drug experience" as follows: "any adverse event associated with the use of a drug in humans, whether or not considered drug related, including the following: an adverse event occurring in the course of the use of a drug in professional practice; an adverse event occurring from drug overdose, whether accidental or intentional; an adverse event occurring from drug abuse; an adverse event occurring from drug withdrawal; and any significant failure of expected pharmacological action."[5] The WHO defines an ADR as "one which is noxious and unintended, and which occurs at doses normally used in man for the prophylaxis, diagnosis, or therapy of disease, or for the modification of physiological function."[6]

Adverse drug reactions can range from relatively minor to severe reactions. Depending on whether the ADR's are predictable or unpredictable toxicity, they are classified as Type A or Type B.[7] *Type A reactions* entail an exaggerated or unexpected extension of the primary or secondary pharmacological activity of the drug such as diuretic-induced hypokalemia or propranolol-induced heart block. These reactions are frequently dose-dependent and may be due to a concomitant disease, drug-drug, or drug-food interactions.[7,8] Type A reactions are responsible for 70 percent to 80 percent of ADR's and are rarely life-threatening, although they can produce significant disability in patients.[1] These known preventable reactions often respond to changes in dosage or schedule of administration and represent the greatest opportunity for decreasing morbidity and mortality. *Type B reactions* include idiosyncratic reactions and immunologic or allergic reactions. The allergic reactions entail the following types: Type I, anaphylactic or immediate; Type II, cytotoxic; Type III, serum sickness; Type IV, delayed allergic. Examples of an idiosyncratic reaction include aplastic anemia with chloramphenicol or Stevens-Johnson syndrome with phenytoin. These reactions are rare, unpredictable, and potentially serious. They are not an extension of the pharmacological activity of the drug and are generally independent of the dose and route of administration.[1,7,8]

It appears that certain drug categories are routinely associated with ADR's. Both the Boston Collaborative[9] and the Caranasos et al.[10] studies found that digoxin, aspirin, warfarin, and prednisone were the agents most frequently associated with ADR's. The 1986 National Adverse Drug Reaction Surveillance Report found that "53 percent of the ADR's reported to the FDA involved only seven categories of drugs" (table 26-1).

Table 26-1. Adverse drug reactions by type of suspect drug[11]

Drug	*Reaction (% administered doses)*
CNS agents	11.9
Antibiotics	10.4
Hypotensive agents	6.9
Nonsteroidal antiinflammatory agents	6.3
Diagnostic agents	6.2
Hormones	5.9
Cardiac drugs	5.0
All others	47.4

Reprinted with permission from Faich GA, Dreis M, Tomita D: National Adverse Drug Reaction Surveillance, 1986. *Arch Intern Med* 148:785-787, 1988.

EPIDEMIOLOGY OF ADR's

The actual frequency of occurrence of ADR's varies widely depending on the population studied, the study methods, and the definition of an ADR used in the study. A definition that includes minor ADR's, drug abuse, or therapeutic failures would identify a greater number of ADR's. Intensive study methods or focusing on a population at risk would also increase the frequency of ADR identification.

More than 70 studies have been published during the last 30 years which examine ADR's.[12-14] These studies attempted to determine (1) the incidence of hospital admissions resulting from ADR's, (2) the frequency of ADR's occurring during hospital admission, (3) the mortality associated with ADR's, (4) the risk factors for developing an ADR, and (5) whether the ADR's were avoidable.

Manasse[13] reviewed D'Arcy[12] and Nolan and O'Malley's[14] summaries of the ADR literature and determined that the "average" of all hospital admissions caused by a drug misadventure may be as high as 10 percent. From 1 to 44 percent of patients experience an ADR during their hospital admission, with the majority of studies reporting an incidence of 10 to 20 percent.[12-14] Although the ranges of ADR incidence from these studies are impressive, because of the variations in the definition of an ADR, the populations studied, and the study methods, they cannot be extrapolated to all hospitals. A summary of several ADR studies is displayed in table 26-2.

Caranasos et al.[10] reviewed all patients admitted or transferred to a medical service over a 3-year period and found that 2.9 percent were admitted because of an ADR. The definition in this study did not include minor ADR's, drug abuse, or suicide attempts.

The Boston Collaborative Drug Surveillance Program[9] monitored 7,017 patients and found that 3.7 percent of hospital admissions were caused or strongly influenced by an adverse reaction to drugs taken in normal doses and used appropriately. An additional 0.5 percent of patients were admitted as a result of adverse events attributed to illicit drugs and 0.7 percent to accidental or intentional overdoses.

In a more recent study of 834 admissions to a medical service, Lakshmanan et al.[3] found a 4.2 percent incidence of hospital admission due to an ADR. Adverse effects related to intentional overdose or intoxication were not included in the study.

Trunet et al.[4] reviewed the reason for admission of patients to an intensive care unit over the course of a year. They found that ADR's resulted in admission in 23 cases (7.1 percent) of the 325 patients observed.

Ives et al.[15] conducted a 12-month study of 293 patients admitted to a family medicine inpatient service and identified 45 (15.4 percent) admissions as drug related. An analysis of the nature of the drug-related admissions revealed that 17 (37.8 percent) of these admissions were classified as adverse drug reactions, 14 (31.1 percent) were the result of drug abuse, 10 (22.2 percent) were attributed to noncompliance with medication regimens, and 4 (8.9 percent) patients were admitted for treatment of intentional overdose.

Hurwitz and Wade[16] found ADR's in 10.2 percent of the 1,268 patients whom they kept under surveillance throughout their hospital stay. Only 4 reactions were considered life-threatening; however, the majority (80 percent) of the 129 observed reactions were of moderate severity.

Bergman et al.[17] reviewed all discontinued medication orders for a medical ward for 6 months and identified 70 ADR's involving 49 patients, 21.4 percent of the total number of patients. They found that 14 patients (6.1 percent) had more than one ADR. The only correlation identified with the development of an ADR was the number of drugs taken by the patient during his or her hospital stay. The risk of development of an ADR was greater than 1 in 3 if a patient received 13 or more drugs during the hospital stay.

Leape et al.[18] reviewed 30,195 randomly selected hospital records and found 1,133 patients (3.7 percent) with disabling injuries caused by medical treatment. Drug complications were the most common (19 percent) type of adverse effect. Eighteen percent of the 178 ADR's were attributed to negligence, and 14 percent resulted in serious disability. Antibiotics (16.2 percent) accounted for more adverse effects than any other drug class, and marrow suppression (16.3 percent) was the drug-related complication most often identified.

The incidence of ADR's also reflects the population of patients studied. It is estimated that elderly patients have a two- to threefold increase of risk for ADR's.[19] This is attributed to a variety of factors including the altered pharmacokinetics and pharmacodynamics of aging as well as multiple drug therapies and disease pathology.[14,19]

The described studies required a considerable commitment of resources to determine the frequency of ADR's at the participating institutions. Regardless of the differences in population and the ADR definition used, these statistics are not duplicated by routine ADR monitoring methods in the majority of health care institutions. An aggressive, ongoing, pharmacy-based ADR monitoring program reported that less than 1 percent of admissions were associated with ADR's and only as many as 2.2 percent of the hospitalized population experienced an ADR.[20]

MORTALITY AND COSTS OF ADR's

In 1972, Talley and Laventurier[21] estimated the mortality due to ADR's to be between 60,000 and 140,000 deaths annually. This is based upon the mortality incidence identified in Caranasos et al.[10] and the Boston Collaborative Studies,[22] 0.18 percent and 0.44 percent, respectively, extrapolated to the number of patients hospitalized annually. This estimate may be high because these studies were based upon medical services and extrapolated to all hospital admissions; however, a substantial number of hospital admissions are to nonmedical services, and the incidence may be lower in these groups.

More recently, Wise et al.[23] reviewed all of the U.S. death certificates for a series of "drug-related" International Classification of Disease (ICD)-9 codes. They identified 11,310 drug-related deaths in 1984. This study would include deaths caused by drugs of abuse and intentional overdoses but may actually underestimate mortality caused by ADR's because it depends upon death certificate coding.

Manasse[13] mentioned the 12,000 ADR-associated deaths reported to the FDA in 1987 and the significance of underreporting of ADR's, possibly as low as 10 percent. He also discussed the difficulties of extrapolating any of the incidence or mortality data to national proportions.

Table 26-2. ADR incidence and mortality

Authors/year (ref no.)	Methods	Total patients in survey	Patients who developed a reaction: In hospital #	In hospital Rate (%)	Requiring admission #	Requiring admission Rate (%)	Degree of ADR: Minor #	Minor Rate (%)	Moderate #	Moderate Rate (%)	Severe #	Severe Rate (%)	Lethal #	Lethal Rate (%)	Avoidable #	Avoidable Rate (%)
Hurwitz & Wade, 1969[16]	Prospective surveillance	1,268	129	10.2	—	—	22	17.0	103	80.0	4	3.0	0	0.0	—	—
Gardner & Watson, 1970[60]	Prospective alerting orders	939	99	10.5	48	5.1	63	27.5	112	49.0	46	20.0	8	3.5	—	—
Bergman et al., 1972[17]	Concurrent alerting orders	229	49*	21.4	—	—	—	—	—	—	—	—	—	—	—	—
Caranasos et al., 1974[10]	Prospective surveillance	6,003	—	—	170†	2.9	—	—	50	28.2	116	65.6	11	6.2	—	—
Miller 1974[9]	Prospective surveillance	7,017	—	—	260	3.7	—	—	—	—	—	—	—	—	—	—
Trunet et al., 1980[4]	Prospective surveillance	325	11	3.0	12	4.0	—	—	14	61.0	7	30.0	2	9.0	14	61.0
Lakshmanan et al., 1986[3]	Retrospective	834	—	—	35	4.2	—	—	—	—	—	—	—	—	19	54.0
Ives et al., 1987[15]	Retrospective	293	—	—	17	6.0	—	—	—	—	—	—	—	—	2	11.8
Leape et al., 1991[18]	Retrospective	30,121	178	0.6	—	—	—	—	—	—	25	14.1	—	—	31	17.7‡

*49 patients experienced 70 ADR's.
†170 patients experienced 177 ADR's.
‡Attributed to negligence.

Although the true incidence of mortality resulting from ADR's is unknown, it is probably somewhere between the extrapolated estimate and the number of reports to the FDA and the death certificate study.

In 1974, Smith and Visconti[24] estimated the cost of an ADR resulting in hospitalization to be $116,835.[24] This includes the direct costs of detection, treatment, and avoidance and the indirect costs of premature death, loss of work, and permanent disability. In 1988, the annual cost of drug-related morbidity in the U.S. was estimated to be as high as $7 billion.[25]

The actual incidence, costs, and mortality of ADR's may be established through the efforts of pharmacoepidemiologists who apply epidemiologic methods to the study of drug exposure in a population. They identify ADR's as part of postmarketing surveillance of drugs.[26-31] Based upon this information, the benefit-to-risk ratio of specific drug therapies can be determined and weighed against alternative drug therapies.

REQUIREMENTS AND OBLIGATIONS FOR MONITORING ADR's

In 1962, the FDA contracted with a number of hospitals throughout the country to report ADR's to FDA. These contracts expired, but the responsibility for ADR's has evolved from mere external reporting to active internal monitoring and expanded from these select hospitals to all types of health care facilities. Since then, the Joint Commission for Accreditation of Healthcare Organizations (JCAHO) and American Society of Hospital Pharmacists (ASHP) have developed requirements and guidelines for monitoring of ADR's.

JCAHO Requirements

Although pharmacists have monitored ADR's for at least 25 years, the JCAHO requirements are responsible for the implementation of many new ADR monitoring programs.[32] The JCAHO has established concurrent ADR monitoring as a function of both the pharmacy and therapeutics (P&T) committee and the pharmacy department.[33] The JCAHO's pharmacy standard is as follows:

> Medication errors and adverse drug reactions are reported immediately in accordance with written procedures.
>
> - This requirement includes notification of the practitioner who ordered the drug.
> - An entry of the medication administered and/or the drug reaction is properly recorded in the patient's medical record.
> - Hospitals are encouraged to report any unexpected or significant adverse reactions promptly

to the Food and Drug Administration and to the manufacturer.[33]

The JCAHO defines the medical staff's responsibility for ADR's with the following standard for the P&T committee: "The definition and review of all significant untoward reactions."[33] The JCAHO describes a system that would fulfill these standards in its drug usage evaluation handbook.[34]

Based on the definition of a significant adverse drug reaction, the specific types of reactions to be considered, and indicators used for screening, a working system should be in place through which nurses, pharmacists, laboratory staff, and other appropriate personnel report the symptoms, signs, or laboratory test results indicating a possible adverse drug reaction. The system should include clear lines of communication and authority for action.

ASHP Guidelines

The ASHP encourages pharmacists to take an active role in monitoring ADR's. It has published comprehensive and clear guidelines for ADR monitoring.[35] The following is a summary of those guidelines.

1. The ADR identification methods should be ongoing and concurrent and include:
   a. Spontaneous notification of a suspected ADR by health care professionals;
   b. Surveillance of drugs or patients with a high risk of ADR's;
   c. Monitoring of "tracer" drugs.
2. Prescribers should be notified of the suspected ADR.
3. The pharmacy should collect all of the relevant data.
4. The causes of the suspected ADR should be evaluated.
5. The description and the outcome of the ADR should be documented in the patient's medical record.
6. Serious or unexpected ADR's should be reported to the FDA and the drug's manufacturer.
7. All ADR's should be reviewed and evaluated by the P&T committee.
8. ADR report information should be used for educational purposes while patient confidentiality should be maintained.
9. ADR findings should be incorporated into the institution's quality assessment program.

The ASHP guidelines provide a more comprehensive course of action than the JCAHO requirements for ADR monitoring. They incorporate features of a drug usage evaluation (DUE) program into an ADR monitoring program. The ongoing nature of such a thorough program complements the risk management and DUE activities of the facility and assists with compliance of JCAHO requirements.

FDA REPORTING

The populations of patients studied in premarketing clinical trials are limited in size and nature. For this reason, the FDA depends upon spontaneous reporting to enhance its postmarketing surveillance data base.[11,26-31,36-39] The FDA is interested in receiving reports of (1) all ADR's associated with a product marketed within the last 3 years, (2) serious ADR's not listed in the product's package insert, and (3) serious ADR's listed in the insert but occurring with increased frequency.[36-38,40]

The FDA has no interest in reports of inappropriate drug use, or of prescribing or administration errors.[36] Incidents of this nature should be reported and evaluated within the institution under the auspices of the risk management and quality assessment programs (table 26-3).

Table 26-3. Overview of hospital drug surveillance

Type of observation	*Internal report*	*Hospital action*	*External report**
Defective product	Yes	Removal	USP or FDA (DQRS)
Suboptimal use	+/-	+/-	No
Misadministration	Yes	Depends	No
Minor ADR	+/-	Depends	No
Serious ADR	Yes	Depends	FDA if new

*DQRS = Drug Quality Report System.
Unpublished material. The author wishes to thank Gerry Faich, M.D., of the FDA, for his permission to use the table.

The FDA's description of a "serious" reaction is one that results in death, hospitalization or prolonged hospitalization, or permanent or severe disability.[36-40] Reports of overdose, cancer, and congenital anomaly are also considered serious.[37] It should be noted that the ADR's the FDA wants reported are actually a subset, serious and unexpected reactions, of the ADR's that the JCAHO and ASHP want monitored.[33,35]

There remains a lot of confusion among health care professionals over the assessment of an ADR and the criteria for forwarding it to the FDA. The FDA no longer requires a causality assessment of the reaction before it is sent a report.[36] Its position is that if there is reasonable suspicion of a serious reaction, it should be submitted to the FDA. The FDA does not want the determination of causality to be an obstacle to detecting new and/or unexpected reactions. Submission of an ADR report to the FDA does not mean that the drug definitely caused the adverse effect.[36,37]

Each submission will be individually reviewed and assessed for severity and probability. If the reaction is serious and unlabeled, the FDA's computer file will be searched for similar reactions. Detailed analysis, incorporating the adverse reaction and the use profiles of the drug, may be pursued.[27,37]

Reporting ADR's to the FDA is a moral obligation of health care professionals and is endorsed by both the JCAHO requirements and the ASHP guidelines. This can be accomplished by completing the FDA's 1639 form or the "short" (1639a) form and sending it directly to the FDA, to the drug's manufacturer, or to both (figure 26-1). The drug manufacturers are required to forward all reports of ADR's to the FDA, and their submissions account for 90 percent of all FDA ADR reports.[26,27,37,38]

Rogers et al.,[41] in a survey of 1,121 community physicians, found that only 57 percent were aware of the FDA's reporting system. The reasons these responding physicians cited for not reporting ADR's to the FDA include the trouble or the unavailability of forms, the fact that the event was already documented or was a minor or expected side

DEPARTMENT OF HEALTH AND HUMAN SERVICES
PUBLIC HEALTH SERVICE
FOOD AND DRUG ADMINISTRATION (HFN-730)
ROCKVILLE, MD 20857

ADVERSE REACTION REPORT
(Drugs and Biologics)

Form Approved: OMB No. 0910-0230.

FDA CONTROL NO.

ACCESSION NO.

I. REACTION INFORMATION

1. PATIENT ID/INITIALS *(In Confidence)*
2. AGE YRS.
3. SEX
4.-6. REACTION ONSET — MO. DA. YR.
7. DESCRIBE REACTION(S)
8.-12. CHECK ALL APPROPRIATE:
- ☐ PATIENT DIED
- ☐ REACTION TREATED WITH Rx DRUG
- ☐ RESULTED IN, OR PROLONGED, INPATIENT HOSPITALIZATION
- ☐ RESULTED IN PERMANENT DISABILITY
- ☐ NONE OF THE ABOVE

13. RELEVANT TESTS/LABORATORY DATA

II. SUSPECT DRUG(S) INFORMATION

14. SUSPECT DRUG(S) *(Give manufacturer and lot no. for vaccines/biologics)*
15. DAILY DOSE
16 ROUTE OF ADMINISTRATION
17. INDICATION(S) FOR USE
18. DATES OF ADMINISTRATION *(From/To)*
19 DURATION OF ADMINISTRATION
20. DID REACTION ABATE AFTER STOPPING DRUG? ☐ YES ☐ NO ☐ NA
21. DID REACTION REAPPEAR AFTER REINTRODUCTION? ☐ YES ☐ NO ☐ NA

III. CONCOMITANT DRUGS AND HISTORY

22. CONCOMITANT DRUGS AND DATES OF ADMINISTRATION *(Exclude those used to treat reaction)*
23. OTHER RELEVANT HISTORY *(e.g. diagnoses, allergies, pregnancy with LMP, etc.)*

IV. ONLY FOR REPORTS SUBMITTED BY MANUFACTURER

24. NAME AND ADDRESS OF MANUFACTURER *(Include Zip Code)*

24a. IND/NDA. NO. FOR SUSPECT DRUG

24b MFR. CONTROL NO.

24c. DATE RECEIVED BY MANUFACTURER

24d. REPORT SOURCE *(Check all that apply)* ☐ FOREIGN ☐ STUDY ☐ LITERATURE ☐ HEALTH PROFESSIONAL ☐ CONSUMER

25 15 DAY REPORT? ☐ YES ☐ NO

25a. REPORT TYPE ☐ INITIAL ☐ FOLLOWUP

NOTE: Required of manufacturers by 21 CFR 314.80

V. INITIAL REPORTER *(In confidence)*

26.-26a. NAME AND ADDRESS OF REPORTER *(Include Zip Code)*

26b. TELEPHONE NO. *(Include area code)*

26c. HAVE YOU ALSO REPORTED THIS REACTION TO THE MANUFACTURER? ☐ YES ☐ NO

26d. ARE YOU A HEALTH PROFESSIONAL? ☐ YES ☐ NO

Submission of a report does not necessarily constitute an admission that the drug caused the adverse reaction.

FORM FDA 1639 (7/86) PREVIOUS EDITION MAY BE USED

Figure 26-1. FDA's 1639 form

effect, liability concerns, and dislike of interacting with the government.

In an effort to stimulate voluntary ADR reporting, the FDA implemented pilot programs in several States: Maryland, Rhode Island, Mississippi, Massachusetts, and Colorado (shown in order of program implementation). The goals of these programs are to increase physician awareness of the need and the mechanism of ADR reporting and to allay their liability-related fears.[42] Fincham[43] discusses the fourfold increase in ADR reporting in Mississippi and the important role pharmacists have in reporting ADR's to the FDA.

ADR MONITORING PROGRAMS

As a result of their indepth knowledge of pharmacology and their increased participation in clinical functions, pharmacists are in an excellent position to implement and manage ADR monitoring programs. A survey conducted by Case and Guzzetti[44] of hospitals with ASHP-accredited residencies found that of the 76 responders, the majority had concurrent ADR monitoring programs. However, the effectiveness of the programs is uncertain because 58 percent of them had fewer than seven ADR's reported over 6 months.

Although an institution may have a policy and procedure on ADR monitoring consistent with the JCAHO guidelines, if the program is not effective in identifying ADR's as determined by annual yields, it may be cited as a deficiency by JCAHO surveyors. The success of a program depends upon whether it remains passive in the policy and procedure manual or whether it is actively promoted.

There are a variety of methods to assist with program management in identifying ADR's. Some programs use computerized screening and analysis; others enlist the assistance of several departments within the institution. It is necessary to tailor the program to the needs and resources of the institution. The following sections provide a description of the essential developmental steps of an ADR monitoring program, which include:

1. Assign responsibility for coordination of ADR monitoring.
2. Develop a definition of an ADR.
3. Promote awareness of consequences of ADR's.
4. Establish mechanisms for identifying and reporting ADR's.
5. Review ADR's for patterns or trends.
6. Develop preventive interventions.

Assign Responsibility

It is important that the individual responsible for this program possess the clinical background to evaluate an ADR and the administrative skills to coordinate a program that should involve the entire facility.[45] Large or teaching institutions often designate this responsibility to the clinical coordinator or the drug information service.[46,47] Smaller facilities may incorporate the responsibility into the duties of the pharmacy's administrative staff. A pharmacy-coordinated ADR team or committee consisting of a physician, nurse, administrator, and pharmacist may provide the most comprehensive approach to surveillance and has been proven successful.[33,47-49]

Develop a Definition

Each institution needs to develop its own definition of an ADR and present it for approval to the P&T committee. Provide a definition that is simple and clear, will minimize confusion, and will not discourage reporting. Include in the definition "any unintended or undesired effect of a drug" and then further narrow it by adding one or more qualifiers such as "resulted in the discontinuation of the drug," "required additional treatment," "required or prolonged hospitalization," or "resulted in death or disability."[34,35,45]

Many institutions adopt or adapt the WHO[6] or the Karch and Lasagna[50] definition of an ADR. According to the latter, an ADR is "any response to a drug that is noxious and unintended, and that occurs at doses used in humans for prophylaxis, diagnosis, or therapy, excluding failure to accomplish the intended purpose."

Most monitoring programs do not usually include intentional overdose, drug abuse, or routine therapeutic failures in their institution's definition of an ADR. However, an unexpected and clinically important failure to achieve the desired pharmacologic effect should be evaluated and considered an ADR.

Promote Awareness

It is important to publicize the consequences of ADR's and the significance of monitoring them. This can be accomplished through newsletters, bulletins, and in-service education. At least one institution developed a videotape on various types of ADR's and circulated it among its clinical staff.[51] Another institution successfully promoted awareness through a system of financial reward.[52] Members of the house staff were paid a $5 bounty for each ADR they reported. This resulted in the medical staff's identifying 70 percent of the ADR's.

The promotion of ADR awareness and reporting should include the institution's definition of ADR's, the mechanism for reporting them, and clear examples of ADR's, particularly from the institution. Physicians and nurses are most likely to discover ADR's and should be primary target groups for ADR awareness promotion. It is also important to reinforce the ADR awareness message through periodic updates.

Establish Mechanisms

Health care professionals need procedures for identifying and reporting ADR's. The focus of a successful program is identifying the ADR's. This encompasses both retrospective and concurrent methods of identifying ADR's. Although total reliance on a retrospective program would not comply with JCAHO standards, a retrospective program could be used to complement the efforts of a concurrent program. Concurrent monitoring consists of three components—spontaneous reporting, alerting orders, and screening of high-risk patients or drugs—which in turn complement each other for thorough ADR identification.

Retrospective Reporting Programs

These programs offer the advantage of being effective in identifying ADR's with use of limited resources. These programs can be implemented with the assistance of the medical records department and/or the quality assessment department. One example of such a program uses a "face sheet."[49] Every patient's chart includes a sheet inquiring whether the patient experienced an ADR during hospitalization. The patient's physician is required to complete the form, and the chart is not considered complete until this is done. The medical records staff members collect the forms and forward them to the ADR committee, which in turn reviews them. Another method of retrospective ADR reporting employs a specially trained technician or the skills of the quality assurance reviewers to screen the charts of discharged patients for clues that may signal a suspected adverse reaction.[20,53]

Although retrospective screening techniques identify ADR's, the quality of the information is inconsistent because of lack of documentation concerning the sequence of events. More important, the opportunity is lost for intervention in the therapy of the patient to minimize the impact of the ADR. For these reasons, retrospective screening programs do not comply with the JCAHO requirements or the ASHP guidelines.

Concurrent Reporting Programs

These programs rely primarily upon voluntary or spontaneous reporting by health care professionals to the ADR program coordinator. The success of the program varies with the institution's method of promoting spontaneous reporting. The ASHP guidelines, however, suggest that spontaneous reporting be included as one of the three components for ADR identification.[35] Monitoring high-risk patients or drugs and using tracer agents constitute the second and third elements of ADR identification as recommended by the ASHP.

Two recent studies identified the inadequacies of spontaneous voluntary reporting and reinforced the necessity for active ADR monitoring.[54,55] Berry et al.[54] determined the sensitivity and specificity for three methods of concurrent ADR detection. During the study phase, no ADR's were spontaneously reported; however, the screening of lab values was the most sensitive method, and the screening of medical orders was very selective. Vorce-West et al.[55] found that even after active promotion of the voluntary reporting mechanism, only 8 percent of the ADR's detected retrospectively were reported under the voluntary system.

Spontaneous reporting depends on someone identifying an ADR and then reporting it. This type of reporting provides a relatively inexpensive and less labor-intensive monitoring system than formal screening programs. Spontaneous reporting frequently identifies serious and unusual ADR's and has proven to be a successful system for the FDA.[27,36,37]

However, the yield of a spontaneous reporting program is usually low. Physician guilt about harm to the patient, liability concerns, the severity of the reaction, and the certainty of the attribution of the reaction to the drug have also been cited as factors affecting reporting of ADR's.[56,57] Because reporting is sporadic, identifying routine problems becomes difficult, and predicting the frequency of occurrence associated with the ADR is impossible.

Nurses and physicians in close contact with patients continue as the most beneficial source of spontaneously reported ADR's.[52,58] Quality utilization nurses have also been incorporated into the concurrent ADR monitoring process by the inclusion of ADR's as one of their monitoring parameters.[47,59]

Once the members of the clinical staff are aware of the importance of identifying ADR's, it is essential that the reporting mechanism be easy and convenient for them. One suggestion is a 24-hour hotline to the pharmacy.[46,55] If ADR reporting forms are used, they need to be uncomplicated and available at all nursing stations (figure 26-2).[20,32,58] Other methods to encourage spontaneous reporting include distributing ADR reporting cards to the medical residents and placing ADR forms on the patients' charts.[45,48] Regardless of the ADR notification method, the overall objective is to use the frontline patient care professionals to activate the spontaneous ADR monitoring program. This will allow for followup of the initial reports in greater detail.

Each suspected ADR should be investigated, and the institution's standard ADR report form should be completed. The form should include all of the information necessary to assess the causality of the suspected ADR (figure 26-3).

Alerting orders are the nonrounding pharmacist's clue that an ADR may have occurred. These orders include the discontinuation or decrease in dosage of a drug, along with the ordering of a laboratory test and/or an "antidote" or "tracer" agent, which is a drug that is commonly used to treat ADR's (table 26-4). Following up on alerting orders may actually be secondhand ADR identification, since the physician or nurse has usually identified the ADR and initiated treatment. However, once symptoms have resolved, the physician is less likely to report it, if an ADR has indeed occurred.[39] If, on the other hand, the pharmacist has identified the ADR through an alerting order, he or she can follow up the documentation and outcome of reaction. Gardner and Watson[60] established the effectiveness of a pharmacist-based system of monitoring drug discontinuation, dose reduction, or antidote drug orders in an elegant study conducted over 10 months in 1969.

Table 26-4. Alerting orders

Abrupt dosage reduction
Abrupt discontinuation
Therapeutic drug level orders
Stat orders for tracer agents
- Atropine
- Corticosteroids
- Dextrose
- Diazepam
- Diphenhydramine
- Epinephrine
- Glucagon
- Hydroxyzine
- Lidocaine
- Naloxone
- Phenytoin
- Phytonadione
- Protamine
- Na polystyrene sulfonate
- Vancomycin (oral)

The tracer agents are the most frequently used of the alerting orders. Some ADR monitoring programs depend on the pharmacist to identify the tracer agents during routine processing of medication orders or daily patient medication review.[60-62] At least two recently published programs

Imprint patient data below.

NORTH MISSISSIPPI MEDICAL CENTER

Nursing Adverse Drug Reaction Form

Suspected Drug:______________________

Place the date and time beside the reaction you suspect may be related to this patient's drug therapy.

(1) Central Nervous System

- ________ Anxiety
- ________ Depression
- ________ Drowsiness
- ________ Extrapyramidal
- ________ Fatigue
- ________ Hallucination
- ________ Headache
- ________ Hyperactive
- ________ Imbalance
- ________ Insomnia
- ________ Malaise
- ________ Nervousness
- ________ Nightmares
- ________ Pain
- ________ Tinnitus
- ________ Vertigo
- ________ Other

(2) Respiratory System

- ________ Bronchospasm
- ________ Nasal Congestion
- ________ Depression
- ________ Other

(3) Gastrointestinal System

- ________ Nausea
- ________ Vomiting
- ________ Diarrhea
- ________ Constipation
- ________ Indigestion
- ________ Cramping
- ________ Dry Mouth
- ________ Anorexia
- ________ Flatulence
- ________ Jaundice
- ________ Hematemisis
- ________ Ascites
- ________ Other

(4) Cardiovascular System

- ________ Angina
- ________ Arrythmia
- ________ C.H.F.
- ________ Irreg. Pulse
- ________ Hypertension
- ________ Hypotension

(4) Cardiovascular System, continued

- ________ Shock
- ________ Palpitations
- ________ Syncope
- ________ Other

(5) Dermatologic System

- ________ Rash
- ________ Itch
- ________ Hives
- ________ Flushing
- ________ Perspiration
- ________ Other

(6) Genitourinary System

- ________ Altered Renal Status
- ________ Hematuria
- ________ Difficult Voiding
- ________ Other

(7) Hematologic System

- ________ RBC Changes
- ________ WBC Changes
- ________ Platelets
- ________ Other

(8) Sensory System

- ________ Altered Taste
- ________ Altered Vision
- ________ Altered Hearing
- ________ Other

(9) Musculoskeletal System

- ________ Myalgia
- ________ Arthralgia
- ________ Other

(10) Miscellaneous

- ________ Superinfection
- ________ Fever
- ________ Electrolytes
- ________ Other

____
L.P.N. or R.N. identifying ADR

Please place in the Pharmacy courier box.

Figure 26-2. Nurses' ADR form

ADVERSE DRUG REACTION PROGRAM

Drug Collection Form

ALLERGIES:

Patient's Name:

Patient's ID Number: Admission Date:

Room Number: Admitting M.D.:

Patient's Age: Gender: Admitting Diagnosis:

Initiation of ADR Detection: Pharmacy __________ Nursing __________ M.D. __________

Background of Patient:

Describe Suspected ADR (include pertinent lab values):

Patient's Current Medications:

Drug(s) Suspected of ADR:

Management of ADR:

Comments: ADR yes __________ no __________

Reviewing Pharmacist ______________________________ Date ____________

Figure 26-3. ADR reporting form

employed the pharmacy's computer to screen for the tracer agents.[20,63]

Screening high-risk patients or drugs offers the best opportunity for immediate intervention and prevention of ADR's.[35,64] This entails the institution's identification of the patient populations and drugs at high risk for ADR's and the cooperation of several departments within the institution (table 26-5). Laboratory reports can be screened for elevated serum drug concentrations, altered blood chemistries, and organisms causing superinfections. With the assistance of the data-processing personnel, the pharmacy's computer can readily identify specific patient populations at risk, such as renal failure or geriatric patients on imipenem. One screening program successfully monitors chemistry laboratory reports of drug concentrations and microbiology laboratory reports of positive *Clostridium difficile* toxins to identify patients at risk for an ADR.[20] Berry et al.[54] found the screening of laboratory reports along with the screening of medication orders for dosage reduction or discontinuation to be an effective combination for identifying ADR's.

Table 26-5. Patients and drugs at high risk of an ADR

Drugs	*Patients*
Aminoglycosides	Pediatric
Amphotericin	Elderly
Chemotherapy	Hepatic failure
Corticosteroids	Renal failure
Digoxin	Polypharmacy
Heparin	
Lidocaine	
Phenytoin	
Theophylline	
Thrombolytic agents	
Warfarin	

Because specialists are often consulted on patients whose differentials include an ADR, one university hospital ADR monitoring program enhanced its ADR identification by regularly checking with the various medical consult services for new ADR's.[65]

Although the screening of high-risk patients or drugs is not specifically incorporated into many ADR monitoring programs, it is, in fact, done by many institutions through their current clinical pharmacy programs. Therapeutic drug monitoring through pharmacokinetic dosing, drug interaction screening, allergy screening, or drug therapy protocols not only screens high-risk drugs and patients but prevents the occurrence of many adverse episodes.

Establish a Procedure for Evaluation of the ADR

Several algorithms exist that standardize the assessment of the relationship between the adverse event and a suspected causal agent. Michel and Knodel[66] performed a study comparing the Naranjo et al.,[67] Kramer et al.,[68] and Jones[69] algorithms. They found that the agreement between the Naranjo and Kramer algorithms was high but the Naranjo algorithm, with its point system, was simpler to use (figure 26-4).

Algorithms can be very time consuming and their use may impede reporting. For this reason, the FDA no longer requires a causality assessment before an ADR is submitted. Some ADR monitoring programs may elect to approach evaluation pragmatically by asking the following questions of each suspected ADR.[34,67-70]

1. Is there a temporal relationship to the onset of the drug therapy and the ADR?
2. Is there a dechallenge, i.e., did the signs and symptoms of the ADR subside when the drug was withdrawn?
3. Can the signs and symptoms of the ADR be explained by the patient's disease state?
4. Are there any laboratory tests that support the ADR?
5. What is the previous general experience with the drug?

A positive rechallenge is the most conclusive evidence linking a drug to an adverse effect. Rechallenges, however, are rarely intentionally done and should not be considered necessary for a strong link of an agent to an adverse effect.

Routinely Review ADR's

All ADR's should be reviewed periodically to determine if patterns or trends for their occurrence exist. This may be as simple as manually preparing a spreadsheet that examines the types and frequency of the ADR's documented.[20] It can be much more thorough with the use of a computer program.[47,52,59,71] One institution is using a data base spreadsheet that is able to track the prescribing physicians and nursing units where the ADR's occurred, as well as the types and frequencies of ADR's.[56] Maliekal and Thornton[71] successfully used a data base software program to store, sort, and retrieve ADR's as well as generate reports. Computer programs for ADR reporting and tracking are now commercially available. A regular review of routinely identified ADR's can not only help to identify areas of potential intervention but can also determine the impact of the interventions.

Develop Preventive Interventions

A well-organized, concurrent ADR monitoring program offers the opportunity for immediate interventions in addition to preventive measures. Pharmacists are routinely involved in ADR prevention when they screen patients' drug regimens for drug interactions, drug allergies, correct dosages, therapeutic duplications, or contraindications.

An institution can use ADR information to focus attention on preventive programs, such as drug use evaluation (DUE) and the formulary revision process.[35] In addition, the medical and nursing staffs will more likely comply with a program they perceive as relevant to them.

Drug interactions are estimated to be the cause of 7 percent of all ADR's.[72] Pharmacists should routinely monitor for drug interactions, through a computerized program or manual review of patient medication profile.[33,73] Pharmacy notification to the medical or nursing staff of a drug interaction has been demonstrated to be effective in stimulating actions that avoid ADR's.[74,75]

Pharmacists can tailor their drug interaction screening program by monitoring interactions known to be occurring

SUSPECTED ADR FORM

ADR Probability Scale*

To assess the adverse drug reaction, please answer the following and give the pertinent score.

	Yes	No	Do not know	Score
1. Are there previous conclusive reports on the reaction?	+1	0	0	______
2. Did the adverse event appear after the suspected drug was administered?	+2	−1	0	______
3. Did the adverse reaction improve when the drug was discontinued or a specific antagonist was administered?	+1	0	0	______
4. Did the adverse reaction reappear when the drug was readministered?	+2	−1	0	______
5. Are there alternative causes (other than the drug) that could on their own have caused the reaction?	−1	+2	0	______
6. Did the reaction reappear when a placebo was given?	−1	+1	0	______
7. Was the drug detected in the blood (or other fluids) in concentrations known to be toxic?	+1	0	0	______
8. Was the reaction more severe when the dose was increased, or less severe when the dose was decreased?	+1	0	0	______
9. Did the patient have a similar reaction to the same or similar drugs in any previous exposure?	+1	0	0	______
10. Was the adverse event confirmed by any objective evidence?	+1	0	0	______

Key

Total Score ≥ 9 Highly probable _____ Total Score = 0 Possible _____

Total Score = 5–8 Probable _____ Total Score ≥ 0 Doubtful _____

Pharmacist Completing Report: ______________________________ Date __________

Figure 26-4. Naranjo's ADR algorithm

Reprinted from Naranjo, CA et al: *Clin Pharmacol Ther* 1981; 30:239-45.

at their institution. An example of this would be to start screening for patients on ciprofloxacin and theophylline after identifying a case of theophylline toxicity resulting from the interaction.

Drug allergy screening has proven effective in the prevention of ADR's. Every new order should be compared to the patient's medication allergy record. If a drug allergy is present, the pharmacist should contact the physician or nurse. As allergic reactions occur, they should be well documented in the patient's chart and added to the allergy profile. The allergy screening program can be enhanced through a review of ADR's of an allergic nature that might have been previously screened.

Therapeutic drug monitoring for high-risk drugs or patients is essential. This encompasses not only therapeutic drug monitoring of the well-established high-risk agents and/or patient populations but also agents or patients identified as particular problems.

Patient counseling programs can be employed to reduce the risk of ADR's to the patients after discharge.[76] Moss et al.[77] surveyed 120 physicians and found that they will accept pharmacists counseling patients about ADR's. Patient counseling programs are particularly useful for patients using agents with narrow therapeutic indices such as digoxin and warfarin. Patient education efforts should focus on those agents suspected as the cause of ADR-related admissions among patients of that institution.

BENEFITS AND FUTURE OF ADR MONITORING

The two most obvious benefits of an ADR monitoring program are (1) that the institution is in compliance with the JCAHO's standards and (2) that the FDA's postmarketing surveillance data base is enhanced. The institution and its staff benefit from a decrease in liability as a result of proper documentation of the prompt recognition and treatment of ADR's. An ADR monitoring program also complements the institution's risk management activities by identifying agents or patients at high risk for ADR's and minimizing the risks.

The less readily apparent but even more important factors are the improved quality of care and the acquisition of knowledge to benefit the public welfare, and specifically, the institution's patients. ADR monitoring programs should lead to early identification, and optimally the subsequent prevention, of ADR's, which will improve standards of patient care. The resulting decrease in morbidity and mortality, associated with a shortened length of stay in the hospital, is sufficient financial justification for such a program. Hepler and Strand[2] have identified pharmacists' efforts in preventing, detecting, and resolving drug-related problems as "pharmacy's mandate and mission for the 21st century."

The future of ADR monitoring depends not only on pharmacists establishing the infrastructure for detection and reporting within a health care institution but also on increased recognition and reporting of ADR's by health care professionals. Education regarding "drug-induced diseases" is essential in the basic training of physicians as well as the basic concept that an ADR be considered whenever a hospitalized patient develops a new problem.

REFERENCES

1. Linkewich JA: Adverse effects of drugs. In Osol A (ed): *Remington's Pharmaceutical Sciences, 17th ed.* Easton, PA, Mack Publishing Co., pp 1321-1335, 1985.
2. Hepler CD, Strand LM: Opportunities and responsibilities in pharmaceutical care. *Am J Hosp Pharm* 47:533-543, 1990.
3. Lakshmanan MC, Hershey CO, Breslay D: Hospital admissions caused by iatrogenic diseases. *Arch Intern Med* 146:1931-1934, 1986.
4. Trunet P, Le Gall J, Lhoste F, et al: The role of iatrogenic disease in admissions to intensive care. *JAMA* 244:2617-2620, 1980.
5. Department of Health and Human Services: New drug and antibiotic regulations; section 314.80 postmarketing reporting of adverse drug experiences. *Fed Reg* 50(30):7500-7501, 1985.
6. *Requirements for Adverse Reaction Reporting*. Geneva, Switzerland, World Health Organization, 1975.
7. Rawlins MD: Adverse reactions to drugs. *Br Med J* 282:974-976, 1981.
8. Lambert D: ADR reporting and education: Proposed solutions—Maine Medical Center. *Hosp Formul* 25:209-211, 1990.
9. Miller RR: Hospital admissions due to adverse drug reactions: A report from the Boston Collaborative Drug Surveillance Program. *Arch Intern Med* 134:219-223, 1974.
10. Caranasos GJ, Stewart RB, Cluff LE: Drug-induced illness leading to hospitalization. *JAMA* 228:713-717, 1974.
11. Faich GA, Dreis M, Tomita D: National adverse drug reaction surveillance 1986. *Arch Intern Med* 148:785-787, 1988.
12. D'Arcy PF: Epidemiological aspects of iatrogenic diseases, 3rd ed. Oxford, Oxford University Press, 1986.
13. Manasse JR: Medication use in an imperfect world: Drug misadventuring as an issue of public policy, part 1. *Am J Hosp Pharm* 46:929-944, 1989.
14. Nolan L, O'Malley K: Prescribing for the elderly, part I: Sensitivity of the elderly of adverse drug reactions. *J Am Geriatr Soc* 36:142-149, 1988.
15. Ives TJ, Bentz EJ, Gwyther RE: Drug-related admissions to a family medicine inpatient service. *Arch Intern Med* 147:1117-1120, 1987.
16. Hurwitz N, Wade OL: Intensive hospital monitoring of adverse reactions to drugs. *Brit Med J* 1:531-536, 1969.
17. Bergman BD, Aoki VS, Black HJ, et al: Advantages of a unit dose distribution system in surveillance of adverse drug reactions. *Clin Toxicol* 5:405-417, 1972.
18. Leape LL, Brennan TA, Laird NM, et al: Nature of adverse effects in hospitalized patients: Results of the Harvard Medical Practice Study II. *N Engl J Med* 324:377-384, 1991.
19. Montamat SC, Cusack BJ, Vestal RE: Management of drug therapy in the elderly. *N Engl J Med* 321(5):303-309, 1989.
20. Koch KE: Incorporation of standardized screening procedures into a pharmacy-based adverse drug reaction monitoring program. *Am J Hosp Pharm* 47:1314-1320, 1990.
21. Talley RB, Laventurier MF: Drug-induced illness. *JAMA* 229(8):1043, 1974.
22. Boston Collaborative Drug Surveillance Program. *JAMA* 216:467-472, 1971.
23. Wise RP, Tsong Y, Gerstman BB, et al: U.S. mortality related to medications. *J Clin Res Drug Dev* 2:181-182, 1988.
24. Smith MC, Visconti JA: On the "costs" of the 1962 drug amendments. *Inquiry* XI:61-64, 1974.
25. Southwick K: A prescription for trouble: Drugs to counteract drugs. *Health Week* 2(Aug 8):1,12, 1988.
26. Michel DJ, Dahl JM, Campbell HE, et al: Postmarketing surveillance of drugs: An overview. *J Pharm Prac* 11:231-238, 1989.
27. Faich GA: Adverse-drug-reaction monitoring. *N Engl J Med* 314:1589-1592, 1986.
28. Strom BL, Niettinen OS, Melmon KL: Post-marketing studies of drug efficacy: How? *Am J Med* 77:703-708, 1984.
29. Strom BL, Melmon KL, Miettinen OS: Post-marketing studies of drug efficacy: Why? *Am J Med* 78:475-480, 1985.
30. Edlavitch SA: Postmarketing surveillance methodologies. *Drug Intell Clin Pharm* 22:68-78, 1988.
31. Grasela TH, Schentag JJ: A clinical pharmacy-oriented drug surveillance network: I. Program description. *Drug Intell Clin Pharm* 21:902-908, 1987.
32. Jacinto MS, Kleinmann K: Hospital pharmacy program for reporting adverse drug reactions. *Am J Hosp Pharm* 40:444-445, 1983.
33. *Accreditation Manual for Hospitals*. Chicago, Joint Commission on Accreditation of Healthcare Organizations, 1989, pp 121,180.
34. *Examples of Drug Usage Evaluation, 1989*. Chicago, Joint Commission on Accreditation of Healthcare Organizations, 1989, p 26.
35. ASHP guidelines on adverse drug reaction monitoring and reporting. *Am J Hosp Pharm* 46:336-337, 1989.
36. Pearson KC, Kennedy DL: Adverse drug reactions and the Food and Drug Administration. *J Pharm Prac* 11:209-213, 1989.
37. Sills JM, Tanner LA, Milstien JB: Food and Drug Administration monitoring of adverse drug reactions. *Am J Hosp Pharm* 43:2764-2770, 1986.
38. Kennedy DL, Goetsch RA, Dreis MW: Use and reported adverse effects of new chemical entities. *Am J Hosp Pharm* 46:558-565, 1989.
39. Edlavitch SA: Adverse drug event reporting—Improving the low US reporting rates. *Arch Intern Med* 148:1499-1503, 1988.
40. *Guidelines for Post-Marketing Reporting of Adverse Reactions.* Rockville, MD, Center for Drugs and Biologics, Division of Drug and Biological Product Experience. 1985, Docket No. 85 D-0249.
41. Rogers AS, Israel E, Smith CR, et al: Physician knowledge, attitudes, and behaviour related to reporting adverse drug events. *Arch Intern Med* 148:1596-1600, 1988.

42. Fincham JE: Pilot projects to stimulate adverse drug reaction reporting. *J Clin Pharm Ther* 12:243-247, 1987.
43. Fincham JE: A statewide program to stimulate reporting of adverse drug reactions. *J Pharm Pract* 11(4):239-244, 1989.
44. Case RL, Guzzetti PJ: A survey of adverse drug reaction reporting programs in select hospitals. *Hosp Pharm* 21:423-434, 1986.
45. Miwa LJ: Implementing a hospital-based adverse drug reaction reporting program. *J Pharm Pract* 11:214-220, 1989.
46. Michel DJ, Knodel LC: Program coordinated by a drug information service to improve adverse drug reaction reporting in a hospital. *Am J Hosp Pharm* 43:2202-2205, 1986.
47. Keith MR, Bellanger-McCleery RA, Fuchs JE: Multidisciplinary program for detecting and evaluating adverse drug reactions. *Am J Hosp Pharm* 46:1809-1812, 1989.
48. Kimelblatt BJ, Young SH, Heywood PM, et al: Improved reporting of adverse drug reactions. *Am J Hosp Pharm* 45:1086-1089, 1988.
49. Nelson RW, Shane R: Developing an adverse drug reaction reporting program. *Am J Hosp Pharm* 40:445-446, 1983.
50. Karch FE, Lasagna L: Adverse drug reactions—a critical review. *JAMA* 234:1236-1241, 1975.
51. Morgan SA, Frank JT: Improved reporting of adverse drug reactions using an educational videotape. *Am J Hosp Pharm* 47:1340-1342, 1990.
52. Gilroy GW, Scollins MJ, Gay GA, et al: A pharmacy-coordinated adverse drug reaction surveillance program using physician reimbursement as an incentive to report. *Am J Hosp Pharm* 47:1327-1333, 1990.
53. Canada AT: Adverse drug reaction reporting: A practical program. *Am J Hosp Pharm* 26:18-20, 1969.
54. Berry LL, Segal R, Sherrin TP, et al: Sensitivity and specificity of three methods of detecting adverse drug reactions. *Am J Hosp Pharm* 45:1534-1539, 1988.
55. Vorce-West TE, Barstow L, Butcher B: System for voluntary reporting of adverse drug reactions in a university hospital. *Am J Hosp Pharm* 46:2300-2303, 1989.
56. Inman WHW (ed): The United Kingdom. In *Monitoring for Drug Safety*, Lancaster, England, MTP Press Ltd., 1980.
57. Koch-Weser J, Sidel VW, Sweet RH, et al: Factors determining physician reporting of adverse drug reactions. *N Engl J Med* 280:20-26, 1969.
58. Kehoe WA: A multidisciplinary approach to monitoring adverse drug reactions in a long-term care facility. *Hosp Pharm* 20:518-525, 1985.
59. Johnston PE, Morrow JD, Branch RA: Monitoring adverse drug reactions—the Vanderbilt University Hospital program. *Am J Hosp Pharm* 47:1321-1326, 1990.
60. Gardner P, Watson J: Adverse drug reactions: A pharmacist-based monitoring system. *Clin Pharm Ther* 11:802-807, 1970.
61. Powell SH, Schwartz PA, Rayment CM, et al: Pharmacy-based adverse drug reaction surveillance program. *Am J Hosp Pharm* 39:1963-1964, 1982.
62. Kilarski DJ, Ziegler B, Coarse J, et al: Adverse drug reaction reporting system: Developing a well-monitored program. *Hosp Formul* 21:949-952, 1986.
63. Chatas CA, Vinson BE: Program for improving adverse drug reaction reporting. *Am J Hosp Pharm* 47:155-157, 1990.
64. Savitsky ME: Recognizing hospital adverse drug reactions. *J Pharm Pract* 11:203-208, 1989.
65. Gibson GG, Strom BL: (Personal communication). Hospital of the University of Pennsylvania.
66. Michel DJ, Knodel LC: Comparison of three algorithms used to evaluate adverse drug reactions. *Am J Hosp Pharm* 43:1709-1714, 1986.
67. Naranjo CA, Busto U, Sellers EM, et al: A method for estimating the probability of adverse drug reactions. *Clin Pharm Ther* 30(2):239-245, 1981.
68. Kramer MS, Levanthal IM, Hutchinson TA, et al: An algorithm for the operational assessment of adverse drug reactions. *JAMA* 242:623-632, 1979.
69. Jones JK: Adverse drug reactions in the community health setting: Approaches to recognizing, counseling and reporting. *Fam Comm Health* 5:58-67, 1982.
70. Spitzer WO: Importance of valid measures of benefit and risk. *Med Toxicol* 1:74-78, 1986.
71. Maliekal J, Thornton J: A description of a successful computerized adverse drug reaction tracking program. *Hosp Formul* 25:436-442, 1990.
72. Boston Collaborative Drug Surveillance Program: Adverse drug interactions. *JAMA* 220:1238-1239, 1972.
73. Shinn AF, Hogan MJ, Zucchero FJ: Drug interactions in perspective. *J Pharm Prac* 11:221-230, 1989.
74. Garabedian-Ruffalo SM, Syrja-Farber M, Lanius PM, et al: Monitoring of drug-drug and drug-food interactions. *Am J Hosp Pharm* 45:1530-1534, 1988.
75. Davidson KW, Kahn A, Price RD: Reduction of adverse drug reactions by computerized drug interaction screening. *J Fam Pract* 25:371-375, 1987.
76. Wiser TH: Patient counseling: Adverse drug reactions. *U.S. Pharmacist* May:48-54, 1988.
77. Moss RL, Garnett WR, Steiner KC: Physician attitudes toward pharmacists counseling patients on adverse drug reactions. *Am J Hosp Pharm* 37:243-246, 1980.

CHAPTER 27

Controlled Substance Surveillance

SARA J. WHITE

The purposes of controlled substance surveillance are threefold: (1) to ensure compliance with State and Federal laws and institutional pharmacy practice standards such as American Society of Hospital Pharmacists' (ASHP) Technical Assistance Bulletin on Institutional Use of Controlled Substances,[1] (2) to prevent diversion of these drugs into illicit markets,[2] and (3) to provide a practical system for controlled substances dispensing and accountability within the institution. Strict compliance with the applicable laws and regulations is necessary for the institution to maintain its controlled substances registration. Without the use of controlled substances, many institutional therapies and procedures such as surgery would be impossible.

The Drug Enforcement Administration (DEA) does not provide a detailed protocol on how to maintain a controlled substances system. Instead, it offers a framework that each institution can use as a basis for designing its control system in conjunction with individual State laws and regulations.[3] These control systems must have ample checks, balances, and documentation that involves several people, each performing only the functions assigned to them with appropriate paper trails.[4,5] If one person performs all the functions in the system, it would be theoretically possible for that individual to alter the records and divert controlled substances. Once controlled substance systems are established, they must be continually monitored by pharmacy management to ensure that all procedures are being followed. Examples of ways to ensure that all procedures are followed are to have personnel not involved in the system conduct spots audits, unannounced total inventory audits, and reconciliations with the records; review the records for completeness; and maintain documentation of these activities. This monitoring should include verification that all reports are accurate and are being maintained for the 2-year requirement.[6,7] If the DEA visits the institution, the pharmacist must be able to produce ordering and disposition records for all controlled substances that have been received and are not currently in stock. The pharmacist should also be responsible for seeing that nursing procedures are appropriate for recording, storing, administering, and charting controlled substances.

Procedures will vary from institution to institution as do State laws. Some institutions may choose to control some drugs as if they were Federal scheduled items. Each institution should have a policy on random drug testing of employees. Areas that use large quantities of controlled substances, such as the operating rooms, may require intensive surveillance. Technology such as cameras and identification badge access should be used as appropriate.

Since pharmacists have to deal with two groups of federally controlled substances, Schedule II items and Schedule III-V items, this chapter deals with only inpatient use and has been divided into two sections. Within each section, the steps involved from the time the drug is ordered through its administration to patients are discussed.

SCHEDULE II CONTROLLED SUBSTANCES

Ordering and Receiving

To order controlled substances, the pharmacy must maintain its current annual registration with the DEA. To register, it is necessary to request the original form (available from the regional office or Registration Branch, DEA, Box 28083, Washington, DC 20005). Schedule II items require the use of the triplicate DEA order form 222. These order forms must be carefully filled out, because any strikeovers, erasures, or other mistakes void the form. The pharmacist should store the unused blank forms in a locked place. Access to and the ability to sign these forms should be restricted to one or two pharmacists to prevent possible diversion of the forms. The order forms may be signed only by the person whose signature is on the original registration form. Power of attorney may be given to another pharmacist to sign the forms.

An institutional purchase order will also have to be completed. The top two copies (brown and green) are sent to the manufacturer, and the last copy (blue) is maintained by the pharmacy as record of ordering the items. These blue copies are official records and should be maintained in a secure place by the pharmacist. The pharmacy's copy of the purchase order should be placed in a date-reminder file by anticipated arrival date. By checking the file, the pharmacist will be alerted if the orders are late so the manufacturer can be contacted, since these drugs may be diverted during shipping. At the end of each month, the manufacturer sends the green copy to the DEA, giving DEA a record of each institution's Schedule II purchases.

Most institutions have a receiving dock area where all shipments are delivered. Once the receiving dock personnel sign for the package, it is the institution's property. Appropriate procedures must ensure that controlled substances cannot disappear from the dock or during transit to the pharmacy. It is critical that no pharmacy packages stay on the dock overnight, since other personnel may have access to the area.

When pharmacy packages are received in the pharmacy, those containing controlled substances must be opened immediately and the packing list verified against the contents, purchase order, and pharmacy's blue copy of DEA form 222. Any discrepancies between what was ordered and received must be documented on the paperwork and signed by the person checking the order in. The person receiving must complete the receipt space on the blue DEA form 222, dating and signing it. Once this verification has been completed, the drugs should be immediately taken to the pharmacy's locked storage area. To provide a paper trail, it is a good idea to copy the packing slip and have the pharmacist who puts the items in the locked storage area, as well as the receiving person, sign for the contents. This copy of the signed packing slip can be attached to the purchase order and matched with the invoice for payment. The invoices and completed DEA 222 forms must be stored separately from other files so they can be readily retrieved if a DEA representative arrives. The copy of the packing slip can be used to enter the items received into the perpetual inventory. Again, the purpose is to ensure that controlled substances do not disappear inside the pharmacy. Although pharmacy hires only trusted employees, they should not be provided with an opportunity to divert controlled substances. From time to time, other employees such as housekeeping, maintenance, etc., will be in the pharmacy and can, unnoticed, remove controlled substances in trash bags if they are accessible.

Storing and Dispensing in Pharmacy

Schedule II items must be in a locked area inside the pharmacy. This locked area can vary from a locked, substantially constructed cabinet to a locked room (vault), with inside locked cabinets.

Schedule III-V items may be stored in a securely locked, substantially constructed cabinet or may be dispersed throughout the stock of noncontrolled substances. The abuse potential and need for dose-by-dose accountability of Schedule II items seem to warrant their being locked up. Determining who has access to the key to the cabinet or vault and inside cabinets and where the key is kept is a very important control mechanism. There should be only one set of keys accessible to the staff pharmacist. They should not be easily duplicated, and should always be carried by a pharmacist. Neither the institution's security personnel nor anyone else in the institution should have a key to the storage area. The storage area key should never be left in an unlocked box or drawer. A combination-lock box mounted on a wall could be used as a place to leave the keys overnight or a backup key when no pharmacist is on duty during the midnight shift or weekend hours.

It may be desirable to have only one small stock available to which the staff pharmacist has access for dispensing drugs to nursing units. The rest of the locked storage cabinet could be accessible only to one or two pharmacists or technicians who are responsible for the controlled substance system. This one dispensing small stock cabinet approach allows for frequent inventories against dispensing records, thereby enabling diversion to be quickly and easily detected.

The required DEA biennial inventory assessment must indicate the time of day it was taken. This inventory for Schedule II items must be an exact count, whereas Schedule III-V drugs can be an estimate of broken packages of 1,000 units or less. The Schedule II inventory record must be a separate document, but Schedule III-V drugs can be interspersed with normal inventory records, provided they are readily retrievable. The pharmacist taking the inventory must sign, date, and time it. The DEA does not require that any reconciliation of the physical and perpetual inventory be done or documented, but it is good practice to do so. The higher the number of controlled substances that are dispensed each month, the more prudent frequent total vault inventories should be.

The pharmacist must notify the regional DEA office of the wish to dispose of packages of controlled substances that are outdated, contaminated, broken, etc. This notification is made in triplicate, using form 41 and listing each item held for destruction. The DEA regional office will instruct the pharmacist in the manner to be used for destruction. A copy of each form 41 must be maintained for 2 years as proof of the disposition of the items.

The pharmacy may transfer controlled substances to another registered practitioner, provided that no more than 5 percent of the dosage units dispensed per registration year are transferred. To transfer controlled substances other than on a prescription written for a specific patient, a DEA Schedule II order form (DEA form 222) must be used. This situation arises when a pharmacist is out of stock, physicians want to stock their offices, or local ambulances that bring patients to the institution's emergency room want to replace their stock. The address preprinted on the 222 form must be where the drugs will be stored and used. At the end of the month, the pharmacist must send the DEA the green copy and retain the brown copy as proof of the disposition of the drugs.

Nursing Units

For inpatients, the physician writes medication orders in the patient's medical record (chart). The physician does not need to record his or her DEA registration number on inpatient orders for controlled substances; however, a list of registration numbers and signatures of all physicians who practice in the institution must be maintained in the pharmacy. The physician's original order or direct copy should be reviewed by the pharmacist prior to the administration of the controlled substance. There are no specific Federal labeling requirements for inpatient use.

Because of the need for dose-by-dose accountability, it is prudent to dispense single-use syringes or vials. These packages should be tamper evident; e.g., they might have a hard plastic outer container that allows the removal of only one syringe at a time. If the syringes are not so protected, the drug may be pulled out by inserting a needle through the back of the syringe or through the needle hub and refilling it with another clear liquid such as hydroxyzine, water, or normal saline. Obviously, vials need similar protection, since the rubber top can be entered with a needle or syringe and an exchange made. With tablets and capsules, individually packaged ones in reverse-numbered rolls or card packages are helpful. With rolled packages, a method of visually inspecting the remaining doses (clear window in the side of the package) is important. It is possible to remove doses at the beginning or middle of a roll and put the roll back in the box with the final number being visible, indicating a full box. Drugs that are not commonly used in the patient care areas should be returned to pharmacy as soon as the order is discontinued.

For practical reasons and emergency situations, most institutions maintain a small (24-hour) supply of needed Schedule II drugs as floorstock in locked boxes or cabinets on each nursing unit. A paper record system for pharmacy dispensing and signing out each item is needed that includes the drug, dosage form, strength, number dispensed, and signature of those who dispensed it, delivered it, and received it on the nursing unit. This information may be incorporated into the records that nurses use on the unit to indicate (in addition to charting) who received each dose (figure 27-1). Numerous systems exist such as signout logs, shingle sheets, and "no carbon required" (NCR) copies of medication administration records for keeping a perpetual inventory on the nursing unit as a "proof-of-use" or "certificate of disposition" system. A system must be in place to document (and have a second nurse cosign) any wastage. These records must be kept by pharmacy to account totally for each dose. Just as in pharmacy, key control is critical to preventing diversion.

A system for replacing the nursing unit's used stock and a documentation procedure for unaccounted-for doses must exist. Two examples of how unit stock can be replaced are (1) the nurse brings the completed proof-of-use sheet to pharmacy and is issued another supply or (2) pharmacy personnel inventory each unit daily and restock items used during the previous 24 hours. To handle the documentation of unaccounted-for doses on the units, a discrepancy form is generally used (figure 27-2). This form documents what the substance is, the fact that the nursing unit has attempted to account for the dose, and what administrative action has been taken. The DEA requires that substantial losses be reported using DEA theft or loss form 106.

Records

For Schedule II drugs, all records must be maintained for at least 2 years; some States may require a longer storage period. The information needed is:

1. The name of the substance.
2. A description of each product in finished dosage form and the number of units or volume of finished form in each commercial container.
3. The number of commercial containers of each such finished form received from other persons, including the date of receipt, number of containers in each shipment, and the name, address, and registration number of the person from whom the containers were received.
4. The number of units or volume of products in finished form dispensed, including the name of the person to whom it was dispensed, the date of dispensing, the number of units or volume dispensed, and the written or typewritten name or initials of the individual who dispensed or administered the substance on behalf of the dispenser.
5. The number of units or volume of product in finished form and/or commercial containers disposed of in any other manner by the registrant, including the date of disposal and the quantity of the substance in finished form disposed.

Many institutions use computers to maintain these records, provided that the specific information on scheduled drugs can be readily retrieved from the data banks and the information is stored, by tape, disc, or any other means, for 2 years.

Records that must be maintained are: (1) used DEA order forms; (2) receiving records and invoices; (3) biennial inventories; (4) proof-of-use disposition records (including DEA order forms used to purchase or transfer drugs from pharmacy); (5) destruction, waste, theft, discrepancy records; (6) physician's original orders (medical records for inpatients and prescriptions for outpatients); and (7) policy and procedure manuals (both pharmacy and nursing).

SCHEDULE III-V CONTROLLED SUBSTANCES

Ordering and Receiving

Schedule III-V drugs can be ordered the same way as any other pharmaceutical, provided the controlled substances are readily identifiable. Similar procedures as for Schedule II drugs should be used with regard to date-reminder files, receiving dock, processing once inside pharmacy, and documenting any discrepancies between what was ordered and received. The invoices for these drugs must be kept separate, since they form the basis of receipt for DEA purposes. Agents in these schedules (Tylenol® No. 3, Valium,® Halcion,® etc.) are better known by name than the Schedule II agents because of their wide use; hence, they are just as subject to diversion as Schedule II drugs. Even though the law does not specify locked storage of drugs other than Schedule II drugs in the pharmacy, the intent is that diversion be prevented.

Storing and Dispensing

Many institutions have chosen to control some or all of these agents as they do Schedule II drugs, whereas other institutions control only the more common ones. It is prudent to at least keep the back stock of these agents locked up, if not in the vault, then in locked storage areas. Quantities of these drugs on open shelves provide the opportunity to divert. The dispensing supply may either be interspersed with the other stock or kept in a separate area under the vision of pharmacists, e.g., in a unit dose cart. The dispensing stock should be kept to a minimum so any diversion would be evident.

Records

For Schedule III-V drugs, the following records must be maintained for at least 2 years: (1) invoices, (2) biennial inventory, (3) proof-of use disposition records, (4) physician's original order (patient's chart or prescription), and (5) policy and procedure manuals (pharmacy and nursing).

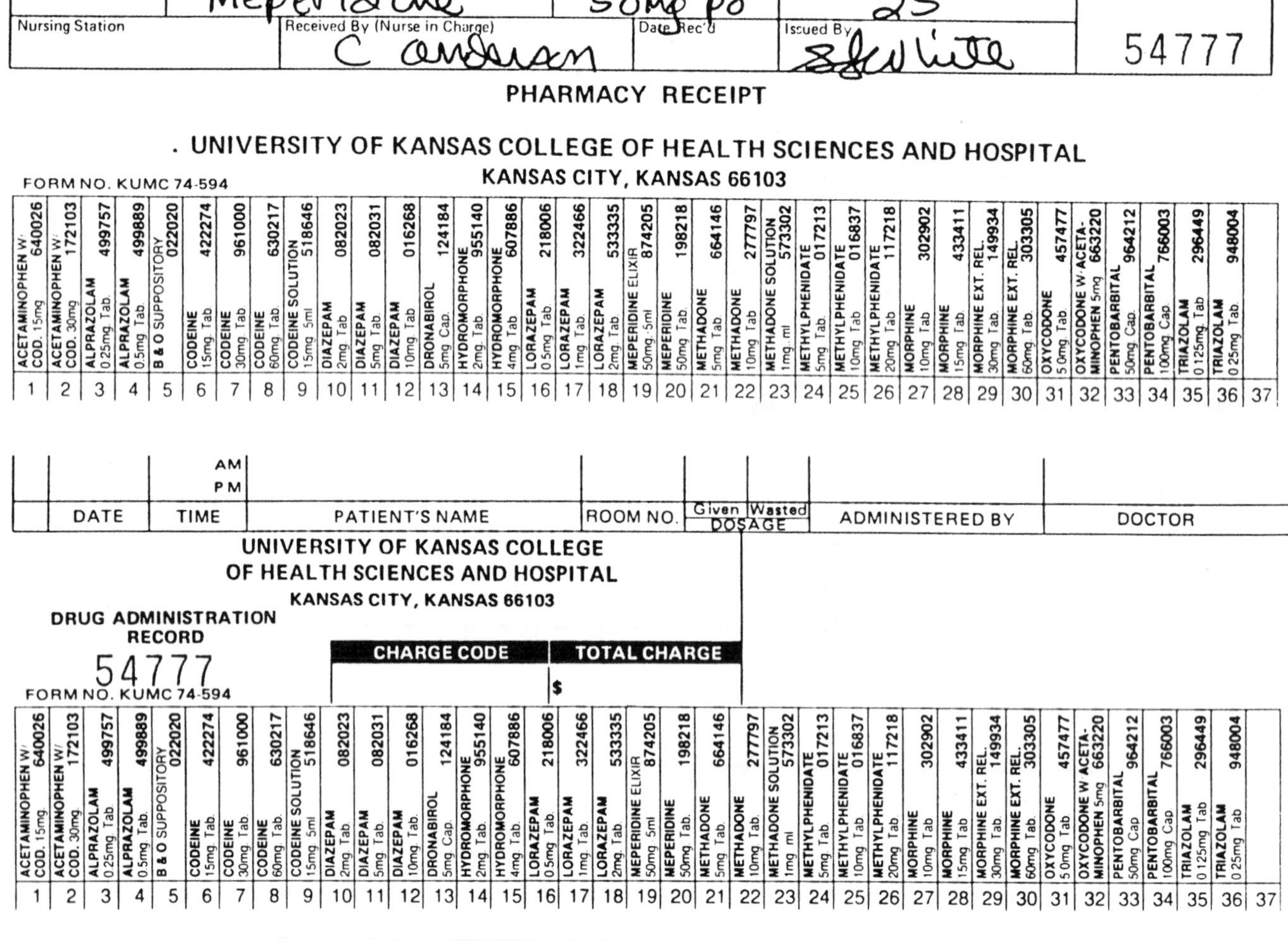

Date	Drug	Strength	Quantity	CONTROL NO.
	Meperidine	50mg po	25	54777
Nursing Station	Received By (Nurse in Charge)	Date Rec'd	Issued By	

PHARMACY RECEIPT

. UNIVERSITY OF KANSAS COLLEGE OF HEALTH SCIENCES AND HOSPITAL
KANSAS CITY, KANSAS 66103

FORM NO. KUMC 74-594

No.	Drug	Code
1	ACETAMINOPHEN W/ COD. 15mg	6400026
2	ACETAMINOPHEN W/ COD. 30mg	1721103
3	ALPRAZOLAM 0.25mg. Tab.	4999757
4	ALPRAZOLAM 0.5mg. Tab.	4999889
5	B & O SUPPOSITORY	0222020
6	CODEINE 15mg. Tab.	4222274
7	CODEINE 30mg. Tab.	9610000
8	CODEINE 60mg. Tab.	6302217
9	CODEINE SOLUTION 15mg. 5ml	5186646
10	DIAZEPAM 2mg. Tab	0820023
11	DIAZEPAM 5mg. Tab.	0820031
12	DIAZEPAM 10mg. Tab	0162268
13	DRONABIROL 5mg. Cap.	1241184
14	HYDROMORPHONE 2mg. Tab.	9551140
15	HYDROMORPHONE 4mg. Tab.	6077886
16	LORAZEPAM 0.5mg. Tab.	2180006
17	LORAZEPAM 1mg. Tab.	3224466
18	LORAZEPAM 2mg. Tab.	5333335
19	MEPERIDINE ELIXIR 50mg.·5ml	8742205
20	MEPERIDINE 50mg. Tab.	1982218
21	METHADONE 5mg. Tab.	6641146
22	METHADONE 10mg. Tab	2777797
23	METHADONE SOLUTION 1mg..ml	5733302
24	METHYLPHENIDATE 5mg. Tab.	0172213
25	METHYLPHENIDATE 10mg. Tab	0168837
26	METHYLPHENIDATE 20mg. Tab	1172218
27	MORPHINE 10mg. Tab	3029902
28	MORPHINE 15mg. Tab.	4334111
29	MORPHINE EXT. REL. 30mg. Tab.	1499934
30	MORPHINE EXT. REL. 60mg. Tab.	3033305
31	OXYCODONE 5.0mg. Tab.	4574477
32	OXYCODONE W/ ACETA-MINOPHEN 5mg	6632220
33	PENTOBARBITAL 50mg. Cap.	9642212
34	PENTOBARBITAL 100mg. Cap.	7660003
35	TRIAZOLAM 0.125mg. Tab	2964449
36	TRIAZOLAM 0.25mg. Tab.	9480004
37		

DATE	TIME (AM / PM)	PATIENT'S NAME	ROOM NO.	DOSAGE Given	DOSAGE Wasted	ADMINISTERED BY	DOCTOR

UNIVERSITY OF KANSAS COLLEGE
OF HEALTH SCIENCES AND HOSPITAL
KANSAS CITY, KANSAS 66103

DRUG ADMINISTRATION RECORD

54777

FORM NO. KUMC 74-594

CHARGE CODE	TOTAL CHARGE
	$

No.	Drug	Code
1	ACETAMINOPHEN W/ COD. 15mg	6400026
2	ACETAMINOPHEN W/ COD. 30mg	1721103
3	ALPRAZOLAM 0.25mg. Tab.	4999757
4	ALPRAZOLAM 0.5mg. Tab.	4999889
5	B & O SUPPOSITORY	0222020
6	CODEINE 15mg. Tab.	4222274
7	CODEINE 30mg. Tab.	9610000
8	CODEINE 60mg. Tab.	6302217
9	CODEINE SOLUTION 15mg. 5ml	5186646
10	DIAZEPAM 2mg. Tab	0820023
11	DIAZEPAM 5mg. Tab.	0820031
12	DIAZEPAM 10mg. Tab	0162268
13	DRONABIROL 5mg. Cap.	1241184
14	HYDROMORPHONE 2mg. Tab.	9551140
15	HYDROMORPHONE 4mg. Tab.	6077886
16	LORAZEPAM 0.5mg. Tab.	2180006
17	LORAZEPAM 1mg. Tab.	3224466
18	LORAZEPAM 2mg. Tab.	5333335
19	MEPERIDINE ELIXIR 50mg.·5ml	8742205
20	MEPERIDINE 50mg. Tab.	1982218
21	METHADONE 5mg. Tab.	6641146
22	METHADONE 10mg. Tab	2777797
23	METHADONE SOLUTION 1mg..ml	5733302
24	METHYLPHENIDATE 5mg. Tab.	0172213
25	METHYLPHENIDATE 10mg. Tab	0168837
26	METHYLPHENIDATE 20mg. Tab	1172218
27	MORPHINE 10mg. Tab	3029902
28	MORPHINE 15mg. Tab.	4334111
29	MORPHINE EXT. REL. 30mg. Tab.	1499934
30	MORPHINE EXT. REL. 60mg. Tab.	3033305
31	OXYCODONE 5.0mg. Tab.	4574477
32	OXYCODONE W/ ACETA-MINOPHEN 5mg	6632220
33	PENTOBARBITAL 50mg. Cap.	9642212
34	PENTOBARBITAL 100mg. Cap.	7660003
35	TRIAZOLAM 0.125mg. Tab	2964449
36	TRIAZOLAM 0.25mg. Tab.	9480004
37		

Figure 27-1. Proof of use system

CONCLUSION

Controlled substances surveillance involves having a control system that has built-in checks to prevent any diversion and maintains all the records required by the DEA. Any system must be constantly monitored to ensure that all the procedures are being followed and the records are complete. Pharmacists must assume the responsibility for the total system, including the nursing unit's drug administration to patients. Pharmacy, in conjunction with nursing, must develop nursing unit procedures and ensure their compliance for controlled substances. Controlled substances are essential for institutions and must be appropriately handled to prevent diversion or abuse.

REFERENCES

1. ASHP technical assistance bulletin on institutional use of controlled substances, In *Practice Standards of ASHP 1989-1990*, Bethesda, MD, American Society of Hospital Pharmacists, 1990, pp 152-160.
2. Title 21, C.F.R. section 1300 to end.
3. Hoover RC, McCormick WC, Harrison WF: Pilferage of controlled substances in hospitals. *Am J Hosp Pharm* 38:1007-1010, 1981.
4. Matanin D, McGuire W, McCombs C: Quality distribution for controlled substances. *U.S. Pharmacist* 12:H2-H14, 1987.
5. Woller TW, Roberts MJ, Ploetz, P: Recording Schedule II drug use in a decentralized drug distribution system. *Am J Hosp Pharm* 44:349-353, 1987.

6. Bergemann DE: Checklist for evaluating management of controlled substances. *Am J Hosp Pharm* 37:1299-1300, 1980.

7. Prosnick JJ: Evaluation of hospital controlled substance distribution systems. *Am J Hosp Pharm* 32:606-608, 1975.

CHAPTER 28

Contract Pharmacy Services

FREDERIC R. CURTISS and HARLAN C. STAI

Hospital officers are turning increasingly to outside contractors to manage certain hospital departments. Food service is more likely to be contracted than any other hospital department, followed closely by housekeeping. Comparing 1988 to 1987, the total number of departments and management contracts increased by 5.3 percent to 4,563. The number of hospital clients using pharmacy management companies in 1988 was 379, up only 1.3 percent from 1987.[1] At a total number of 379 contracts nationwide, pharmacy departments in hospitals are as likely to be managed by an outside contractor as the laundry, plant operations/maintenance, cardiopulmonary diagnostics, and respiratory therapy departments.

Pharmacy management companies are relatively limited in number, with a total of only six companies in 1988. Three companies dominate the market, possessing 84 percent of the pharmacy contracts. The largest, Owen Healthcare, Inc., held 42 percent of all pharmacy contracts in 1988, and the second largest pharmacy contract company, HPI Health Care Services, Inc. (formerly HPI Hospital Pharmacies), held 28 percent of all pharmacy contracts. Therefore, the two largest pharmacy contract companies held 70 percent of all hospital pharmacy management contracts in 1988.[1]

BACKGROUND

Hospital pharmacy practice has evolved rapidly in the last three or four decades. Prior to the discovery of antibiotics and other major therapeutic advances in the 1930's and 1940's, the role of drug therapy in hospital care was relatively unimportant. As drug therapy became a more significant part of patient care, the role of the hospital pharmacist also became more important. Correspondingly, by the 1950's, pharmacy departments became more common in hospitals; 59 percent of hospitals maintained a pharmacy department in 1956.[2] By 1975, two-thirds of U.S. hospitals maintained a pharmacy department with a (full-time) registered pharmacist.[3] The evolution of the hospital pharmacist's role was summarized by the Study Commission on Pharmacy in 1975: pharmacy practice had evolved into a "knowledge system"; many of drug compounding and preparation functions had been assumed by the pharmaceutical industry, and the pharmacists were increasingly involved in direct patient care, including communication of drug information and education of physicians.[4] Pharmacists became more responsible for the oversight and performance of the entire *drug use process:* (1) identifying the patient's problem; (2) determining the patient's history of drug use; (3) prescribing; (4) selecting drug product; (5) dispensing drugs; (6) educating and counseling the patient; (7) administering drugs; (8) monitoring drug therapy; (9) reviewing drug use; and (10) conducting drug education of health professionals.[5]

Comprehensive Services

By the late 1970's, "comprehensive hospital pharmacy services" had come to mean pharmacist involvement in the entire drug use process and implementation of specific systems and services:[6] (1) unit dose drug distribution systems, (2) centralized intravenous (IV) admixture programs, and (3) clinical pharmacy services.

With the use of more potent drugs through the 1950's and greater use of the IV route of drug administration in the 1960's and 1970's, it became increasingly apparent that comprehensive pharmacy services were not a luxury in hospitals but a necessary part of patient care. Published reports of medication errors began appearing in the 1950's.[7-9] Later research studies showed that even patients in university teaching hospitals were not protected from medication errors and that one in every six doses was administered in error.[10,11] Another study reported a medication error rate of 18 percent, which reached 31 percent when wrong time of administration was counted as an error.[12] Subsequent studies confirmed the high incidence of medication errors in hospitalized patients.[13-16]

In addition to the medication error rates that established the need for greater control of drug distribution systems by pharmacists, the need for comprehensive pharmacy services was further evidenced in studies examining adverse drug reactions. "Adverse drug reactions" are defined as the unintended and undesirable, noxious effects of drugs used for diagnostic, prophylactic, or therapeutic purposes. A summary report of nine studies conducted over a 15-year period showed that up to 7 percent of all hospital admissions were caused by adverse reactions, and as many as one in five patients experience an adverse drug reaction while hospitalized.[17] More recently, adverse drug reactions have been found to be the most common type of iatrogenic illness in hospitalized patients.[18] (See also chapter 26 in this handbook.)

The need for comprehensive pharmacy services, including more active pharmacist involvement in drug use monitoring, has been underscored by several studies that found less than optimal prescribing decisions to be common: widespread use of largely ineffective drugs,[19] irrational dosage amounts or combination therapy,[20-22] and a preference for newer agents of greater expense and sometimes higher toxicity but not necessarily higher efficacy.[23] Unnecessary, costly, and dangerous prophylactic antibiotic use in hospitalized patients has been documented, with only 10 percent of patients receiving appropriate prophylactic antibiotic therapy.[24] Further evidence of misprescribing was found in a study of 10,700 prescriptions, which revealed 1,130 errors and a physician noncompliance prescribing rate of 14.38 percent.[25]

Several factors conspired to highlight the need for and functioning of the pharmacist as the watchdog of drug prescribing. Accordingly, pharmacist responsibility expanded beyond drug distribution to direct patient care services now described as "clinical pharmacy." "Comprehensive hospital pharmacy services" now denote (1) a complete unit dose drug distribution system, (2) a pharmacy-based IV admixture program, (3) a pharmacy quality assurance program, (4) clinical pharmacy services, and (5) full-time pharmacist and pharmacy management services.

WHY CONTRACT PHARMACY SERVICES?

Personal familiarity of the authors with more than 700 hospital pharmacy contracts and a review of the literature show that hospitals contract with pharmacy management companies for many reasons besides achieving implementation of comprehensive pharmacy services in a timely and efficient manner.

The most common reasons that cause hospital officers to look to outside contractors for assistance in managing their pharmacy departments can be divided into three categories:

1. Staffing/personnel
2. Cost
3. Service

Several specific reasons can be articulated under each of these three categories.

1. Staffing/personnel
   a. Shortage of hospital pharmacists, particularly in remote geographic areas
   b. Difficulty in retaining competent pharmacy personnel and achieving continuity in pharmacy department services
   c. Insufficient hospital pharmacy knowledge and experience among available pharmacy personnel
   d. Inadequate management training among available hospital pharmacists
   e. Unsatisfactory performance of in-house staff in achieving pharmacy department objectives
   f. Personality conflicts and organizational dynamics
   g. Specific hospital personnel management objectives such as evaluation of staff performance or termination of certain personnel
   h. Need for reallocation of available in-house management resources to other responsibilities and problem areas in the hospital
2. Cost
   a. Pressure for cost reduction and cost management, since Medicare reimbursement is not keeping up with the increases in drug costs and the gap is widening between Medicare costs and Medicare revenues
   b. Need for better financial performance of the pharmacy department, including reduction in lost charges and greater control of acquisition costs
   c. Insufficient capital to purchase new fixtures, purchase new equipment, or otherwise modernize the pharmacy department
3. Service
   a. Accreditation, certification, and other regulatory pressures
   b. Need for greater drug use control to contain drug diversion or reduce medication dispensing and administration errors
   c. Physician demands for certain clinical pharmacy services such as pharmacokinetic dosing, patient education, and drug information services
   d. Hospital administration demands for drug formulary development
   e. Response to nursing staff demands relating to a need for greater confidence in the pharmacy department and drug distribution responsibilities
   f. Purchase of certain specialized technical and professional services unavailable elsewhere
   g. Unavailability of sufficient nursing staff
   h. Need for computerization

Staffing and Efficiency

Trained and experienced hospital pharmacists are in short supply, and many hospitals located in remote geographic areas have no access to hospital pharmacists at all. Disregarding aspects of education, training, and experience of pharmacist manpower, the Department of Health and Human Services (DHHS)[26] reported that in 1978 approximately 3,000 counties in the United States had fewer pharmacists than the number required to serve the population. Estimates of available pharmacy manpower using government data range from 118,000 to 172,000, a 31 percent discrepancy. The high-end estimate is a result of multiple-State licensure; the current estimate of 117,182 active, practicing pharmacists indicates that the shortage of pharmacists today is in the range of 25,000 to 40,000.[27]

Hospitals in many remote areas have experienced difficulty in recruiting and retaining competent hospital pharmacists. Often, small hospitals have had to turn to local community pharmacists to perform drug purchasing, manage inventory control, and oversee the drug distribution process on a part-time basis. Generally these community pharmacists lack sufficient hospital pharmacy knowledge and experience. Even if a community pharmacist is otherwise competent in pharmacy and clinical practice, comprehensive hospital pharmacy systems and services require the participation and oversight of a full-time pharmacist, properly trained in hospital pharmacy practice. Contract companies make available to the pharmacist multiple career paths and opportunities for continued training and education that may not be available from individual hospitals or, indeed, even from multihospital organizations.

Pharmacy management companies are also attractive to some hospitals seeking to meet certain personnel management objectives such as performance evaluation of pharmacy personnel. Pharmacy management companies have the necessary resources to evaluate staff performance and productivity and can make specific recommendations to hospital officers. These studies can be used to make informed personnel changes and to justify these changes. Less often, a hospital may enter a pharmacy contract in part to terminate certain personnel or otherwise carry out difficult personnel management decisions that it might not otherwise achieve.

Resolving personality conflicts and dealing with organizational dynamics are an important part of the successful management of any organization. Hospital care is not immune from personal ego needs, personality conflicts, professional "turf," and other problems of a more emotional rather than rational nature. Although we might all hope that patient care needs and the desire to deliver effective medical services in an efficient manner would transcend such emotional factors, this is not always the case. Indeed, territorial battles are almost guaranteed in an industry in which functional areas are protected by licensure and other certification mechanisms, down to specific and discrete patient care tasks. Territorial conflicts and other emotional factors can so embroil pharmacists that they become incapable of achieving objectives such as implementing a complete unit dose drug distribution system and other comprehensive pharmacy services. Pharmacy management companies have a distinct advantage in overcoming these obstacles via a broad knowledge and experience base in personnel management and the ability to tap an extensive personnel resource pool. Conflict situations can be analyzed and personalities assessed to best match pharmacy personnel with the needs in any given hospital. Perhaps a pharmacist or support person of a different age, sex, ethnicity, training and experience, personality type, communication skills, or other factor may be able to mesh better with nonpharmacy personnel in the hospital to resolve the conflict and to achieve objectives in a timely manner.

Myriad other human resource factors may contribute to a decision to contract with a pharmacy management company. For example, perhaps a relatively acute need arises within a given hospital to focus existing in-house management resources. A pharmacy management contract removes responsibility for day-to-day management from hospital officers and thereby permits concentration of available in-house management resources to other responsibilities and problem areas. Also, some small hospitals may simply be unable to attract sufficient management talent to oversee all hospital operations. A contract with a pharmacy management company can ameliorate a management shortage at levels above the pharmacy department.

Whether full-time or part-time, the pharmacy staff in a given hospital may exhibit unsatisfactory performance in achieving certain pharmacy department objectives, be they financial, drug use control, clinical, or other. Certainly, the implementation of comprehensive pharmacy services in hospitals is still incomplete, with many hospitals not reaching this professional practice standard. As late as 1987, only 57 percent of all hospitals had both unit dose drug distribution systems and pharmacy-based IV admixture programs. Only 5 percent of all U.S. short-term hospitals had implemented full-scope, comprehensive pharmacy services, including at least five clinical pharmacy programs.[28] Inadequate training of pharmacists in hospital practice and a lack of management expertise appeared to be the most important obstacles to the implementation of comprehensive pharmacy services in U.S. hospitals.[29]

Small hospitals are particularly prone to incomplete implementation of necessary pharmacy services. The Council on Professional Affairs of the American Society of Hospital Pharmacists (ASHP) addressed the poor quality in scope of pharmacy services in many small hospitals and concluded, "A primary cause of this problem was the inadequate understanding of hospital pharmacy practice by administrators and pharmacists in these facilities."[30]

The need for greater control of the entire drug use process and the adoption of broader standards and practice recommendations for hospital pharmacy have put further strain on the already short supply of trained hospital pharmacists. Practice standards require the pharmacy to evaluate the appropriateness of prescribed drug therapy, including analysis of the effectiveness of drug therapy and drug use evaluation (DUE), as well as consultation with physicians, nurses, and other health practitioners.[31] Other minimum standards require maintenance of a medication profile for each patient, pharmacist review of the appropriateness of all physician medication orders prior to dispensing, preparation of all sterile products (including IV admixtures, piggybacks, and irrigating solutions) by pharmacy personnel, provision of drug information to patients as well as staff, preparation of an operations manual governing all pharmacy functions, development and maintenance of a drug formulary for the hospital, etc. Moreover, the same pharmacy standards apply to all hospitals, regardless of size. Accreditation, certification, and other regulatory demands relating to these practice standards have, in many cases, precipitated hospital contracts with pharmacy management companies in order to correct deficiencies quickly and efficiently.

Pharmacy management companies have developed particular proficiency in implementing complete unit dose and IV admixture systems in hospitals. The companies typically operate "implementation teams," which have the necessary experience and capability to implement these complete drug distribution systems within 4-6 weeks of the start of the contract. These teams are not as encumbered as in-house pharmacy staff when implementing changes in drug and IV distribution systems and in the pharmacy department. Implementation teams can achieve in a matter of days what may take years to accomplish by in-house staff pharmacists. Experts cite examples of in-house pharmacists needing up to 2 years merely to obtain approval from hospital administrators to *begin* implementation of a unit dose system or a pharmacy-based IV admixture program.[32]

Financial Performance

The financial performance of the pharmacy department is a major factor in many hospital pharmacy contracts. For the year 1989, the drug cost component of the cost index upon which hospitals' Medicare reimbursement is based increased at approximately twice the rate of the overall index. Therefore, drug costs are becoming a much larger piece of overall hospital costs. Pharmacy management companies can, through guaranteed fee arrangements, curb the increase in pharmacy costs and at the same time maintain a (contractually) specified level of service. Additionally, for the approximately 50 percent of patients who are not covered by public programs (Medicare or Medicaid), the profitability of the pharmacy department (i.e., excess revenue over department expense) can be improved dramatically by a pharmacy management company, simply through a reduction in lost patient charges. Reconciliation of the pharmacy dispensing record with the nursing medication adminstration record (MAR) and the patient billing document on a regular and timely basis ensures that all doses are accounted for and charged properly and that each patient is charged only for those doses actually administered. Greater pharmacy department productivity, reduction in drug costs associated with drug diversion resulting from pilferage, and reduced drug acquisition costs can further improve the financial performance of the pharmacy department under a management contract. Finally, the pharmacy management companies have considerable experience in the development of drug formularies, which have financial implications for hospitals as well as a salutary effect on patient care through more appropriate drug prescribing.

Large pharmacy management companies are proprietary organizations with greater access to capital than most community, nonprofit hospitals. New hospitals and hospitals short of cash or otherwise experiencing difficulty in obtaining affordable debt financing can still modernize the pharmacy department via a management contract. Capital costs incurred by the contractor in purchasing equipment, replacing fixtures, and modernizing the pharmacy department are amortized over the term of the contract and financed via pharmacy revenues. Also, when the management contract includes complete control of the hospital's drug inventory, the hospital can benefit from an immediate cash infusion upon valuation of the drug inventory and its purchase by the contractor.

Service and Quality

Once complete drug and IV distribution systems are operational and other management controls are in place, the pharmacy department operations are typically turned over to a director of pharmaceutical services employed by the management company to operate the pharmacy under the terms of the contract. Since the drug and IV distribution systems are operated under specific policies and procedures and according to performance standards, dramatic changes can occur in the correction of former problems having to do with drug diversion, medication administration errors, etc. Pharmacist reconciliation of the drug dispensing record with the medication administration record helps detect, correct, and often prevent medication administration errors and requires accountability for all drug doses that leave the pharmacy. Pharmacist reconciliation of the dispensing record and MAR to the patient billing document helps to further control drug loss due to waste, as well as virtually eliminate lost charges and thereby improve the financial performance of the pharmacy.

Aside from the need for hospitals to implement comprehensive pharmacy services, sometimes made more acute as a result of deficiencies identified by regulatory agencies, hospitals may turn to pharmacy management companies to satisfy physician or nursing staff demands. Nurses may demand greater confidence in the pharmacy department in its performance of drug distribution tasks. Physicians may demand clinical pharmacy skills in pharmacokinetic dosing, patient education, or drug information. A pharmacy contract may also be consummated as a result of a shortage of nursing staff. A complete unit dose system and centralized IV admixture program can save as much as 14-17 minutes or more of nursing time per patient day (0.23-0.28 nursing hours per patient) compared to traditional drug distribution and IV admixtures prepared by nurses.[33]

Computerization, either the need to implement a new system or evaluate an existing one, can often cause hospitals to seek input from pharmacy management companies. Input from companies that are exposed to a number of pharmacy computer systems in multiple locations is of definite value in reviewing the capabilities of an existing system or an anticipated purchase.

Finally, large and small hospitals alike may at times experience the need for certain specialized technical or professional services that may not be readily available elsewhere. By virtue of shared resources and economies of scale, a pharmacy management company can attract leaders in various fields and those individuals with the greatest expertise. These individuals may be involved in the development and provision of the most progressive services such as comprehensive quality assurance programs[31] and clinical pharmacy certification programs.[34] This level of expertise would simply be unavailable to most hospitals except through such a management contract with a large company.

CONTRACT TERMS AND SCOPE OF SERVICE

A pharmacy management company has the capability to implement comprehensive and progressive pharmacy services in a rapid but orderly and nondisruptive manner. Indeed, most hospital pharmacy contracts specify the timeframe for implementation of specific services, usually no more than 60 days from initiation of the contract. Contractors usually guarantee certain performance standards for various systems and services in the terms of the contract.

Most pharmacy contracts involve "full-scope" comprehensive services. However, sometimes hospitals will purchase discrete, limited, or "unbundled" services, and the contract terms will vary accordingly. For example, a hospital may contract with a management company to perform an analysis and evaluation of the hospital's current drug delivery system and pharmacy operations. The contractor may be responsible only for identifying deficiencies and making specific recommendations for correction of the deficiencies. The service would probably be performed within a specified timeframe for a fixed-fee amount, like any other consultant-management service. The fee would generally be paid to the contractor in one lump sum on completion of the study and submission of a written report. Alternatively, portions of the fee may be paid at various stages of the study or in part at periodic reevaluation points such as every 6-12 months.

Limited-scope contracts may involve the purchase of one or more specific services, such as:

1. Personnel search and successful placement of the director of pharmacy services, other staff pharmacists, or support personnel
2. Backup support services to ensure continuity of service, particularly in small hospitals in remote areas, during times of illness or unexpected leaves of absence of existing pharmacy personnel, or to protect against other threats to continuity of pharmacy service
3. Productivity and efficiency studies and evaluations
4. Drug formulary development
5. Development of policy and procedure manuals for pharmacy operations
6. Drug purchasing
7. Inventory control
8. Drug information and/or staff (and "in-service") education
9. Pharmacy quality assurance programs, including periodic assessment and evaluation
10. Retrospective drug utilization review (DUR) studies
11. Analysis of lost pharmacy charges or other financial performance of the pharmacy department
12. Analysis of drug diversion within the hospital

Generally, the term "limited-scope" pharmacy contracts is now used to refer to relationships between hospitals and community pharmacists in which the community pharmacist is employed by the hospital for a few hours each week to do such things as check inventory, purchase and stock drugs, and otherwise meet minimum accreditation standards. In some small hospitals, community pharmacies may be involved in certain drug distribution responsibilities, including, in some cases, actually dispensing medications to hospital patients from the community pharmacy. These arrangements may not involve formal contracts and are more commonly referred to as "consultant pharmacist services."

Limited-scope pharmacy contracts are held by both large and small companies. Most full-scope pharmacy contracts are held by large pharmacy management companies, but small companies may also provide full-scope pharmacy services and, in a few instances, a hospital will contract with a second hospital for limited- or full-scope pharmacy services.

Comprehensive pharmacy systems and services require the participation and oversight of a full-time pharmacist, properly trained in hospital pharmacy practice. Full-scope pharmacy contract services would include most or all of the following:

1. Complete unit dose drug distribution system
2. Complete pharmacy-based IV admixture program
3. Comprehensive quality assurance program
4. Daily reconciliation of patient charges with the pharmacy drug dispensing profile and the nurses' MAR
5. In-service education of nurses, physicians, and other health professionals
6. Concurrent monitoring of patient drug profiles to check for drug interactions, adverse drug reactions, and inappropriate drug prescribing
7. Complete pharmacy staffing, including personnel recruitment, selection, education, training, and fringe benefit expenses
8. Professional and technical support, including backup pharmacists and technicians to ensure continuity of services
9. Management and supervisory support services provided by regional and home office personnel
10. Research and development, including innovations in drug delivery, electronic data processing, and clinical pharmacy services such as pharmacokinetic analyses and drug dosing
11. Purchase of entire pharmacy department inventory and remodeling of fixtures to permit implementation of unit dose and IV admixture programs
12. Management training and education programs for staff pharmacists and support personnel
13. Drug information services, including periodic newsletters
14. Full-time pharmacist service, including 24-hour on-call coverage
15. Periodic management reports to hospital administration
16. Development of hospital-specific pharmacy policy and procedure manuals
17. Pharmacist participation in hospital committees such as the pharmacy and therapeutics (P&T) committee and utilization and review committee
18. Retrospective DURs
19. Drug therapy consultations with nurses and physicians
20. Management of all computer-related and data management requirements of the pharmacy department.

Each of the services identified above may be specified to varying degrees in the contract. Alternatively, each service is explained in greater detail in the management company's "proposal for services." This document is generally prepared following an onsite analysis and evaluation of the hospital's present drug distribution system and pharmacy operations. Following the onsite visit, often referred to as a "feasibility study," the proposal is prepared, including an explanation of the deficiencies and/or opportunities detected and the proposed systems and services to take advantage of the opportunities or to correct the deficiencies. A contract may be negotiated between the management company and the hospital subsequent to presentation of the results of the onsite study and analysis of the proposal for services. Elsewhere, Fink[35] has described some of the liability and other legal issues associated with hospital pharmacy contracts. Under the terms of the full-scope pharmacy contracts, the management company assumes responsibility for essentially all pharmacy services and department operations. However, the hospital cannot abrogate ultimate responsibility for the quality of care rendered to patients in the hospital, and, by necessity, must provide certain services and facilities necessary for complete pharmaceutical services. As with the responsibilities of the pharmacy contractor, the responsibilities of the hospital should also be specified in the contract and may include the following:

1. Nursing staff responsibilities, including the actual administration of drug to patients, updating patient MAR's, and cooperation with the pharmacy department in reconciling the dispensing record to the MAR
2. Allocation of physical space for the pharmacy department, unit dose cabinets, and exchange carts in the nursing units and other parts of the hospital and space requirements for the night drug storage locker

3. Billing and collecting of pharmacy charges and handling of deductions from revenue associated with contractual allowances to third-party payers and bad debts
4. Preparation of appropriate claim forms, cost reports, and other documents for third-party payers and any other necessary interactions with these parties
5. Day-to-day housekeeping and other maintenance services of the pharmacy department and related space operated by the contractor in the hospital
6. Local telephone, power, and other utility services
7. Receiving and storage space and perhaps some limited services associated with these functions of the contractor in managing pharmacy inventories
8. Payment to the contractor

Compensation

Pharmacy management companies are compensated for their services in several ways, ranging from fixed annual management fees, generally paid in monthly amounts, to a fee per item, usually linked to the cost of the item dispensed. Although most hospital-pharmacy management company financial arrangements will involve one of the following methods, some contracts may incorporate two or more of these methods:

1. *Unit service charge* (SC), in which the hospital is charged for each unit dose dispensed by the pharmacy to patients or to the nursing unit. The SC amount is usually calculated from some multiple factor times the cost of the medication, e.g., 1.2 times average wholesale price (AWP).
2. *Management fee with a passthrough* of drug costs to the hospital. The cost passthrough may be calculated from the management company's actual acquisition costs (AAC's), AWP, discounted AWP's such as estimated acquisition costs (EAC's), or via some other price schedule.
3. *Annual management fee*, including all drug costs, salary, and other operating expenses.
4. *Management fee tied to hospital census or volume of activity*, e.g., management fee per patient day, per patient case, per diagnosis-related group (DRG).

A hospital's pharmacy price schedule is independent of the financial arrangement with the pharmacy contractor. Most hospitals finance pharmacy services through a mark-up on the cost of medication actually dispensed to the patient, using the AAC, AWP, EAC, or some similar basis. Customary mark-up multipliers range from 2.5 to 4.0 times the drug cost. These drug cost "multiples" are generally supplemented by minimum patient charges such as $1.00 for an oral solid unit dose, $1.50 for an oral solid controlled substance, and $4.00 for an injectable medication. The minimum amount is charged to the patient when the cost of the medication, times the multiplier, is less than the minimum amount. "Minimum" patient charges are conceptually sound, since this method recognizes that there is a service cost associated with dispensing each unit dose of medication, and this service cost is relatively fixed and independent of the actual product cost of the medication.

Regardless of the type of financial arrangement between the pharmacy management company and the hospital, the patient price schedule should be determined by the hospital without any element of control by the contractor. However, the pharmacy management company will generally have responsibility for maintaining the patient price schedule and for updating the schedule periodically.

The precise terms of a contract will be unique to a given hospital management company arrangement. The financial arrangement and scope of services of the contract will result from negotiations between the management company and the hospital. Depending on the unique circumstances in a given hospital, the pharmacy management company may assume certain financial risks in providing pharmacy services to the patients and staff of the hospital. For example, with the annual management fee arrangement specified, a pharmacy management company would assume a considerable degree of risk having to do with drug utilization, including the use of expensive medications. In this arrangement, the pharmacy management company may limit its risk through certain conditions, specified in the contract, such as adjustment for fluctuating patient case mix (or severity of illness) or a maximum aggregate drug cost as a percentage of the total fee paid by the hospital to the contractor, e.g., 50 percent of the management fee.

The hospital retains a degree of risk associated with the total cost of the pharmacy contract in the unit service charge arrangement. In this case, the total amount paid to the pharmacy management company would depend on drug utilization, determined by drug prescribing, and the possible use of expensive medication. A hospital may try to limit this element of financial risk by specifying certain conditions in a contract, such as a maximum amount to be paid to the contractor, determined on a per patient day or per patient case basis, e.g., up to but not more than $40 per patient day.

Other terms of the financial arrangements between hospitals and pharmacy management companies may include provisions such as a cash discount for prompt payment by the hospital to the contractor, an adjustment factor for third-party contractual allowances to the hospital, or other deductions from revenue such as bad debts, as well as myriad other factors. The management company may also specify a minimum profit amount to the hospital such as $10 per patient day or $70 per patient case. This amount would be calculated from the average amount of pharmacy revenue per patient day less the average amount paid to the management company per patient day, perhaps less the amounts having to do with deductions from revenue. For example, a pharmacy contract guarantees a minimum pharmacy department gross margin of $40 per patient day for the hospital. Actual total pharmacy revenue from patient charges for a given fiscal period equals $1 million divided by 12,500 total patient days, yielding $80 per patient day. Pharmacy service charges for the same fiscal period totaled $600,000, or $48 per patient day. In this example, the pharmacy management company would be obligated to return $100,000 to the hospital ($8 per patient day times 12,500 patient days) under this financial guarantee.

It is possible for a hospital to retain a pharmacy management company to implement full-scope pharmacy services and finance these services without raising its patient prices, solely through gaining control of lost pharmacy charges.[36] Inadequate record keeping and insufficient reconciliation result in lost patient charges of as high as 30 percent. Additionally, patient revenue may be enhanced without increasing patient prices through (1) updating drug costs in a more timely manner, (2) improving consistency in patient pricing, and (3) reducing interdepartmental transfers of medications, i.e., drugs incorrectly charged to nursing units rather than to individual patients.

GOVERNMENT REGULATIONS AFFECTING PHARMACY MANAGEMENT CONTRACTS

All Medicare and Medicaid regulations that affect hospital operations and the provision of patient care may affect directly or indirectly the management of the pharmacy department by a contractor. Also, State and Federal regulations regarding drug distribution and controlled substances are generally recognized as the responsibility of the pharmacy management company. However, the following five regulations are of particular note and are discussed here:

1. Medicare Conditions of Participation
2. Maximum allowable cost (MAC) limits
3. Prudent buyer concept
4. Prohibition against revenue-sharing arrangements
5. Access to books and records of subcontractors

The Medicare Conditions of Participation affect pharmacy contractors and in-house pharmacy services alike. The conditions are those requirements that hospitals must meet in order to participate in the Medicare and Medicaid programs (Titles XVIII and XIV of the Social Security Act). These conditions were first published in 1966, and changes in Medicare Conditions of Participation are made periodically.

The Conditions of Participation are used by Medicare intermediaries to accredit approximately 1,500 of the 6,700 short-term hospitals in the United States. Most of these are small, rural hospitals. The rest of the 6,700 hospitals are accredited by the Joint Commission on Accreditation of Healthcare Organizations (JCAHO), and JCAHO standards supersede the Medicare Conditions of Participation for accreditation purposes. In 1983, the Health Care Financing Administration (HCFA) published proposed rules that granted hospitals greater flexibility in meeting the Medicare standards for accreditation.[37] The proposed changes included relaxation of standards for pharmaceutical services.

Part 19 of the Code of Federal Regulations (C.F.R.) has to do with maximum costs that may be paid for the acquisition of drugs, particularly the Federal "Maximum Allowable Cost" program. Although less important with the advent of the Medicare Prospective Payment System (PPS), which replaced cost-based Medicare reimbursement, the rules still exist and are applicable for PPS-exempt hospitals. The rules specify that the cost of drugs and related medical supplies furnished by providers to Medicare beneficiaries "shall not exceed the amount a prudent and cost-conscious buyer would pay for the same item."[38] This reasonable cost limitation is generally referred to as "the prudent buyer concept." Part of the prudent buyer regulation states that for purchases made on or after the effective date of the final "MAC" determinations, the allowable cost for any multiple-source drug for which a MAC has been established may not exceed the lowest of: (1) the actual cost, (2) the amount that would be paid by a prudent and cost-conscious buyer for the drug if obtained from the lowest priced source that is widely and consistently available within a provider's service area, whether sold by generic or brand name, or (3) the MAC. The only exception to the MAC limitation occurs when a physician certifies that in his or her medical judgment, a specific brand name drug is medically necessary for a particular patient. The patient's name and the particular drug prescribed must be clearly identified and the certification made in the physician's own handwriting. There is also one *exemption* to the MAC regulations for unit dose drug distribution systems, including pharmacy-based medication dispensing records and profile monitoring, when operated by a pharmacy management company.[39] Hospital drug distribution systems overseen and otherwise managed by community pharmacies are not included in this exemption.

Therefore, MAC price limits on prescription drugs today are important primarily for community pharmacies (for Medicaid program reimbursement) and have less application to the hospital industry. The Medicare Prospective Payment System, which reimburses hospitals at a prospective fixed price per DRG (per Medicare discharge), was implemented with each hospital's new cost-reporting period beginning on or after October 1, 1983. The Medicare DRG prices are paid by HCFA without regard to actual costs of the provider institution or actual patient charges. Hence, determination of "reasonable costs" by Medicare intermediaries is no longer necessary, since hospitals now have a strong financial incentive to be "prudent" in purchasing products and services, including drugs and medical supplies, in order to control their costs at a level less than or equal to the DRG prices.[40]

Two other Federal regulations have some relevance to hospital pharmacy departments operated by management companies. Section 109 of the Tax Equity and Fiscal Responsibility Act (TEFRA) passed by Congress in 1982 prohibited payment for services provided to hospitals (or hospital patients) by contractors and paid by hospitals on the basis of "a percentage (or other proportion) of the provider's charges, revenues, or claim for reimbursement."[41] This provision of TEFRA excluded percentage contracts and revenue-sharing arrangements between hospitals and contractors, including pharmacy management companies. However, as a result of language in the statute having to do with exceptions to this prohibition, HCFA encountered difficulty in writing regulations to implement this section of TEFRA. Also, new financial incentives inherent in the Medicare Prospective Pricing System supersede the perceived need for HCFA to police the cost-control behavior of hospitals. Consequently, regulations to implement the prohibition of revenue-sharing arrangements were not written by HCFA, and although the prohibition is technically not enforceable, revenue-sharing agreements between hospitals and contract management companies have virtually disappeared from the marketplace.

Section 952 of Public Law 96-499, the Omnibus Reconciliation Act of 1980, required HCFA to write regulations prohibiting reimbursement for the cost of services provided to hospitals by subcontractors unless the contract included a clause allowing the Secretary of Health and Human Services and the comptroller general "... access to the contract and to the subcontractor's books, documents, and records necessary to verify the costs of the contract."[42] Final regulations published on December 30, 1982, made this requirement retroactive to all contracts entered into or renewed after December 5, 1980. The access clause requirement pertains to all contracted services, including legal services, management and consultant services, etc., wherein the annual cost of the contract is $10,000 or more. The $10,000 threshold amount may be increased to $50,000.[43]

As with other HCFA regulations pertaining to most "reasonable cost" determinations by Medicare intermediaries, the perceived need for monitoring and enforcement of the access to subcontractors' records was transcended by the Medicare Prospective Pricing System.

SUMMARY

Contract pharmacy services fill an important need for professional services and drug and IV distribution systems in many hospitals nationwide. From trained personnel to tried and proven drug and IV distribution systems and competent financial management and clinical pharmacy services, pharmacy management companies provide many hospitals with resources and services that may not be otherwise available. And pharmacy management companies represent a desirable career alternative for pharmacists and pharmacy technicians by providing expanded opportunities for advancement, management experience and training, and geographic mobility and flexibility.

REFERENCES

1. Lutz S: Contract management survey. *Mod Healthcare* (Aug 25): 47-56, 1989.
2. *Hospitals* (Guide Issue) 31 (Aug):399, 412, 1957.
3. Stolar MH: National survey of selected hospital pharmacy practices. *Am J Hosp Pharm* 33:225-230, 1976.
4. American Association of Colleges of Pharmacy: *Pharmacists for the Future*. Ann Arbor, MI, Health Administration Press, 1975, pp 49-59.
5. McCleod DC: The drug use process. In McCleod DC, Miller A (eds): *The Practice of Pharmacy*. Cincinnati, OH, Harvey Whitney Books, 1981, pp 11-15.
6. Tanner DJ: Comprehensive pharmaceutical services in an 85-bed hospital: A one-year evaluation. *Am J Hosp Pharm* 34:486-490, 1977.
7. Byrne AK: Errors in giving medications. *Am J Nurs* 53:829-831, 1975.
8. Schlosberg E: Sixteen safeguards against medication errors. *Hospitals* 32:62, 1958.
9. Safren MS, Chapanis A: A critical incident study of hospital medication errors. *Hospitals* 34:32-34, 1960.
10. Barker KN, McConnell WE: The problems of detecting medication errors in hospitals. *Am J Hosp Pharm* 19:360, 1962.
11. Barker KN, Heller WM: The development of a centralized unit dose dispensing system for UAMC. Part VI: The pilot study—medication errors and drug losses. *Am J Hosp Pharm* 21:609, 1964.
12. Barker KN: The effects of an experimental medication system on medication errors and costs. *Am J Hosp Pharm* 26:388-397, 1969.
13. Parker PF: Unit dose systems reduce error, increase efficiency. *Hospitals* 42:65, 1968.
14. Owyang E, Miller RA, Brodie DC: The pharmacist's new role in institutional patient care. *Am J Hosp Pharm* 25:316, 1969.
15. Best DF Jr: An integrated pharmacist-nurse approach to the unit dose concept. *Am J Hosp Pharm* 25:397-407, 1968.
16. Smith WE, Mackewicz DW: An economic analysis of the PACE pharmacy service. *Am J Hosp Pharm* 27:123-126, 1979.
17. Stewart RB: Adverse drug reactions in hospitalized patients. Pharm Intern 1:77-79, 1980.
18. Steel K, Gertman PM, Crescenvi C, et al: Iatrogenic illness on a general medical service at a university hospital. *N Engl J Med* 304:638-642, 1981.
19. Temin P: *Taking Your Medicine: Drug Regulation in the United States*. Cambridge, MA, Harvard University Press, 1980.
20. Castle M, Wilfert CM, Cate TR, et al: Antibiotic use at Duke University Medical Center. *JAMA* 237:2819-2822, 1977.
21. Scheckler WE, Bennett JV: Antibiotic usage in seven community hospitals. *JAMA* 213:264-267, 1970.
22. Stewart RB, Cluff LE, Philip JR (eds): *Drug Monitoring: A Requirement for Drug Use*. Baltimore, Williams & Wilkins, 1977.
23. Maugh TH II: A new wave of antibiotics builds. *Science* 214:1225-1228, 1981.
24. Fry DE, Harbrecht PJ, Polk HC: Systemic prophylactic antibiotics. *Arch Surg* 116:466-469, 1981.
25. Ingrim NB, Hokanson JA, Guernsey BG, et al: Physician noncompliance with prescription writing requirements. *Am J Hosp Pharm* 40:414-417, 1983.
26. Anon: *Supply and Characteristics of Selected Health Personnel*. DHHS Publication No. (HRA) 81-20. Hyattsville, MD, Health Resources Administration, Division of Health Professions Analysis, Bureau of Health Professions, June 1981.
27. Manasse HR: Pharmacy's manpower: Is our future in peril? *Am J Hosp Pharm* 45:2183-2191, 1988.
28. Stolar MH: National survey of hospital pharmaceutical services—1987. *Am J Hosp Pharm* 45:801-818, 1983.
29. Haas M: Comprehensive pharmacy services in the small hospital. In McCleod DC, Miller WA (eds): *The Practice of Pharmacy*. Cincinnati, OH, Harvey Whitney Books, 1981, pp 440-457.
30. Anon: Report of the Council on Pharmaceutical Affairs of the American Society of Hospital Pharmacists. *Am J Hosp Pharm* 38:1207, 1981.
31. Coe CP: *Preparing the Pharmacy for a Joint Commission Survey*. Bethesda, MD, American Society of Hospital Pharmacists, 1987, pp 61-81.
32. Chase P: Assessment of pharmaceutical services in the small hospital. *Am J Hosp Pharm* 39:864-865, 1982.
33. Marshall G: Clinical program may effect savings. *Hospitals* 48 (Dec):79, 80, 102, 1974.
34. Talley CR: Certification program for clinical services developed by HPI Hospital Pharmacies. *Am J Hosp Pharm* 38:1418-1420, 1981.
35. Fink JL: Liability issues relating to contract pharmaceutical services. *Am J Hosp Pharm* 40:2188-2190, 1983.
36. Anon: Why some hospitals are turning to contract pharmacies. *Am Druggist* 175(2):21-25, 1977.
37. Medicare and Medicaid Programs. Conditions of Participation for Hospitals. 42 C.F.R. Parts 405, 480, 482, 483, 484, 485, 487, 488. Proposed rule. *Fed Reg* 48(2):299-315, 1983.
38. Cost of drugs and related medical supplies. *Provider Reimbursement Manual*, Part I, Section 2119. *Medicare and Medicaid Guide*, Paragraph 5923, vol. 1. Chicago, Commerce Clearing House, pp 1951.6-1952.
39. Methodology for comparing prices: Unit dose. *Provider Reimbursement Manual*, Part I, Section 2119, *Medicare and Medicaid Guide*, Paragraph 5923.61, vol 1. Chicago, Commerce Clearing House, pp 1951.14, 1951.15.
40. Medicare Program: Prospective payment for Medicare inpatient hospital services. Final rule. *Fed Reg* 49(1):233-339, 1984.
41. H.R. 4961, Tax Equity and Fiscal Responsibility Act of 1982, Medicare and Medicaid Spending Reductions, as passed by Congress August 19, 1982. *Medicare and Medicaid Guide*, extra edition No. 361. Chicago, Commerce Clearing House, August 24, 1982.
42. Medicare Program: Access to books, documents, and records of subcontractors. Final rule. *Fed Reg* 47(251):58260-58270, 1982.
43. Regulation Section 420.300-304, Subpart D: Access to books and records of subcontractors. *Medicare and Medicaid Guide*, Paragraph 20,906G. Chicago, Commerce Clearing House, pp 8361.14-8363.

CHAPTER 29

The Literature of Pharmacy

WILLIAM A. ZELLMER

It is early Monday morning, and the pharmacy staff at Community Hospital has just concluded its weekly meeting. There was a lot to discuss this week, which is often the case when the pharmacy prepares for the next monthly session of the pharmacy and therapeutics (P&T) committee. Another big topic today was the need for a renewed hospital initiative on drug use evaluation.

While other staff members hasten to their regular duties, pharmacists Keene and Joffery remain for several minutes to review with the pharmacy director the assignments she has given them. Keene has been asked to prepare a report that will be distributed to the P&T committee in advance of its reconsideration of thrombolytic agents in the formulary. Joffery's challenge is to map out a strategy for building support for ongoing pharmacy-based drug use evaluation.

After 10 minutes of discussion, Keene and Joffery leave the room with clear plans for tackling their assignments. Although each exercise is quite different, both pharmacists start by doing the same thing: checking the literature.

INTRODUCTION

As reflected in the scenario above, the literature of institutional pharmacy is an inherent part of institutional pharmacy practice. It is hard to imagine being an institutional pharmacist without regularly reading and consulting the literature.

The literature of institutional pharmacy is the body of written work produced and used by practitioners, educators, and researchers in this field. That literature includes this handbook, for example, as well as any other printed information that institutional pharmacists use in their practices. The literature could be defined to include unpublished manuscripts and documents. However, such informal publications are beyond the scope of this chapter, which is limited to the literature that is readily accessible by virtue of its formal publication.

Just as *institutional pharmacy* is a component of the broader profession of *pharmacy*, so the *literature of institutional pharmacy* is a component of the *pharmacy literature*. The pharmacy literature, in turn, is a component of the biomedical literature, which is a subcategory of the scientific literature. Some literature used in institutional practice is quite specific to this area of the profession (e.g., an article on inpatient drug distribution). However, a large part of the literature that is applied in institutional practice is the same as that used in other parts of the profession (e.g., a reference book on drug interactions.)

The balance of this chapter discusses the link between the literature and the profession, uses of the literature, categories of literature, periodicals used in institutional pharmacy, use of periodicals for current awareness, computer-based literature retrieval services, books used in institutional pharmacy, contributing to the literature, the journal peer-review process, and controversies related to the literature. This chapter looks at the literature largely from the vantage point of general practitioners and managers in institutional pharmacy. Other perspectives might well produce a substantially different picture. For example, if the interests of the drug information specialist had been the focus, this chapter would have dealt more heavily with sources of clinical information, methods of literature retrieval, and techniques for evaluating published research.

THE LINK BETWEEN THE LITERATURE AND THE PROFESSION

Many pharmacists take the literature of pharmacy for granted and do not appreciate the vital role that it has played, and continues to play, in shaping the profession. The earliest known form of pharmacy literature is a 4,000-year-old pharmacopoeia written on a clay tablet that documents the preparation of pharmaceutical dosage forms in Sumerian civilization.[1] The vast literature on drug therapy that was generated in Arabian culture between the 9th and 13th centuries is believed to have helped form the basis for pharmacy as an independent profession.[1]

A profession, by definition, cannot exist without its own unique, scientifically based literature. As Starr[2] has indicated, professionals derive their authority from three distinctive claims:

1. That a professional's knowledge and competence have been validated by a community of his or her peers
2. That this validated knowledge and competence rest on rational, scientific grounds
3. That the professional's judgment and advice are oriented toward a set of substantive values, such as health

The "rational, scientific grounds" for pharmacy are expressed through its literature. Further, the values of pharmacy—the things that it stands for as a health profession—

are expressed and clarified through its literature. A career commitment to institutional pharmacy practice implies keeping up with the latest knowledge and thinking in the field, i.e., keeping up with the literature.

One of the ways of defining pharmacy is as a "knowledge system":

> [Pharmacy] is a system which generates or integrates knowledge about man in sickness and in health, takes knowledge from other sciences and arts, criticizes and organizes that knowledge, translates knowledge into technology, uses some knowledge to create products, devices, and instruments, transmits the knowledge through the education of practitioners and dissemination to others, to the end that an individual known as a patient may benefit from the particular knowledge system and its consequent skills. The thread which holds research, education and practice together in a rational system is *knowledge*.[3]

The obvious should be added: this knowledge is expressed through the printed word of the pharmacy literature.

USES OF THE LITERATURE

The literature may be used in three general ways: current awareness, research, and education.

Most practitioners review professional journals primarily for current awareness. One of the thrills of pharmacy practice comes from reading an idea that sparks creative thinking about a problem that the reader is experiencing firsthand. Sometimes a pharmacist will first become aware of an important practice problem through an article in the pharmacy literature. Reading about the problems that other practitioners are facing can give institutional pharmacists a greater sense of community and help establish cohesiveness and *esprit de corps* within the discipline. Many pharmacists take pride in being conversant on contemporary pharmacy issues, and they attain their comfort with the issues of the day by reading the literature.

Whenever a practitioner consults the literature to find out what has been said about a particular subject, the research value of the literature comes to the fore. Use of the literature for research purposes may range from the informal to the formal. For example, one may consult a reference book to determine what package sizes a particular product comes in, or one may look up a journal article that relates to a practice problem. At the other extreme, one may do a comprehensive literature search on a well-defined subject area to prepare for a formal research project or to write a pharmacy and therapeutics (P&T) committee monograph on a new medication.

The literature is used extensively in both the education of pharmacy students and in the continuing education of pharmacists. Continuing education may be planned by a continuing education provider (e.g., a college of pharmacy, a professional society, or a pharmaceutical company) or may be self-directed by the practitioner. In either case, the content of the educational program will have a basis in the literature, the formal repository of the knowledge of the discipline. Many professional journals contain review articles and other content that is written especially for continuing education purposes. Often, those articles may be used to earn credit in those states that require continuing education to maintain a practice license.

CATEGORIES OF LITERATURE

The scientific literature is generally divided into two broad categories. The *primary literature* consists of the original reports of research and innovations in the field, written by the researchers and innovators themselves. The *secondary literature*, which is made up of review articles, reference books, and textbooks, reflects experts' syntheses or overviews of subjects based on the primary literature. Abstracting and indexing services are also considered part of the secondary literature.

This categorization is not entirely satisfactory for the literature of institutional pharmacy, especially with respect to news reports about developments in the profession. A news report in a pharmacy magazine such as *Hospital Pharmacist Report* may be the first occasion for certain information to appear in print. However, such reports are hardly "original reports of research and innovations" in the sense of complete and carefully written articles by the individuals who performed research or developed an innovation. Hence, news would not seem to fit the definition of primary literature. Although news writing is often a synthesis based on observations of many events, the ephemeral nature of most news articles hardly permits them to be placed in the category of "secondary literature." Nevertheless, news reports have some of the characteristics of the secondary literature in that they may be useful in leading one to more complete information about a subject (such as by identifying a person who was interviewed for a story). Perhaps the best solution is to create a separate category for news, such as *current affairs literature*.

The literature may also be classified according to the form in which it is produced. In this chapter, only the main forms are discussed, namely, *periodicals*, *computer-based services*, and *books*. Although not an exhaustive list, the following forms might also be considered by some to be a part of the literature of institutional pharmacy: package inserts; pamphlets and booklets; advertising and other promotional materials; and the scripts for films, videotapes, and audiotapes.

A new form of communication in institutional pharmacy is the electronic bulletin board, such as the American Society of Hospital Pharmacists (ASHP) PharmNet service or the FIX bulletin board produced by a company called The Formulary. The messages on these services are basically electronic forms of correspondence; no permanent record is kept of them, and they are not retrievable after they become "old" (typically within several months), at which point they are removed from the electronic bulletin board. A growing number of pharmacists find these electronic networks informative and entertaining, but the information on an electronic bulletin board, because of its short retrievable life, is not considered a part of the literature of institutional pharmacy.

PERIODICALS USED IN INSTITUTIONAL PHARMACY

The types of periodicals in institutional pharmacy include peer-reviewed journals, abstracting and indexing journals, current affairs publications, newsletters, and company-sponsored publications. Many periodicals are not purely of one type. For example, although the *American Journal of Hospital Pharmacy* is primarily a peer-reviewed journal, it also carries news and occasionally publishes supplementary issues that are, to some extent, company-sponsored publications. It is common for a current affairs magazine such as *American Druggist* and *Drug Topics* to publish review articles that may be used for continuing education. Some company-sponsored publications consist largely of abstracts of articles from the primary literature.

Institutional pharmacists use journals from their own discipline as well as from pharmacy at large, the pharmaceutical sciences, medicine, and health care management. The most important periodicals to institutional pharmacists are listed in Appendix 29-A. Most of these periodicals have archival value. (This means that major libraries keep back volumes, and many subscribers find it useful to save issues for at least several years for future reference.) In addition to these periodicals from the United States, a number of English-language foreign journals are reviewed regularly by some institutional pharmacists. The most notable among these journals are also listed in Appendix 29-A.

Listed in Appendix 29-A are well-established periodicals that are supported through subscription revenue or advertising or both and that are available from bona fide publishers. There has been a proliferation of "throwaway" publications in pharmacy—publications that look like regular journals or newsletters but are funded by a single sponsor, are often produced by an advertising agency, and are distributed free to pharmacists. The sponsor supports the publication for marketing purposes and generally will not make a long-term commitment to its existence. Although many of these periodicals contain information that pharmacists find interesting and useful, their quality varies greatly and they are not considered to be of archival value. Even the most comprehensive health sciences library does not maintain collections of throwaway periodicals.

USE OF PERIODICALS FOR CURRENT AWARENESS

Many pharmacists spend a substantial portion of their time in keeping up with the current literature. It would not be unusual for an ambitious institutional pharmacist to scan regularly all of the periodicals listed in Appendix 29-A (and often additional ones as well). Pharmacists who specialize in a particular area of practice may concentrate their attention on the literature in that area. Some pharmacy departments assign pharmacists to monitor specific journals and to bring to the attention of the whole staff articles that are especially relevant to the department's activities. Some departments conduct a journal club that meets regularly, e.g., monthly, to hear oral summaries by staff members of important articles from the current literature. Some medical journals (e.g., *JAMA*) make suggestions for articles to be discussed by journal clubs. One medical journal (*Annals of Internal Medicine*) has begun publishing a sister journal (*ACP Journal Club*) specifically for this purpose.[4]

International Pharmaceutical Abstracts (*IPA*), pharmacy's only abstracting and indexing journal, has special utility for current awareness. Published twice a month, with coverage of more than 750 journals, *IPA* offers abstracts of articles that are of interest to pharmacy practitioners, educators, students, and researchers. (*IPA* also includes abstracts of most presentations made at the ASHP Annual Meeting and Midyear Clinical Meeting.) Abstracts are grouped in 25 subject areas (such as pharmacy practice; legislation, laws, and regulations; adverse drug reactions; drug evaluations; and pharmaceutical education), which facilitates scanning issues for current awareness. A typical issue contains 650 abstracts. Through its controlled index, *IPA* also offers subscribers a tool for searching for papers on a particular subject. As discussed below, the *IPA* data base may also be searched by computer.

COMPUTER-BASED LITERATURE RETRIEVAL SERVICES

There has been rapid growth over the past decade in computerized searching of the literature. Although the technology and methods to perform automated literature searches have been available for 30 years or more, it took the proliferation of microcomputers in the 1980's to make this practical for pharmacists at any practice site.

To understand this subject, it helps first to think of a secondary literature service, such as *International Pharmaceutical Abstracts*, which has been a printed publication since 1964. In 1970, the production of *IPA* became computerized, and its index and abstracts were made accessible to computer searches through intermediary online data base vendors. These vendors maintain the *IPA* index and abstracts on their computers, and a pharmacist may access those computers remotely with the use of his or her own computer terminal that is equipped with a modem. The local computer terminal dials up the central computer, and after the user is connected, he or she goes through a series of commands to see if the *IPA* file contains any information on the subject in question.[5]

There are several major online data base vendors in the United States of interest to pharmacists (see Appendix 29-B), and each of them carries a number of literature data bases that may be useful to practitioners. After users first register with a vendor, they receive complete instructions on how to access specific data bases. Data base producers and data base vendors offer training seminars on online computer literature searching. Users have an incentive to learn to be efficient in their searches, since most vendors base their charges in part on the length of time of the user's connection with a data base.

A relatively recent development has been the addition of selected reference books and textbooks to the offerings of data base vendors. Books that may be searched by this method include *AHFS—Drug Information*, *Handbook on Injectable Drugs*, *Martindale: The Extra Pharmacopoeia*, *Medication Teaching Manual*, and *USP DI*.

Before microcomputers became so ubiquitous, online literature searching initiated by pharmacists was often actually performed by a medical librarian, who provided this service to all of the health professionals at a particular institution. Now many practitioners themselves dial up a literature data base vendor and do quick, on-the-spot searches.

Currently at the forefront of information-retrieval technology is CD-ROM (compact disk, read-only memory). Through the use of laser encoding technology, a disk the size of a standard CD for recorded music will hold all of the information in several large medical reference books. When a CD encoded with such information is inserted into a CD reader, which is connected to a microcomputer, the user can search the data base in much the same way as with an online service. The CD information product entails a one-time purchase rather than a per-use charge as with online services.

Several CD pharmacy information products are already available (e.g., the Poisindex and Drugdex systems; the index to the Iowa Drug Information Service; and *AHFS — Drug Information* combined with the *Handbook on Injectable Drugs* and *IPA* abstracts published since 1970), and more are likely to be available in the future. As this technology matures, the cost of the products may decline, making their use an increasingly attractive option for pharmacy departments.

It is expected that in many hospitals in the future, CD-ROM information services will be accessible with the computer terminals used for processing medication orders throughout the institution. This will be a major step forward in giving pharmacists and other health professionals immediate access to computer-searchable literature data bases.

BOOKS USED IN INSTITUTIONAL PHARMACY

It is beyond the scope of this chapter to discuss thoroughly the books of institutional pharmacy. Hundreds of books are available that might be of some use in practice, and scores of new ones are published every year. Hence, one has to be selective about new acquisitions. A good way to learn about new books is to read the book review sections of periodicals such as the *American Journal of Hospital Pharmacy* and the *American Journal of Pharmaceutical Education.*

There would probably be strong agreement among institutional pharmacists with respect to a short list of books that should be available in every institutional pharmacy department. Many practitioners would want to own personal copies of some of the books on such a list.

Included on the list would probably be a current medical dictionary, such as Stedman's or Dorland's. This handbook, edited by Thomas R. Brown, would be on the list. Also present would be the current editions of *ASHP Practice Standards, AHFS — Drug Information, Facts and Comparisons, Martindale: The Extra Pharmacopoeia, Physician's Desk Reference, Remington's Pharmaceutical Sciences, U.S. Pharmacopeia/National Formulary, USP DI, USAN and the USP Dictionary of Drug Names, American Drug Index*, and a general medical text such as *Harrison's Principles of Internal Medicine*. Further, Anderson and Knoben's *Handbook of Clinical Drug Data* and Trissel's *Handbook on Injectable Drugs* have become standard institutional pharmacy department reference books.

Beyond this short list of basic books, many others will be found in pharmacy departments to aid them with specific needs related to their scope of services.

CONTRIBUTING TO THE LITERATURE*

It is well within the ability of every institutional pharmacist to write for publication in the pharmacy literature. Further, every practitioner has ideas and makes observations and innovations that are likely to have merit for publication.

There are two categories of reasons why pharmacists should want to contribute to the literature. The first stems from altruistic motives related to a desire to share what one has learned for the benefit of others and to help advance the profession of pharmacy. In the second category are more self-serving reasons relating to personal satisfaction, career development, and recognition. Although there can be some negative aspects associated with the latter reasons, such as submitting the least publishable unit (see section entitled "Controversies Related to the Literature"), vigilant journal editors can control most of them.

Notwithstanding these reasons for writing for publication, the vast majority of pharmacists never contribute to the literature. In part this is true because of some common myths about the publication process. One such myth is that *B.S. degree pharmacists* do not stand much chance of getting anything accepted for publication. If the following are substituted for the italicized words in the preceding sentence, one has a list of other common myths about journal publication: (1) staff pharmacists, (2) pharmacists from small hospitals, (3) pharmacists from nonteaching hospitals, (4) pharmacists who do not belong to ASHP, (5) young pharmacists, and (6) old pharmacists.

There is no objective evidence that such biases exist among the peer-reviewed journals in pharmacy. The primary distinction between papers that are accepted for publication and those that are rejected relates to the quality of writing, including the quality of the ideas expressed. There are very few naturally gifted writers in pharmacy; most authors have to work hard to produce clear, concise copy that holds the reader's interest and conveys a message worthy of the reader's time. In fact, the hard work required to produce a published paper is probably the main reason that most pharmacists do not write for publication in a professional journal.

It would not be unreasonable for a young pharmacist to develop a strategy for becoming a published author. This strategy could be an important component of a plan for building a fulfilling career, which in itself might be a component of an even larger plan for living a balanced, satisfying life. We all require creative outlets for personal growth, and publishing in a professional journal can be an avenue for fulfilling this need.

An early step for a pharmacist in a strategy for becoming a published author should be to build confidence in his or her ability to write. This can be done by taking on writing assignments in the pharmacy department (e.g., preparing meeting minutes, developing policies and procedures) and seeking feedback on performance. Pharmacists who lack academic preparation for good writing might consider taking courses part time at a local college. Many reference books are available on writing, which may be obtained readily at a good public library or a full-service bookstore. The following two are worth adding to a personal library: *The Elements of Style*, 3rd ed.[6] and *Why Not Say It Clearly—A Guide to Scientific Writing.*[7]

Two useful books specifically about writing and publishing papers in the professional literature are *How to Write and Publish a Scientific Paper*, 3rd ed.[8] and *How to Write and Publish Papers in the Medical Sciences*, 2nd ed.[9]

Before beginning to write a piece for publication, be sure that you have something important to say. A high proportion

*A portion of this section was published previously by the author as an editorial in *American Journal of Hospital Pharmacy* 48:687, 1991. These comments relate to writing descriptive (not evaluative) reports and other general interest contributions for publication. For advice on writing research reports, see *Am J Hosp Pharm* 38:545-550, 1981. Advice on preparing review articles may be found in *Am J Hosp Pharm* 44:2264, 1987.

of papers rejected for publication are redundant with material already in the literature or deal with subjects that are deemed of insufficient importance to take up space in a journal.

Your first publication does not necessarily have to be a long article. Many journals like to receive short letters or reports on practical solutions to everyday problems in pharmacy. These short communications are easier to write than full articles and are good confidence builders for the fledgling author. Also, keep in mind that college and residency projects often can be adapted for publication.

After selecting a topic to write about, study the journals that might be interested in your work. Peruse the material in recent issues and look for pieces similar to the one you plan to write. This will give you a model for your own writing and help you select the journal to which you want to submit your work. Keep in mind that some journals, for example, *Topics in Hospital Pharmacy Management*, solicit nearly all of their papers. Unless your topic happens to coincide with a theme issue on the drawing board, such journals are unlikely to accept your paper. (To "solicit" a paper means that the journal staff identifies the topic of a prospective manuscript and recruits an author to write it. "Unsolicited" papers are submitted to journals by the authors without any explicit prompting by the publications.) If you are uncertain about whether a particular journal would be interested in reviewing a paper on your subject, write or call the editor to inquire.

After you have selected the journal, study its requirements for manuscripts carefully, looking at both the general instructions to authors and any special advice for the type of paper you will write. It pays to follow a journal's instructions diligently to avoid delays in its review of your work.

Before beginning to write your manuscript, check to learn if similar papers have already been published, especially within the past 5 years. One of the computerized literature retrieval services discussed earlier will aid this checking process. Cite relevant literature in your paper, but take extreme care not to plagiarize any of the articles you have reviewed.

You are now ready to begin writing. Strive to do an excellent job of organizing your thoughts and expressing them succinctly and clearly. Never submit a first draft to a journal. Even highly experienced authors will prepare three or more drafts before sending a paper to the editor. Have others whose writing ability you respect read and critique your paper when you think it is finished. Evaluate their comments with an open mind and do further revision if indicated. It is a good idea to set aside the finished paper for a few days and then give it one final reading with fresh eyes; this more detached scrutiny will often suggest additional polishing you will want to do. When you finally submit the paper to a journal, be sure to keep a copy for your files.

Most journals acknowledge receipt of a manuscript immediately. Several weeks later (the amount of time will depend on the paper's length and complexity), you will receive comments back from the journal's editorial staff. It is not unusual for the editors, based on their own analysis and the advice of outside reviewers, to ask for clarifications and to make suggestions for revision. Keep in mind that the editors' comments are based on their assessment of the needs of the journal's readers.

If the editors encourage you to resubmit your work, by all means do so, and do it promptly. There is a human tendency to avoid dealing with any type of negative feedback, which sometimes leads a novice author to set aside a returned paper and never get back to it. Recognize that tendency and work hard to overcome it. Although it may seem difficult to believe when you face a blunt list of things wrong with your paper, most editors have an honest desire to help you communicate your ideas in the most effective way. It will almost always be in your best interest to cooperate with the editors toward that end.

You may find that most of the editors' comments or suggestions make sense, and you will want to comply with them. Others may seem of be of borderline wisdom, and you must decide whether to follow them or defend your position. Still other criticisms may be clearly ill founded, in which case you should hold your ground and tell the editors why. After you revise your paper, resubmit it with a cover letter that discusses in detail how you have handled all of the questions, comments, and suggestions.

If a journal rejects your paper, you have the option of submitting it to another publication. If you decide to do so, consider first revising it to take into account any criticisms passed on to you by the first editors. If your paper is not explicitly rejected but you wish to submit it elsewhere anyway (because, for example, it will not be possible for you to accommodate the requests for revision), you must first withdraw the paper from the journal to which you have already submitted it. One of the principles of author ethics is that a paper must not be sent to more than one journal at a time. If you do not respond to a journal's request for revision, the journal will still consider your paper a pending manuscript. If that paper later appears in print elsewhere without having been withdrawn from the first journal, your reputation will be sullied among that journal's editors.

The publication of your first paper in the professional literature will be a thrilling experience. Your family, friends, and boss will be impressed, and colleagues will bestow upon you all manner of flattery, both deserved and undeserved. Before the glow of that experience fades, begin planning your next paper.

THE JOURNAL PEER-REVIEW PROCESS

The steps that journals go through to ensure the quality of what they publish is called the "journal peer-review process." It entails seeking the advice of experts with respect to the paper's merit for publication but also includes the review efforts of the editors themselves. The overall goal of the review process is to evaluate the quality of a manuscript in terms of its organizational structure, clarity of expression, and, fundamentally, contribution to the literature. This last factor means the extent to which a paper adds to the body of knowledge in a field. Papers that are judged to make major contributions in this regard are given high priority for publication. The least meritorious papers are rejected. Most papers fall at various points on the scale between these two extremes.

Reviewers are asked to focus on the heart of a paper's content (writing style and organizational structure are scrutinized carefully by the editorial staff). It is not always possible to find reviewers who are fully knowledgeable in all of the key aspects of a paper. If a manuscript reports a study of the clinical pharmacokinetics of theophylline, for example, it might be necessary to select one or two reviewers who are clinical pharmacokinetics experts and another reviewer who is familiar with the nuances of theophylline therapy. Further, if none of these reviewers has expertise in study design and data analysis, another individual may be asked to analyze those aspects of the paper.

Specialized expertise is required to review the methods of data analysis in research reports. That is why many biomedical journals, including the *American Journal of Hospital Pharmacy* and *Clinical Pharmacy*, retain a statistical consultant, who is usually outside the immediate discipline represented by the journal.

Typically, journal editors will select two outside reviewers for a manuscript. Certain straightforward, brief communications (including letters to the editor) may be reviewed only by the journal's staff. Journals maintain lists of reviewers coded by areas of expertise. They also generally maintain a record of experience with each reviewer that covers, for example, promptness and helpfulness of reviews, to aid the staff in deciding which experts to use in the future. Most editors welcome volunteers for the review process. Reviewers contribute their time without remuneration as a service to the profession. Statistical consultants, however, are usually paid.

As an example of the magnitude of the review process for a large journal office, consider the operations of the American Society of Hospital Pharmacists, which publishes the *American Journal of Hospital Pharmacy* (*AJHP*) and *Clinical Pharmacy* (*CP*) with a consolidated staff for both journals. *AJHP* and *CP* together receive about 600 manuscripts per year. About 50 percent of these papers are eventually published in *AJHP* or *CP*, most of them with substantial revision. Some of the papers published by ASHP are solicited, including most review articles for *CP*. The manuscript review process is handled by six pharmacist editors who are full-time employees of ASHP. (These individuals apply their own expertise—in pharmacy practice as well as editing—in the peer review process, as a complement to the advice of outside reviewers.) A reviewer file of more than 1,000 names is maintained.

The entire process of tracking manuscripts and reviewers at ASHP has been automated. This includes maintaining records on reviewers, searching for appropriate reviewers on a specific topic, tracking a manuscript's progress through the review and editing steps, generating routine correspondence to authors and reviewers, and producing routine reports.

Figure 29-1 is a diagram of ASHP's manuscript review process, tracing the milestones between receipt of a paper and its ultimate publication and showing a timeline for the entire cycle. Most peer-reviewed journals will follow procedures similar to this.

In the case of *AJHP* and *CP*, the average lag time between submission of a paper and its publication is 6 months. As figure 29-1 shows, half of this time is consumed by the review and revision process and half is consumed by the steps necessary to put the final manuscript in the pages of a journal.

There is substantial variability among journals in how they handle some of the specific steps in peer review. For example, whereas some pharmacy journals, including *AJHP* and *CP*, mask the reviewers to the identity of the authors, the major medical journals do not, in part because their editors believe that most reviewers would be able to discern the authors' identities or at least their institutional affiliations. Those who mask author identity believe that doing so reduces bias in the review process and is worth the effort for that reason.

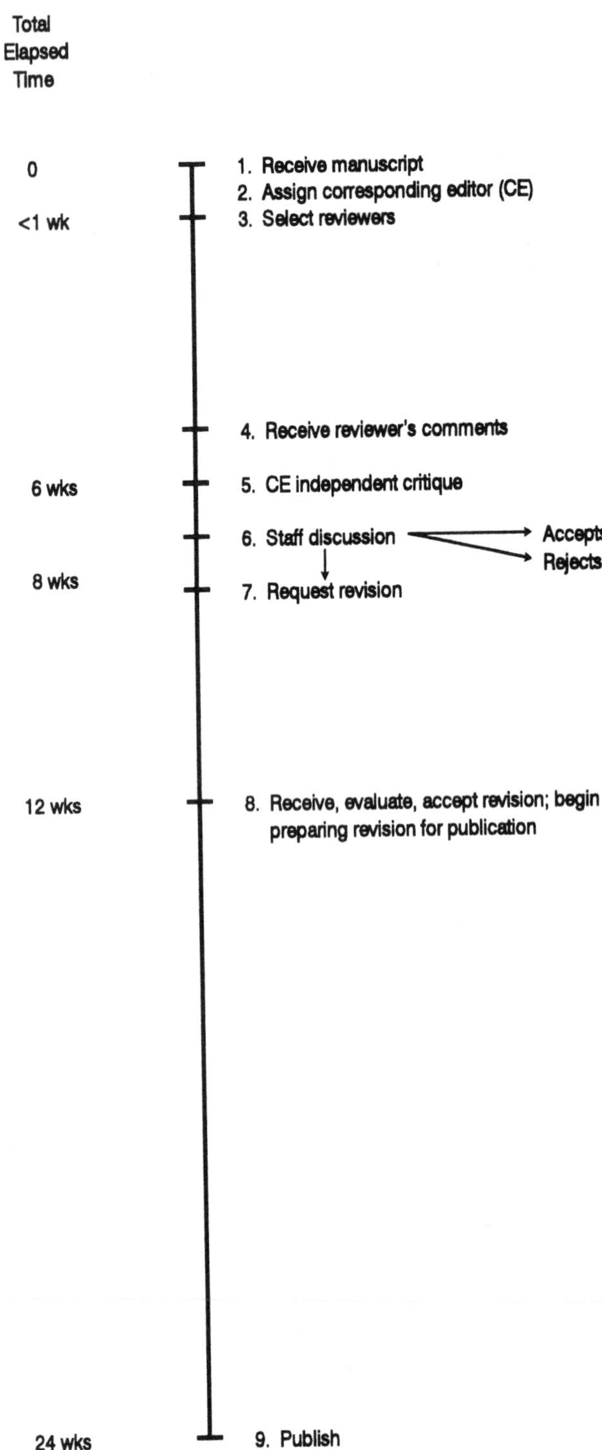

Figure 29-1. ASHP manuscript review process. Diagram of steps in the manuscript review process for journals published by ASHP. On the left is shown typical elapsed time between steps as well as for the total cycle. "Corresponding editor" refers to a pharmacist-editor employed on the staff of ASHP. "Reviewers" are outside experts who are called upon to analyze papers and advise on their merit for publication. At step 6, the entire staff of pharmacists-editors meets to arrive at a consensus on how papers that have gone through the review process should be handled. At step 8, a paper may be rejected if the revision is highly unsatisfactory. Between steps 8 and 9, the author is sent a galley proof for checking, which is the author's opportunity to review and approve editorial changes that have been made.

Most journals mask authors to the identity of the reviewers. However, it is not uncommon for reviewers to ask that their identities be revealed in case the author wishes to contact them for a clarification of their critiques.

Some journals, including *AJHP* and *CP*, exchange critiques among reviewers. By showing each reviewer what the other has said, individual reviewers have a basis for assessing the quality of their work, and they may learn about additional points to cover in future critiques.

Most editors consider the comments of reviewers advisory, not binding. The editors may well pursue a revision of a paper even though all of the outside reviewers are recommending rejection. Conversely, based on their perspective, the editors may reject a paper in the face of unanimous advice to accept. Factors that editors weigh in these decisions, which may not necessarily be points that reviewers considered, include the recent acceptance of other similar papers, the backlog of papers awaiting publication, and an assessment of author or reviewer bias or motive that is inconsistent with the objectives of journal publication. It is not unusual for the editors to be more familiar than outside reviewers with the literature in a particular area and for this to weigh heavily in the final decision. Further, if a paper has extraordinary problems in structure and writing style, the editors may decide that they cannot afford to devote the resources necessary for making it acceptable for publication, even though there may be some germ of merit buried within its pages.

Although it is widely believed that the journal peer-review process improves the quality of the literature, it is not a guarantee of infallibility. Arnold Relman, a former editor of *The New England Journal of Medicine*, has made this point well:[10]

> Papers that pass the peer-review process must not be assumed to have received editorial endorsement or some sort of scientific seal of approval. Publication of a manuscript in the most selective and carefully edited of journals does not guarantee its validity or durability. Reviewers and editors, however capable and conscientious, make mistakes and may overlook serious flaws. Furthermore, new evidence may soon invalidate or modify even a flawless study. All that a good peer-reviewed journal can do is make reasonable efforts to winnow out unsound work and repair correctable defects. But readers of the literature should understand that scientific journals are records of work, not of revealed truth. The better the journal, the better—and the more worthy of reading—the published work is likely to be.

CONTROVERSIES RELATED TO THE LITERATURE

Those who read and contribute to the literature should be aware of the major controversies associated with journal publishing. The debate on these issues has been going on for quite some time and is not likely to be resolved soon.

Perhaps the biggest concern about the literature relates to its proliferation. One analyst of the situation has made the following observation:[11]

> For more than 300 years, the pace of growth in quantity of all learned literature has been maintained at a compound interest, with an exponential increase of about 6 to 7 percent each year, a doubling in size every 10 to 15 years, and a tenfold increase in every generation of 35 to 50 years. It is spectacular and unprecedented that year after year such a growth can be steadily maintained. The sustained growth is no sudden explosion or any sort of crisis, but each and every generation has seen its libraries grow by a mighty factor.

Institutional pharmacy has had its own literature explosion, although it probably has not been at the same rate as the expansion of the literature throughout civilization as a whole.

The development of computerized literature searching services has been in direct response to the expansion of the primary literature and the overwhelming difficulty that individuals have in keeping up with all of the information published in their fields. The problem is compounded by the publication of information relevant to a particular discipline in the journals of other specialized fields.

This growth in the literature is related largely to genuine expansion of knowledge and the need to disseminate that knowledge. However, there are also abuses of the publishing enterprise that contribute to the growth of the literature. Because of the limited resources available for publishing, steps are being taken to curb those abuses.

The most prominent abuse stems from pressure on individuals, particularly those in academia, to publish more in order to advance their careers—the "publish or perish" phenomenon. Sometimes researchers will divide a project into several small aspects and attempt to publish a paper on each facet. Or they may take the ethically repugnant course of publishing the same work in more than one journal. The practice of writing up the least publishable unit has been referred to disparagingly as "salami slicing." Sometimes individuals may be listed as coauthors, even though they had virtually nothing to do with writing the paper, solely because of the power they hold over the primary author.

Some academic institutions have made an important reform in their promotion and tenure systems in an effort to counter the pressure to publish many papers. Rather than weigh the number of publications of someone up for promotion, those institutions evaluate the quality of just a few publications selected by the candidate.

The journal peer-review process has been criticized on many fronts.[12] The objects of this criticism include the biases of reviewers, failure of the system to keep marginal papers from being published, and failure to detect errors and improprieties that wind up in print. There is a concerted effort underway by editors of biomedical journals to better understand issues such as these through educational conferences and research.

The research literature, including that of institutional pharmacy, has been criticized often for use of faulty statistical methods. As stated earlier, some journals have instituted expert statistical review of manuscripts to deal with this problem. A fundamental resolution of this issue would come from an upgrading of the statistical knowledge of researchers.

CONCLUSION

The strength and vibrancy of institutional pharmacy is explained by many factors, not the least of which is the literature of institutional pharmacy. This sector of the profession has been guided by a distinct literature separate from that of the rest of pharmacy for 40 years or more. This has helped create a strong identity for institutional pharmacy and has been an instrument for leadership and development of the discipline.

Use of the literature is a primary skill for practitioners of institutional pharmacy. In addition, many practitioners will want to plan to contribute to the literature as an aspect of their career development and self fulfillment.

REFERENCES

1. Sonnedecker G: *Kremers and Urdang's History of Pharmacy*, 4th ed. Philadelphia, Lippincott, 1976, pp 3-36.
2. Starr P: *The Social Transformation of American Medicine*. New York, Basic Books, 1982, p 15.
3. *Pharmacists for the Future: The report of the study Commission on Pharmacy*. Ann Arbor, MI, Health Administration Press, 1975, p 13.
4. Anon: ACP Journal Club. *Ann Intern Med* 114:165, 1991.
5. Tousignaut DR: Online literature-retrieval systems: How to get started. *Am J Hosp Pharm* 40:230-239, 1983.
6. Strunk W Jr, White EB: *The Elements of Style*, 3rd ed. New York, Macmillan, 1979.
7. King LS: *Why Not Say It Clearly—A Guide to Scientific Writing*. Boston, Little, Brown, & Co., 1978.
8. Day RA: *How to Write and Publish a Scientific Paper*, 3rd ed. Philadelphia, ISI Press, 1990.
9. Huth EJ: *How to Write and Publish Papers in the Medical Sciences*, 2nd ed. Baltimore, MD, Williams & Wilkins, 1990.
10. Relman AS: Journals. In Warren KS (ed): *Coping with the Biomedical Literature—a Primer for the Scientist and the Clinician*. New York, Praeger, 1981, pp 67-78.
11. Price DD: The development and structure of the biomedical literature. In Warren KS (ed): *Coping with the Biomedical Literature—a Primer for the Scientist and the Clinician*. New York, Praeger, 1981, pp 3-16.
12. Lock S: *A Difficult Balance—Editorial Peer Review in Medicine*. Philadelphia, ISI Press, 1986.

ACKNOWLEDGMENT

Appreciation is expressed to the following individuals for their assistance in developing this chapter: C. Richard Talley, Catherine Nichols Klein, Jane L. Miller, Guy R. Hasegawa, Cheryl A. Thompson, Dwight R. Tousignaut, and Michaelene W. Morgan.

Appendix 29-A

PERIODICALS IMPORTANT TO INSTITUTIONAL PHARMACISTS

The publisher's name and address are given below each journal's name. Each publication's emphasis, from the perspective of practicing pharmacists, is categorized according to this schema:

A—frontline pharmacy practice
B—pharmacy practice management
C—professional issues
D—pharmaceutical sciences
E—pharmaceutical education
F—drug therapy
G—current affairs
H—abstracting-indexing service

Institutional Pharmacy Journals

American Journal of Hospital Pharmacy (A,B,C,D,G)
American Society of Hospital Pharmacists
4630 Montgomery Avenue
Bethesda, MD 20814

Clinical Pharmacy (F)
American Society of Hospital Pharmacists
4630 Montgomery Avenue
Bethesda, MD 20814

DICP Annals of Pharmacotherapy (A,C,F)
Harvey Whitney Books Company
P.O. Box 42696
Cincinnati, OH 45242

Hospital Formulary (B,F)
Modern Medicine Publications, Inc.
7500 Old Oak Boulevard
Cleveland, OH 44130

Hospital Pharmacy (A,B,C,F)
J.B. Lippincott Company
1143 Wright Drive
Huntingdon Valley, PA 19006

International Pharmaceutical Abstracts (H)
American Society of Hospital Pharmacists
4630 Montgomery Avenue
Bethesda, MD 20814

Journal of Pharmacy Practice (A,B,C,F)
W.B. Saunders, The Curtis Center
Independence Square West
Philadelphia, PA 19106-3399

Pharmacotherapy (F)
Pharmacotherapy Publications, Inc.
11 Nassau Street
Boston, MA 02111

The Consultant Pharmacist (A,B,C)
American Society of Consultant Pharmacists
2300 Ninth Street, South, Suite 515
Arlington, VA 22204

Topics in Hospital Pharmacy Management (B)
Aspen Publishers, Inc.
7201 McKinney Circle
Frederick, MD 21701

U.S. Pharmacist (Hospital Edition) (A,F)
Jobson Publishing Corporation
352 Park Avenue South
New York, NY 10010

General Pharmacy Periodicals

American Pharmacy (A,B,C,G)
American Pharmaceutical Association
2215 Constitution Avenue, N.W.
Washington, DC 20037

Pharmacy Times (A,B,C)
Romaine Pierson Publishers, Inc.
80 Shore Road
Port Washington, NY 11050

Pharmaceutical Sciences Journals

Journal of Pharmaceutical Sciences (D)
American Pharmaceutical Association
2215 Constitution Avenue, N.W.
Washington, DC 20037

Pharmaceutical Research (D)
Plenum Publishing Corporation
233 Spring Street
New York, NY 10013

Pharmaceutical Education Journals

American Journal of Pharmaceutical Education (E)
American Association of Colleges of Pharmacy
1426 Prince Street
Alexandria, VA 22314-2841

Journal of Pharmacy Teaching (E)
The Haworth Press, Inc.
10 Alice Street
Binghamton, NY 13904-1580

Current Affairs Periodicals

American Druggist (G)
The Hearst Corporation
959 Eighth Avenue
New York, NY 10019

ASHP Newsletter (G)
American Society of Hospital Pharmacists
4630 Montgomery Avenue
Bethesda, MD 20814

Drug Topics (G)
Medical Economics Publishing Company
680 Kinderkamack Road
Oradell, NJ 07649

F-D-C Reports (The Pink Sheet) (G)
F-D-C Reports
5550 Friendship Boulevard, Suite 1
Chevy Chase, MD 20815

Hospital Pharmacist Report (G)
Medical Economics Company
680 Kinderkamack Road
Oradell, NJ 07649

Weekly Pharmacy Reports (The Green Sheet) (G)
F-D-C Reports
5550 Friendship Boulevard, Suite 1
Chevy Chase, MD 20815

Medical Periodicals

Annals of Internal Medicine (F)
American College of Physicians
Independence Mall West, Sixth Street at Race
Philadelphia, PA 19106-1572

Journal of the American Medical Association (JAMA) (F)
American Medical Association
515 N. Dearborn Street
Chicago, IL 60610

The Medical Letter on Drugs and Therapeutics (F)
The Medical Letter, Inc.
56 Harrison Street
New Rochelle, NY 10801-6588

New England Journal of Medicine (F)
Massachusetts Medical Society
10 Shattuck Street
Boston, MA 02115-6094

Health Care Management Periodicals

Hospitals (B,G)
American Hospital Publishing, Inc.
211 East Chicago Avenue
Chicago, IL 60611

Modern Healthcare (B,G)
Crain Communications, Inc.
740 Rush Street
Chicago, IL 60611

English-Language Foreign Journals

Canadian Journal of Hospital Pharmacy
Canadian Society of Hospital Pharmacists
123 Edward Street, Suite 603
Toronto, Ontario, M5G 1E2
Canada

The Australian Journal of Hospital Pharmacy
Society of Hospital Pharmacists of Australia
P.O. Box 72
Abbostford, Victoria, 3067
Australia

The Pharmaceutical Journal
Royal Pharmaceutical Society of Great Britain
1 Lambeth High Street
London, SE1 7JN
England

Drugs
ADIS Press Limited
41 Centorian Drive, Private Bag
Mairangi Bay, Auckland 10
New Zealand

The Lancet
Williams & Wilkins
428 E. Preston Street
Baltimore, MD 21202-3993

Appendix 29-B

MAJOR ONLINE VENDORS OF LITERATURE-RETRIEVAL SYSTEMS IN THE UNITED STATES

BRS Information Technologies
8000 Westpark Drive
McLean, VA 22102
(800) 289-4277
(703) 442-0900

Data-Star
485 Devon Park Drive, Suite 110
Wayne, PA 19087
(800) 221-7754
FAX (215) 687-0984

DIALOG Information Services, Inc.
3460 Hillview Avenue
Palo Alto, CA 94304
(415) 858-2700
Telex 334499 (DIALOG)

MEDLARS Management Section
National Library of Medicine
8600 Rockville Pike
Bethesda, MD 20894
(301) 496-6193

CHAPTER 30

Literature Evaluation

HAZEL H. SEABA

Clinical studies, surveys, and reviews are the primary resources used by pharmacists to provide information for rational drug prescribing and effective drug use. Once the primary literature for any topic is identified and retrieved, the next step, evaluation, is often approached with hesitancy. Whatever the source of this hesitancy and whatever the strengths of one's educational background, evaluation can be accomplished with skill by all pharmacists. Literature evaluation is approaching published studies, surveys, and reviews with the goal of understanding what the research or review accomplished and concluding how this knowledge relates to current therapeutics.

Published studies and reviews should bring the reader logically through the rationale for the study or review, the protocol (plan) under which the research or review was executed, the results of the study or review and the significance of those results. The reader must give attention to each part of the study or review, and final assessment is based on his or her judgment of the reasonableness of each part.

BASIC ELEMENTS OF CLINICAL STUDIES

Objective and Purpose

Investigators begin research with an objective to be achieved or a question to be answered. The research objective may involve describing a situation of interest, e.g., describing the clinical course of a disease process or characterizing the attitude of a group of individuals. Alternatively, the investigator's purpose may concern analytical research. Analytical research investigates cause-effect relationships.[1] Regardless of the purpose of the research, the investigator's objective needs to be clearly stated. If a research report does not state the objective in the introduction or purpose section, the reader may find it embedded in the summary or the conclusion.

If a cause-effect relationship is to be investigated, the researcher should clearly state the problem to be addressed in the investigation. Following statement of the problem, the specific question or questions to be answered are identified. Clearly stating the question is an important step that sets the clinical stage for decisive answers.[2] The reader's overall responsibility in literature evaluation is to determine how well the author realized the objective or answered the question.

The diagnostic and prognostic parameters of the population to whom the research is targeted are specified in the objective; thus, the reader is provided with a statement of who should be represented in the study. The objective for analytical research further describes the treatment, therapy, or procedure to be applied to that part of the population participating in the research. The indicators that the investigator uses to observe and measure the treatment outcome are identified and correlated with the population's original characteristics. Last, the outcome which the investigator hopes to achieve is stated.

In the objective, the investigator hypothesizes the relationship between the treatment and the outcome. He or she then tests the relationship and (it is hoped) discovers the true influence of the treatment (cause) on the subject's outcome (effect). To quantitate the relationship and provide a means for analyzing the outcome, a statistical hypothesis is used. Clinical investigators frequently express the statistical hypothesis in the form of a null hypothesis. The null hypothesis states there is no value, worth, or difference between the tested situations. The investigator, through experimental and mathematical methods, generates data that will allow him or her either to concede or reject the null hypothesis.

Population and Sample

Simply stated, the population is the group of patients or items to which the investigator wishes to apply the research results. The entire population can rarely, if ever, be studied. Thus, the investigator has to choose a limited number of individuals from the entire population to study, i.e., a sample. If the research results are to be applied to the population, the sample must be a reliable substitute for the larger population. Investigators, then, are confronted with some risk of making a sampling error, the difference between how the entire population responds and how the sample responds. The population must be clearly defined, and the sample must adequately represent the entire population. The reader thereby knows the targeted population by the characteristics that describe the sample.

With the targeted population in mind, the sample is selected; however, not all selection factors are completely under the investigator's control. In clinical research, selection control can be particularly difficult to achieve. Individuals have diverse reasons for seeking medical care, choosing a specific doctor or hospital, and consenting to participate in a research study. If the investigation depends on referrals from other doctors or hospitals, many factors determine who is referred. Surveys may depend on medical records for their population sample. Retrieval factors, such as completeness of the medical record data base, access to the data base, and completeness of the information in the record determine the representativeness of a medical record sample. These subject selection factors are potential sources of selection bias.

To control bias (prejudice that causes the sample to be different from the defined population), the sample must be selected by diagnostic inclusion criteria that are appropriate for the condition or disease. When the study involves prevention or prophylaxis, each member of the sample must be susceptible to and be exposed to whatever situation the researcher wanted to prevent. Subject characteristics such as sex, age, weight, economic and geographic status, coexisting diseases, use of other treatments or drugs, and the severity, extent, and duration of the disease may influence the patient's response to the investigative treatment. As potential prognostics, these characteristics must be considered at the time the target population is identified and the sample eligibility established. The sample is most likely to truly represent the population if it is randomly chosen, i.e., if all members or items of the population have some chance of being chosen.

The investigator may not have access to the entire population and, therefore, cannot choose a random sample. If the investigator does not choose a probability (nonzero chance of being selected) sample, bias may enter the study. A "chunk" sample describes a nonrandom sample convenient for the investigator's research. The "chunk" sample individuals are members of the population who are available for research, but may not represent the population. A "volunteer" sample (self-selecting) also is a convenient group to study but may not indicate how the nonselecting group would respond to the same investigation. The reader, through pharmaceutical and medical judgment, must determine how closely the sample will predict the response of the targeted population.

The number of individuals or items selected for the sample is determined by several factors, including the amount of risk the investigator is willing to take that whatever is measured could occur by chance; the magnitude of the difference between treatments or situations to be measured (the smaller the difference, the larger the sample size must be); and the amount of assurance that the investigator wants that the research will show valid, statistically significant results. The appropriate sample size can be fixed at the start of the study or can be determined at some point during the research when the investigator has enough data to reach a reasonable conclusion (sequential design).

Design, Sample Allocation, and Control

Clinical studies may be described as being prospective (start and look forward) or retrospective (start and look backward). These adjectives apply to two separate aspects of clinical investigation. First, how the subject data are collected may be prospective or retrospective. If the investigator designs the procedure by which the data are recorded and controls its collection, the study data are prospective. If the investigator collects the data from records that were compiled independently prior to the study, the study data collection is retrospective. Second, the group to be studied may be observed either prospectively or retrospectively in time. In a prospective study the subjects are chosen, the treatment is applied, and the observable events are then followed, such as cure or incidence of side effects. In a retrospective design, the subjects exhibiting the effect, cure, or side effect are chosen and the investigator then determines which subjects had the disease or used the treatment. The first observes cause-to-effect and the last observes effect-to-cause. Patients who are followed prospectively have been called "cohorts" and those who are followed retrospectively have been called "cases" or "trohocs."

The retrospective trohoc study design (case control study) is more vulnerable to reliability and validity threats than prospective cause-to-effect studies. The reader's judgment of the retrospective case control study should be based on the study's ability to show convincingly whether or not the cause (disease, drug, etc.) has been used by the subjects and whether or not the subjects are a representative sample of the total population. The control group (discussed below) should be selected with specified inclusion criteria.[3,4]

Control is basic to scientific research, and several different concepts of control have been developed. Feinstein[5] has outlined three: regulation, the control period, and comparison. Regulation control distinguishes a clinical trial or experiment from a survey, cohort study, and case control study. In a survey or cohort study, the investigator does not decide what treatment the subjects will undergo, whereas in an experiment, the investigator does decide. Thus, in the clinical trial, the investigator controls allocation of the sample members to the study treatments. In the survey or cohort study and the case control study, sample members either have been allocated to the treatment groups before the study begins or are allocated to the treatment groups by someone other than the investigator. Quality control, as applied to the production of pharmaceuticals, is a regulatory control. Controlling the environment of the research study is also regulatory control; not losing patients for followup and maintaining patient compliance are environmental controls. Second, the control period describes the qualification period during which subjects are tested or interviewed for their ability to meet the criteria of the study. The stabilization period, which may be used to record baseline test values, is a control period. A "washout control period" occurs between treatment periods in a crossover design study. The washout period provides time for study subjects to return to their pretreatment status before entering the second treatment period. The investigator should explain to the reader the length of the washout period and the choice of using or not using a placebo during this period. The third concept, control as a comparison, is necessary for the investigator to conclude that the treatment, prophylaxis, or procedure was responsible for the observed effect. Comparison controls available to the researcher are discussed below.

1. *No treatment.* The treated group is compared to a group that is the same in every respect except that it receives no treatment. This study design demands that there be no measurable placebo effect associated with the treatment.
2. *Patient as own control.* Patients serve as their own controls when they are observed for a time and then the experimental treatment or procedure is applied. The pretreatment state is then compared to the treated

state of the patient. Unless the treated or posttreated state is a high-order pharmaceutical or medical breakthrough, the study results are suspect. Subjects used as their own controls cannot substitute for a true control.

3. *Intrasubject control.* In some clinical studies, it is possible to compare treatments or compare treatment to placebo in the same patient. Comparing different treatments in corresponding areas of the body (finger joints, eyes, ears, etc.) may be possible if the areas are equally diseased and the treatment affects only the local area.
4. *Placebo.* The comparison group receives a "treatment" identical in all respects to the real treatment except that it is inactive. A treatment placebo must resemble the active dosage form in all characteristics that the subject can discern, such as taste, color, odor, and appearance. The placebo, inactive pharmacologically, elicits psychological and physiological responses.
5. *Active treatment.* Active treatment controls are used when it is impossible or unethical not to treat a group of subjects. Comparative efficacy information for a new drug is obtained by using an older standard drug as an active control.
6. *Case control or matched control.* In retrospective studies, in which patients who already exhibit some effect are followed in search of a cause, the subjects are matched with a control who does not exhibit the effect. The investigator seeks a control for each subject who is comparable both demographically and clinically. The goal is to establish comparable susceptibility to the effect in the subjects and controls. The controls are often chosen to match subject demographic variables such as age, sex, socioeconomic class, and race. Clinical variables, such as family history, medication history, health status, hospitalization, or ambulatory status, should be considered for matching.[6]

   Matching may also be used to select controls for surveys or cohort studies. To improve the comparability among the study's treatment groups, the investigator may seek a matched control for each member of the intervention group. Again, both demographic and clinical characteristics are considered for matching. Generally fewer than four variables are matched.
7. *Historical control.* The historical control is data generated at a previous time. Historical controls have been employed in studies of diseases or conditions that are predictable in their natural history, signs, symptoms, and mortality rate. The ability of the historical control to describe the current group in all respects except treatment is often open to doubt. The major concerns are changes wrought by time and the reliability of the original recorded data. Time influences the population susceptible to and exposed to diseases and the diagnostic and health care available. Medical records suffer changes in disease classification schemes and completeness of patient prognostic data. Despite the problems inherent with the historical control, under circumstances in which the disease condition is rare or there is pressure to quickly obtain comparative efficacy information for a promising new treatment, it may be used.[7,8] When compared with the results of randomized controlled clinical trials, the historical control trial appears to have some bias in the direction favoring the experimental treatment over the control treatment.[9,10]
8. *Crossover design control.* Crossover exists when one group of subjects receives sequential treatments and another group receives the same treatments in the opposite order. All subjects receive both the experimental treatment and the control treatment in sequence. If there is not an adequate washout period between the treatments, the patients will not return to baseline status, and bias may influence the study's outcome as a result of carryover effects. The time between treatments has to be short enough not to allow a change in the natural course of the disease or subject parameter being measured but long enough to allow the pharmacological, physiological, and psychological effects of each treatment to disappear.

   As crossover designs compare the outcome of each treatment on each subject, the precision of the outcome measurements is greater than that obtained from a parallel group study. This crossover design feature is particularly advantageous for comparative bioavailability studies of healthy subjects. Use of the crossover design to assess drug efficacy in diseased subjects, however, requires justification. This is done by showing that the subjects return to baseline status before each treatment period, and there was no carryover effect from one treatment period to the next.[11]
9. *Strata control.* Qualitative comparability of the study groups may be improved with strata control. Before the subjects are assigned to groups, they are stratified for subject variables that are capable of influencing the results of the investigation. The individuals in each stratum are assigned to the treatment groups. Each treatment group is thus ensured an adequate representation from each stratum. Age, sex, weight, and severity of disease may be stratified when they are known to affect the outcome of a disease process (prognostic stratification).

The reader may wonder how to judge the appropriateness of the investigator's choice of a control. The logic employed to determine which control is appropriate is based, according to Feinstein,[12] on four factors: potency, relativity, multiplicity, and concurrence of the treatment and the control.

For drug studies the choice of the drug's dosage and administration rate is a *potency* decision. The dosage regimen should be reasonable to test the relationships stated in the study's objective. If the investigation involves a comparison, the three other factors are also of concern.

Relativity of the investigation considers to what control the treatment should be compared. An efficacy study requires a placebo or no-treatment control, whereas an efficiency study requires that the treatment be compared to an established or standard treatment. Constituents, those ingredients that are administered with the active treatment, are also of concern in a comparison study. For pharmaceuticals, the constituents are the "inactive" ingredients that are present in the dosage form. For drug comparisons, the constituents should be the same for each treatment group. The environment in which the treatments or procedures are delivered should be the same for all groups. "Environment" describes the care and attention the groups receive from the investigators.

Multiplicity considers the number of treatments to be compared and also influences the choice of a control. For example, a study comparing an oral drug preparation to an intramuscular drug preparation may require a control (placebo) for both the oral and the intramuscular preparation. A combination investigational treatment consisting of two active drugs may require an active control for each drug.

Concurrence, or whether or not the study subjects received their individual treatments at the same time, affects the comparability of the treatment groups. Crossover studies, studies in which treatments are employed in stages, and studies in which treatments are separated by long time periods may not be able to ensure treatment group comparability. These studies require justification that one treatment does not affect the success of the next and that the disease state of the subjects has not changed with time.

After choice of control, the next concern is the method by which treatments or procedures are assigned to members of the study sample. In patient-as-own-control studies, case control studies, cohort or survey studies, and historical control studies, the assignment has been made by someone other than the investigator. Other study designs provide the investigator with more opportunities for ensuring the comparability of the treatment groups and thus improving the study's validity. Randomized allocation to the treatment and control groups provides the investigator with several advantages.[13] "Randomized allocation" means that each subject in the study has a nonzero and independent chance of receiving the study treatments. Randomized assignment of sample subjects to various treatment groups provides the best assurance that no treatment group is biased with subjects having particular characteristics. The treatment groups are also more likely to be balanced for subjects with various prognoses. Some of the prognostic indicators may be known and some may not. Last, randomization of subjects to the groups ensures the validity of employing statistically significant tests to compare the treatment results. The randomized clinical study is useful to determine the efficacy of a treatment or the relative efficiency of more than one therapeutic treatment. However, some therapeutic questions cannot use this powerful design. Studies concerning the treatment of rare disease states do not lend themselves to randomization, as there are too few individuals available for research. Also, ethical considerations preclude randomized clinical trials to determine adverse events such as teratogenicity or carcinogenicity.

Adaptive allocation methods may also be used to determine which treatment a subject receives.[14,15] In contrast to fixed randomized allocation, adaptive allocation procedures change the subject's probability of being assigned to the treatment groups as the study progresses. In an adaptive design study, the treatment that a newly recruited subject receives is dependent upon the subjects already in the study. Assignment of the subject's treatment is determined either by the balance of subjects already in treatment groups (baseline adaptive allocation) or by the response of individuals who entered the study first (response adaptive allocation). The response adaptive allocation design assumes that all subjects who enter the study have the same characteristic responses to the treatments. This design hopes to give the largest number of subjects the best treatment. Since the responses of previous subjects must be known before the next subject can be allocated, the design suffers when the subjects' responses do not occur within a short time. Also, the design demands that only one response be measured to determine how successful the treatments are before the next subject is admitted.

The investigator has to be concerned not only with the initial comparability of the treatment groups but also with the comparability of the treatment groups throughout the study. To this end, the investigator has to ensure that all the participants will remain available for observation or examination at the times specified in the protocol and for the necessary duration of time. Subjects in the comparative groups should be examined or observed with equal regularity and duration, so that all events have the same opportunity for detection. Both the sample subjects and the investigator or observer should adhere to the study regimen of treatment, observation, examination, and data collection.

Data Collection

Before collecting any data, the investigator must clearly define what is to be measured or observed. These definitions are necessary so that problems associated with choosing, observing, and classifying the study events are controlled.[16] This control allows the study data to be assessed and validated and the results reproduced.

The quantity that is actually measured or observed is called a "variable." As its name implies, the value of a variable can vary. Several different scales are available to assign measurement values to a variable. "Metric" or "interval variables" are ranks with equal intervals between the ranks, e.g., 1, 2, 3. "Ordinal variables" are graded ranks with an unequal interval between the ranks, e.g., mild, moderate, severe. "Nominal variables" are not graded or ranked, e.g., eye color, hair color. "Existential variables" describe the presence or absence of an item or are expressed as yes or no.

The evidence or data collected may be termed "hard" or "soft." "Hard" data describe measurements or observations that can be made with little subjective judgment. "Soft" data require subjective judgment and interpretation. Because of their objectivity, it is easier to establish the reliability of hard data. Although the hard data measurements may be preferred because they can be evaluated with greater confidence, the importance of soft data measurements such as pain relief or quality of life is not diminished.

The most important evidence or data collected by the investigator is an index to the research and is called the "index variable(s)." Index variables may be used to determine sample eligibility. The study's results are an analysis of the index variables. An index variable may be expressed numerically (metric) or further categorized to an expression with clinical meaning, e.g., ordinal variables such as abnormally high, normal, or too low. The investigator should inform the reader if a measurement reflects a single observation or if multiple observations were averaged or summed. The conclusion of the study may be based on the outcome of a single index variable, or index variables may be combined to express a more complex total situation. The combination of index variables may consider each variable equal and combine the variables with Boolean logic (and, or, not). Alternately, the variables may be weighted and the combination index is a sum of individual weighted variables.

Combining variables requires sound clinical judgment and logic. The reader has to determine the physiological and clinical relevance of the variables. Because hard data are more easily defended and considered more reliable, the investigator may choose index variables that, although reliable, may not directly reflect the objective of the study. The index variables should be suitable for the objectives of the study and measure what the investigator wanted to measure.

How data are collected also influences the reliability of the results. The investigator is obligated to show that the methods of observation or measurement are standard throughout the study and reproducible. Bias can be generated by both the individual responsible for measurement and by study subjects. The best attempts to be objective can become unknowingly biased if either the subject or the observer knows which treatment the subject is receiving. A double-blind study, in which both the subject and the observer do not know which treatment the subject is receiving, eliminates this bias. If possible, separate individuals should administer the treatments and execute the measurements or observations. If only the subject is blinded, the study is single-blind.

After the study is underway and data are being collected, events do not always happen as planned. If the subject has to administer a treatment or make an observation, the possibility of noncompliance exists. Whether or not missed doses and lost observations are included in the raw data is a matter requiring the investigator's judgment. The treatment or procedure may cause unexpected adverse effects in individual subjects. Subjects with disease conditions may experience serious decline in their health. In these two instances, ethical considerations prevent further participation, and the subjects may be withdrawn from the study. Particularly in studies of long duration, subjects may drop out on their own accord and be "lost to followup." Prophylaxis is the best management of this data loss, and efforts should be taken to find these individuals. Although the investigator cannot protect the protocol from all interruptions or collect perfect data, the interruptions and imperfect data should be pointed out to the reader and the manner in which these factors are handled in the analysis explained.

Data Analysis

The objective of research is to observe and measure changes or differences that occur in the index variables because of the treatment under study. Measurement of change over time requires pretreatment data collection. Data collected during and after the treatment or procedure can be contrasted to pretreatment data and the change expressed in several ways. Change expressed as trend is plotting the data measurements and fitting a line or curve to the data points. Variables with graded ranks (ordinals) may be used to compare the pre- and posttreatment results in clinical terms, such as better, worse, or the same. In comparison studies, the change measured in the treatment group is compared to the change occurring in the control group. If the investigator is interested only in the difference between the index variable outcome of the treatment group and the control group, then pretreatment measurements are not needed.

The analysis of the results of a clinical study commonly consists of a descriptive statistical analysis and an inferential statistical analysis. First, the data are summarized by descriptive statistics. Descriptive statistical analysis presents the central tendency of the data (mode, median, mean) and the dispersion of the data (range, percentile, standard deviation). The measurement scale of the variables (metric, ordinal, nominal, existential) dictates which measure of central tendency or dispersion is appropriate. Descriptive statistical analysis characterizes either the difference between the change in the treatment group and the control group or the difference between the outcome variable of the treatment group and the control group. Descriptive statistical analysis is an evaluation of the data for the study groups only.

Inferential statistical analysis is an extrapolation of the study results to the larger target population. Inferential statistical analysis allows the reader to evaluate the "generalizability" of the research results. So far, the analysis of clinical studies and surveys has not required a knowledge of statistics. Statistical manipulation cannot rectify errors made in the design and execution of the research. Thus, clinical knowledge, logic, and judgment applied to evaluation of research are extremely valuable. The knowledge required to determine the most appropriate statistical test to apply to the data is beyond the scope of this chapter. However, knowledge of basic terms and definitions can provide insight to these mathematical manipulations.

Many inferential statistical tests are based on the criterion that the sample is a random sample of the population. If the sample was not or could not be chosen randomly, statistical tests requiring random samples cannot be used for analysis. Another assumption common to many statistical tests is normal (Gaussian) distribution of the data. As normal distribution may not occur in patient-related data, the investigator may try to "normalize" the data via a mathematical transformation or use another method of analysis (nonparametric) that does not require the assumption of normality.

Earlier, the null hypothesis was presented as a tool for testing the hypothesis of a study. The null hypothesis states that the treatment is of no value or there is no difference between treatments.[17,18] The null hypothesis may be either true or false and the investigator, after the analysis of the data, will either concede or reject the hypothesis (table 30-1).

Table 30-1. Null hypothesis decision table

Investigator's decision	*Null hypothesis*	
	True	*False*
Concede	No error	Type II error or β
Reject	Type I error or α	No error

The opportunity exists for making two different errors: type I or type II. The probability for making a type I error is called alpha (α), and the probability for making a type II error is called beta (β). If a type I error is made, the null hypothesis is rejected when indeed it was true. This means a worthless treatment has been declared useful. A type II error means a treatment that is truly useful has been declared worthless. Type I errors are most detrimental to ethical professional practice; however, they cannot be completely eliminated, as the null hypothesis would have to be conceded each time to have zero type I errors. The probability (*P* value) of making a type I error is calculated, and the decision to concede or reject the null hypothesis is based on the magnitude of this probability. Thus, the lower the α value

(P value), the lower the probability of making a type I error. Frequently, α values of P less than or equal to 0.01 or 0.05 are used to declare the results of the study statistically significant. Mainland[19] suggests a working definition of significance of "probably indicating something that would rarely occur as the result of chance alone." Thus, if the difference between the treatment group outcome and the control group outcome is statistically significant, the null hypothesis is rejected and it is concluded that the difference is probably real and would rarely occur as a result of chance alone.

When the null hypothesis cannot be rejected, i.e., the calculated P value is greater than the established α, the reader needs to evaluate β.[20,21] Conceding the null hypothesis does not mean that the comparison treatments are equivalent. It only means that this particular research study failed to find a difference between the treatments. Whereas "negative" trials (P value > 0.05) can mean there is very little difference between the treatments tested in the trial, it can also mean that a type II error has occurred. Several factors contribute to the probability of making a type II error. The ability of a clinical trial to find delta (Δ), a difference between treatments of a given size, is partially dependent upon the size of the trial sample. Thus, "negative" trial results may be caused by an inadequate sample size.

Deciding upon and recruiting an adequate sample size are important steps for investigators. Before beginning a trial, the investigators choose α and β levels and establish Δ, the smallest clinically important difference between treatments that they want to detect. With these values, the appropriate sample size is calculated. If the calculated sample size is not achievable, a greater risk of making a type II error may be accepted and/or a larger Δ adopted.

As with all methods of analysis, the null hypothesis is not without problems and criticisms.[17,18] It can be used to determine the significance of only one objective, be it an objective based on a single variable or several variables. To achieve the single index for analysis, the combination of variables may sometimes appear contrived from the viewpoint of clinical judgment. By its definition, the null hypothesis shows only differences in treatments or procedures, not similarities. Assigning 0.05 or less as the significant P value is common but still an arbitrary cutoff point. We might consider whether or not results with P values greater than 0.05 are clinically useful.

Pharmacists whose curriculum did not include basic statistics and who wish to evaluate further the statistical analyses used in clinical research may be guided by surveys describing the relative frequency of use of statistical tests in pharmacy and medical journals.[22-25] The results of these surveys suggest that the descriptive statistical procedures of mode, median, mean, and range, percentage, standard deviation, and inferential statistical procedures of t test and X^2 (Chi square) account for approximately 75 percent of the statistical analyses found in pharmacy and medical journals. An understanding of these procedures would provide a reasonable background for evaluation of statistical analyses by pharmacists.

Conclusion

The final obligation of the investigator is to draw a conclusion from the research that allows the research to make a contribution to pharmaceutical and medical practice. The reader's responsibility is to evaluate the conclusion with respect to the entire study.

Clinical and statistical significance deserve careful consideration by both investigators and readers. Anello,[26] in his discussion of this topic, said, "Statistical significance tells nothing about the quality of planning or execution of an experiment, nothing about the biological or clinical meaning of difference in numbers, and nothing about whatever was alleged to cause the difference." Statistical significance is not a direct measure of clinical significance. The application of research results to practical, therapeutic situations should be made with this distinction in mind.

Federal drug legislation requires that drug therapies be proved safe and efficacious prior to marketing. Pharmacists' literature evaluation is frequently concerned with safety and efficacy. Although the Food and Drug Administration has defined its interpretation of "adequate and well-controlled clinical investigations,"[27] we do not have a definition of what constitutes "safety and efficacy." As pointed out by Feinstein,[28] our problems with these two concepts are multiple and not easily solved. The possibility of statistically significant results not being clinically significant has already been mentioned. Delta, the clinically significant difference between treatments in comparative studies, is determined by judgment. To obtain an overall picture of efficacy, it may be important to consider the effect of drug therapy on several signs and/or symptoms of a disease process. However, statistical tests can assess the response of only one variable or index. If multiple variables are combined to generate a single index variable, the combination must withstand close clinical scrutiny. With pharmaceutical agents, we need to consider not only pharmacological efficacy but also therapeutic efficacy. Demonstration of pharmacological efficacy by itself does not allow for the deduction of therapeutic efficacy. Also, the interaction of a patient with health care professionals is complex and cannot or may not be clearly distinguished from the patient's interaction with drug therapy. The common expression of safety — "Do the benefits outweigh the risks?" — does not provide firm direction for literature evaluation.

BASIC ELEMENTS OF CLINICAL REVIEWS

The function of literature evaluation is not only to judge the validity and generalizability of individual clinical studies but also to integrate the knowledge gained from separate studies into a coherent overview of the topic. Individual clinical research studies generate pieces of knowledge that must be combined in some fashion to provide a global representation of the topic for use by clinical practitioners making patient care decisions. Establishing and maintaining current, comprehensive consensus of the research literature is a significant challenge for health care professionals. For many years, the traditional published review of the literature, coupled with an individual's informal review and evaluation of the literature, served the need for a global perspective of therapeutics. As a consensus process, traditional narrative literature reviews can be subjective. Alternatively, meta-analysis offers systematic procedures to combine clinical trial results. Meta-analysis increases the confidence with which we can view a summary conclusion drawn from the results of separate clinical trials. Glass[29] in 1976 named and defined meta-analysis as "the statistical analysis of a large collection of results from individual studies for the purpose of integrating the findings." Meta-analysis is a strategy to pool clinical data from individual research studies. Although there is a standard structure for the overall process, there is no single recommended meta-analysis method or meta-analysis statistical technique.[30]

The structure of meta-analysis reports is analogous to that of clinical trials, but instead of individual subjects being selected to form the study sample, individual clinical trials are chosen to form the meta-analysis study group. The authors of a meta-analysis report have the same obligation as other clinical investigators to state their hypothesis (purpose) and adequately present their protocol for executing the analysis.[31] The following structural guidelines by Mulrow et al.[32] for review articles provide an evaluation structure for meta-analysis reports: (1) purpose, (2) data identification, (3) study selection, (4) data extraction, (5) results of data synthesis, and (6) conclusions.

Purpose

The overall purpose of all meta-analyses is to aggregate individual studies into a general conclusion. Each meta-analysis also has its own specific objective. The specific objective may concern quantitating the effect of an individual drug regimen or a class of drugs for a given disease condition or identifying a subgroup of patients who respond uniquely to a treatment regimen. Meta-analysis is particularly useful for estimating the size of a treatment effect when individual studies have shown only moderate or equivocal treatment effects. Similarly, a subgroup effect may be more convincing when quantitated from an analysis of many studies.

Data Identification

The data identification section of the report informs the reader of the thoroughness with which the authors went about finding studies that were pertinent to the meta-analysis objective. For the analysis to present an aggregate conclusion, all studies relevant to the topic must be found and considered. The search for articles should include a manual and/or computer-assisted search of appropriate indexing and abstracting services, clinical trial registries, and textbook collections. The bibliographies and/or references of relevant studies frequently identify further reports. Expanding the search to recover unpublished studies remains controversial.[30,31,33] Unpublished trials may be of such poor quality that they were denied publication. As their poor quality may detract from the accuracy of the meta-analysis, they are considered inappropriate by some investigators for inclusion. Publication bias, on the other hand, may keep some good trials with negative results from being published.[34] Exclusion of negative-result trials from the meta-analysis may distort the outcome.

Study Selection

Once suitable studies have been identified, they are evaluated against inclusion and exclusion criteria. These criteria are determined primarily by the objective of the meta-analysis; however, authors may also use selection criteria to set a quality standard that studies must meet to be included in the analysis. Quality standards frequently include assessment of design features, e.g., randomization, inclusion of all subjects in the analysis ("intent to treat" principle), or consideration of only studies with sample sizes of a predetermined number. There are no standard meta-analysis inclusion criteria. As part of their justification of the study inclusion criteria, the authors may present a sensitivity analysis consisting of two analyses: one analysis of all studies identified in the literature search and another of just those studies that meet the inclusion criteria.

Data Extraction

Data extraction or collection methods determine which key descriptive and treatment result data are obtained from the selected studies. This process involves interpretation and judgment. To control bias in interpretation and documentation of study data, several blinded observers can collect data and the interobserver agreement can be assessed. Another responsibility of investigators is to ensure that subject data are counted only once. Results of small trials or results from a single location of a multicenter study are sometimes published, and then the same data are combined with other data in a subsequent publication.

Before statistically combining the results of the clinical trials, the investigators must decide whether or not the trials are enough alike (homogeneous) to permit pooling of their results. If the variability in the results of the separate clinical trials can be reasonably explained by sampling error, the trials are considered homogeneous.[35] Statistical tests for homogeneity can be used. If the trials' results vary enough that the homogeneity test value is significant, proceeding further with the meta-analysis should be justified by the investigators and explained to the reader.

Results of Data Synthesis

Several statistical models are available for combining data from clinical trials.[34,36] The simplest method is to combine the data from each study into a single data set for analysis. Although this kind of lumping is used to analyze the separate data sets in multicenter clinical trials, the known and unknown differences among the individual clinical trials of a meta-analysis are recognized to be too large to justify combining raw data into a single data set. The statistical technique used depends on the number of studies to be combined, the intended use of the results, and the kind of data to be analyzed. For binomial data (data with only two outcomes, e.g., success or failure, dead or alive) some investigators choose to calculate the odds ratio (OR) and its 95 percent confidence interval for each study and plot these on a graph. The graph visually presents the size of each study's odds ratio (OR = 1 means no effect) and how they compare to one another. The analysis may be taken one step further and a summary odds ratio representing all the studies calculated.

A single summary statistic can be generated by a method to average P values or to add Z values. Otherwise, methods that combine the magnitude of the effect of the treatment being considered (i.e., the difference between treated and control group for each study) can be selected. Estimation of effect size is useful for continuous or quantitative data.[31,37] Meta-analysis of the same studies using different statistical methods can show different results. Some investigators recommend that more than one statistical method be applied to the studies considered in a meta-analysis. If different analyses show the same result, more confidence can be placed in the conclusion. Statistical techniques that weigh individual trials (e.g., take into account the sample size of each study) and that consider differences or variability between the trial results (heterogeneity) are also preferred.[30,31]

The resulting summary significance level (*P* value) must be interpreted with the same, if not greater, care than that used to interpret the significance level in individual clinical trials. A cautious approach suggests that the *P* value necessary to conclude statistical significance for a meta-analysis be fixed at a lower level than that generally used for clinical trials. As with clinical trials, the *P* value to be considered significant should be set prior to the actual meta-analysis of the data.

Conclusions

Conclusions drawn from a meta-analysis reflect an overall data review, not just a final *P* value. The quality of the individual studies combined, the variability of important clinical prognostic factors (e.g., disease severity, subject age), variability of the treatments (e.g., dose, duration of treatment), and agreement between outcome variable(s) in each study are all important considerations. A discussion of clinical consistency, clinical significance, and clinical application of the results belongs in the conclusion.[31]

A positive meta-analysis outcome adds to the confidence placed in the treatment under study. However, meta-analysis alone cannot be used to make medical treatment decisions. Nor can meta-analysis of individual clinical trials replace our need for well-constructed, randomized controlled clinical trials with sample size adequate to determine the medical value of a treatment. Meta-analysis improves our understanding of the quality of clinical studies and the magnitude and variability of the aggregated effect calculated from the individual studies.

Traditional narrative reviews of the literature document and describe the evidence to support a treatment regimen or the data associating a therapy with adverse effect(s). The evaluation structure of Mulrow et al.[32] used to discuss meta-analysis is also particularly useful to evaluate narrative reviews. A reader can expect a narrative review to (1) state its purpose; (2) describe how articles for review were found (data identification); (3) list the inclusion and exclusion criteria applied to select studies; (4) identify who and what standards were used to abstract pertinent information from each study (data extraction); (5) present the results of the data synthesis, which for a narrative review may use only descriptive statistics; and (6) derive a conclusion from the review that discusses the clinical usefulness of the therapy under review and justifies any recommendations.

QUALITY OF PUBLISHED THERAPEUTIC RESEARCH

It is impossible to achieve perfect design, data, analysis, and conclusions in the real world of pharmacy and medicine. The goal is evaluation of research with guidance from sound clinical judgment and common sense. The responsibility of the reader to judge the reliability and validity of clinical research reports and to evaluate the generalizability of research results cannot be abrogated to journal editors, referees, or authors of review articles. There has been substantial evidence, beginning in 1951 and continuing into the present, that research reports with incomplete documentation, poor design, questionable data collection methods, inappropriate statistical analyses, or indefensible conclusions are published.[4,21,38-89] There have been more than 35 separate evaluations of the methods employed in medical and pharmacy studies. Whereas earlier evaluations tended to consider any therapeutic study or report that appeared in selected journal issues, recent studies have concentrated on specialty journals, e.g., acute care,[85] dermatology,[57] psychiatry,[59] surgery,[52] or on a specific topic in therapeutics, e.g., cancer therapy,[46,63,64,72] therapy for pregnant women and newborn infants,[51,56,62] otitis media,[48] congestive heart failure,[68] or on specific drug classes, e.g., antibiotic prophylaxis,[53,60] corticosteroids,[44] new drugs,[58] contrast media.[70] Other topics studied include adverse drug reactions,[49] drug analysis methods,[67] diagnostic tests,[55] and case control studies.[4,71]

The research reports from investigators evaluating the validity of medical and pharmacy literature have, themselves, been evaluated, e.g., articles assessing the scientific accuracy of medical literature[65] and meta-analyses.[66] Sources of the articles evaluated were primarily U.S., Canadian, or British journals. The majority of the evaluation studies used a checklist of important design and/or analysis criteria to judge the acceptability of the reports and studies. Methods used in these various evaluation studies are different, and the operational definitions of an acceptable or valid clinical study are also different. Despite these limitations, the results from these studies are presented in table 30-2.

The statistical analyses performed in the articles have also been assessed. More than 15 evaluations of the appropriateness of statistical analyses in clinical trials have been published.[74-89] These authors found that 9-83 percent of journal articles (table 30-3) that used descriptive and/or inferential statistical analyses had at least one error of commission or omission in the statistical analysis. Most of these evaluations reported an unacceptability rate of 50-60 percent for the statistical analyses. Glantz[76] reported the use of the *t* test as inappropriate in 69 percent of studies. Godfrey[82] considered the use of tests to compare the means of several groups, multiple *t* tests primarily, and found them used inappropriately in 54 percent of articles. Fisher's exact test was not completely described in 59 percent of studies assessed by McKinney et al.[88] Even the number of statistical tests employed by investigators to analyze the results of a clinical trial has been considered inappropriately high; Pocock et al.[84] reported a median number of eight tests per trial and concluded that this led to reports that were biased toward an exaggeration of treatment differences.

Studies with "negative" (not statistically significant) outcomes have also been evaluated for the appropriateness of the conclusions. Freiman et al.[21] and Reed and Slaichert[77] evaluated the ability or power of negative outcome clinical trials to support the negative outcome. Freiman et al.[21] found that about 69 percent of the 71 randomized controlled trials evaluated had a greater than 20 percent risk of missing a true, 50-percent therapeutic improvement. Reed and Slaichert[77] found that between 60 and 84 percent of the 2,619 tests in 355 articles from 6 journals had a greater than

Table 30-2. Results of therapeutic literature evaluation studies

Study	*Results*
1951 Ross[38]	63% of 100 articles had no or inadequate control.
1961 Badgley[39]	41.5% of 103 articles had a problem(s) with derivation of conclusion.
1964 Mahon and Daniel[40]	94.6% of 203 articles did not meet all 4 validity criteria.
1966 Schor and Karten[41]	47.5% of 295 articles were judged not acceptable.
1968 Reiffenstein et al.[42]	83.1% of 367 articles did not meet all 4 validity criteria.
1970 Lionel and Herxheimer[43]	32.6% of 141 articles were judged not acceptable.
1974 Weitzman and Berger[44]	64% of 8 standards were not adhered to in 32 studies of the effect of corticosteroids on bacterial infections.
1978 Ambroz et al.[45]	66% of 172 randomized controlled trials were judged less than well executed.
1979 Horwitz and Feinstein[4]	46% of 85 case controlled studies were not adequately compliant with 12 methodologic criteria.
1980 Mosteller et al.[46]	76% of 132 randomized controlled trials in cancer did not adequately report on 5 important pieces of information.
1982 DerSimonian et al.[47]	44% of 67 comparative trials did not adequately report on 11 criteria.
1982 Marchant and Shurin[48]	39% of 13 standards in 25 trials of otitis media treatment were poorly adhered to or inadequately described.
1982 Venulet et al.[49]	39% of 5,737 adverse drug reaction articles did not provide information to calculate incidence of adverse reactions.
1983 Smith et al.[50]	80% of 96 trials did not give information on agents of all study subjects.
1983 Tyson et al.[51]	90% of 86 studies in perinatal therapeutics did not fulfill criteria to justify their treatment/management conclusions.
1984 Emerson et al.[52]	41% of 84 surgical clinical trials omitted or ambiguously reported on at least 1 of 11 criteria.
1984 Evans and Pollock[53]	80% of 45 studies of antibiotic prophylaxsis of abdominal surgical wound infections articles were judged to have doubtful clinical significance.
1984 Meinert et al.[54]	50% of 113 clinical trials did not report on 5 major evaluation criteria.
1984 Sheps and Schechter[55]	74% of 129 diagnostic test evaluation trials were missing 3 or more of 7 important criteria.
1984 Thomson and Kramer[56]	69% of 16 studies of early contact on subsequent maternal-infant behavior were missing 4 or more of 11 methodologic standards.
1985 Bigby et al.[57]	59% of 13 methodologic items in 62 dermatology articles were not reported.
1985 Bland et al.[58]	98% of 80 trials of 7 new drugs introduced in U.K. in 1978-1979 gave no information on criterion for choice of trials' sample size.
1985 Edlund et al.[59]	57.1% of 84 treatment studies in 3 psychiatric journals did not mention informed consent, and none of the trials mentioned the number or characteristics of patients who refused to enter trials.
1985 Evans and Pollock[60]	62% of design and conduct points, 53% of analysis points, and 75% of presentation points adhered to 33 methodologic standards in 56 trials of prophylaxis of surgical abdominal wound infections
1985 Kelen et al.[61]	60%, 59%, and 65% of 11 methodological criteria were not clearly reported in 45 trials from 3 acute-care journals.
1986 Bauchner et al.[62]	70% of 20 cohort or case control studies assessing the protective effect of breast-feeding did not meet even 3 of 4 methodological standards.
1986 Liberati et al.[63]	Mean overall quality score for 63 randomized controlled trials of primary breast cancer was 50% on 100-point scale.
1986 Marsoni et al.[64]	85% of 27 randomized controlled trials of advanced ovarian cancer used incorrect randomization process; in 81% of trials, the sample size would detect differences only in response rate >50%.
1986 Williamson et al.[65]	15% of 33 studies that assessed the scientific adequacy of medical literature were judged to have weakly substantiated results.
1987 Sacks et al.[66]	72% of 86 meta-analyses did not satisfactorily address all of 6 major methodological areas. Mean number of 23 individual items satisfactorily addressed was 7.7 per meta-analysis.
1988 Eggers and Bircher[67]	51% of 357 investigations concerning plasma concentration of drug or other substance did not report test's precision; 79%, 47%, and 84% did not report test's accuracy, sensitivity, or specificity, respectively.
1988 Marantz et al.[68]	55% of 51 randomized placebo-controlled congestive heart failure trials did not specify criteria to diagnose congestive heart failure.
1989 Neihouse and Priske[69]	31% of 99 references were inappropriately quoted in drug therapy review articles.
1989 Powe et al.[70]	Mean overall quality score was 39 (maximum 100) for 100 randomized controlled trials comparing low- to high-osmolality contract media.
1989 Shapiro[71]	78% of 9 case control postmarketing surveillance studies from record linkage data bases judged not to fulfill 8 standard validity criteria.
1989 Zola et al.[72]	43% of 11 quality standards judged inadequately met in 70 multiseries studies on primary treatment of early cervical cancer.
1990 Evans et al.[73]	36% of 150 citations in 3 surgery journals were in error; 29% of 137 quotations in same journal issues were considered quotation errors.

20 percent risk of missing a relatively large treatment difference. The possibility that a clinical trial with negative results had a sample size inadequate to detect even a relatively large difference between treatments should always be considered.

Overall, criteria used to judge clinical studies may have become more stringent over the years; however, the results of these evaluations are still disheartening. Clinical study results are the foundation of therapeutic decisions. The shortcomings of clinical research identified by these studies should alert health professionals to the care required in all literature evaluation activities.

REFERENCES

1. Feinstein AR: Clinical biostatistics, XLIV. A survey of the research architecture used for publications in general medical journals. *Clin Pharmacol Ther* 24:117-125, 1978.
2. Fredrickson DS: The field trial: Some thoughts on the indispensable ordeal. *Bull NY Acad Med* 44:985-993, 1968.
3. Feinstein AR: Clinical biostatistics, XX. The epidemiologic trohoc, the ablative risk ratio, and "retrospective" research. *Clin Pharmacol Ther* 14:291-307, 1973.
4. Horwitz RI, Feinstein AR: Methodologic standards and contradictory results in case-control research. *Am J Med* 66:556-564, 1979.

Table 30-3. Results of evaluations of statistics used in therapeutic studies

Study	Results
1977 Gore et al.[74]	52% of 62 analytic articles contained at least 1 error when judged by 5 statistical criteria.
1978 Freiman et al.[21]	70% of 71 "negative" randomized controlled trials had a >10% risk of missing a 50% improvement.
1979 White[75]	34% of 139 articles were found to have at least 1 major error as judged by 5 statistical criteria.
1980 Glantz[76]	69% of 52 articles using the *t* test used the test inappropriately.
1981 Reed and Slaichert[77]	335 articles with "negative" results had a mean probability of detecting a medium improvement (effect size of d = .50) of 0.387 (power of 0.80 recommended).
1982 Hall et al.[78]	78% of 91 analytical trials in Australasian surgical journal contained errors in usage of inferential statistical techniques.
1983 Gardner et al.[79]	67% of 12 published articles were considered statistically unacceptable for publication by 9 statistical assessment criteria.
1984 Felson et al.[80]	60% of 94 articles from 1967-1968 had 1 or more error, 66% of 119 articles from 1982 had 1 or more error as judged by 6 statistical error criteria.
1985 Avram et al.[81]	9% of descriptive, 83% of parametric, and 61% of nonparametric inferential statistical tests appearing in 243 anesthesiology articles had errors.
1985 Godfrey[82]	54% of 50 articles used inappropriate statistical methods to analyze the difference between group means.
1985 Thorn et al.[83]	63% and 80% of statistical methods in 29 articles from 2 pharmacy journals were judged incorrect or incomplete; 29% and 39% of methods in 91 articles from 2 medical journals were judged incorrect or incomplete.
1987 Pocock et al.[84]	Median number of significance tests in 45 comparative trials was 8; conclusion was that reporting of clinical trials appears to be biased toward exaggeration of treatment differences.
1988 Klein[85]	35% of 43 trials of irritable bowel syndrome therapy used inappropriate statistical methods.
1988 Morris[86]	54% of 24 studies on bone or joint surgery topics used inappropriate or unclear statistical techniques.
1988 Murray[87]	39% of 28 studies on surgery topics contained statistical errors.
1989 McKinney et al.[88]	59% of 56 studies from 6 medical journals did not specify the "sideness" (1- or 2-sided) of Fisher's exact test.
1990 Gardner and Bond[89]	15% of 45 articles from 1 journal were judged not to be of an acceptable statistical standard using a 24-point checklist.

5. Feinstein AR: Clinical biostatistics, XIX. Ambiguity and abuse in the twelve different concepts of "control." *Clin Pharmacol Ther* 14:112-122, 1973.
6. Hayden GF, Kramer MS, Horwitz RI: The case-control study, a practical review for the clinician. *JAMA* 247:326-331, 1982.
7. Gehan EA: Comparative clinical trials with historical controls: A statistician's view. *Biomedicine* (special issue) 28:13-19, 1978.
8. Cranberg L: Do retrospective controls make clinical trials "inherently fallacious"? *Br Med J* 2:1265-1266, 1979.
9. Sacks H, Chalmers TC, Smith H: Randomized versus historical controls for clinical trials. *Am J Med* 72:233-240, 1982.
10. Sacks HS, Chalmers TC, Smith H: Sensitivity and specificity of clinical trials, randomized v historical controls. *Arch Intern Med* 143:753-755, 1983.
11. Hills M, Armitage P: The two-period cross-over clinical trial. *Br J Clin Pharmacol* 8:7-20, 1979.
12. Feinstein AR: Clinical biostatistics, III. The architecture of clinical research. *Clin Pharmacol Ther* 11:432-441, 1970.
13. Byar DP, Simon RM, Friedewald WT, et al: Randomized clinical trials, perspectives on some recent ideas. *N Engl J Med* 295:74-80, 1976.
14. Simon R: Adaptive treatment assignment methods and clinical trials. *Biometrics* 33:743-749, 1977.
15. Hill C, Sancho-Garnier H: The two-armed-bandit problem a decision theory approach to clinical trials. *Biomedicine* (special issue) 28:42-43, 1978.
16. Feinstein AR: Clinical biostatistics, IV. The architecture of clinical research (continued). *Clin Pharmacol Ther* 11:595-610, 1970.
17. Feinstein AR: Clinical biostatistics, V. The architecture of clinical research (concluded). *Clin Pharmacol Ther* 11:755-771, 1970.
18. Mainland D: Statistical ward rounds - 17. *Clin Pharmacol Ther* 10:714-736, 1969.
19. Mainland D: Statistical ward rounds - 18. *Clin Pharmacol Ther* 10:867-900, 1969.
20. Feinstein AR: Clinical biostatistics, XXXIV. The other side of "statistical significance": Alpha, beta, delta, and the calculation of sample size. *Clin Pharmacol Ther* 18:491-505, 1975.
21. Freiman JA, Chalmers TC, Smith H, et al: The importance of beta, the type II error and sample size in the design and interpretation of the randomized control trial, survey of 71 "negative" trials. *N Engl J Med* 299:690-694, 1978.
22. Feinstein AR: Clinical biostatistics, XXV. A survey of the statistical procedures in general medical journals. *Clin Pharmacol Ther* 15:97-107, 1974.
23. Moore R, Smith MC, Liao W, et al: Statistical background needed to read professional pharmacy journals. *Am J Pharm Educ* 42:251-254, 1978.
24. Hayden GF: Biostatistical trends in pediatrics: Implications for the future. *Pediatrics* 72:84-87, 1983.
25. Emerson JD, Colditz GA: Use of statistical analysis in The New England Journal of Medicine. *N Engl J Med* 309:709-713, 1983.
26. Anello C: Considerations of significance—clinical and statistical. In McMahon FG (ed): *Importance of Experimental Design and Biostatistics.* Mount Kisco, NY, Futura Publishing Company, Inc., 1974, pp 5-14.
27. U.S. Food and Drug Administration: Hearing regulations and regulations describing scientific content of adequate and well-controlled clinical investigations. *Fed Reg* 35:7250-7253, 1970.
28. Feinstein AR: Clinical biostatistics, IX. How do we measure "safety and efficacy"? *Clin Pharmacol Ther* 12:544-558, 1971.
29. Glass GV: Primary, secondary and meta-analysis of research. *Educ Res* 5:3-8, 1976.
30. L'Abbe KA, Detsky AS, O'Rourke K: Meta-analysis in clinical research. *Ann Intern Med* 107:224-233, 1987.
31. Boissel J-P, Blanchard J, Panak E, et al: Considerations for the meta-analysis of randomized clinical trials. *Controlled Clin Trials* 10:254-281, 1989.
32. Mulrow CD, Thacker SB, Pugh JA: A proposal for more informative abstracts of review articles. *Ann Intern Med* 108:613-615, 1988.
33. Einarson TR, McGhan WF, Bootman JL, et al: Meta-analysis: Quantitative integration of independent research results. *Am J Hosp Pharm* 42:1957-1964, 1985.
34. Dickersin K: The existence of publication bias and risk factors for its occurrence. *JAMA* 263:1385-1389, 1990.
35. Halvorsen KT: Combining results from independent investigations, meta-analysis in medical research. In Bailar JC, Mosteller F (eds): *Medical Uses of Statistics.* Waltham, MA, NEJM Books, 1986, pp 392-416.

36. DeMets DL: Methods for combining randomized clinical trials: Strengths and limitations. *Stat Med* 6:341-348, 1987.
37. Teagarden JR: Meta-analysis: Whither narrative or review? *Pharmacotherapy* 9:274-284, 1989.
38. Ross OB: Use of controls in medical research. *JAMA* 145:72-75, 1951.
39. Badgley RF: An assessment of research methods reported in 103 scientific articles from two Canadian medical journals. *Can Med Assoc J* 85:246-250, 1961.
40. Mahon WA, Daniel EE: A method for the assessment of reports of drug trials. *Can Med Assoc J* 90:565-569, 1964.
41. Schor S, Karten I: Statistical evaluation of medical journal manuscripts. *JAMA* 195:1123-1128, 1966.
42. Reiffenstein RJ, Schiltroth AJ, Todd DM: Current standards in reported drug trials. *Can Med Assoc J* 99:1134-1135, 1968.
43. Lionel NDW, Herxheimer A: Assessing reports of therapeutic trials. *Br Med J* 3:637-640, 1970.
44. Weitzman S, Berger S: Clinical trial design in studies of corticosteroids for bacterial infections. *Ann Intern Med* 81:36-42, 1974.
45. Ambroz A, Chalmers TC, Smith H, et al: Deficiencies of randomized control trials (abstract). *Clin Res* 26:280A, 1978.
46. Mosteller F, Gilbert JP, McPeek B: Reporting standards and research strategies for controlled trials, agenda for the editor. *Controlled Clin Trials* 1:37-58, 1980.
47. DerSimonian R, Charette LJ, McPeek B, et al: Reporting on methods in clinical trials. *N Engl J Med* 306:1332-1337, 1982.
48. Marchant C, Shurin PA: Antibacterial therapy for acute otitis media: A critical analysis. *Rev Infect Dis* 4:506-513, 1982.
49. Venulet J, Blattner R, von Bulow J, et al: How good are articles on adverse drug reactions? *Br Med J* 284:252-254, 1982.
50. Smith C, Ebrahim S, Arie T: Drug trials, the "elderly," and the very aged (letter). *Lancet* 2:1139, 1983.
51. Tyson JE, Furzan JA, Reisch JS, et al: An evaluation of the quality of therapeutic studies in perinatal medicine. *Obstet Gynecol* 62:99-102, 1983.
52. Emerson JD, McPeek B, Mosteller F: Reporting clinical trials in general surgical journals. *Surgery* 95:572-579, 1984.
53. Evans M, Pollock AV: Trials on trial, a review of trials of antibiotic prophylaxis. *Arch Surg* 119:109-113, 1984.
54. Meinert CL, Tonascia S, Higgins K: Content of reports on clinical trials: A critical review. *Controlled Clin Trials* 5:328-347, 1984.
55. Sheps SB, Schechter MT: The assessment of diagnostic tests, a survey of current medical research. *JAMA* 252:2418-2422, 1984.
56. Thomson ME, Kramer MS: Methodologic standards for controlled clinical trials of early contact and maternal-infant behavior. *Pediatrics* 73:294-300, 1984.
57. Bigby M, Stern RS, Bigby JA: An evaluation of method reporting and use in clinical trials in dermatology. *Arch Dermatol* 121:1394-1399, 1985.
58. Bland JM, Jones DR, Bennett S, et al: Is the clinical trial evidence about new drugs statistically adequate? *Br J Clin Pharmacol* 19:155-160, 1985.
59. Edlund MJ, Craig TJ, Richardson MA: Informed consent as a form of volunteer bias. *Am J Psychiatry* 142:624-627, 1985.
60. Evans M, Pollock AV: A score system for evaluating random control clinical trials of prophylaxis of abdominal surgical wound infection. *Br J Surg* 72:256-260, 1985.
61. Kelen GD, Brown CG, Moser M, et al: Reporting methodology protocols in three acute care journals. *Ann Emerg Med* 14:880-884, 1985.
62. Bauchner H, Leventhal JM, Shapiro ED: Studies of breast-feeding and infections, how good is the evidence? *JAMA* 256:887-892, 1986.
63. Liberati A, Himel HN, Chalmers TC: A quality assessment of randomized control trials of primary treatment of breast cancer. *J Clin Oncol* 4:942-951, 1986.
64. Marsoni S, Liberati A, Farina ML, et al: Quality analysis of randomized control trials (RCTs) of the treatment of advanced ovarian cancer (AOC) (abstract). *Controlled Clin Trials* 7:239, 1986.
65. Williamson JW, Goldschmidt PG, Colton T: The quality of medical literature: An analysis of validation assessments. In Bailar JC, Mosteller F (eds): *Medical Uses of Statistics.* Waltham, MA, NEJM Books, 1986, pp 370-391.
66. Sacks HS, Berrier J, Reitman D, et al: Meta-analyses of randomized controlled trials. *N Engl J Med* 316:450-455, 1987.
67. Eggers RH, Bircher J: Inadequate reporting of analytical quality control in the clinical pharmacological literature. *Eur J Clin Pharmacol* 34:319-321, 1988.
68. Marantz PR, Alderman MH, Tobin JN: Diagnostic heterogeneity in clinical trials for congestive heart failure. *Ann Intern Med* 109:55-61, 1988.
69. Neihouse PF, Priske SC: Quotation accuracy in review articles. *DICP* 23:594-596, 1989.
70. Powe NR, Kinnison ML, Steinberg EP: Quality assessment of randomized controlled trials of contrast media. *Radiology* 170:377-380, 1989.
71. Shapiro S: The role of automated record linkage in the postmarketing surveillance of drug safety: A critique. *Clin Pharmacol Ther* 46:371-386, 1989.
72. Zola P, Volpe T, Castelli G, et al: Is the published literature a reliable guide for deciding between alternative treatments for patients with early cervical cancer? *Int J Radiat Biol* 16:785-797, 1989.
73. Evans JT, Nadjari HI, Burchell SA: Quotational and reference accuracy in surgical journals, a continuing peer review problem. *JAMA* 263:1353-1354, 1990.
74. Gore SM, Jones IG, Rytter EC: Misuse of statistical methods: Critical assessment of articles in BMJ from January to March 1976. *Br Med J* 1:85-87, 1977.
75. White SJ: Statistical errors in papers in the British Journal of Psychiatry. *Br J Psychiatry* 135:336-342, 1979.
76. Glantz SA: Biostatistics: How to detect, correct and prevent errors in the medical literature. *Circulation* 61:1-7, 1980.
77. Reed JF, Slaichert W: Statistical proof in inconclusive "negative" trials. *Arch Intern Med* 141:1307-1310, 1981.
78. Hall JC, Hill D, Watts JM: Misuse of statistical methods in the Australasian surgical literature. *Aust NZ J Surg* 52:541-543, 1982.
79. Gardner MJ, Altman DG, Jones DR, et al: Is the statistical assessment of papers submitted to the "British Medical Journal" effective? *Br Med J* 286:1485-1488, 1983.
80. Felson DT, Cupples LA, Meenan RF: Misuse of statistical methods in Arthritis and Rheumatism, 1982 versus 1967-68. *Arthritis Rheum* 27:1018-1022, 1984.
81. Avram MJ, Shanks CA, Dykes MHM, et al: Statistical methods in anesthesia articles: An evaluation of two American journals during two six-month periods. *Anesth Analg* 64:607-611, 1985.
82. Godfrey K: Comparing the means of several groups. *N Engl J Med* 313:1450-1456, 1985.
83. Thorn MD, Pulliam CC, Symons MJ, et al: Statistical and research quality of the medical and pharmacy literature. *Am J Hosp Pharm* 42:1077-1082, 1985.
84. Pocock SJ, Hughes MD, Lee RJ: Statistical problems in the reporting of clinical trials, a survey of three medical journals. *N Engl J Med* 317:426-432, 1987.
85. Klein KB: Controlled treatment trials in the irritable bowel syndrome: A critique. *Gastroenterology* 95:232-241, 1988.
86. Morris RW: A statistical study of papers in The Journal of Bone and Joint Surgery [Br] 1984. *J Bone Joint Surg* [Br] 70-B:242-246, 1988.
87. Murray GD: The task of a statistical referee. *Br J Surg* 75:664-667, 1988.
88. McKinney WP, Young MJ, Hartz A, et al: The inexact use of Fisher's Exact Test in six major medical journals. *JAMA* 261:3430-3433, 1989.
89. Gardner MJ, Bond J: An exploratory study of statistical assessment of papers published in the British Medical Journal. *JAMA* 263:1355-1357, 1990.

ADDITIONAL READING

Bulpitt CJ: *Randomised Controlled Clinical Trials.* The Hague, Martinus Nijhoff, 1983.

Fletcher RH, Fletcher SW: Clinical research in general medical journals, a 30-year perspective. *N Engl J Med* 301:180-183, 1979.

Friedman LM, Furberg CD, DeMets DL: *Fundamentals of Clinical Trials,* 2nd ed. Littleton, MA, PSG Publishing Company, Inc, 1985.

Gehlbach SH: *Interpreting the Medical Literature, Practical Epidemiology for Clinicians,* 2nd ed. New York, Macmillan Publishing Company, 1988.

Horwitz RI, Feinstein AR: Methodologic standards and contradictory results in case-control research. *Am J Med* 66:556-564, 1979.

Ingelfinger JA, Mosteller F, Thibodeau LA, et al: *Biostatistics in Clinical Medicine,* 2nd ed. New York, Macmillan Publishing Company Inc, 1987.

Riegelman RK: *Studying a Study and Testing a Test, How to Read the Medical Literature,* 2nd ed. Boston, Little, Brown & Company, 1981.

CHAPTER 31

Drug Information Services

ANN B. AMERSON

In the introduction to the American Society of Hospital Pharmacists (ASHP) Guidelines on Minimum Standards for Pharmacies in Institutions,[1] three prominent components of pharmaceutical services are identified. One of these concerns the evaluation and dissemination of comprehensive information about drugs and their use to the institution's staff and patients. Another addresses the monitoring, evaluation, and assurance of the quality of drug use. Of the six standards listed in the document, Standard IV (Drug Information) and Standard V (Assuring Rational Drug Therapy) both address philosophies and functions that encompass drug information services.

With the emphasis placed on drug information-related activity by the standards, it was surprising to review the results of the 1987 survey of hospital pharmaceutical services. Of the 609 responding hospitals, 81.8 percent characterized their drug information services as limited.[2] This meant that the drug information library was modest and that drug information was supplied on an ad hoc basis by most staff. Only 5.6 percent of all hospitals rated their drug information services as extensive, which meant ready access to extensive drug information and provision of a formal service with at least one full-time equivalent pharmacist position. The remaining institutions (12.6 percent) fell in between. Of hospitals with greater than 400 beds, 15 (37.5 percent) characterized their drug information services as extensive, and a similar number characterized them as limited. For 124 hospitals (200-399 beds), 72.6 percent had limited drug information services.

As indicated by the survey, a limited number of institutions choose to establish a formal drug information center. This concept, first developed in 1962, remains a viable, useful approach to accomplishing the responsibilities of drug information provision. It implies a physically separate location with dedicated personnel to conduct the program. The origin, growth, and development of drug information centers have been reviewed.[3] Other institutions integrate drug information services into other departmental activities and involve many individuals within the department. This chapter describes drug information services that may be provided and discusses considerations in their development.

DEFINING DRUG INFORMATION SERVICES

Examining the current practice is one way to define drug information services. Drug information centers provide a number of different services that are now well established. Table 31-1 depicts the services that deserve discussion.

Table 31-1. Drug information services

1. Response to questions
2. Pharmacy and therapeutics committee activity
   a. Development of drug use policies
   b. Formulary considerations
3. Publications: newsletters, bulletins, journal columns
4. Education: in-service programs, students
5. Drug usage evaluation
6. Investigational drug activity
7. Coordination of reporting programs
8. Poison information

Response to Questions

Provision of drug information on demand is one of the first services usually considered. Such a service allows the inquirer to have specific information needs met in a timely fashion. Information resources can be concentrated in a central, accessible location with personnel available for answering questions. Although some investment is required to establish this service, centralizing resources avoids unnecessary duplication. The expertise of the personnel involved may be more fully developed and efficiently used when they are routinely involved in providing the service. The number and types of questions and callers often are used as a measure of success of the center and its activities and require appropriate documentation.

Pharmacy and Therapeutics Committee Activities

The pharmacy and therapeutics (P&T) committee is a committee of the medical staff with the director of pharmacy (or his or her designee) usually serving as secretary. Representatives from nursing and hospital administration are included as well as other pharmacy representation such as the drug information center director. Active participation in this committee is vital to pharmacy's role and influence in the drug use process within the institution. The secretarial function of preparation of agendas and minutes provides an opportunity for input into committee activities and the evolution of a leadership role. This needs to be supported by excellent information in the form of drug monographs and other background material for committee deliberations. These can be prepared adequately by a drug information service or center. With the current environment of cost containment and the continuing availability of new, often high-tech drugs, the need for evaluative information is essential in making P&T and formulary decisions.

Monographs provide an objective overview and evaluation of the information on a drug and should assist the P&T committee in its decision making. A standard format is desirable with a section to discuss special considerations for given drugs. Minimally, monographs might summarize important information in the package insert. Ideally, the monograph should provide an evaluation of the clinical drug literature available on the product in question compared to previously available agents. The ASHP has published guidelines for information that should be considered for inclusion.[4] When this list was used to evaluate monographs prepared by different institutions, a significant amount of variation in content was noted.[5] None of the reports contained all of the elements listed in the guidelines, but 80 percent summarized more information than provided in the package insert.

Institutions with a relative lack of formulary control have recognized the necessity of greater selectivity and are moving to develop or improve formularies. Once a formulary is developed, maintenance is required. Formulary maintenance includes a process of continuing revision by review of drug classes and specific agents as well as updating, printing, and distribution. These functions are a component of P&T committee activities and provide a continuing avenue of needed communication to the medical staff. Availability of a current formulary should facilitate appropriate use of drugs within the institution. (For further discussion of formulary development, see chapter 8 of this handbook.)

Publications

Efforts to communicate information regarding drug use policies and current developments that influence drug selection are an important component of drug information services. Most often, newsletters are published to accomplish this goal, but other techniques have been used to convey certain kinds of information. For example, pocket-sized cards can be developed that focus on a class or group of agents. Examples of topics that might be covered on such cards are antimicrobial selection, appropriate use and dosing of the preferred H_2 receptor antagonist, or cost considerations for particular classes of agents (e.g., thrombolytics, antimicrobials). These allow ready access to information important in the prescribing process and assist in implementing drug use policies. Where a significant change in drug use is being made in an institution, the drug information service can serve a coordinating function to ensure thorough communication of the impending change prior to implementation. Effective communication is important to complete a cycle of discussion, decision, communication, and implementation of drug use policies.

Factors to consider in developing the publication are the intended audience, the needs of the audience, and the desired goals. Defining these factors will indicate individuals whose input should be sought in development and approval and identify appropriate content for the audience. Some institutions, for example, elect to have a separate newsletter for physicians and nurses because of different audience needs for drug information and different desired goals of communication. In designing the newsletter, requesting and reviewing copies of newsletters published at other institutions will aid in decisions regarding content and format.

Issues relating to content and format need to be thoroughly addressed for a successful newsletter. Content issues relate to the practicality and tone. Topics often considered for regular inclusion are: (1) drug reviews; (2) abstracts of current literature; (3) announcements regarding new procedures, P&T committee decisions, and programs; (4) drug use evaluations including results of reviews conducted as well as information from the literature; (5) drug information requests received; and (6) adverse drug reaction reports summarized from the institution's reports and/or literature. Information addressing these topics should be targeted to the audience, address practical issues, and not lecture.[6,7]

Format issues involve the appearance and editorial management. The newsletter should have an eye-catching, yet professional, appearance. In the masthead, the name usually reflects the content with the publisher (pharmacy department, P&T committee) clearly identified. Considerations in formatting include the use of regular columns or features to provide consistency from issue to issue. Headlines and subtitles assist in clearly presenting the information. Colored paper can add identity to the newsletter, but brilliant or offensive colors that detract from readability should be avoided. The final editing process must pay close attention to correction of misspellings, typographical errors, and content errors. Such uncorrected problems convey a poor image. The editor should seek to achieve clarity and simplicity in presentations of content.[6,7]

The wide availability of desktop publishing technology offers assistance in addressing format issues.[8] Many pharmacy department drug information centers have most or all of the computer hardware to support the software. Costs for software (e.g., Pagemaker, Ventura) are around $800. The initial investment in desktop publishing will be offset by later savings in costs for typesetting and layout. Once initiated, the newsletter should be published regularly and contain timely information for greatest benefit.

Dissemination of information outside the institution is important. Exchange of newsletters with other hospitals facilitates communication of differing approaches to the same problems and promotes information sharing. Publishing columns in State and national pharmaceutical journals is another means of sharing information as well as providing publicity to the hospital and the pharmacy.

Education

Involvement in education may vary considerably depending on the resources within the institution and whether it is a teaching facility. Since the minimum standards for institutional pharmacies identify a responsibility to both health professionals and patients regarding drug information, needs and resources for both groups should be evaluated and ranked by priority. Whether the programs are centralized through a drug information service or decentralized may depend on the availability of clinical practitioners. A program for development and dissemination of information for discharge counseling would be an example of a drug information service for patients. In-service programs for various groups can be coordinated through a drug information service and may help develop visibility for the service. In a teaching institution, training pharmacy students and other health professionals is an important responsibility that should involve the drug information center.

Drug Usage Evaluation

Of increasing importance is the relationship between drug use evaluation (DUE) and P&T committee activities. A successful DUE program requires planning, coordination, and involvement by the medical staff, particularly in the view of the standards of the Joint Commission on Accreditation of Healthcare Organizations (JCAHO). Drug information service involvement can include development of a yearly plan, provision of the literature support for development or refinement of criteria or indicators, and participation in data gathering and analysis. (A thorough discussion of this activity is provided in chapter 24 of this handbook.)

Investigational Drugs

In a facility in which investigational drugs are regularly used, sufficient emphasis must be given to providing appropriate information to all health professionals involved with their use. Various approaches to provide this service depend on the resources of the institution. The drug information service can provide the necessary liaison between the institutional review board, the P&T committee, and the pharmacy. The responsibility of coordinating the acquisition, development, and dissemination of appropriate information for investigational drugs lies with a drug information service. (For further information on investigational drugs, see chapter 23 of this handbook.)

Coordination of Reporting Programs

National programs like the Food and Drug Administration (FDA) Adverse Drug Reaction Reporting Program and the Drug Product Quality Reporting Programs (U.S. Pharmacopeia and FDA) depend primarily on the initiation of reports by individuals. Institutions should participate and coordinate this process from a central location to facilitate consistency and completeness in reporting and appropriate review before dissemination. Since these programs involve drugs, this function should be included as a drug information service. (The current emphasis of the JCAHO on adverse drug reaction reporting warrants the more detailed discussion of this process presented in chapter 26 of this handbook.)

Poison Information

This area may be viewed as a specialized component of drug information that has different requirements. (A decision to provide this service requires substantial commitment of resources, personnel, and time for an effective program and is described fully in chapter 32 of this handbook.)

The combining of drug and poison information functions into one center deserves comment. This has been mandated by statute in a few States. The 1986 survey of drug information centers showed a decline from previous surveys in the number affiliated with a poison control program. The combination of two such services has advantages and disadvantages. The obvious advantages for both programs include reduced space requirements. As discussed by Troutman and Wanke,[9] in the combined program, the drug information service will usually benefit from the communication and data management equipment as well as the increased staffing of the poison center. The poison center benefits from the literature search and evaluation skills of the drug information specialist.

Potential disadvantages in combining services include lack of development of maximal skills of staff members in either discipline and possible disputes over areas of responsibility. Since poison information calls usually require more immediate response, drug information inquiries may be unduly neglected unless appropriate priority is identified for staff. Poison information providers, particularly nonpharmacists, may feel added pressure in having to respond to drug information inquiries. The potential disadvantages to both services can be avoided with appropriate recognition and action.

Drug information services are defined primarily from a functional viewpoint. Inclusion of all or most of these functions should result in a total program as provided by a drug information center. However, certain drug information functions can be identified, developed, and implemented as part of a pharmacy service without a formally established drug information center. Two surveys of drug information centers provide a useful perspective on the kinds of services most often provided.[10,11]

In the environment in which a formal drug information center or service exists, all proposed functions should be integrated into a program with stated goals and common philosophy. If the resources cannot be committed to a complete program, certain functions may be identified and incorporated as part of the pharmacy service. The next section will discuss the development of a comprehensive drug information service. The same principles of development can be applied to the initiation of a specific function if resources or need do not exist for a comprehensive service.

CONSIDERATIONS IN DEVELOPING A PROGRAM

Careful, thoughtful identification of the goals of the program are required. Factors to consider include the areas of activity (service, education, research), the needs and priorities of the facility in establishing the program, the intended audience and its geographic location, and whether it will be a center or simply serve a single function.

Drug information programs may differ in their focus of activity. Each program desirably should encompass aspects of service, education, and research; however, the degree of emphasis will depend on the needs and priorities of the institution supporting the program. In a community hospital, service activities would likely receive the most emphasis, with education next, and probably limited activity in research. In a university teaching hospital, an equal balance among the three areas might be expected.

The needs of the institution for drug information services must be identified and priorities established, since it is unlikely, and probably unwise, for all activities to be initiated simultaneously. Need considerations may include a determination of the magnitude of formulary assistance required, the emphasis placed on drug use evaluation, and the current state of adverse drug reaction reporting. Another factor in addressing needs and priorities involves the existence and activity of clinical pharmacy practitioners. The support of clinical practitioners is an important priority for a drug information center. The breadth and depth of service may also be delineated by identifying the consumer services provided by the center. The geographic area to be served is also a part of this consideration. These decisions will assist in determining whether the focus will be institutional or regional and whether it will be only health professionals or involve information for consumers.

Finally, priorities of the personnel involved in determining the goals may differ. The drug information specialist, the pharmacy director, and the hospital administrator may not always agree on the top priority and each party should recognize this. For example, the drug information director may feel that day-to-day information requests should be the top priority. For the pharmacy director and hospital administrator, information provided to the P&T committee for developing a formulary or a drug use evaluation program may have a higher priority. Recognizing that compromise may be required, the drug information and pharmacy directors should work together to establish priorities and schedules for implementation. Certainly, the pharmacy director will have to support the proposed services when seeking resources to implement from administration.

JUSTIFICATION

Once the goals have been developed, justification for implementation is required. This applies whether it is a totally new program or whether it is a new service of an existing program. In preparing justification, support from the potential consumers of the service should be assessed to confirm the anticipated needs. Medical staff and/or nursing support is crucial for services initiated within an institution and should be solicited.

Another source of justification may be formal statements or guidelines adopted by such groups as the American Society of Hospital Pharmacists. Currently, statements exist on the formulary system, the pharmacy and therapeutics committee, and guidelines for formularies.[1] Recognition of services by national organizations can be used as an additional source of support. Requirements imposed by the JCAHO also provide justification, via its standards regarding desirability of a drug information center, drug use evaluation, and adverse drug reaction reporting.

Financial resources are important to the justification. Financial assistance may be available from a single group such as the hospital, or there may be joint partners involved such as the hospital and a college of pharmacy or a medical library. Where more than one group provides financial support, the relative contributions of the respective parties should be identified. Depending on the programs planned, outside sources of funding may be sought such as State support or third-party payers. These sources often support poison information services.

In general, most aspects of drug information services are viewed as a non-revenue-generating component of the pharmacy department. The acquisition and maintenance of the resources require a continuing budgetary commitment in addition to personnel and operating expenses. Budgets reported by centers have varied widely and probably depend on a number of site-specific factors.[11] However, opportunities for the service to generate revenue should be assessed. This could result from fee-for-service, provision of investigational drug services, outside consulting, or subscription services to other institutions.[3] In general, these charges do not generate sufficient revenue to support the total costs of the service.

Another method used for cost justification is the examination of potential dollar savings resulting from the activities of the service. Savings resulting from rational formulary decisions based on drug information center information should contribute to significant savings and result in meaningful cost justification.

RESOURCES

Developing a budget proposal requires assessment of needs for space, personnel, equipment, and information sources. In an existing facility, requirements for space should be estimated, even though space for operation may be identified only after the program is approved. Any anticipated renovation costs should be included in the budget. For a new facility, renovation cost is unnecessary, but the space requirements must still be identified.

Some considerations in identifying a desirable location include the work environment, accessibility to the medical library, and availability of teaching programs. Hospital-based centers are most common. The majority of centers (60 percent) are located in hospital pharmacy departments with others (13 percent) located in other areas of the hospital.[11] About 14 percent of centers are located in colleges of pharmacy and another 9 percent are located in medical libraries. The center should be located outside the mainstream of pharmacy operations where the environment is conducive to information retrieval and evaluation. Accessibility to medical library services is an important consideration where choice of space is available. A medical library may provide a desirable location in some settings. More space will be required if teaching is a primary function.

Tatro[12] has recommended guidelines that consider the number of people staffing the center and space requirements for information storage and retrieval. A drug information center staffed by one full-time equivalent pharmacist and a secretary should contain a minimum of 840 square feet.

Factors to consider in estimating personnel requirements include the scope of services expected. Where several functions are initiated and particularly if a significant educational component is involved, commitment of at least one individual's time is necessary. For the function of answering questions, it is important to have someone available to respond to calls during the hours of operation. Unless combined with a poison center, most centers operate on a standard daytime, weekday schedule with coverage provided after hours through a 24-hour pharmacy service or on-call personnel. Arrangements for additional coverage may include use of staff pharmacists, residents, and/or students. These individuals require appropriate training and orientation. Adequacy of secretarial services can be determined by the scope of services proposed.

Equipment needs include office furniture (desks, chairs, files, and shelving). If students use the resources, other work areas such as a table or counter may be needed. Shelving and file cabinets should be selected so that they can accommodate adequate expansion over a period of years. Computer equipment (hardware and software) is essential for use of commercial data bases and the creation of internal systems. A computer for word processing must be available to the secretary. A sufficient number of telephone lines and other telecommunication equipment requires careful evaluation. Minimally, two lines are needed, particularly if online computer literature searching is anticipated. Microfiche equipment may be considered, although trends have evolved more toward use of online computer or compact disk systems.

Factors important in selecting information sources include the scope of references needed, existing resources, and monetary resources available. Information resources can be divided into three categories: reference (tertiary), journals (primary), and indexing and abstracting (secondary) literature sources. Each component requires startup costs as well as annual recurring fees. With primary and secondary literature, these costs are likely to be the same with need to accommodate price increases. The startup cost for tertiary literature is likely to be higher because the whole reference is purchased, whereas the annual fee involves paying for supplements to some of the references.

Each component must be evaluated against existing resources. The institutional library services should be evaluated, exploring the opportunity for cooperation in resource acquisition as well as identifying the kinds of library services available (e.g., reprints, current awareness program, computer retrieval service). A readily available (within walking distance) medical library can reduce the need for certain types of resources such as journals and secondary literature sources. Some references may also be acquired by the library that will not need to be duplicated in the drug information center (e.g., references dealing with foreign products). Computer retrieval services are generally available through medical libraries, and needs for this resource should be evaluated. Development of a close working relationship with library personnel will provide mutual benefits for both parties.

The most recent surveys of drug information centers provide lists of the most popular information sources in each of the three categories.[10,11,13] Because of continual changes in price (usually higher), development of different features (e.g., supplements, availability on compact disk), and the availability of new references, these lists provide a starting point to evaluate the selection of resources.

The use of one or more computerized retrieval systems for secondary literature is essential for today's practice. More than 60 percent of centers used online computer searching in 1985.[13] With more systems available through online vendors and further development of compact disk technology, easy access to primary literature is a reality and should be used. A general discussion of online information retrieval in pharmacy, including considerations and approaches, may be helpful.[14] The cost of implementing and using online retrieval has been evaluated in some settings and was found beneficial.[15,16] Comparison of a pharmacist versus a medical librarian in doing literature searching for drug information requests has found the pharmacist's searches to be as useful.[17]

Opportunities exist to acquire certain resources on a no charge basis. For example, a number of publishers generously provide complimentary copies of certain journals to the drug information service and/or the pharmacy director. Pharmaceutical companies may also be a source for certain reference texts.

Each center or service must establish files. The degree to which this is done may vary greatly, depending on philosophies and the surrounding resources. The philosophies at two extremes might be to copy drug-related articles from an extensive number of journals and file these versus searching for information only after it is requested. Most approaches are a compromise of the two. The first scenario involves time, personnel (could be student or volunteer help), and expense (photocopying). Some of the articles may never be used. The second scenario avoids most of these factors, but the lag time with some literature sources becomes more of a problem in finding answers. The decision about what approach to take will be influenced by the library resources readily available and the location of the service. Most centers will probably employ a selective approach to filing and indexing of requests for retrieval.

PLANNING FOR IMPLEMENTATION

Once approval is obtained and an implementation date is set, policies and procedures for operation should be developed and/or refined. This includes a statement of the general philosophy of the service and identification of the specific role in various activities within the department. Procedures for handling phone calls should be developed, along with forms for documentation, particularly if several people will be involved in providing this service. A sample of some of the information that should be documented is provided in Appendix 31-A. A training program, encompassing both competence in use of resources and procedural matters, will help ensure consistency. Notifying the target audience about implementation of the service, particularly the function of answering questions, is a key element. Mechanisms to announce the new service might include a newsletter (if already established), separate and specially printed announcements distributed, posted, and/or mailed letters to key individuals, and in-service programs to groups within the target audience.

If the decision was made to implement a large-scale service with a variety of activities, priorities on the order of implementation also are needed. Assessment of the most pressing needs may indicate that the formulary/P&T committee aspect requires immediate priority with a newsletter to physicians to communicate the ongoing activities in this area. Implementation of other services may have to wait until these activities are established.

DOCUMENTATION AND QUALITY ASSURANCE

In the present environment of cost containment, documentation and evaluation of the service's activity, quality, and cost benefit are essential. This is especially important where new services are being extended to complement existing services. Continuing evaluation and documentation of established programs must be undertaken to justify the benefit of the program and to demonstrate the quality and cost benefit of proposed new services. Useful documentation includes the number and kinds of consumers, their location, and the nature of requests. A form that documents the nature of requests must be developed. These requests and responses should be indexed and/or filed for retrieval in response to similar questions in the future. Other documentation of the level of activity is provided by copies of newsletters or publications, copies of the formulary and P&T committee information, the number of adverse drug reaction reports, and the DUE activity. The number of calls provides an indication of growth (in a new service) or stability (in an established service) but does not measure total productivity.[3,12,18] Other statistics, such as the number of monographs prepared for the P&T committee, help reflect a broader scope of activity.

Some method for measuring outcome of services will likely be required. As with any service, quality or outcome measures are an important consideration. There are structure, process, and outcome elements of a drug information service. Approaches to a quality assurance program for the major activities in a drug information center have been described.[19,20] The programs described relied heavily on elements of structure and process with some elements of outcome. Assessment of outcomes regarding the impact of drug information services is difficult to accomplish objectively because of the presence of many other variables. The indicator log presented by two facilities may provide assistance to those developing quality assurance activities.[19,20] Several quality assurance programs have focused on the process of answering questions and reported different approaches to evaluating process and outcome.[21-24] Methods include user assessment of the impact of the information on patient care[21] and process evaluations including review by drug information specialists,[22] use of an external committee,[23] and anonymous test questions.[24] Good objective methods of assessment are difficult to design.

FUTURE DRUG INFORMATION PRACTICE

Drug information centers have not yet reached their maximum potential for development.[18,25] Regionalization of services provided by drug information centers is a viable approach to improving availability.[26,27] Opportunity exists for institutions to develop specific services even if a center is not feasible. Specific drug information functions such as P&T committee support are important in the institutional setting, and pharmacists, in general, should improve their ability to perform some of these functions.

The Specialty Practice Group on Drug Information of the ASHP provides an opportunity for interaction of practitioners who have a drug information focus. This group replaced the Special Interest Group, which addressed a number of drug information practice issues. The Special Interest Group developed criteria for a specialty residency in drug information, which was approved by the ASHP Board of Directors.[28] This training program will supply a core of individuals with specialized training in the area. The Special Interest Group activities addressed other areas, such as minimum standards and quality assurance. Minimum standards for personnel, physical facilities, organization, resources, and services were discussed by the Special Interest Group and have been incorporated as the basis for qualification of the site for residency training. Quality assurance guidelines (not an official ASHP guideline) were developed by the Special Interest Group in 1980 to offer technical assistance to ASHP members. Continued activities of this nature to be considered by the Specialty Practice Group will provide the leadership needed for a maturing drug information practice.

In the future, the number of drug information centers will likely increase and the opportunity and/or demand for some drug information services should be greater. The latter, particularly, provides for a more active role in determining drug use policy and an opportunity to fulfill some of the responsibilities identified in the minimum standards. Services provided by centers will undergo needed reevaluation and possible reorganization to better meet changing needs. Drug information services remain an important component of pharmacy practice.

REFERENCES

1. *Practice Standards of ASHP, 1989-90*. Bethesda, MD, American Society of Hospital Pharmacists, 1989, p 27-30.
2. Stolar MH: ASHP national survey of hospital pharmaceutical services, 1987. *Am J Hosp Pharm* 45:801-818, 1988.
3. Amerson AB, Wallingford DM: Twenty years' experience with drug information centers. *Am J Hosp Pharm* 40:1172-1178, 1983.
4. ASHP technical assistance bulletin on the evaluation of drugs for formularies. *Am J Hosp Pharm* 45:386-387, 1988.
5. Majerick PL, May JR, Longe RL, et al: Evaluation of pharmacy and therapeutics committee drug evaluation reports. *Am J Hosp Pharm* 42:1073-1076, 1985.
6. Almquist AF, Wolfgang AP, Perri M: Pharmacy newsletters—the journalistic approach. *Hosp Pharm* 23:974-975, 1988.
7. Murdoch L: Newsletters with impact. *Can J Hosp Pharm* 42(1):1, 1989.
8. Utt JK, Lewis KT: Using desktop publishing to enhance pharmacy publications (letter). *Am J Hosp Pharm* 45:1863-1864, 1988.
9. Troutman WG, Wanke LA: Advantages and disadvantages of combining poison control and drug information centers. *Am J Hosp Pharm* 40:1219-1222, 1983.
10. Rosenberg JM, Martino FP, Kirschenbaum HL, et al: Pharmacist-operated drug information centers in the United States, 1986. *Am J Hosp Pharm* 44:337-340, 1987.
11. Dombroski SR, Visconti JA: National audit of drug information centers. *Am J Hosp Pharm* 42:819-826, 1985.
12. Tatro DS: Establishing a drug information service. *Top Hosp Pharm Mgt* 2(1):74-86, 1982.
13. Michel DJ, Knodel LC: Use of bibliographic, abstracting and computer resources in drug information centers. *Am J Hosp Pharm* 45:624-625, 1988.
14. Perry CA: Online information retrieval in pharmacy and related fields. *Am J Hosp Pharm* 43:1509-1524, 1986.
15. Schneiweiss F: Use and cost analysis of online literature searching in a university-based drug information center. *Am J Hosp Pharm* 40:254-256, 1983.
16. Souney PF, Churchill WW, Kaul AF: Cost of implementing and maintaining a hospital-pharmacy-based online literature search system. *Am J Hosp Pharm* 42:2496-2498, 1985.
17. Wanke LA, Hewison NS: Comparative usefulness of MEDLINE searches performed by a drug information pharmacist and by medical librarians. *Am J Hosp Pharm* 45:2507-2510, 1988.
18. Amerson AB: Effectiveness of drug information centers. *CRC Crit Rev Med Informatics* 1:135-148, 1986.
19. Park BA, Benderev KP: Quality assurance program for a drug information center. *Am J Hosp Pharm* 42:2180-2184, 1985.
20. Moody ML: Revising a drug information center quality assurance program to conform to Joint Commission standards. *Am J Hosp Pharm* 47:792-794, 1990.
21. Repchinsky CA, Masuhara EJ: Quality assurance program for a drug information center. *Drug Intell Clin Pharm* 21:816-820, 1987.
22. Wheeler-Usher DH, Hermann FF, Wanke LA: Problems encountered in using written criteria to assess drug information responses. *Am J Hosp Pharm* 47:795-797, 1990.
23. Smith CJ, Sylvia LM: External quality assurance committee for drug information services. *Am J Hosp Pharm* 47:787-791, 1990.
24. Woodward CT, Stevenson JG, Poremba A: Assessing the quality of pharmacist answers to telephone drug information questions. *Am J Hosp Pharm* 47:798-799, 1990.

25. Rosenberg JM: Drug information centers: Future trends. *Am J Hosp Pharm* 40:1213-1215, 1983.
26. Skoutakis VA, Wojciechowski NJ, Carter CA, et al: Drug information center network: Need, effectiveness, and cost justification. *Drug Intell Clin Pharm* 21:49-56, 1987.
27. Golightly LK, Davis AG, Budwitz WJ, et al: Documenting the activity and effectiveness of a regional drug information center. *Am J Hosp Pharm* 45:356-361, 1988.
28. ASHP supplemental standard and learning objectives for residency training in drug information practice. *Am J Hosp Pharm* 39:1970-1972, 1982.

Appendix 31-A

SAMPLE DOCUMENTATION FORM FOR A DRUG INFORMATION SERVICE

Drug Information Request
Drug Information Center

( ) Medical Center　　( ) Phone　　( ) Mail
( ) Nonmedical Center　　( ) Personal Visit

Request # ____________
Date: ____________
Time: ____________
By: ____________

Inquirer ____________
Address ____________

Phone ____________

RPH　　Student
MD　　Consumer
RN　　Other ____________
Dentist

Question (include patient information and/or background)

Response (continue on back if necessary)

References used to access information (include all references searched)

Disposition　　Estimated time in preparation ____________

Date: ____________　( ) Phone Call
Time: ____________　( ) Mail
By: ____________

Materials Sent:
( ) Reprints　　( ) Letter
( ) Abstracts　　( ) Bibliography

Classification of Request　　Index Term ____________

( ) Identification
( ) Availability
( ) Pharmacokinetics
( ) Pregnancy/Nursing
( ) Interactions
( ) Formulation
( ) Other ____________
( ) Adverse Reactions/Side Effects
( ) Toxicity/Poisoning
( ) Dosage/Administration
( ) Therapeutic Use/Efficacy
( ) Compatibility/Stability

Drug Information Center Request:

CHAPTER 32

Poison Centers

GARY M. ODERDA

A mother finds her 2-year-old child with a bottle of children's vitamins with iron. Tablets are spread all over the floor. There are tablet fragments in the child's mouth, and she has some in her hand.

A young woman stops by her mother's house on her way home from work. The mother takes aspirin for chronic arthritis. She appears confused and has an elevated respiratory rate.

A young man has been welding galvanized metal at work. He began feeling ill during the afternoon. At home after work, he develops symptoms he thinks are the "flu."

What do these people have in common? What should they, or their caretakers, do?

These are three examples of the types of calls received every day by poison centers across the United States. Each caller has an acute need for information. Health professionals who work at poison centers are trained to take a history by telephone, consult information sources, assess the situation, and make recommendations to the caller. In many cases, no treatment is required. In some, home treatment is appropriate. In the remainder, treatment in a health care facility is necessary.

POISON EPIDEMIOLOGY

When most people think of poisoning, they think of children. Although children are the most common victims of unintentional poisonings, most serious poisonings, and most poisoning deaths, are in adults. The American Association of Poison Control Centers (AAPCC) maintains a voluntary national data collection system. The system began collecting data in 1983 with 16 pilot centers. In 1989, 70 centers participated and reported 1,581,540 poison exposures.[1] These centers served 182.4 million people, or 73 percent of the population of the United States. Extrapolating from this percentage, approximately 2.1 million poisonings were reported to poison centers in 1989.[1] The percentage of actual poison exposures that are reported to poison centers varies from center to center, and it is difficult to estimate.

Most poison exposures are in children. During 1989, 61.1 percent were 5 years of age and under.[1] Almost all of these are unintentional. Poisonings are also common in older children and adults. The percentage of intentional poison exposures, such as suicide and drug abuse, increases in older age groups. Most poisonings occur in the home (91.9 percent) and involve one substance (93.7 percent).[1]

When one thinks of poisoning, oral exposures come to mind. AAPCC data show that poisonings occur from a variety of other routes such as dermal (7.0 percent), ophthalmic (5.9 percent), inhalation (5.5 percent), and parenteral (0.3 percent).

Most poison exposures require no treatment or can be treated at home; approximately one poison victim in four requires treatment in a health care facility. Overall, 72.2 percent of poison exposures were treated in a non-health-care facility; 25.3 percent did require health care facility treatment, and in the remaining 2.5 percent, the treatment site was unknown.[1]

If poison centers did not exist, many of these patients would likely use emergency transportation and an emergency room. These unnecessary emergency room visits would result in significant additional health care costs. Poison centers save far more than their annual operating costs from health care savings in preventing unnecessary emergency room visits alone. In a recent study, King and Palmisano[2] measured the impact of closing a regional poison center on health care expenditures. The Louisiana Poison Center closed on October 31, 1988, as a result of significant cutbacks in available funding. Minimal poison information was provided by the Children's Hospital of Alabama in Birmingham until June 30, 1989. Before the Louisiana center closed, triage patterns in Louisiana and Alabama were almost identical. After the closing, self-referral to emergency rooms for poisoning increased fourfold in Louisiana compared to Alabama, whereas the home management rate in Louisiana was half that in Alabama. Charges for health care were estimated to be between $300,000 and $1,400,000 depending on the model employed; the savings from closing the center was $400,000.

Fortunately, most poison exposures do not result in significant morbidity or mortality, as evidenced in table 32-1.

Classification into "unknown-nontoxic" and "unknown-potentially toxic" is done by the person answering the call. These two classifications are used when followup data are not obtained to determine the outcome with certainty. Unknown-nontoxic is used when no toxic effects are expected. Unknown-potentially toxic is used when toxic effects are anticipated.

The types of agents commonly ingested are those most commonly found around the home. These include prescription and nonprescription drugs and a variety of other agents. The top 16 categories of agents for 1989 are shown in table 32-2.

Table 32-1. Medical outcome of human poison exposures

Medical outcome	*No. of cases*	*% of cases*
No effect	519,891	32.9
Minor effect	369,331	23.4
Moderate effect	37,685	2.4
Major effect	4,509	0.3
Death	590	0.0
Unknown—nontoxic*	505,955	32.0
Unknown—Potentially toxic†	103,661	6.6
Unrelated effect	37,893	2.4
Unknown	2,025	0.1
Total	1,581,540	100.0

*No followup provided because exposure was assessed as nontoxic.
†Patient lost to followup. Exposure was assessed as potentially toxic.

Table 32-2. Categories of poisonings

Category	*No. of Exposures*	*Percentage of exposures*
Cleaning substances	160,652	10.2
Analgesics	160,951	10.2
Cosmetics	130,207	8.2
Cough and cold preparations	90,798	5.7
Pesticides	60,045	3.8
Bites/Envenomations	58,750	3.7
Hydrocarbons	58,616	3.7
Topicals	56,920	3.6
Foreign bodies	56,356	3.6
Chemicals	53,011	3.4
Sedative hypnotics/Antipsychotics	50,883	3.2
Antimicrobials	50,236	3.2
Food poisoning	48,336	3.1
Alcohols	43,549	2.8
Vitamins	40,922	2.6

Both tables reprinted with permission from Litovitz TL, Schmitz BF, Baily KM: 1989 annual report of the American Association of Poison Control Centers National Data Collection System. *Am J Emerg Med* 8:394-442, 1990.

POISON CENTER HISTORY AND REGIONALIZATION

The first poison center was established in Chicago in 1953 by the Illinois chapter of the American Academy of Pediatrics. The purpose of the center was to provide product formulation information to pediatricians who were treating poisoned children. Prior to that time, no resource was available that maintained formulations of commercial products. Information was provided only to physicians. During the 1950's and 1960's, poison centers rapidly proliferated. By the mid-1960's, there were approximately 600 poison centers in the United States. Most had no staff, no budget, and limited resources. Distribution of poison centers was inconsistent. Illinois alone had more than 100 centers. To avoid unnecessary duplication of services and to develop significant expertise within the centers, a move toward regionalization of poison centers occurred during the 1970's and 1980's.

The goal was to produce a national network of approximately 100 poison centers across the United States. Each center would serve between 1 and 10 million people. The service area would be as small as a single city in densely populated areas, such as New York City, or multiple States in less densely populated areas. Each of these centers would maintain a professional staff of health professionals, provide 24-hour service, and would have adequate resources to provide a quality service.

A recent survey of poison centers was conducted by the American Association of Poison Control Centers.[3] A total of 350 possible centers was identified, and a survey was mailed to each one; 277 centers returned the completed survey. An initial analysis indicated that many of these centers provided minimal service. From this study, however, came a list of centers that met the following criteria: (1) regional poison centers meeting the AAPCC criteria, (2) nonregional centers handling more than 5,000 human exposure cases annually, or (3) AAPCC member centers handling fewer than 5,000 calls per year. A total of 104 centers met one of these inclusion criteria. Of these, questionnaires were complete enough to allow analysis in 99 cases; 36 of these centers were certified regional centers. Table 32-3 summarizes the differences between regional and nonregional centers.

Table 32-3. Comparison of regional and nonregional centers

	Regional centers, No.	*Nonregional centers, No.*
Population served, range	1.1 - 17 million	0.1 - 7.5 million
No. of human exposures handled in 1988, range	12,931 – 63,488	399 – 50,333
Mean No. of poison information specialists	9.48	3.44
Mean amount of direct State support	$318,387	$193,178
Mean total center budget	$633,983	$233,512
Mean cost per human exposure call answer	$20.58	$19.45
Mean penetrance, No. of human exposure cases/1,000 population served	20.58	9.37

Adapted with permission from Manoguerra AS: The status of poison control centers in the United States—1989: A report from the American Association of Poison Control Centers. *Vet Hum Toxicol* 33:131-150, 1991.

REGIONAL VERSUS NONREGIONAL CENTERS

One important consideration in the development of a regional poison center is the impact on quality. Regional poison centers manage a larger volume of cases and have dedicated staff with better access to resources that should allow a regional poison center to do a better job of providing information. This hypothesis was tested in a study conducted by Thompson et al.[4] A pseudorandom sample of 15 regional centers and 15 nonregional centers was selected. Informed consent for the study was obtained from each of the centers. Two calls were made to each center. One was made between 10 a.m. and 2:00 p.m. and the other between 10:00 p.m. and 2 a.m. A standard question was developed that required probing by the poison center staff to obtain all necessary information. An expert panel was used to provide a consensus of all information that needed to be obtained before the call was answered. In this test situation, the patient had ingested 220 mg/kg of aspirin, an amount that requires treatment. Information was provided by the centers as shown in table 32-4.

Table 32-4. Responses to test question[4]

Recommendation	*Regional poison centers, No. of calls (%)*	*Nonregional poison centers, No. of calls (%)*
Treatment	28 (93.3)	20 (66.7)
No treatment	2 (6.7)	4 (13.3)
No decision	0 (0)	6 (20)

The correctness of the information provided was also evaluated, as depicted in table 32-5.

Table 32-5. Evaluation of responses[4]

Management	*Regional poison centers, No. of calls (%)*	*Nonregional poison centers, No. of calls (%)*
Correct	28 (93.3)	12 (40)
Incorrect	2 (6.7)	18 (60)

It can be seen that there is a risk of obtaining incorrect information. Other differences were noted in the amount of history obtained, the proficiency in obtaining the history, and the likelihood that a followup call would be made. Some nonregional centers recommended ineffective or potentially dangerous procedures to induce vomiting, including mechanical stimulation, raw eggs, mustard water, and saltwater.

POISON CENTER SERVICES

Poison centers provide a variety of services to the communities they serve. First and most important, they respond to questions about poisoned patients 24 hours per day. These include calls from both health professionals and the general public. Calls from health professionals generally involve patients who are already being treated in the health care system. The caller usually wants information on product ingredients, expected toxic effects, and recommendations for treatment. Calls from the general public require the specialist in poison information to take a history over the telephone, consult information sources, assess the toxicity of the case, and make recommendations. These recommendations may include doing nothing, home therapy such as ipecac syrup, or treatment in a health care facility. When patients are referred to a health care facility, the poison center calls the hospital to provide information on expected toxicity and recommended treatment.

Poison centers provide a significant role in education. This includes education of health professionals and the general public. Health professional education is provided by teaching courses for health professional students and continuing education for practicing health professionals. Educational experiences for the general public are generally aimed at teaching poison prevention and increasing awareness of the poison center and its services. Poison centers use a variety of mechanisms to educate the general public, including face-to-face presentations, distribution of brochures and other materials, and use of the media to deliver their message.

STAFFING

The key to providing quality service is a core of well-trained health professionals who serve as specialists in poison information. Pharmacists, nurses, or physicians can function in this role. Most centers use either pharmacists or nurses, or a combination of the two. The AAPCC maintains certification programs for specialists in poison information. Pharmacists, nurses, or physicians working as specialists in poison information who have at least 1 year of experience and have answered at least 2,000 calls may sit for the exam. All poison centers should have at least one certified specialist in poison information on duty at all times. A minimum of five or six full-time specialists in poison information are required to provide 24-hour per day single coverage. Many centers use other poison information providers to ensure additional telephone coverage. These individuals can be health professional students or others not qualified to become specialists in poison information. Other poison information providers work under the direct supervision of specialists in poison information.

Medical control for poison center services is provided by a medical director. The medical director must be a physician with a demonstrated interest and expertise in medical toxicology. At a minimum, duties include protocol review and approval, audit of poison center recommendations, and availability for consultation on difficult cases. Medical directors should provide at least a 25 percent commitment of their effort to poison center activities.

An administrative director must be available to provide overall direction of the program. The medical director may also serve as the administrative director. In many cases, pharmacists, and particularly those with a Pharm.D. degree and specialized training, serve as directors or administrative directors of poison centers.

All poison centers must provide a public education program. For these programs to function efficiently, a public education coordinator should be available. In many cases, a specialist in poison information can fulfill this function. Background as a health professional is not essential. It is more important that this individual have an excellent background in education, including development of objectives and materials, and the interest and skills to be a good teacher.

BUDGET AND ADMINISTRATIVE LOCATION

Most commonly, poison centers function as administrative components of a hospital. They may be a part of an emergency medicine program or a service offered by the hospital pharmacy. A variety of other possible administrative structures exist. A few poison centers are freestanding, nonprofit corporations. Some are divisions or departments of pharmacy schools. Poison centers should be designated by an appropriate health agency, such as a State or local health department.

Budgets vary widely, depending on the size of the program, but are generally at least $400,000 and may be in excess of $1,000,000. It is essential that a stable source of continued funding be identified. Many poison centers have significant funding difficulty. This takes considerable energy of center personnel that can be more productively used. A recent survey by the AAPCC identified that the average cost of answering a call was approximately $20.50. The volume of calls reported to poison centers that participate in the AAPCC data collection system ranged from 202 to 66,417 in 1989, with a mean of 22,593.[1]

DATA COLLECTION

The AAPCC maintains a voluntary national data collection system. The system is flexible in that it allows participating poison centers to submit data in a variety of ways. Most centers use a combined form that contains a medical record and a scannable data entry form. Data are entered on the forms using a special high-carbon, ink felt tip pen. These forms are then scanned by an optical scanner, which creates an electronic file on diskette. The scanning process includes error-checking routines to ensure that data were accurately entered. Once scanned, the data are available for local analysis and are submitted to the AAPCC to be entered into the national data base.

The AAPCC data base is used in several ways. It describes the national experience with poisoning. A summary report is published each fall in the *American Journal of Emergency Medicine*.[1] The data set is a powerful research tool. Companies can purchase data describing the poisoning experience of their products. (For further information on this data base, contact the AAPCC at 202-784-4666.)

Several systems are currently available that allow direct entry of poison center cases by using a computer. These systems have the advantage of eliminating the form bubbling and scanning steps. All data entered are instantly available for analysis. The software then abstracts the information entered and produces a file that is AAPCC-compatible. Using technology for this purpose offers significant promise for the future. At present, these programs are still being evaluated and tested. Their overall utility will be shown as they enter wider use.

Poison center forms are considered medical records and must be stored and protected in a manner consistent with requirements for other medical record storage. Once forms are completed by poison center staff, they are audited as part of a quality assurance program by administrative staff and/or the medical director. They must be filed so they can be located when needed. This may be necessary to evaluate protocols, for research purposes, or for medicolegal reasons. Poison center call volume is generally large; storage of forms can present a significant problem. At an annual call volume of 50,000, a center will fill two four-drawer file cabinets each year. The length of time forms must be stored differs from State to State. The most restrictive require that medical records be stored for 7 years after the patient reaches the age of majority. Since more than half of poison center patients are under the age of 5, this means that forms must be stored, and be locatable, for 20 to 25 years. Because this volume of paper becomes unmanageable, most poison centers use alternative means of storage. Microfilming has been the standard. New devices that scan the forms and write the data onto compact disks have become available and are ideal for this purpose.

POISON CENTER CERTIFICATION

The AAPCC provides a program that certifies regional poison centers. This process ensures that certified centers meet minimum criteria as designated by the association. The criteria address the following major areas:

1. Designation by appropriate public health officials (e.g., State health department) to serve the designated region.
2. Demonstration that the center is used appropriately throughout the region.
3. Adequate staffing by specialists in poison information. At least one specialist in poison information (pharmacist, nurse, or physician) must be present in the center at all times. An adequate number of staff must be available to adequately answer all incoming calls. The call volume per available full-time equivalent (FTE) staff member should not exceed 5,500. The minimum number of staff needed to answer a volume of up to 30,000 calls per year is 5.4 FTE.
4. Demonstration of the role of the physician medical director in the operation of the center. The medical director should devote 0.5 FTE to toxicology, of which at least 10 hours per week of effort must be devoted to poison center activities.
5. Adequate training and experience of an administrative director or managing director, and demonstrated responsibility for operation of the center.
6. Demonstration of adequate programs in professional and public education.
7. A good working relationship with all treatment facilities in the center's region, an understanding of analytical toxicology services, and description of the patient transportation system available in its area.
8. Participation in the AAPCC data collection system. Appendix 32-A describes certified regional centers by State as of May 1, 1990.

DEVELOPING A POISON CENTER

The most important step in determining if a poison center should be developed is determining if there is a need. If a certified regional center already exists in the target area, there should be no need to start an additional center. If a noncertified regional center or a local poison center is present, it may make sense to work collaboratively to gain the additional resources necessary to improve the existing program, rather than start a new center. If a need exists, a coalition of key players necessary to put the program together should be developed. This would include representatives from health departments, professional groups (e.g., medical society), schools of pharmacy and medicine, the hospital administrator, and chiefs of hospital departments that may be involved (pharmacy, medicine, pediatrics, emergency medicine). This group is responsible for providing advice for proceeding with the development of a poison center and developing a process for implementation. A budget must be developed, and a stable funding source, or group of funding sources, must be identified. Poison centers are expensive. Without a long-term funding commitment, the poison center will struggle for survival from year to year. This seriously erodes the time and energy necessary to build and maintain a quality program.

SUMMARY

Poison centers play an important role in the health care system. In addition to promoting optimum care for poisoned patients, they save health care dollars by preventing unnecessary emergency room visits. Poison centers also have significant involvement in prevention efforts, education, and research. Pharmacists play an important role in the operation and staffing of poison centers.

REFERENCES

1. Litovitz TL, Schmitz BF, Bailey KM: 1989 annual report of the American Association of Poison Control Centers National Data Collection System. *Am J Emerg Med* 8:394-442, 1990.
2. King WD, Palmisano PA: Poison control centers: Can their value be measured? *Southern Med J* 84:722-726, 1991.
3. Manoguerra AS: The status of poison control centers in the United States - 1989: A report from the American Association of Poison Control Centers. *Vet Hum Toxicol* 33:131-150, 1991.
4. Thompson DF, Trammel HT, Robertson NJ, et al: Evaluation of regional and non-regional poison centers. *New Engl J Med* 308:191-194, 1983.

Appendix 32-A

REGIONAL CENTERS BY STATE

State	City	Center name	Emergency phone numbers
Alabama	Tuscaloosa	Alabama Poison Center	205-345-0600 800-462-0800 (AL only)
	Birmingham	Children's Hospital of Alabama Regional Poison Center	205-939-9202 205-933-4050 800-292-6678
Arizona	Tucson	Arizona Poison and Drug Information Center	800-362-0101 (AZ only) 602-626-6016
	Phoenix	Samaritan Regional Poison Center	602-253-3334
California	Fresno	Fresno Regional Poison Control Center	209-445-1222
	Los Angeles	Los Angeles County Medical Association Regional Poison Center	213-664-2121 213-484-5151
	San Diego	San Diego Regional Poison Center	619-543-6000 800-876-4766
	San Francisco	San Francisco Bay Area Regional Poison Center	415-476-6600 800-523-2222 (CA only)
	Sacramento	UC Davis Regional Poison Control Center	916-734-3692 800-342-9293
Colorado	Denver	Rocky Mountain Poison Center	303-629-1123 800-332-3073 (CO only) 800-442-2702 (WY only) 800-525-9083 (MT only)
Florida	Tampa	The Florida Poison Information Center	813-253-4444 800-282-3171 (FL only)
Georgia	Atlanta	The Georgia Poison Control Center	404-589-4400
Kentucky	Louisville	Kentucky Regional Poison Center of Kosair Children's Hospital	502-589-8222 800-722-5725
Maryland	Baltimore	Maryland Poison Center	301-528-7701 800-492-2414 (MD only)
Massachusetts	Boston	Massachusetts Poison Control System	617-232-2120 800-682-9211
Michigan	Grand Rapids	Blodgett Regional Poison	800-632-2727
	Detroit	Children's Hospital of Michigan Regional Poison Center	315-745-5711 800-462-6642 (MI only)
Minnesota	Minneapolis	Hennepin Regional Poison Center	612-347-3141
	St. Paul	Minnesota Regional Poison Center	612-221-2113
Missouri	St. Louis	Cardinal Glennon Children's Hospital	800-392-9111 800-366-8888 314-772-5200
Nebraska	Omaha	Mid-Plains Poison Center	402-390-5555 800-955-9119
New Jersey	Newark	New Jersey Poison Information and Education System	800-962-1253
New Mexico	Albuquerque	New Mexico Poison and Drug Information Center	505-843-2881 800-432-6866
New York	East Meadow	Long Island Regional Poison Control Center	516-542-2323
	New York	New York Poison Control Center	212-340-4494

State	City	Center name	Emergency phone numbers
Ohio	Columbus	Central Ohio Poison Center	800-682-7625 614-221-2672
	Cincinnati	Regional Poison Control System and Cincinnati Drug and Poison Information Center	513-558-5111
Oregon	Portland	Oregon Poison Center	503-494-8968 800-452-7165
Pennsylvania	Philadelphia	Delaware Valley Regional Poison Control Program	215-386-2100
	Pittsburgh	Pittsburgh Poison Center	412-681-6669
Rhode Island	Providence	Rhode Island Poison Center	401-277-5727
Texas	Dallas	North Texas Poison Center	214-591-5000 800-441-0040
	Galveston	Texas State Poison Center	409-765-1420 713-654-1701 800-392-8548 (CA only)
Utah	Salt Lake City	Intermountain Regional Poison Center	800-456-7707 (UT only) 801-581-2151
Washington, D.C.	Washington, D.C.	National Capital Poison Center	202-625-3333
West Virginia	Charleston	West Virginia Poison Center	304-348-4211 800-642-3625 (WV only)

Reprinted with permission from Manoguerra AS: The status of poison control centers in the United States — 1989: A report from the American Association of Poison Control Centers. *Vet Hum Toxicol* 33:131-150, 1991.

CHAPTER 33

Clinical Services

PAMELA A. PLOETZ and LARRY E. BOH

HISTORICAL BACKGROUND

The early concept of clinical pharmacy services was embedded in the philosophy that pharmacists should use their professional knowledge to foster the safe and appropriate use of drugs in and by patients while working with other members of the health professions.[1] This concept has been supported in the literature since the 1960's with extensive documentation of various types of clinical activities and services of pharmacists. The early documentation included examples of the pharmacist's role in solving medication errors or adverse drug reactions, detecting drug-drug or drug-laboratory interactions or IV admixture incompatibilities, and drug-induced diseases.[2] At this time, much of the enthusiasm for "patient-oriented practice" focused on what Brodie[3] termed "drug-use control." This led many practitioners to advocate their role in terms of a product and not necessarily for the welfare of patients.

Subsequently, the literature reported on the expansion of the pharmacist's clinical role to include therapeutic drug monitoring, pharmacokinetic dosing, patient education, and medication counseling, medication histories, drug utilization review, emergency medical care, and provision of drug information to other health professionals.[4] Finally, recognition of the pharmacist's clinical role in these activities followed, as evidenced by reports of acceptance by physicians, nurses, and even the reimbursement agencies in the private and public sector.[4,5]

To further foster the "clinical pharmacy" movement, the American Society of Hospital Pharmacists (ASHP) Research and Education Foundation and ASHP conducted a national consensus conference, commonly referred to as the "Hilton Head Conference," in February 1985. The conference objectives were (1) to explore the extent to which the profession of pharmacy has established goals with respect to clinical practice, (2) to assess the current status of the clinical practice of pharmacy and pharmacy education, and (3) to identify practical ways for advancing clinical practice.[6] Participants included pharmacy practitioners and educators with observers from medicine, nursing, and hospital administration. A major outcome of this conference was a consensus that the goals of "clinical pharmacy" are indistinguishable from those of "pharmacy" and that pharmacy should be thought of more in terms of a responsibility for patient care outcomes than specific functions.[6]

Members in attendance at this conference also identified a variety of barriers to providing effective clinical pharmacy services. There was general consensus that many pharmacy directors are unable to provide effective leadership to their staff. At the same time, there was agreement that the practice of pharmacy lacks an agreed-upon philosophy of the practice of pharmacy and what the standards of pharmacy practice are. This poor understanding by the profession was also felt to be extended to the consumer, who had a poorer understanding of the services that could be offered by pharmacists. This perspective is critical, since there was also a consensus that the pharmacist's self-image is a barrier to effective clinical practice.[6] Together, these and the other barriers are important to understand as we seek to foster the advancement of the clinical pharmacy philosophy.

PREVENTION OF DRUG MISADVENTURES

To achieve this goal, *all* pharmacists who provide clinical pharmaceutical services were encouraged to focus their attention on *patient care outcomes*. To do this, practitioners were encouraged to assume a "patient advocacy role" in ensuring that patients receive the maximal benefit from their medications while minimizing the drugs' harmful effects. These harmful effects, termed "drug misadventures" by Manasee,[7] can include drug interactions (e.g., antacids-antibiotics, digoxin-quinidine); excessive therapeutic effects (e.g., hypoglycemic coma from insulin, major bleeds from heparin or warfarin therapy); pathologic reactions that are either allergic or nonallergic (e.g., teratogenic, carcinogenic, mutagenic); unwanted pharmacologic effects (e.g., diarrhea, constipation, dry mouth, blurred vision, abdominal pain); or superinfections that occur with antibiotic therapy.[7-9]

PHARMACEUTICAL CARE

To encompass pharmacy's traditional role as a dispenser of medications and this new philosophy termed "clinical pharmacy," which advocates the practitioner's role in enhancing patient care outcomes, Hepler[10,11] proposed the concept of "pharmaceutical care." This term was intended to define the relationship *between* the pharmacist and the patient. Within this framework, the pharmacist accepts responsibility and accountability for the drug use control functions and provides services for the purpose of achieving specific and definite outcomes that improve the patient's health and, ultimately, quality of life.[11] These outcomes can be broadly thought of as (1) preventing drug misadventures, (2) minimizing or eliminating patient symptoms, (3) modifying or curing a disease process, or (4) identifying and resolving drug-related problems.

Pharmaceutical care is a process that involves the pharmacist's participation and cooperation with a patient, health care providers, and other professionals. To be effective and successful, it cannot be performed without these individuals' involvement. Pharmacists must define and redefine their role to focus on assisting in designing, implementing, and monitoring a therapeutic plan. The plan should not be diagnostic but medication based and directed at achieving specific therapeutic outcomes for the patient. The three major functions of pharmaceutical care are (1) to identify potential and actual drug-related problems, (2) to resolve actual drug-related problems, and (3) to prevent potential drug-related problems.[12]

TYPES OF DRUG-RELATED PROBLEMS

In providing pharmaceutical care, pharmacists must constantly focus attention on drug-related problems, which have the potential to occur in an institutional setting whenever a medication is prescribed. These problems, which can or actually do occur, ultimately interfere with the patient in achieving optimum therapeutic benefit from the medication. To assist the practitioner who provides pharmaceutical care with recognition of medication-related problems, Strand and colleagues[13] have identified eight categories:

1. *Untreated indications.* The patient's medical condition requires drug therapy but he or she is not receiving a drug for that indication. An example of this may include a patient who has hypertension or glaucoma but is taking no medications for this problem.
2. *Drug therapy used when not indicated.* The patient is receiving a medication for a medical condition that does not require drug therapy, such as obesity.
3. *Improper drug selection.* Drug therapy is indicated but the patient receives the wrong medication. The most common example is a patient with a bacterial infection that is resistant to the medication the patient was prescribed.
4. *Subtherapeutic dose.* The medical condition requires drug therapy and the patient receives the correct medication, but the dose is subtherapeutic, as may be observed with too low an insulin dose.
5. *Failure to receive drug.* The patient's medical condition requires drug therapy, but for pharmaceutical, psychological, sociological, or economic reasons, the patient does not get the medication. The most common example is noncompliance with hypertensive therapy.
6. *Overdose or toxic dose.* The patient has a medical problem that is being treated with too much of the correct drug (toxicity). Common examples include fluid overload secondary to intravenous fluid replacement, or hyperkalemia from too much potassium.
7. *Adverse drug reaction.* The patient has a medical problem that is the result of an adverse drug reaction or side effect. The reaction, whether expected or unexpected, such as a gastric ulcer secondary to anti-inflammatory medications or a rash with an antibiotic, requires the patient to seek medical attention.
8. *Drug interaction.* The patient has a medical problem that is the result of a drug-drug, drug-food, or drug-laboratory interaction. Most common are intravenous incompatibilities such as those that occur in total parenteral nutrition solutions or intravenous (IV) fluids.

These eight examples are not intended to be all inclusive, but with this list of potential problems, practitioners interested in providing quality pharmaceutical care can begin to focus their efforts.

COMPONENTS OF A PATIENT DATA BASE

These clinical services, which are based on influencing patient outcomes, should be viewed as *independent* of the type of patient, practice area, site, or location of the service provided. The provision of clinical services to pediatric and geriatric patients or hospitalized and ambulatory patients still relies on the same critical elements of an accurate and complete patient data base. This data base must contain, at a minimum, patient information in the following areas:

1. *Allergic or adverse drug reaction history.* An accurate and complete history of allergic or adverse reactions to medications or foods to which the patient has been exposed. Exposure to the commonly used medications such as penicillin, sulfas, aspirin, local anesthetics, iodine, narcotics, and radiocontrast dyes should be identified. Additionally, information on the type of reaction, when the reaction occurred, how it was managed, and if the patient has been rechallenged must be documented.
2. *Medical and medication history.* This should include a brief but complete listing of past and current medical problems that require medication therapy. Medication therapy (prescription and nonprescription) used in the past and currently should also be documented.
3. *Renal function.* Identification of the status of the patient's renal function using serum creatinine to calculate creatinine clearance or using an actual measured creatinine clearance is critical for providing dosing adjustments. Information on whether the renal function is stable or changing will also provide useful information for dosing guidelines.
4. *Hepatic function.* Generally, laboratory tests commonly referred to as "liver enzymes" provide a poor indication of function, and they should be used in concert with the patient's medical history or signs of liver dysfunction observed during the physical examination. These data are especially important for providing dosing information on medications that undergo extensive hepatic metabolism (e.g., theophylline) or first-pass metabolism (e.g., propanolol).
5. *Weight and height.* These data are critical for providing dosing information and calculation of renal function (e.g., creatinine clearance).
6. *Age.* The patient's chronological age and estimated physiologic age are important in identifying changes that may occur with the disposition of medications and disease state manifestations.
7. *Insurance information.* The pharmacist's awareness of a patient's insurance carrier is rapidly becoming important, since issues of reimbursement may ultimately influence the patient's compliance with the prescribed regimen.

Once the data base information becomes documented and assessments are made, the pharmacist must determine how the data base will be continually updated. This updating is critical since data base information changes with time and as the patient's therapeutic regimen becomes modified. Therefore, decisions on how to update this data base must be individualized and not performed according to a predetermined schedule. Regardless, the data base must remain current and accurate in order to be valid and useful for providing clinical services.

CLASSIFICATION OF CLINICAL PHARMACY SERVICES

Since clinical pharmacy services or programs offered by an institutional pharmacy program are embedded in the concept of pharmaceutical care, they must be aimed at meeting various societal needs.[11,14] Specifically, the clinical service should positively alter a patient's drug therapy outcome. To assist practitioners with identifying the types of clinical pharmacy services, the ASHP has issued a position statement on the pharmacist's clinical role.[15] Four groups have been proposed for evaluating clinical pharmacy services.[16] This grouping (see Appendix 33-A), increases in complexity from Class I to Class IV. It requires an increase in the specialization of the practitioners providing them.

Class I clinical services are generally viewed as the foundation of any clinical program. These services are not focused on any particular patient but are embedded in any hospital-wide program that purports to influence the positive outcomes of drug therapy. These programs often are performed by all pharmacists who spend a portion of their time in this area.

Clinical services in Class II are categorized based on their direct role in communication with patients. These activities, whether providing drug histories or performing medication counseling, require interaction with a patient. When performed by practitioners, they provide the most visible contribution to patient care as reflected from the lay public.

In Class III, these services are more formal and structured. They focus on specific patient groups or drug classifications. Pharmacists providing these services are often more specialized.

Finally, the Class IV category of clinical services represents the most specialized type of clinical service. Practitioners in this area are highly trained in a particular area. Preparation for providing these services requires an indepth understanding of pathophysiology and pharmacotherapeutics for the particular disease state or patient type.

STATUS OF CLINICAL PHARMACY SERVICES

Stolar,[17-20] in a series of reports on a national survey of hospital pharmacies, has provided insight into the evolution of the type and extent of clinical pharmacy services offered in the hospital setting that are considered to directly enhance patient care outcomes. In his evaluation, he defined five clinical services, which included (1) preparation of written medication histories; (2) counseling of patients on their medication during their stay or at discharge; (3) monitoring of drug therapy, which includes a review of the patient's chart in conjunction with direct patient observation and oral or written followup of the prescriber; (4) accompanying the medical and nursing staff on rounds; and (5) consultation for pharmacokinetics or nutritional therapy, which highlighted a review of therapy and oral or written followup to the prescriber, as necessary.

Stolar's data demonstrated several interesting observations concerning clinical pharmacy services (see figure 33-1). The percentage of hospitals reporting no clinical pharmacy service declined from 38 percent in 1985 to 24 percent in 1987, whereas the percentage reporting providing any three clinical pharmacy services rose from 3.8 percent to 15.1 percent during the same period. The percentage of hospital pharmacies providing each of the five clinical services has also shown a significant growth from 1978 to 1987. Therapeutic drug monitoring and pharmacokinetic or nutritional consultations are performed in 61 percent and 45 percent of hospital pharmacies. Meanwhile, the performance of drug histories by pharmacists and their participation in rounds with medical and nursing staffs have shown a less rapid growth and appear to value less, since less than 20 percent of the national respondents reported providing these clinical services.

The extent to which clinical pharmacy services are provided also varies with hospital size (figure 33-2). Of the large hospitals (greater than 400 beds), only 15 percent reported providing no clinical pharmacy service compared to almost 25 percent of medium (200-399 beds) and small (fewer than 200 beds) hospitals. Similarly, a greater percentage of large hospitals provided the five clinical pharmacy services compared to the small or medium-sized institutions, except for taking medication histories.

Are clinical pharmacy services provided for all or only a selected number of patients? As shown in figure 33-3, there is a definite difference in the provision of the various clinical services to patients. Hospital pharmacists were more likely to provide clinical pharmacy services to selected than to *all* patients in their institutions. This was especially true for the clinical services of patient discharge counseling, participation at rounds, and medication history interviews. At the same time, therapeutic drug monitoring and performance of pharmacokinetic or nutritional consultations were similar with respect to all or selected patients.

MODELS TO THE PROVISION OF CLINICAL PHARMACY SERVICES

Generalist Model

The provision of clinical pharmacy services aimed at enhancing patient outcomes and preventing misadventures can occur through a variety of models. The two models most recently proposed are the generalist and the specialist model.[21]

The generalist model attempts to coordinate and integrate the distributive or drug use control and clinical service efforts for all patients. This model evolved as hospital pharmacy relocated from the basement of the hospital to the patient care units or wards. This decentralization of pharmacists and pharmacy services resulted in pharmacists continuing their role as dispensers of medication. In addition, these decentralized practitioners began to assume responsibility for a variety of clinical services such as drug therapy monitoring, drug use reviews, quality assurance, participation in

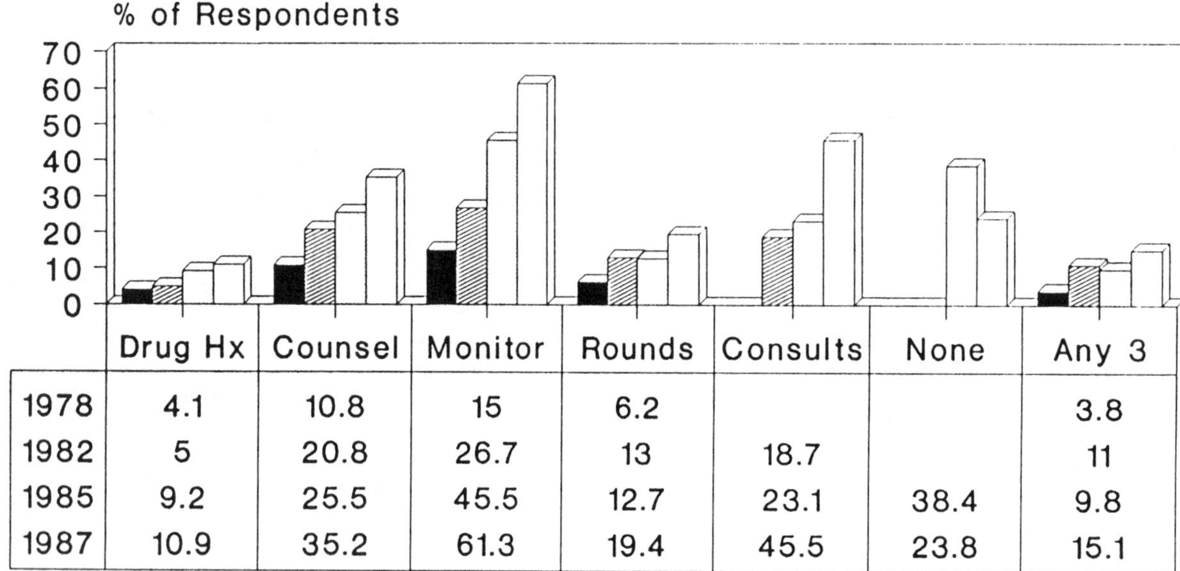

	Drug Hx	Counsel	Monitor	Rounds	Consults	None	Any 3
1978	4.1	10.8	15	6.2			3.8
1982	5	20.8	26.7	13	18.7		11
1985	9.2	25.5	45.5	12.7	23.1	38.4	9.8
1987	10.9	35.2	61.3	19.4	45.5	23.8	15.1

Figure 33-1. Comparison of clinical pharmacy services from 1978-1987

Source: Stolar MH: ASHP National Survey of Hospital Pharmaceutical Services — 1987. *Am J Hosp Pharm* 45:801-818, 1988.

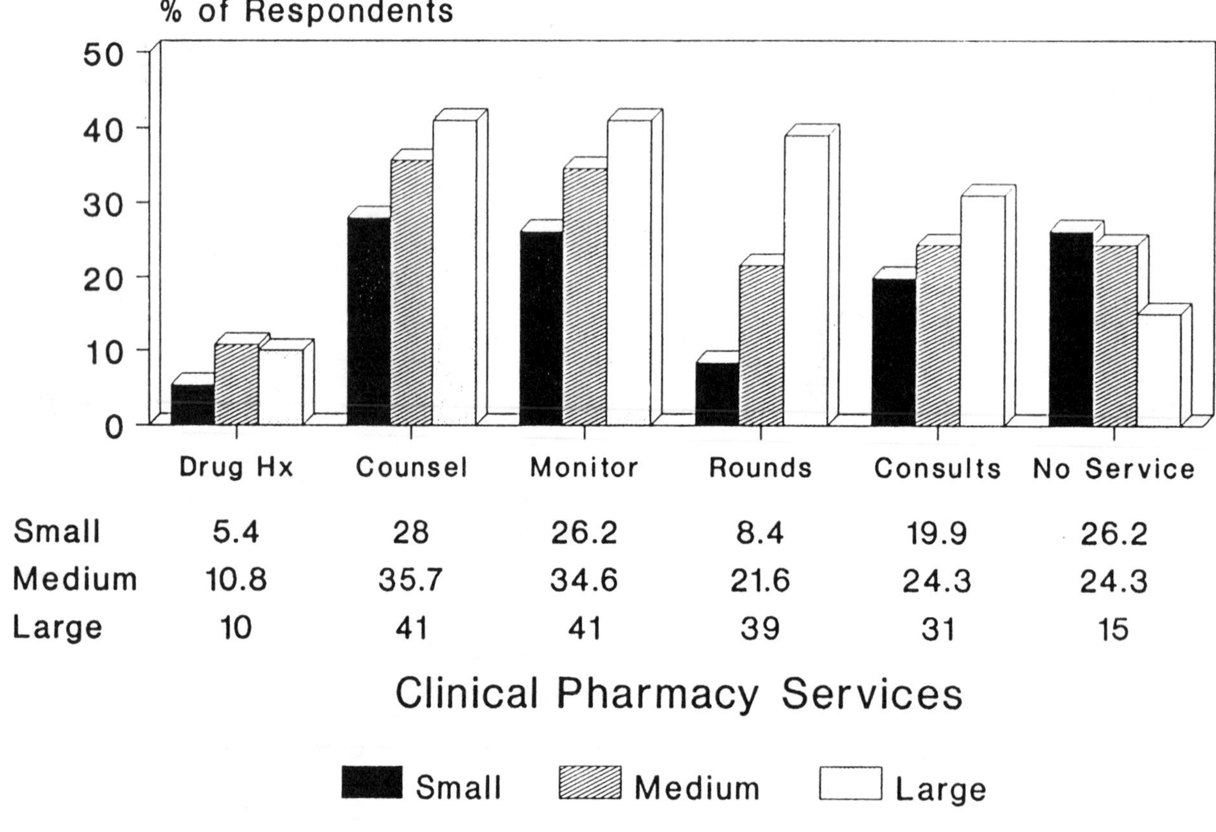

	Drug Hx	Counsel	Monitor	Rounds	Consults	No Service
Small	5.4	28	26.2	8.4	19.9	26.2
Medium	10.8	35.7	34.6	21.6	24.3	24.3
Large	10	41	41	39	31	15

Figure 33-2. Comparison of clinical pharmacy services in 1987 by hospital size

Source: Stolar MH: ASHP National Survey of Hospital Pharmaceutical Services — 1987. *Am J Hosp Pharm* 45:801, 1988.

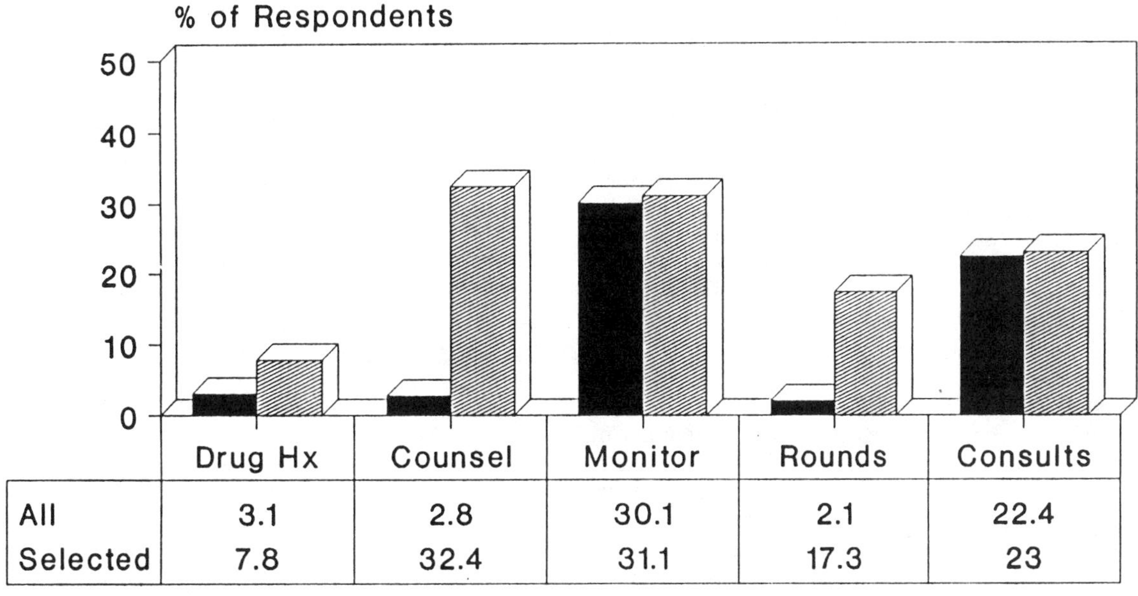

	Drug Hx	Counsel	Monitor	Rounds	Consults
All	3.1	2.8	30.1	2.1	22.4
Selected	7.8	32.4	31.1	17.3	23

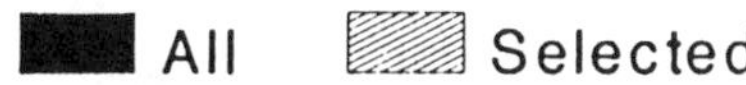

Figure 33-3. Clinical pharmacy services provided to all or selected patients

Source: Stolar MH: ASHP National Survey of Hospital Pharmaceutical Services — 1987. *Am J Hosp Pharm* 45:801, 1988.

cardiopulmonary resuscitation, discharge counseling, and medication history interviews. In this model, all pharmacists working in the decentralized patient care area are accountable for providing an integrated service of clinical and drug use control. Similarly, all patients on the unit, ward, or service will benefit from this integrated approach. If performed in a structured environment with guidelines for practitioners and the necessary administrative support, this model is extremely effective in fostering the concept of pharmaceutical care. It does not lead to a fractionation between the pharmacists who perform only the technical or distributive services and those providing the clinical services. Both responsibilities are performed by the same individual. Unfortunately, many institutions are unable to provide the depth and breadth of clinical services to all patients because of departmental or institutional priorities, budgetary constraints, personnel shortages, or lack of qualified practitioners.

Specialist Model

In the specialist model, selected individuals are identified to provide *only* clinical pharmacy services. These individuals then become responsible for providing only clinical services to all patients or a preselected category of patients. If all patients receive clinical services from this person, the depth and breadth of clinical services often are not comprehensive because of limited human or financial resources. For example, all patients will receive a particular clinical service such as admission medication histories or therapeutic drug monitoring but will not receive discharge medication counseling.

When only selected patients receive a clinical service in the specialist model, the patient must meet predefined criteria or receive a physician-initiated consultation. By choosing selective populations that meet predefined criteria, such as those who are elderly or those with compromised renal or hepatic function, pharmacy departments with limited clinical pharmacy manpower can focus on groups with a high risk of potential medication toxicity, and thereby (potentially) provide a higher quality of clinical service for a limited number of patients. Further, the selective monitoring of medications that have narrow therapeutic windows (e.g., anticoagulants, antibiotics, digoxin, theophylline) can minimize medication toxicity and ensure the appropriate use of these agents.

A physician-initiated consultation for clinical pharmacy services is the second process by which selected patients receive these services. The consultation specifically requests for assistance with a particular patient care problem or issue involving medication. The most common examples of consultations are for providing pharmacokinetic dosing recommendations (e.g., aminoglycosides, vancomycin, theophylline, anticoagulants, digoxin, antiarrythmics, anticonvulsants), admission medication history interviews, medication discharge counseling, or parenteral nutrition monitoring. The pharmacist who performs this consultation provides a written and/or oral recommendation to the physician. The responsibility for implementing the recommendation varies among institutions. Although some pharmacists have prescribing authority, they often do not use it unless requested. Followup on the recommendation is also dependent on the type of consultation requested. Pharmacists who provide the recommendation usually have received specialized training in this area. Their documentation of the recommendation in the patient chart further increases their accountability for assisting and providing patient care, and as such, is viewed as a critical element of clinical pharmacy services.

In the specialist model, the distributive or drug use control efforts are rarely coordinated by this individual but by other practitioners, such as staff pharmacists. Without coordination of effort, the implementation of recommendations or provision of specific clinical services can be significantly hampered. Specific dosing recommendations provided by a pharmacist specialist that are not prepared and administered correctly at the right time by the drug distribution system will minimize the value of recommendation. Other health professionals such as nurses and physicians may also experience difficulty with this system if they are unable to determine who is in charge when they need resolution of medication-related problems. Further, patients also become confused with this system as they try to understand the identity and role of these new practitioners who may identify themselves as pharmacists, clinical pharmacists, or doctors of pharmacy. Finally, the practitioners themselves see a separation of responsibility in providing pharmaceutical care, and conflict between the various specialists and staff pharmacists will occur unless the management system reflects this awareness.

Integrated Patient-Specific Model

Recently, an alternative model termed "integrated patient-specific model" has been proposed.[21] This model defines three major components necessary to the provision of clinical pharmacy services or pharmaceutical care: (1) a mission statement to guide the clinical services that are provided, (2) a description of the clinical and distributive activities that must be accomplished, and (3) a managerial framework that supports and implements the mission statement and activities into actual practice. The integrated aspect of this model seeks to establish a commitment for all activities in the drug use control process; the patient-specific component is aimed at defining the desired patient-centered outcomes of the drug therapy. The end results of this model are the identification and establishment of priorities that guide the patient-centered philosophy for integrating clinical services with the traditional drug distribution system.

Regardless of the type of clinical pharmacy service provided, it is extremely important that an integrated, efficient, and effective drug use control system that includes distribution, purchasing, and administration be present.[14] Without assurances that the patient will receive "*the right drug at the right time*," the clinical services provided to a particular patient may be limited. To maximize the benefits of clinical pharmacy services, administrative support is essential. This includes a mission statement, organizational structure, practice standards, and staff development activities for the clinical pharmacy programs.

VALUE OF CLINICAL PHARMACY SERVICES

The economic value and acceptance of clinical pharmacy have been documented extensively in several review articles.[5,22,23] The studies in many of these reviews have supported the cost savings or cost avoidance that occur when clinical pharmacy services are provided. Unfortunately, these same studies fail to quantify all costs or measures of health outcome. As a result, there remains a need to develop sound research methodologies for conducting cost-benefit studies for clinical pharmacy services. (See chapter 13 and references 4 and 15 for more detailed information.)

Impact of Future Health Care Technology Innovations

In the future, the impact of biotechnology on drug product development and delivery systems (liposomes, implants, and portable pumps) will have a strong effect on how clinical pharmacy services are provided. As a result of monoclonal antibody technologies and recombinant DNA techniques, it will be possible to isolate and produce large quantities of human proteins that have been either difficult or very expensive to produce. We have already seen some of these products, such as human insulin, human growth hormone, interferon alfa, alteplase, muromonab-CD3, and epoetin alfa. These products are just beginning to effect an evaluation of pharmacists' responsibilities related to product evaluation, distribution systems, clinical monitoring, and education of patients and health professionals.[24-27]

Innovative technology has begun to simplify the distributive requirement of providing medications to patients. The use of automated IV solution devices, computers, and robotics will further reduce the pharmacist's involvement in the distributive component. Meanwhile, this technology has begun and will continue to assist with monitoring for patient medication compliance, assisting with detecting drug interactions and incompatibilities, and guiding in the selection of appropriate medications. These changes, coupled with the increased use of technical support personnel, will provide the pharmacist with an increased opportunity to focus on enhancing patient care outcomes.

SUMMARY

In summary, clinical pharmacy services in the institutional setting have evolved from a drug use control perspective to a focus on the role of pharmacy and its practitioners in serving the pharmaceutical care needs of patients and society. In the future, the provision of clinical services will require a continued awareness and implementation of new technology. This awareness is needed to minimize pharmacists' involvement in the technical aspects of pharmacy practice, thereby creating more opportunities for clinical activities that are focused on providing quality care to patients.

REFERENCES

1. Fancke GN: Evolvement of clinical pharmacy. *Drug Intell Clin Pharm* 3:348-353, 1969.
2. Smith WE: Clinical pharmacy in the 1980s. *Am J Hosp Pharm* 40:223-290, 1983.
3. Brodie DC: Drug use control: Keystone to pharmaceutical service. *Drug Intell Clin Pharm* 1:63-65, 1967.
4. Black BL: *Resource Book on Progressive Pharmaceutical Services.* Bethesda, MD, American Society of Hospital Pharmacists, 1986.
5. Willett MS, Bertch KE, Rich DS, et al: Prospectus on the economic value of clinical pharmacy services. *Pharmacotherapy* 9:45-56, 1989.

6. Anon: Directions for clinical practice in pharmacy. *Am J Hosp Pharm* 42:1287-1342, 1985.
7. Manasse HR: Medication use in an imperfect world: Drug misadventuring as an issue of public policy. Part 1. *Am J Hosp Pharm* 46:929-944, 1989.
8. Manasse HR: Medication use in an imperfect world: Drug misadventuring as an issue of public policy. Part 2. *Am J Hosp Pharm* 46:1141-1152, 1989.
9 Kellaway G: The patient. In Inman WHW (ed): *Monitoring for Drug Safety,* 2nd ed. Boston, MTP Press, 1986, pp 637-649.
10. Hepler CD: The third wave in pharmaceutical education: The clinical movement. *Am J Pharm Educ* 51:369-385, 1988.
11. Hepler CD: Unresolved issues in the future of pharmacy. *Am J Hosp Pharm* 45:1071-1081, 1988.
12. Hepler CD, Strand LM: Opportunities and responsibilities in pharmaceutical care. *Am J Hosp Pharm* 47:533-543, 1990.
13. Strand LM, Cipolle R, Morley PC: Drug related problems: Their structure and function. *Drug Intel Clin Pharm* 24:1093-1097, 1990.
14. Brodie DC: Pharmacy's societal purpose. *Am J Hosp Pharm* 38:1893-1896, 1981.
15. ASHP statement on the pharmacist's clinical role in organized health-care settings. *Am J Hosp Pharm* 46:805-806, 1989.
16. McKay AB, Hepler CD, Knapp DA: *How to Evaluate Progressive Pharmaceutical Services.* Bethesda, MD, ASHP Research and Education Foundation, 1987.
17. Stolar MH: ASHP national survey of hospital pharmaceutical services - 1987. *Am J Hosp Pharm* 45:801-818, 1988.
18. Stolar MH: ASHP national survey of hospital pharmaceutical services - 1985. *Am J Hosp Pharm* 42:2667-2678, 1985.
19. Stolar MH: ASHP national survey of hospital pharmaceutical services - 1982. *Am J Hosp Pharm* 40:963-969, 1982.
20. Stolar MH: ASHP national survey of hospital pharmaceutical services - 1978. *Am J Hosp Pharm* 36:316-325, 1979.
21. Strand LM, Guerrero RM, Nickman NA, et al: Integrated patient-specific model of pharmacy practice. *Am J Hosp Pharm* 47:550-554, 1990.
22. Hatoum HT, Catizone C, Hutchinson RA, et al: An eleven-year review of the pharmacy literature: Documentation of the value and acceptance of clinical pharmacy. *Drug Intell Clin Pharm* 20:33-41, 1986.
23. ASHP technical assistance bulletin on assessment of departmental directions for clinical practice in pharmacy. *Am J Hosp Pharm* 46:339-341, 1989.
24. Stewart CF, Fleming RA: The pharmacist as educator in biotechnology: Introduction. *Am J Hosp Pharm* 46(supp 2):S3-S4, 1989.
25. Stewart CF, Fleming RA: Biotechnology products: New opportunities and responsibilities for the pharmacist. *Am J Hosp Pharm* 46(supp 2):S4-S8, 1989.
26. Black CD, Hicks CI, Koeller JM: Impact of biotechnology on pharmacy practice. *Am J Pharm Educ* 54:73-74, 1990.
27. Speedie MK: The impact of biotechnology upon pharmacy education. *Am J Pharm Educ* 54:55-61, 1990.

Appendix 33-A

CLASSIFICATION OF CLINICAL PHARMACY SERVICES[13]

CLASS	DEFINITIONS AND EXAMPLES
I	Services involving hospital-wide programs aimed at selection of drug therapy, drug therapy monitoring, and education. – Pharmacy and therapeutic committee and formulary system activities – Medication error monitoring system – Adverse drug reaction reporting system – Retrospective drug use review – Drug therapy bulletins or newsletters – In-service education programs for pharmacists, nurses, and physicians
II	Services that directly gather information from or provide information to patients. – Medication histories, e.g., selected patient populations – Discharge counseling – Patient education programs, e.g., renal transplant, cardiac rehabilitation, patient-controlled analgesia
III	Formalized hospital-wide services, focusing on patient groups or drug types aimed at improving therapy by educating prescribers or patients. – Drug information centers – Pharmacokinetic dosing services – Nutritional support teams – Investigational drug services – Target drug and disease programs (prospective use review, antibiotics, H_2-antagonists) – Medication monitoring clinics – Medication refill and compliance clinics – Cardiopulmonary arrest programs
IV	Services provided by highly specialized practitioners aimed at select patient populations. – Critical care pharmacy services – Emergency room pharmacy services – Transplant services – Hematology-oncology services – Pharmacist-managed primary-care clinics – Pharmacist-managed specialty clinics

CHAPTER 34

Specialization in Pharmacy

MARIE A. SMITH

"Today the person we call a specialist is the person we used to say had a one-track mind." — Anonymous

INTRODUCTION

Over the past few years, there has been a heightened awareness among the pharmacy profession on issues related to specialization in pharmacy practice. The topic of specialization in pharmacy has evoked intellectual, political, and emotional statements from individual practitioners, pharmacy educators, and organizational representatives. Several events in the last 2 years have contributed to the increased interest in the subject of specialization, including (1) the recognition of two new pharmacy specialties, nutrition support pharmacy practice and pharmacotherapy; (2) the American Council on Pharmaceutical Education (ACPE) declaration of intent on the entry-level degree in pharmacy;[1] and (3) the proceedings of conferences on specialization in pharmacy,[2] and postgraduate pharmacy residency training.[3]

This chapter outlines some of the concepts that are integral to professional specialization, reviews the background of specialization in pharmacy, and discusses the current process for specialty recognition and certification in pharmacy.

BASIC CONCEPTS AND TERMINOLOGY

To understand the concept of pharmacy specialization, one must be able to distinguish between differentiation in practice and pharmacy specialization. The following discussion attempts to clarify the meaning of these terms and to elaborate on these concepts.

Differentiation

Since the 1960's, the pharmacist's role has been expanding, and it continues to evolve. The expansion and evolution of pharmacy practice have led to the differentiation or diversification of practice opportunities for pharmacists. Pharmacy practice differentiation can be attributed to several factors, including the rapid development of new drugs and drug delivery systems, changes in the health care delivery system, an increase in the acuity of illness of institutionalized patients, increased emphasis on patient outcomes and quality of health care, and the rapid proliferation of drug information.

Differentiation occurs when a practitioner concentrates on a specific aspect of practice. It does not imply that a practitioner possesses a highly unique or specialized knowledge or has had formal training in a specific practice area.

In 1975, the Study Commission on Pharmacy characterized pharmacy as a differentiated system in which pharmacists performed specific roles within a health care system.[4] Today, pharmacy practice is highly differentiated; pharmacists have diverse practice roles depending on their place of practice (e.g., community pharmacy, hospital pharmacy, managed-care pharmacy); their primary function (e.g., management, patient care, research); and the level of patient care they provide (e.g., emergency care, long-term care, ambulatory care, acute care, home health care).

In addition to practice differentiation, there has been differentiation in pharmacy education and postgraduate training experiences.[5] Although a vast majority of pharmacists hold only a B.S. degree, there have been recent shifts in educational statistics for the pharmacy work force. In 1979, 1 out of 30 pharmacists had completed a Pharm.D. degree, whereas 1 out of 16 had this degree by 1987. Similarly, in 1979, 1 out of 83 pharmacists had completed a residency or fellowship, whereas 1 in 31 had this postgraduate training in 1987. As schools of pharmacy move toward adoption of the entry-level Pharm.D. degree, it is likely that the rate of differentiation within postgraduate training programs (i.e., residencies and fellowships) will only increase.

The evolution of pharmacy residency training has paralleled changes in pharmacy practice differentiation. Over the past 25 years, there has been steady growth in the number of graduates from accredited pharmacy residency programs.[5] In 1991, a total of 406 residents graduated from 245 residency training programs accredited by the American Society of Hospital Pharmacists (ASHP). ASHP has accredited three types of residency programs: two entry-level residencies—hospital and clinical—and specialized residencies. Originally, hospital residencies focused on pharmacy operations and management training, whereas clinical residencies broadened exposure to patient-care services. In late 1991, a new ASHP accreditation standard was approved for a residency in pharmacy practice (with an emphasis on pharmaceutical care). A residency in pharmacy practice is an organized, directed, postgraduate training program that centers on development of the knowledge, attitudes, and skills needed to pursue rational drug therapy. The new accreditation standard will incorporate elements of the hospital pharmacy and clinical residency accreditation standards. As of July

1992, ASHP will accredit two types of residency programs—pharmacy practice residencies and specialized residencies.

Specialized residencies have developed alongside the differentiation of pharmacy practice. As pharmacy services expanded into discrete patient care areas, there was an accompanying need to train pharmacists with a more focused knowledge base in complex drug therapy management. Specialized postgraduate training is an important element in the development and recognition of pharmacy specialties. In the future, specialized postgraduate training may become an eligibility requirement for certification of pharmacy specialists.

Pharmacy practice has evolved from an era of drug distribution to an era of drug information and clinical pharmacy and is now challenged by an era of pharmaceutical care.[6] Each phase in this evolution has provided opportunities for differentiation in pharmacy practice as well as education and training.

Specialization

One must recognize that differentiation and specialization are not equivalent. Differentiation in pharmacy, as described above, results from a distinction in place of practice, function, or level of patient care. True specialization in pharmacy is based on a unique core of scientific knowledge and practice skills. Specialization is an indicator of professional maturity and growth.

In pharmacy, the specialty recognition process is intended to assure the public that the pharmacy specialist has attained a high level of competence and skill. Another purpose of specialty recognition is to inform other professional colleagues of the pharmacy specialist's educational and training accomplishments, thereby assuring that a patient referred to the specialist will be competently served. Among other aims of specialty recognition are the stimulation of research, enhancement of training programs, and overall advancement of the pharmacy specialty. Pharmacy specialization and specialty recognition are not self-serving efforts to legitimize pharmacy as a clinical profession; rather, they constitute another phase in the evolution of the profession.

Specialized practice areas in pharmacy have developed as a result of practice differentiation. Practitioners with a specific expertise or focus in some differentiated practice areas (e.g., drug information, intravenous (IV) therapy, investigational drugs) are sometimes referred to as "specialists." The use of the term "specialist" is often used to indicate a specific expertise or focus of practice rather than an individual's credential. It is becoming increasingly common to see the term "specialist" used in position descriptions for clinical practice positions regardless of the existence of that practice area as a formally recognized pharmacy specialty. For example, a position listing may seek a "drug information specialist" even though there is no recognized pharmacy specialty in this practice area. This imprecise terminology can be quite confusing and possibly misleading to other health professionals and the public.

Practice differentiation leads to recognition of specialized practice needs. As differentiated practice areas develop a unique knowledge base and skill level, postgraduate training experiences have developed to foster the growth of a specialized practice area. As practitioners in these specialized practice areas conduct research and scholarly activities, they contribute to the further maturation of the specialized practice area. At this point, the specialized practitioners have made significant progress in the development of a specialty and may wish to petition for recognition of the specialized practice area as a formal pharmacy specialty.

CREDENTIALING IN PHARMACY

Various professions have developed specific procedures to grant credentials to individuals or programs in the profession. Credentialing is a process that entitles an individual or program to exercise a certain position or authority. In pharmacy, there are three methods of credentialing.

Licensure

A pharmacy license is granted to an individual by a governmental agency (e.g., State board of pharmacy) to guarantee the public a minimal level of professional competence. A pharmacist receives a license to practice pharmacy upon graduation from an accredited pharmacy program and successful completion of a practice examination. In most states, the board of pharmacy requires its licensed pharmacists to earn a specified number of continuing education (CE) credits—typically 15 per annum—to be relicensed. The credits are usually obtained by attending CE programs or by completing self-study programs provided by accredited CE providers.

Accreditation

Accreditation is a process used to review and evaluate educational or training programs rather than individuals. The process is controlled by the profession and assures the public (as well as the profession) that the program has met established standards for producing a high-quality learning experience.

Examples in pharmacy include the accreditation of (1) pharmacy degree programs and continuing education programs by the ACPE and (2) pharmacy residency programs and technician training programs by ASHP.

Certification

Certification is the process of credentialing an individual in a recognized practice area or pharmacy specialty. Certification is usually controlled by the profession, and is a mechanism for recognizing an individual who has met the eligibility requirements, passed an examination, and is competent to practice in the specified area. The certification body for pharmacist specialists is the Board of Pharmaceutical Specialties (BPS). The specialty recognition and certification process for pharmacists is discussed in the next section of this chapter.

Certification of a pharmacy specialty or individual specialists should not be confused with pharmacy certificate programs. Although the terms are similar, certificate programs are a specific type of continuing education programs. Certificate programs usually follow a planned curriculum, have a didactic and experiential component, teach new practice skills, enable new practice competencies, and qualify for continuing education and/or academic credit.[7] The certification process for a pharmacy specialty encompasses a greater scope and depth of knowledge and practice than that covered in certificate programs.

SPECIALTY RECOGNITION AND CERTIFICATION

A formal process to recognize pharmacy specialties and certify pharmacy specialists has existed since 1976. At that time, the BPS was created to serve as the certification agency for the pharmacy profession. The BPS was born as a result of recommendations made by the American Pharmaceutical Association (APhA) Task Force on Specialties in Pharmacy. In its final report,[8] the task force concluded that (1) pharmacy specialties may exist in the future, (2) an official board with independent decision-making authority should be established, and (3) this board should be empowered to certify individuals as specialists.

The task force emphatically stated its belief that a specialty certification process should exist for the benefit of society, not for the mere benefit of the pharmacy profession. To ensure this belief, the task force drafted a set of criteria that should be met by any group seeking the recognition of a specific practice area as a pharmacy specialty. These criteria are delineated later in this discussion. In addition, the task force outlined an organizational structure and certification process that are nearly identical to those of the BPS today.

The BPS is an independent organizational body that is governed and financed by the APhA. Its purposes are (1) to grant recognition of pharmacy specialties, (2) to establish standards for the certification and recertification of pharmacy specialists, (3) to certify and recertify qualified individuals as pharmacy specialists, and (4) to serve as an information source for pharmacy specialties and specialists. The BPS is composed of nine members appointed by the APhA Board of Trustees—six members are pharmacists, two members represent other health care professions, and there is one public member.[9]

Current Specialties

In 1978, the BPS approved nuclear pharmacy practice as the first specialty in pharmacy. This petition was developed by the APhA Academy of Pharmacy Practice, Section on Nuclear Pharmacy. There was a hiatus in the development of pharmacy specialties until 1986, when the Committee on Clinical Pharmacy as a Specialty [supported by the American College of Clinical Pharmacy (ACCP)] submitted a petition to recognize clinical pharmacy as a specialty. After considerable review, the BPS rejected the petition, stating that "clinical pharmacy practice is too broad and too general to be recognized as a specialty."[10] In late 1987, the American Society for Parenteral and Enteral Nutrition (A.S.P.E.N.) and ASHP cosponsored and submitted a petition to BPS requesting recognition of nutritional support pharmacy practice as a specialty. A few months later, ACCP submitted a petition to recognize pharmacotherapy as a specialty. Both petitions were approved in October 1988, and pharmacy now has three specialties—nuclear pharmacy, nutrition support pharmacy, and pharmacotherapy.

In late 1990, ASHP sponsored and submitted a petition to the BPS requesting the recognition of psychopharmacy practice as a specialty. The petition is currently under review by BPS.

Specialty Petition Development

Any individual or group may petition the BPS to recognize a specific area of pharmacy practice as a specialty. The BPS has seven criteria with guidelines that must be met in the petition. The intention is to give the petitioner an opportunity to state clearly that the proposed area of specialty practice meets the criteria and merits specialty recognition.

The criteria[8] that must be met in the petition are:

1. *Demand.* The demand for the proposed specialty is characterized by statements of pharmacy and nonpharmacy leaders and estimates of filled and unfilled positions in the proposed specialty area.
2. *Need.* The need for the proposed specialty is established by examining the public health or patient care needs that are best met by pharmacists in the proposed specialty area. In addition, there must be documentation that public health and welfare may be at risk if the services of the proposed specialists are not provided.
3. *Number and time.* There must be a reasonable number of individuals who devote a significant amount of time in their practice to the proposed specialty area.
4. *Specialized knowledge.* Documentation is provided to demonstrate that the proposed specialty area has a unique body of knowledge that is based in the biological, physical, pharmaceutical, and behavioral sciences.
5. *Specialized functions.* Documentation is provided to demonstrate the specialized functions and skills required by a practitioner in the proposed specialty area.
6. *Education and training.* The type of education and training programs that are necessary to produce practitioners in the proposed specialty are described.
7. *Transmission of knowledge.* Documentation is provided to demonstrate that there is a transmission of knowledge in the proposed specialty through the professional, scientific, and technical literature, and professional or scientific meetings.

The BPS also solicits comments from pharmacists and other health professionals on the merit of each petition. After careful consideration, the BPS either approves or rejects the petition to recognize a pharmacy specialty.

BPS is currently conducting a self-study process, including a thorough review of the specialty recognition process. It is possible that this review could change the processes outlined above.

Specialty Certification

Once a specialty is recognized, the BPS establishes a specialty council with the input of the petitioners or the sponsoring organization. The specialty council comprises pharmacists in the recognized specialty and pharmacists who are considered generalists (not practicing in the recognized specialty area). The charges of the specialty council are: (1) to recommend standards and requirements for certification and recertification of pharmacists in the specialty, (2) to develop and administer specialty certification examinations, and (3) to recommend qualified individuals to the BPS for certification or recertification as specialists.

Two of the major tasks of the specialty council include (1) using the discrete knowledge areas and practice behaviors identified for the specific pharmacy specialist (compared to a general pharmacy practitioner or another pharmacy specialist) to develop the certification examination, and (2) establishing the eligibility requirements for individuals interested in taking the certification examination.

Development of the certification process is comprehensive, rigorous, and time-consuming. It is reasonable to expect a 2-3-year period between recognition of a specialty and administration of the first specialty examination in that area.

SUMMARY

Specialization in pharmacy has stemmed from the differentiation of practice and postgraduate training experiences. It is a natural step in the maturation of a profession. Practice differentiation and specialization will present pharmacists with challenging opportunities to serve as a force in society for the safe, appropriate, and cost-conscious use of medications. Several segments of the pharmacy profession—practitioners, educators, associations, accrediting bodies, and regulatory agencies—must be aware that the role of the pharmacist in providing high-quality, contemporary pharmaceutical care is expanding, and as it does the profession is developing and recognizing pharmacy specialties.

REFERENCES

1. American Council of Pharmaceutical Education: *Declaration of intent: Revision of accreditation standards in 1990s in keeping with changes in pharmacy practice and pharmaceutical education.* Chicago, American Council on Pharmaceutical Education, September 18, 1989.
2. Directions for specialization in pharmacy practice. Proceedings of an invitational conference sponsored by the American Association of Colleges of Pharmacy, the American College of Clinical Pharmacy, the American Pharmaceutical Association, and the American Society of Hospital Pharmacists. *Am J Hosp Pharm* 48:469-500, 691-719, 1991.
3. Directions for postgraduate pharmacy residency training. Proceedings of the 1989 National Residency Preceptors Conference conducted by the American Society of Hospital Pharmacists. *Am J Hosp Pharm* 47:85-126, 1990.
4. American Association of Colleges of Pharmacy: *Pharmacists for the future: The report of the Study Commission on Pharmacy.* Ann Arbor, MI, Health Administration Press, 1975.
5. Knapp KK, Letendre DE: Educational differentiation of the pharmacy work force. *Am J Hosp Pharm* 46:2476-2482, 1989.
6. Hepler CD, Strand LM: Opportunities and responsibilities in pharmaceutical care. *Am J Hosp Pharm* 47:533-543, 1990.
7. Chalmers RK: Chair report of the AACP/ACPE Conference on Certificate Programs. *Am J Pharm Educ* 54:80-83, 1990.
8. Cohelan J, Edwards WJ, Fenninger LD, et al: Final report: APhA task force on specialties in pharmacy. *J Am Pharm Assoc* NS14:618-622, 1974.
9. Board of Pharmaceutical Specialties: *Petitioner's guide for specialty recognition.* Washington, DC, American Pharmaceutical Association, 1989.
10. Board of Pharmaceutical *News Release #87-01*, July 9, 1987.

CHAPTER 35

Home Health Care Services

LARRY D. PELHAM and MICHAEL R. NORWOOD

The growth of our elderly population, coupled with cost-containment in hospitals and limited options in the nursing home care, means increased numbers of patients will now receive health care in their homes. Home health care, enhanced by home infusion therapy, is becoming an integral part of health care delivery, traditionally dominated by hospitals prior to the 1990's. New jobs in home care grew more than 20 percent in 1990, triple the rate of growth for health care industry overall, according to the Bureau of Labor Statistics.[1] Home care programs broadly defined include health-related products or services made available to a patient at home to avoid or minimize institutional care in nursing homes or hospitals. Home care services range from personal care, homemaking, and shopping assistance to high-technology medical care such as renal dialysis and infusion therapy. It also includes medical diagnosis and treatment, physical and speech therapy, the provision of medical supplies and equipment, health aide and homemaker assistance, transportation, mental health care, adult day care, and respite care.

The number of home health agencies (HHA's) providing skilled intermittent, continuous home care, or specialized home infusion therapy increased by 12 percent to 8,105 as of October 1989.[2] Sunbelt states of Texas, Florida, and California experienced the greatest growth. Texas claimed the most HHA's at 796, but Florida experienced the greatest growth (184 percent) in 1989 to a total of 531 HHA's. Diverse growth in home care services is also potentiated by increasing levels of chronic disease and functional disability, consumer preference for home care over nursing home care, increasingly sophisticated medical technology, and changing Federal policies (most notably, the implementation of the Medicare Prospective Payment System) for Medicare reimbursement in 1983 for hospitals. The number of Medicare-certified, hospital-based HHA's tripled between 1981 and 1986, from 432 to 1,260, and then leveled off to a slow steady growth, which reached 1,537 by December 1990. Of the 1,700 hospice agencies in the United States, only 43 percent (724) participate in the Medicare-certified program. Most hospices are based in home health agencies (39 percent), but 33 percent are freestanding, and 27 percent are hospital-based. Skilled nursing facilities account for the remaining 1 percent. Not only is the use of home care as an alternative viable, safe, and cost-effective, but this type of health care is also mutually satisfying to the patient and caregiver.

FEDERAL AND STATE MEDICAL HEALTH CARE PROGRAMS

Coverage of home health care under the Medicare program (Title 18) implemented in 1966 represented a major commitment by the Federal Government to provide an alternative to institutional care. Medicare accounted for 55 percent of all home health revenues in 1989.[3] To qualify as a provider of home health care services under Medicare, a skilled intermittent nursing agency must be approved and certified by the Health Care Financing Administration (HCFA), U.S. Department of Health and Human Services, to bill for Medicare home visits.[4] Even though most home health agencies must be licensed by the State in which they operate, they do not have to become Medicare certified unless they service and bill Medicare beneficiaries for skilled intermittent home visits. Medicare HHA reimbursement is based upon reasonable home care agency costs, not to exceed a specified capitated cost per visit limit. Capitated rates are established annually. Reasonable and allowable costs are submitted annually to a fiscal intermediary payer in the form of a Medicare cost report. Allowable costs primarily include salaries with lesser provisions for supplies and operational expenses. Medicare-certified home care agencies usually provide either short-term intermittent skilled care or private duty staffing services and staffing relief. Once certified as a Medicare home health provider, each agency is authorized to bill designated Medicare fiscal intermediaries (e.g., Blue Cross of California services Washington State hospital-based Medicare agencies) for services provided within an approved geographic area, usually defined by county boundaries.

Medicare Part A home care provides reimbursement for skilled services deemed medically necessary by a prescribing physician for a "home-bound" patient. Medicare-certified home health care services are traditionally categorized as "skilled" and "nonskilled" as illustrated in table 35-1. Under Medicare Part A, a patient must first qualify for one of the primary services of nursing, physical therapy, or speech therapy before being eligible for other benefits in order that other services will be supervised and reimbursed. For example, home health aide visits would be reimbursed by Medicare only if ordered by a physician in conjunction with skilled nursing services, and only if the home health aide functioned under the direction of the skilled home health nurse. The majority of "homebound" patients receive at least

2 to 3 home visits per week for at least 30 days when admitted to service. The typical homebound patient admitted to a Medicare-certified agency received an average of 21 visits per admission. Rogers[5] noted a 22-percent increase in the number of home care referrals after implementation of the Medicare Prospective Payment System initiated in 1983. The Medicare "Conditions of Participation" detail more relevant home health care coverage guidelines.[6]

Table 35-1. Medicare certified home health care service

Skilled services:	Nursing Physical therapy Occupational therapy Speech therapy Social worker services
Nonskilled services:	Homemaker Home health aide

Medicare-covered Part B provides coverage for the provision of medical services that include durable medical equipment (product sales and rentals), prosthetic devices, parenteral, and enteral nutritional products reimbursed at 80 percent of allowable or capitated cost schedules. Presently, intravenous antibiotics and pain management administered without an infusion pump are not reimbursed by Medicare Part B. Part B is voluntary insurance and involves a nominal monthly premium by Medicare beneficiaries. The proposed Medicare Catastrophic Coverage Act of 1988 would have broadened the coverage for outpatient prescription drug benefits, including home intravenous antibiotic services.[7-10] The entire act was repealed November 22, 1989, except for several provisions affecting Medicaid. Hospitals have been providing home health care benefits to Medicare patients since the enactment of the Medicare legislation in 1965.

Medicaid

Medicaid (Title 19) is an entitlement program administered by the State under Federal guidelines providing health care services to the needy. The program encompasses a broad range of joint social welfare programs that are funded through general Federal revenues and in part by State contributions. Since Medicaid programs are State administered, coverage of home health care services varies from one State to another including the level of reimbursement, eligibility, criteria, scope of benefits, services, and administrative procedures for skilled care. For instance, Washington State does not reimburse for social worker visits, whereas Medicare-certified agencies do receive reimbursement. In some States, the level of care extends beyond skilled care to include unskilled care such as nonmedical home care services, including sitter services and homemakers. Drugs and biologicals, including intravenous antibiotics, usually are reimbursed by Medicaid at the *Redbook*[11] average wholesale price plus dispensing fee, whereas Medicare financial coverage is narrowly restricted to home patients on cancer chemotherapy, pain management, enteral, and parenteral nutrition under Part A and Part B, Medicare.

Durable medical equipment and injectable medications pose substantial reimbursement burdens for providers, usually requiring prior approval when covered. Cognitive or clinical monitoring expenses are not reimbursed for pharmacists or nurses when services are based upon patient home infusion therapy needs alone. However, Medicaid skilled intermittent services are billed separately from pharmacy products and usually reimbursed per visit at substantially less than Medicare skilled services. Insufficient reimbursement by Medicaid for total parenteral nutrition (TPN) and home enteral nutrition (HEN) products, services, and supplies based upon product cost plus dispensing fee or minimal fixed rates has resulted in proprietary companies targeting commercial payers in their business growth rather than Medicaid.

Preferred Provider Organizations

The high cost of fee-for-service home health care and initiatives to contain health care premiums has led to the growth in preferred provider organizations (PPO's).[12] As a result, the routing of patients through cost-effective and high-quality home health care providers is rapidly evolving in the health insurance industry, including home health care.

Private insurance for home health services ranges from skilled nursing services provided on a hourly or shift basis to coverage on a per visit basis. Eligibility requirements include physician's order and medical necessity, often emulating Medicare coverages. However, explicit identification of home health services is usually absent from subscriber benefits packages. Home intravenous therapies such as antibiotics, TPN, chemotherapy, pain management, and hydration offer limited reimbursement from commercial payers for pharmacists' cognitive or professional clinical services; therefore, effective negotiation with case managers and insurers should result in reimbursement of clinical services or patient training that would accomplish similar patient outcomes. For example, pharmacists conducting nutritional consults, patient medication training, clinical laboratory monitoring, and coordination of infusion devices could be substituted for the nurse; however, skilled nursing home visits would not be appropriate.

Both per diem flat rates and contracted discounts are being introduced in the daily process of "prior authorization" and negotiation of preferred provider agreements. Most per diem proposals represent significant charge deductions of 5-25 percent off fee-for-service charges and per diem pricing discounts of up to 75 percent below usual and customary fee-for-service charges. This reduced reimbursement is being bundled by payers to cover all pharmacy services and products usually including medical and surgical supplies (central catheter supplies), durable medical equipment (infusion devices), compounding, delivery, and clinical monitoring by pharmacists. Strategic pricing of products must account for provision of clinical monitoring and product (drug) to remain service competitive long term. Skilled intermittent nursing visits for homebound patients are usually reimbursed separate from the infusion vendor's per diem schedules when both a skilled intermittent home health agency and home infusion provider are providing services to the same patient; consequently, home infusion providers may be forced to accept reduced fee-for-service home infusion product reimbursement as patient charges are "unbundled" to distinguish product from service costs, while at the same time learn to negotiate more skilled visits and patient training sessions to offset the unbundling of products with services.

Most payers will not authorize skilled home nursing visits from both the primary (skilled home health) and secondary (home infusion). Usually the skilled intermittent agency serves as the primary patient provider that bills for skilled intermittent visits; the home infusion or durable medical equipment provider bills separately for products and selective services related to the secondary provider's infusion products, supplies, and services.

The influence of PPO's on home health care is becoming a major factor in the growth of home care services and increased patient cost sharing. Historically, a patient was referred to a home health care provider by the physician, nurse, or designated discharge planner; however, today, the referral, which is screened by the private insurer case manager, may redirect the original referral to a PPO for either economic or quality of care reasons. Case managers, usually experienced registered nurses, employed by third-party payers negotiate prices unique to each payer's insurance coverage of products (TPN solutions, antibiotics) and services (skilled nursing, physical therapy). The tendency by some commercial payers has been to select the home care provider based upon least cost to the insurer; however, the pendulum appears to be swinging back to a balance with quality of services at higher reimbursement rates when long-term cost savings rather than short-term cost advantages are realized. Blue Shield of California is negotiating with 300 alternative care organizations to contract as the only designated provider for participants in Blue Shield's PPO plan.[13] Failure by the patient or physician to use the PPO would result in the patient's becoming financially responsible. To curtail suspected abuses in equipment rental and billing practices, Blue Cross and Blue Shield of Illinois have established a similar preferred provider network of home medical equipment, to begin in 1992.[14]

Health Maintenance Organizations

The growth of health maintenance organizations (HMO's) in the 1980's can be attributed to the support of business and industry as a another viable alternative to rising health care costs. HMO's rely primarily upon case management, prior authorization by case managers, and concurrent review to manage home care use. Cost-effectiveness is also essential for survival in this type of managed care. HMO's, in their need to limit financial risk, aggressively control use in fee-for-service contracts, with emphasis on cost-effectiveness for survival. When HHA's receive capitated payments from HMO's, the risk tends to fall on the home health care provider.[15]

HMO's and PPO's may look to comprehensive health care providers to contain rising costs that are thought to be more common when multiple providers are involved (i.e., skilled intermittent home health, hospice, and home infusion provider). For example, pain management for the terminally ill patient usually involves a hospice agency as the primary skilled agency with the home infusion provider the secondary through supplying the portable infusion pumps, pain medications, and catheter supplies for infusions. Consequently, hospital-based home health care programs are a logical component to institutional HMO's and PPO's; those facilities with broad-based programs offering a continuum of care will be in a more competitive position for managed care. The major benefit of this evolving continuum of care comes from consistency between payers and providers to decrease administrative burdens, enhance billing clarity and payment of claims, encourage cost-effective delivery of home care, and target predictability for reimbursement of services. Very few commercial payer contracts with hospitals include a separate recognition or addendum for home health, hospice, or home infusion services. Increasingly, larger HMO's now contract for Medicare reimbursement and develop their own home care programs in an effort to maintain low costs in their overall programs; however, disagreement remains among HMO's and Medicare whether HMO's are responsible for providing beyond skilled intermittent care services to their homebound beneficiaries.

Reimbursement Trends

Competitive and financial pressures that challenge hospitals also characterize home health care reimbursement. Similarly, the terms "managed care," "PPO," and "HMO" are used without regard by many for their specific differences and similarities affecting home care. Most Medicare-certified skilled home health agencies receive 60-80 percent of their revenues from Medicare. In contrast, national home infusion proprietary companies derive only 10-20 percent of their revenues from Medicare because of significantly better reimbursement from commercial HMO, PPO, and private payers, which generate the remaining 80-90 percent. Providing clinical expertise on managing patients in their homes, once the primary challenge, has now become a secondary concern of most providers in comparison to the challenges of reimbursement. The complex reimbursement for home health care services, equipment, and supplies has increased paperwork, administrative burdens, lags in payment, and retroactive denials, which lead to financial failures by providers.[16]

Computerized clinical and billing systems for skilled intermittent home health agencies are increasingly common; however, automated billing and clinical systems unique to home infusion services' needs are extremely rare in both community and hospital-based programs and represent the greatest challenge to successful implementation and maintenance of long-term comprehensive home health care. Home care providers that submit electronic billing claims in the near future may receive priority processing at the expense of those that submit paper claims as a result of Federal cutbacks in payments to fiscal intermediaries. Average payment times of 45-60 days for home health and 70-100 days for home infusion are expected to significantly increase, with paper claims resulting in significant cash-flow problems for many agencies. Most home infusion or home health providers employ 15-20 percent of their staff in the reimbursement area to screen payer mix, private pay creditworthiness, and third-party insurer claims collection.

To enhance reimbursement, home health agencies must develop sophisticated contracts with payers that specify services to be covered, authorization procedures, billing and payment procedures, methods to handle disputes, and responsibilities for continuous quality improvement in patient outcomes. Physician ownership and fee-for-service arrangements between home health providers and physicians have come under close scrutiny in the 1990's, reflecting the fact that the Federal Office of Inspector General is tightening fraud and abuse statutes relating to physician compensation for referral of Medicare patients.[17] Years in development, the final "safe harbor" regulations became effective July 29, 1991, and are intended to clarify application of the Medicare's antikickback statute by defining business practices that will *not* risk Federal prosecution.

Currently, physician compensation for home health agency clinical consultations or updating of patient care treatment plans is minimal for commercial payers and nonexistent for Medicare. Third-party payers have yet to recognize the value of physician's consultation services that result in direct reimbursement so that providers do not have to purchase physician services themselves using fee-for-service or joint ventures. Unfortunately, a select group of providers and physicians have initiated steps to restrict the admission of Medicare and Medicaid beneficiaries to their services because of inadequate reimbursement for services.

LICENSURE

As a result of the rapid growth, Federal and State regulatory agencies have expanded their scrutinizing of home health care. State licensure requirements for home health agencies and home infusion pharmacies vary. Washington State's Board of Pharmacies, unlike most, was timely in adopting the framework of the National Association of Boards of Pharmacies' guidelines to implement home infusion pharmacy licensure requirements.[18] Unfortunately, most State board of pharmacies and department of health agencies have not coordinated with each other on the development of new regulations governing the professional disciplines of pharmacy and nursing in home care. As a result, the professional practice model for the pharmacist is neither recognized nor reimbursed beyond drug dispensing. Depending upon the nature of the primary business, home infusion providers may be licensed as home health agencies specializing in home infusion services or as home health agencies emphasizing skilled intermittent home health care, with the infusion therapy only a secondary emphasis. In either case, Washington State, like most States, requires a home health license for skilled care similar to Medicare-certified agencies when direct patient care or skilled services are provided with infusion products.[19] Numerous small and large home care businesses, such as community pharmacies, durable medical equipment vendors, and home health agencies, have rushed into the home infusion market to compete with large national proprietary companies and hospital-based programs to capture dwindling health care dollars. These agencies now face increasing regulatory and licensure requirements, which increases the startup costs for policy and procedure manuals, human resource management, provider contracts, quality assurance programs, and reimbursement guidelines.

The certificate of need (CON) application process has been a barrier to entry into the home health care field for many potential providers, particularly national proprietary companies in most States. Originally developed to preclude overbidding and to ensure maximum use of all health care resources, the CON has also inhibited the growth of many hospital diversifications nationwide. In those States in which hospitals must go through the CON process for all new services, CON is mandatory for all hospital-based or community-based Medicare providers. Consequently, a new hospital-based program desiring to provide Medicare-certified home health skilled services would be bound by the CON process to gain approval to provide and bill for Medicare Part A skilled home health or a new Medicare provider number. In contrast, a hospital-based home infusion program providing infusion and enteral products under Medicare Part B reimbursement would be exempt if skilled services such as nursing visits were not billed under Medicare. Typically, in this case the hospital-based home infusion program coordinates this skilled intermittent care for homebound Medicare patients to be provided by the local community-based, Medicare-certified agency.

Coordination of care between the hospital-based home infusion nurse specialist or pharmacist and community-based home health agencies remains a significant challenge to providing "high-tech" home care. Areas of responsibilities and coordination of services should be delineated in the patient care record to inform all providers entering the patient's home. The influx of numerous portable infusion devices is one of the most common after-hour patient problems encountered by caregivers and providers when training is insufficient. The term "high-tech" partially relates to the marketing efforts of business-oriented home care organizations that desire to differentiate sophisticated and potentially life-saving infusion therapies from more traditional home care services, such as durable medical equipment and skilled intermittent nursing.

Home Care Accreditation

There are now two major national home care accrediting bodies: the Community Health Accreditation Program (CHAP), a subsidiary of the National League for Nursing, and the Home Care Accreditation Program, a division within the Joint Commission on Accreditation of Healthcare Organizations (JCAHO). CHAP requires agencies to meet standards for accreditation that cover the quality of workers, staff recruitment, patient satisfaction, and types and amount of training required. A strong focus is placed upon management and finances of the surveyed organization.[20] Most hospital-based programs are accountable to JCAHO Home Care Accreditation when the hospital is JCAHO accredited. JCAHO places similar emphasis upon staff quality, training, and policy and procedure reviews as they relate to the coordination of patient care.

From 1968 to 1988, the Joint Commission on Accreditation of Healthcare Organizations offered home care accreditation solely to hospital-based home care services as part of the hospital accreditation process using standards in the JCAHO *Accreditation Manual for Hospitals*.[21] From 1986 to 1988, JCAHO revised and broadened the home care standards and developed a survey process for both community-based and hospital-based home health care programs.[22]

The JCAHO home care survey and accreditation are applicable to those home care programs providing any one of the primary services listed in table 35-2, either directly or through contracts.[23] For example, a community or hospital pharmacy that only dispenses injectable antibiotics, without performing ongoing clinical monitoring in the home with its own or contracted nurses and pharmacists, is not eligible for JCAHO survey and accreditation. The same is true for hospital-based programs limiting their activities to product dispensing only; however, numerous contractual relationships or joint ventures between national proprietary companies and hospitals warrant their own consultation with JCAHO to determine eligibility and responsibility, which might affect the hospital's primary accreditation.

Table 35-2. JCAHO home care program eligibility*

1. Home Health Services:
   physical, occupational, speech, skilled nursing services, skilled infusion and respiratory nursing, in-home respiratory therapists
2. Personal Care and Support Services:
   home health aide, chore services, transportation, adult day care, respite care
3. Pharmaceutical Services:
   intravenous therapy providers, pharmacist dispensing and clinical monitoring, patient medication deliveries and home infusion education and compliance monitoring
4. Equipment Management:
   durable medical equipment, portable infusion pumps, enteral feeding pumps, neonatal phototherapy equipment, oxygen equipment, blood glucose monitoring devices

*JCAHO Home Care Accreditation is applicable to home care programs providing primary services either directly or through contracts.

Hospital-based programs that choose to directly provide all of these services and products themselves are considered secondary services in the survey of the hospital or parent organization. When two or more sets of Joint Commission standards are applicable to an organization, two accreditation team surveyors combine to survey in a "tailored" survey process. For example, for an acute-care hospital that provides home infusion therapy services, both a JCAHO home care nurse and pharmacist surveyor/consultant from the Home Care Accreditation Program coordinate with the Hospital Accreditation Program survey team. One program's accreditation is contingent upon on the other's performance. Since the same is true for contracted providers, most providers contract with JCAHO-accredited providers to avoid future accreditation problems. On June 1, 1988, the Joint Commission began conducting nationwide surveys of home care programs, focusing on compliance with standards on policies, procedures, and written documentation to ensure that processes are in place that enhance positive patient outcomes.[24] Based upon the survey experiences of the first JCAHO Home Pharmacist Consultant surveyors from 1988-1990, revised and more advanced standards for clinical pharmacy monitoring of home infusion therapies received high priority to become effective with the new July 1991 JCAHO Home Care Pharmacy Chapter Standards.[25] This date coincides with the 3-year resurvey or accreditation cycle and should pose a significant challenge to those providers accredited since 1988 that have not integrated therapeutic drug monitoring into their service's patient outcomes in a planned, systematic, and ongoing manner.

On July 1, 1991, JCAHO completed its first home care 3-year accreditation cycle for more than 2,000 home care providers. Based upon the first 2 years of surveying, the services provided by the first 1,000 JCAHO-accredited home care organizations were home health (70 percent), durable medical equipment (45 percent), clinical respiratory (25 percent), infusion services (35 percent), and private duty (55 percent).[26] Nationally, 66 of the 100 top home care companies in 1991 have achieved JCAHO home care accreditation, demonstrating that home care industry has shown substantial compliance with national standards that address quality patient care.[27]

JCAHO accreditation remains voluntary for community-based providers. For hospital-based programs, accreditation is mandatory for the hospital's overall JCAHO accreditation. CHAP has been accrediting home care organizations since 1965. Accreditation by JCAHO or CHAP may also weigh heavily in reducing the risk of liability by providers that have chosen to undertake accreditation to ensure that their services meet the national standards of practice. On September 5, 1991, CHAP became the first private accrediting body to be recommended for "deemed status" by the U.S. Department of Health and Human Services (JCAHO is pending). "Deemed status" means that home health agencies that meet either CHAP or JCAHO accreditation standards will be considered to have met HCFA "conditions of participation" in Medicare. CHAP's survey process includes annual unannounced site visits by two surveyors, usually lasting 4 days for the first survey and 2 days in subsequent years, like JCAHO. If history serves as a guide, submission to JCAHO or CHAP accreditation may soon become mandatory as a prerequisite for Medicare- and Medicaid-sponsored programs.

Patient Referral

Traditionally, home health care is viewed as an extension of hospitalization. This is supported by national trends demonstrating that approximately 7 percent of all hospital patient admissions result in a home health care referral. More recently, an increasing number of patients are initiated on home infusion therapies or home health care services directly from physicians' offices, nursing homes, outpatient clinics, and outpatient surgery centers without being admitted to the hospital. In either case, the home health care process begins with a referral from a discharge planner, clinic nurse, or physician while the patient is either hospitalized or under the care of a physician. The patient's clinical assessment by a qualified home health nurse should be the initial and most important step during the referral process.[28] Subsequently, the collaboration and assessment of other interdisciplinary team members is initiated to ensure that the appropriateness of therapies and other involvement of professional disciplines is identified.

Unfortunately, for some providers, the first steps in the assessment include a review of each individual's insurance coverage. Frequently, agencies will deny or delay the admission process if sufficient insurance coverage is lacking. Increasingly, the payer's case manager must be negotiated with to demonstrate how cost savings can be realized by supporting home care. Clinically oriented case managers for most payers now assist in the decision-making process of medical necessity, which has overcome many of the earlier problems of payers employing clerks with no medical background to authorize the level and intensity of patient care services requested by the home health care patient assessment.

The next step is to collaborate with skilled nursing and the referring physician to ensure that the patient meets home care admission criteria. Review of the medical chart, consultation with floor nurses, physicians, patient care area pharmacists, and a discharge planning conference with patient and family should be accomplished within 24 hours of referral.

For home intravenous (IV) patients, if the patient and his or her caregivers agree to receive home infusion therapy, an appointment to orient the patient on aseptic techniques, actions and side effects of medications, preparation for infusion, troubleshooting infusion devices, and inspection of products and labels is scheduled promptly. Additionally, patients are taught central catheter care, needle and syringe care, and aseptic manipulation of infusion extension tubing with catheter tip. Usually, the nurse demonstrates most of these procedures, referring to a written step-by-step patient instruction sheet that will remain with the patient. Patient-specific instruction sheets differ in some therapies, but generally include a list of catheter supplies, how to assemble the infusion equipment, administration techniques, and signs or symptoms of potential adverse reactions.

New technology has allowed many more patients to become home infusion candidates.[29-31] The development of programmable portable infusion pumps allows patients to carry medications that are infusing with them at all times.[32] An important aspect of the patient assessment is to check the patient's home environment to ensure access to emergency services, transportation, electrical safety, telephone rates for handicapped persons, and refrigerated storage of medications or nutritional solutions. Hospital-based programs should encourage admission to service regardless of ability to pay for patients being discharged from their institutions as a cost avoidance strategy.[33] Typical hospital IV therapy daily rates are usually four times higher than home health care.[34]

An advantage of having both Medicare-certified skilled intermittent home health service and home infusion service as hospital based, is that it enables a program to admit and bill a Medicare-certified homebound patient for skilled services while the patient's need of intravenous antibiotics that are not covered by Medicare Part A or B remains uncompensated. Without these combined services, most patients remain hospitalized for their therapy, whereas here, the skilled intermittent visits can be reimbursed even if the drug costs are not reimbursed. Selected arrangements by hospitals with community-based agencies can also minimize these unnecessary delays in the patient's care resulting from reimbursement problems.

QUALITY ASSURANCE IN HOME HEALTH CARE

Measuring and monitoring quality in home health care have rapidly become major issues among HHA's, researchers, JCAHO, and State and Federal regulators as a result of mounting cost pressures, new technological advances in the scope of medical care, and the influence of case management. The Office of Technology Assessment defines quality as "the degree to which the process of care increases the probability of outcomes desired by patients, and reduces the probability of undesired outcomes given the state of medical knowledge."[35] Traditional home health quality continues to be defined as a "paper compliance" with Medicare regulations through medical record charting and documentation audits that have achieved minimal success in measuring the quality of patient care outcomes.

Focus on the patient is a critical component of the broader and longer view of quality, as is the belief that quality improvement is itself the driving force, rather than merely a way of complying with regulatory requirements (e.g., Medicare, JCAHO, State government, board of pharmacy). The Joint Commission is phasing in "continuous quality improvement" (CQI) as the replacement for these methods. The premise of CQI is that processes can be continually improved and patient outcomes are improved as a result.[36]

To track a home health care agency's CQI performance, key indicators that will affect outcomes need to be identified and monitored over time. An indicator is a quantitative measure that can be used as a guide to monitor and evaluate the quality of patient care.[37] Indicators are one of three types: structure, process, and outcome (see table 35-3). Indicators should alert the HHA of a potential problem with an outcome or process. Model indicators and training programs to teach health care professionals how to use them are in the process of being developed by JCAHO, Federal and State governments, private foundations, and professional organizations, including the American Society of Hospital Pharmacists (ASHP). Home health agencies are becoming selective in contracting with higher quality community HHA's that view improvement as not a one-time effort. Ongoing improvement requires the commitment of management and dedication of staff. Participative management is critical to determine causes and make suggested changes.[38]

Table 35-3. JCAHO home infusion therapy quality indicators

Structure Indicators
Infusion devices (e.g., time certification, inspection)
Medical equipment (e.g., laminar flow-hood inspection, cleaning, temperature logs)
Staff qualifications (e.g., licensure, certification)
Process Indicators
Clinical assessments (e.g., physical, nutritional)
Care or treatment plan (e.g., documentation compliance)
Technical aspects of care (e.g., R.Ph. validating orders)
Management of complications (e.g., infusion site pain, phlebitis, catheter occlusions, adverse reactions)
Outcome Indicators
Infusion therapy complications (e.g., extravasation)
Adverse events (e.g., patient falls due to dehydration, drug toxicity, catheter-related sepsis)
Patient satisfaction (e.g., access to care, interpersonal and technical skills of personnel, home delivery)
Short-term patient treatment results
Long-term patient functional status

Reprinted with permission from St. Joseph Home Health Care, Tacoma, WA.

Hospital-Based Home Health Care Services

With the onset of the hospital prospective payment system in the early 1980's, hospitals entered a home health marketplace that traditionally had been dominated by voluntary, community-based, not-for-profit organizations. The trend toward shorter hospital stays and capitated inpatient reimbursement has encouraged several acute-care hospitals to either establish their own hospital-based service or to contract with commercial vendors.[28,33,39,40] Hospital-based providers, the fastest growing segment of home health providers, have cited a variety of objectives in entering the home health business, among them: (1) to promote continuity of care; (2) to increase visibility of the hospital in the community; (3) to control patients indirectly in the health care delivery channels; (4) to provide cost-containment and case management alternatives; (5) to offer diverse health care product lines; and (6) to provide a limited contribution of profit to offset non-revenue-generating services to the community. Table 35-4 identifies a wide array of products and services offered in the home.

Table 35-4. Reimbursable home care products and services

Services	*Products*
Skilled nursing	Infusion devices, pumps
Social work services	Renal dialysis (e.g., peritoneal)
Physical therapy	Drug therapy
Occupational therapy	Enteral feedings
Speech therapy	Medical/surgical supplies
Home health aides	Oxygen/respiratory equipment
Private duty nursing	Self-diagnostic devices

The personnel services side of home care industry accounts for approximately 70 percent of industry revenues; the product or drugs and supplies account for the remaining 30 percent. Determining whether the hospital's HHA should be developed as an independent provider, a collaborative provider, or perhaps not developed at all requires careful consideration, since the implementation of a hospital-provided HHA may not only be a financial risk but also an issue of community relations. Hospitals acknowledge that their relationships with other provider organizations in the community will change as their business ventures evolve. Few community-based programs have the financial resources to extend themselves to meet the increasingly complex uncompensated care needs of hospital-discharged patients. In contrast, hospital-based HHA revenues may be used to offset bad debt, increase contractual allowances, or purchase more sophisticated home care capital equipment such as portable infusion devices.

Reimbursement remains the most difficult aspect of initiating a successful hospital-based home infusion service. Most hospital-based infusion programs either fail or marginally exist because of their lack of reimbursement expertise unique to home care. In contrast, hospital-based, Medicare-certified home health services, which are reimbursed under allowable costs under Part A reimbursement, are much more straightforward with the use of Medicare cost reports and annual audits. By contracting with commercial vendors, hospitals may establish earlier access to limited reimbursement trends, capital, professional marketing, clinical monitoring expertise, and sales capabilities. Some hospitals have gained experience in this manner and then ventured out on their own, either through a for-profit subsidiary or through retaining complete responsibility for their own hospital-based nonprofit program.

Hospital- and community-based programs have significantly increased their depth in clinical expertise, as an increasing number of home care pharmacy specialists have advanced their technical expertise in parenteral therapeutics to complement their strong clinical or patient care-oriented backgrounds. Minimal success in today's complex in-home infusion programs can be expected when home care agencies restrict the pharmacist's role to providing only the purchasing and compounding of intravenous admixture services rather than expanding their role to coordinating patient care with nursing and direct patient interactions to include drug therapy education, compliance monitoring, and home visits.

Ten Years' Experience: St. Joseph Hospital Home Health Care Services

St. Joseph Home Health Care Services were initiated in 1981 by the department of pharmacy and IV therapy services as a diversification strategy into home care.[41] During the first 3 years, selected inpatient pharmacists and registered IV therapy nurses identified, trained, and facilitated discharge planning for inpatient candidates to home parenteral nutrition and intravenous antibiotics. Inpatient staff also monitored drug therapy, infusion devices, and central catheter care, managed reimbursement, and provided direct patient deliveries in the home while maintaining a 20-hour on-call responsibility to patients.

As the program grew, additional staff and resources were allocated to the pharmacy-based home infusion service. In 1983, one full-time equivalent (FTE) nurse clinician was totally dedicated to the service. One year later, two additional FTE's (nurse clinician and pharmacist specialist) were included. The key element of success was establishing a "vested" participation of professional and technical staff in the pharmacy and IV therapy services. Interested consumers of these new home health services included hospital administration, medical staff, nursing, financial services, discharge planners, case managers, payers, and existing specialty services such as oncology, infectious diseases, and nephrology services. In 1985, nursing services initiated a Medicare-certified skilled intermittent home health agency under a separate ambulatory service.

In 1988, JCAHO accredited the home care program against national standards as described by Bing.[42] In July 1989, both home care programs were organizationally reassigned to a new product line of home health care services. Four months after the combining of both the Medicare-certified and home infusion services, a hospice (non-Medicare-certified) program was initiated to enhance the continuum of care for terminally ill oncology, AIDS, cardiology, nephrology, and pulmonary patients.

Each home health care program operates financially as a separate cost center with unique revenue and cost allocations. Separate budgets, monthly financial statements, personnel, and productivity standards are responsible to each program's director, who reports to the home health care administrator. In June 1990, a separate home infusion satellite was established 30 miles to the north in the Seattle area to provide home infusion services to a large teaching medical center. Concurrently, a separate pharmacy license, Drug Enforcement Agency number, purchasing contracts, and home health agency license were established to manage this new entrepreneurial venture. As a separate cost center, a unique budget was developed to provide management, professional, technical, and reimbursement staff. Six months later, a previously existing clinical dietary home tube feeding program consisting of three clinical dietitians was integrated under the umbrella of "home health care services" (figure 35-1). Since July 1989, home care staffing has grown from 22 FTE's to more than 80 FTE's by late 1991, proportionate to the growth of home health services. The multidisciplinary staff consists of 41 nurses, 7 pharmacists, 4 home health aides, 3 clinical dietitians, 5 pharmacy technicians, 3 social workers, 5 physical, speech, and occupational therapists, 7 managers/directors, and 9 reimbursement/secretarial (figure 35-2).

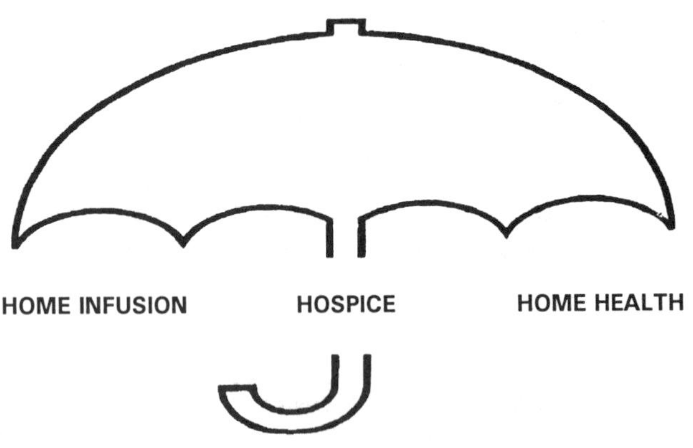

Figure 35-1. St. Joseph Home Health Care services

Approximately 5 percent of St. Joseph's Medicare homebound patients also receive home infusion services in which all supplies, professional services, intravenous drug or nutritional admixtures, and reimbursement services are directly coordinated by hospital-based services.[28,33] Similarly, only about 5 percent of this program's home infusion patients are also receiving skilled intermittent care from the home health service. With the addition of hospice care, primarily for the oncology population, typically 10-15 percent of the hospice patients receive high-tech injectable or epidural pain management.[43,44] In each case, the patient's care is coordinated among hospice, home infusion, and home health staff to ensure that continuity of care is synchronized with the patient ambulatory oncology clinic and inpatient treatments.

Many of the aspects of care presented here are applicable to community-based home health care programs; however, coordination of care among multiple providers such as hospice and home infusion or home health and home infusion agencies is often problematic as a result of the increasing complexity of home care, decreasing reimbursement, or evolution of regulatory agencies slowly adjusting to the growth of home health care.

The opportunities for pharmacists frequently evolve from the home infusion or high-tech home health care alternatives, either in the hospital or in community-based programs. Klotz[45] demonstrated that decentralization of high-tech care into the patient's home presents major challenges and opportunities to all health care professionals. Other community-based agencies and outpatient clinics have provided extensive reviews of parenteral antineoplastic and antibiotic therapies in the home through conventional and unusual delivery methods with moderate success.[46-51] Total parenteral nutrition and intravenous antibiotics, the fastest growing sector, accounted for more than 65 percent of home infusion revenues according to a 1989 Prudential Bache report. Several other therapies, once more high risk, are now being performed routinely outside the hospital or clinic environment by specialized home infusion professionals.[52-56] Home infusion pharmacists have developed specialized expertise in their clinical skills of pain assessment, drug information, infusion catheters, and portable infusion devices to complement the hospice services provided to the terminally ill.[57-61]

PATIENT SERVICES

Hospital pharmacies directing intravenous therapy teams have successfully implemented hospital-based programs using inpatient pharmacists and nurses motivated to provide skilled care in the patient's home 24 hours per day, 7 days per week. Attempts by pharmacy departments to depend upon emergency room nurses or clinic nurses to provide after-hour injections are seldom customer driven and cannot survive in a competitive marketplace unique to home care. Increases in home care staffing were justified through variable workload measurements adapted from inpatient services.[33,41] As the number of patients and revenues increased, commensurate salary and nonsalary expenses were adjusted. Twenty-four-hour backup for both pharmacy and nursing infusion services are accomplished through on-call personnel and 24-hour inpatient pharmacy and intravenous therapy team services. Inpatient pharmacists, IV nurses, and support personnel were cross-trained to be responsible for home IV admixtures and clinical management to minimize fixed staff costs. The cross-training of inpatient staff incorporates depth and breadth in experience to meet the growing needs of home care services. Gradually, full-time nurse specialists and pharmacists can be employed to coordinate all aspects of home care, including patient screening for admission to service, education and training of patients and families, admixture compounding, home delivery of nutritional solutions and medications, clinical management, and reimbursement services.

The eventual success of a program depends heavily on attracting highly motivated managers and professional staff in addition to establishing strong referral networks with local physicians, hospital discharge planners, insurance case managers, and other health care professionals in the community.

Combining three home health programs certified annually by Medicare, licensed annually by the State Department of Health and Washington State Board of Pharmacy, and accredited by JCAHO every 3 years creates a dynamic atmosphere for continually orienting staff and advancing patient care standards amid varying expectations of regulatory agencies. In October 1991, St. Joseph Home Health Care Services were JCAHO reaccredited based upon the new enhanced 1991 JCAHO home care standards, which represent the most advanced national pharmaceutical care standards in home care. Commendations to the service were given to recognize excellence in the following standards, which are typically major compliance problems nationally: (1) initial and ongoing clinical monitoring by pharmacists, specifically documentation, (2) ongoing processes for integrating laboratory results with prescribed therapies, (3) therapeutic appro-

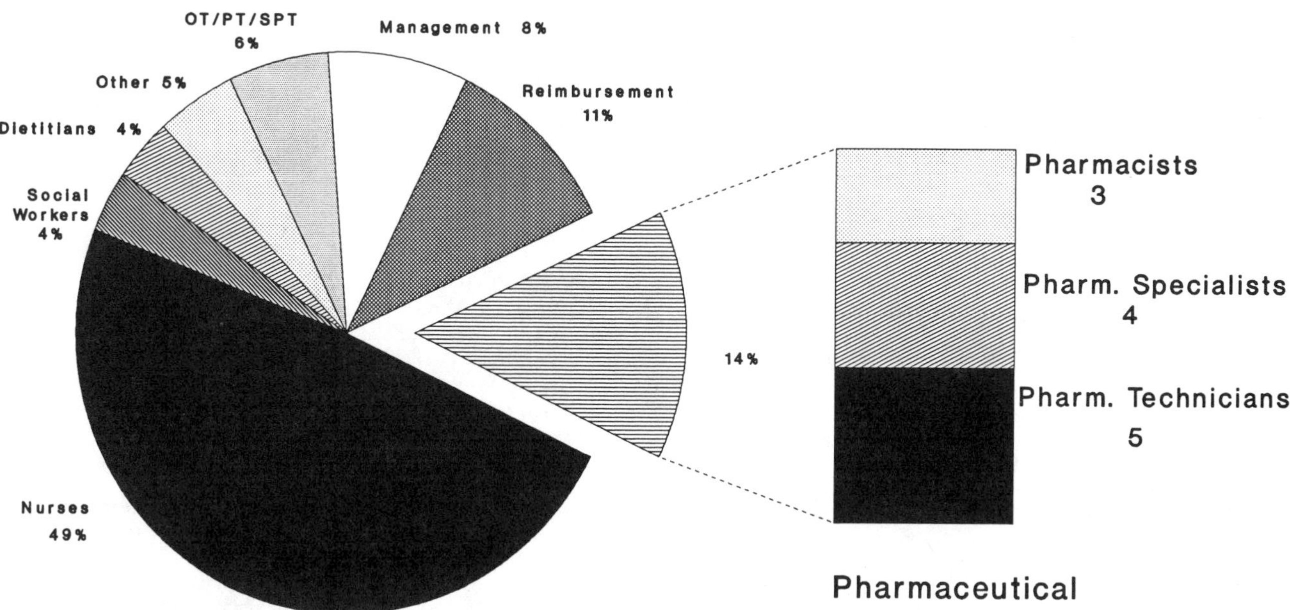

Figure 35-2. St. Joseph Home Health Care services (multidisciplinary staff)

priateness and response to drug treatment, (4) monitoring and reporting of adverse side effects, and (5) coordination and communication with prescribing physicians and home health nurses coordinating the patient's care.

In comparison to earlier JCAHO national survey results, a sample of 147 home infusion therapy providers surveyed by the earlier, less stringent pharmacy standards in 1990 found that 63 percent of the providers had compliance problems in drug monitoring; 33 percent in pharmacy monitoring and evaluation; 24 percent in care or service planning, and 24 percent in treatment planning.[62]

Significant differences in exceeding national standards can be attributed to integrating nurses, pharmacists, and other members of the home health care team from home infusion, home health, and hospice into an interdisciplinary approach to patient care. St. Joseph's continued success with integrating these combined home health care programs has resulted in its developing a consultation service to assist other institutions that desire to expand the continuum of patient care into the home during economically challenging times.

CONCLUSION

Home health care comprises the medical and social or "custodial" services available to recovering, disabled, chronically ill, and terminally ill people. A number of interrelated forces have changed the home health care market, namely, the growth of HMO's and PPO's, implications of diagnostic-related groups (DRG's), reinterpretation of Medicare reimbursement polices, increasing technical sophistication of home care, and the proliferation of home care agencies.

There is little doubt that as consumers become better educated and as the health care market continues to change, all parties will be forced to seek cost-effective alternatives to hospitalization, including home health care services.

REFERENCES

1. Verespej M: It's time to cure the patient. *Industry Week* 240(11): 55-62, 1991.
2. Curtiss F: Hospices participate in medicare. *Reimbursement Update* 31:31-32, 1989.
3. Health Care Financing Administration, Office of the Actuary: Data from the Office of National Cost Estimates, Washington DC Government Printing Office, Baltimore, MD, 1990.
4. Sawyer D: The Medicare and Medicaid Data Book. Baltimore, MD, Health Care Financing Administration pub no. 03156, December 1984.
5. Rogers P: The demand and intensity of home health services following prospective payment. *Home Health Care Quarterly* 10(1/2):49-60, 1989.

6. Medicare Program; Home health agencies: Conditions of participation and reduction in recordkeeping requirements. *Fed Reg* 54:33354-33373, 1989.
7. Medicare Program: Catastrophic outpatient drug benefit. *Fed Reg* 54:37190-371208, 1989.
8. Medicare Program: Conditions of participation for home intravenous drug therapy providers. *Fed Reg* 54:37220-37238, 1989.
9. Medicare Program: Outpatient prescription drugs: List of covered home IV drugs. *Fed Reg* 54:37239-37421, 1989.
10. Medicare Program: Coverage of home intravenous drug therapy services. 54:37422-37438, 1989.
11. Cardinale VA: *Drug Topics Redbook, 1991.* Oradell, NJ, Medical Economics Company, 1991.
12. Christiansen L: The highs and lows of PPO's. *Business and Health* 9(9):72-77, 1991.
13. Coile RC: Housecalls, innovation, and alternate care. *Healthcare Forum J* 2(Mar/Apr):48, 1990.
14. Oakland K: Illinois Blues form preferred-supplier network. *Homecare* 13(10)(Oct):144, 1991.
15. McNiff ML: HMOs and a VNA's Experience. *Caring* (May) 30-33, 1986.
16. Curtiss FR: Reimbursement dilemma regarding home health care products and services. *Am J Hosp Pharm* 41:1548-1554, 1984.
17. Lepper GJ, Swoboda J: Narrow harbors. *Health Progress* (Dec): 44-47, 1991.
18. Parenteral products for nonhospitalized patients. Washington State Administrative Code, Chapter 360-16A WAC,1990.
19. Home Health Agency Rules and Regulations. Washington State Administrative Code, Chapter 248-27 WAC, July 1989.
20. Mitchell M: Community Health Accreditation Program Manual. New York, NY, National League for Nursing, 1991.
21. *Accreditation Manual for Hospitals, vol. 1, Standards.* Oakbrook Terrace, IL, Joint Commission on Accreditation of Healthcare Organizations, 1991.
22. *Accreditation Standard for Home Care.* Oakbrook Terrace, IL, Joint Commission on Accreditation of Healthcare Organizations, 1988.
23. *Key To Quality: A Guide to Joint Commission Home Care Survey and Accreditation. Scoring Guidelines For Home Care Standards.* Oakbrook Terrace, IL, Joint Commission on Accreditation of Healthcare Organizations, 1989.
24. *Accreditation Manual for Home Care, vol. 1, Standards.* Oakbrook Terrace, IL, Joint Commission on Accreditation of Healthcare Organizations, 1991.
25. Boesch D: Meeting Joint Commission Standards: Pharmacists and home care agencies. *Consult Pharm* 5:437-446,1990.
26. Rooney A: Personal communication: Joint Commission on Home Care surveyors conference. Oakbrook Terrace, IL, May 1990.
27. Watson L, Samaripa J: Top 100 companies to watch aim for business expansions, new product areas. *Homecare* 13(12):46-75, 1991.
28. Pelham LD, Bushaw KE, Norwood MR, et al: Operational issues for hospital-based home infusion pharmacies. *J Pharm Pract* 4:11-18, 1990.
29. Baptista RJ, Mitrano FP: Home intermittent amrinone infusions in terminal congestive heart failure. *Drug Intell Clin Pharm* 23:59-62, 1989.
30. Chattopadhyay T, Catania P, Mergener M: Outcome of intravenous antibiotic therapy for hospitalized and home care osteomyelitis patients. *Consult Pharm* 6:45-48, 1991.
31. McPherson ML: Management of AIDS and infectious complications. *J Home Health Care Prac* 3(2):17-24, 1991.
32. Kwan J: High-technology i.v. infusion devices. *Am J Hosp Pharm* 48(suppl):S36-S51, 1991.
33. Linggi AJ, Pelham LD, Norwood MR, et al: Home health care: Pharmacy involvement. *Am J Hosp Pharm* 43:392-396, 1986.
34. Toon S: The rise of home infusion therapy. *Continuing Care* Jan 19-36, 1991.
35. U.S. Congress, Office of Technology Assessment: *Quality of Medical Care: Information for Consumers.* Publication OTA-H-386. Washington, DC, Government Printing Office, June 1988.
36. *Primer on Indicator Development and Application: Measuring Quality of Health Care.* Oakbrook Terrace, IL, Joint Commission on Accreditation of Healthcare Organizations, 1990.
37. *Guide to Quality Assurance.* Oakbrook Terrace, IL, Joint Commission on Accreditation of Healthcare Organizations, 1988.
38. Walton M: *The Deming Management Method.* New York, Doss Mead, 1986, pp 96-118.
39. Galt MA, Galt KA: Pharmaceutical services in hospital-based home health care agencies. *Am J Hosp Pharm* 41:285-291, 1982.
40. Burgess-Bishop J, Dunlap ST: Medical center diversification into the home infusion therapy market. *Home Care Econ* 1:72-79, 1987.
41. Linggi A, Pelham LD: Strategic planning for clinical services, St. Joseph Hospital and Health Care Center. *Am J Hosp Pharm* 43(9):2164-2168, 1986.
42. Bing C: Integration of standards into high-tech home care pharmacy practice. *J Pharm Pract* 1(1):45-52, 1988.
43. Shafer A, Donnelly AJ: Management of postoperative pain by continuous epidural infusion of analgesics. *Clin Pharm* 10:745-764, 1991.
44. Norwood MR: Homecare of the terminally ill. *Am J Hosp Pharm* 47(suppl):S23-S26, 1990.
45. Klotz R: Opportunities for progressive pharmacy practice in homecare. *J Pharm Pract* 4:19-27, 1990.
46. Bennett MA, Allen R: High-technology home pharmacotherapy, I: An overview of antiinfective and antineoplastic therapies. *J Pharm Pract* 4:34-39, 1990.
47. Brown R: Home intravenous antibiotic therapy. *Infect Dis Pract* 11(1):1-8, 1987.
48. Goldenberg R: Pitfalls in the delivery of outpatient intravenous therapy. *Drug Intell Clin Pharm* 19:293-296, 1985.
49. Rehm S, Weinstein A: Home intravenous antibiotic therapy—a team approach. *Ann Intern Med* 99:388-392, 1983.
50. Balinsky W, Nesbitt S: Cost-effectiveness of outpatient parenteral antibiotics: A review of the literature. *Am J Med* 87:301-305, 1989.
51. McPherson ML: Monitoring home IV antibiotic therapy. *J Home Health Care Prac* 2(4):69-77, 1990.
52. Martin JK, Norwood MR: Pharmacist management of antiemetic therapy under protocol in an oncology clinic. *Am J Hosp Pharm* 45:1322-1328, 1988.
53. Mitchell MM, Higginbotham PL: Care of the elderly patient receiving continuous 5-fluoruracil at home. *J Home Health Care Prac* 2(4):46-51, 1990.
54. Santiago OL: Establishing a community-based home transfusion program. *J Home Health Care Prac* 2(4):21-28, 1990.
55. Bennet MA, Allen RD: High-technology home pharmacotherapy, II: An overview of the newest home therapies. *J Pharm Pract* 3(1):40-47, 1990.
56. Gorski LA, Schmidt TB: Home dobutamine therapy. *J Home Health Care Prac* 2(4):11-20, 1990.
57. Arter SG, Lipman AG: Hospice care: A new opportunity for pharmacists. *J Pharm Pract* 3(1):28-33, 1990.
58. Lipman AG: Pain management in the home-care and hospice patient. *J Pharm Pract* 3(1):48-59, 1990.
59. Kerr IG, Sone M, DeAngelis C, et al: Continuous narcotic infusion with patient controlled analgesia for chronic cancer pain in outpatients. *Ann Intern Med* 108:554-557, 1988.
60. Littrell RA: Epidural analgesia. *Am J Hosp Pharm* 48:2460-2474, 1991.
61. Podell LB: Medicare coverage of hospice care. *Am J Hosp Pharm* 41:942-944, 1984.
62. Schneider P: JCAHO completes first home care accreditation cycle. *Nutrition in Clin Pract* 6:127, 1991.

ADDITIONAL READING

Catania PN, Rosner MM (eds): *Home Health Care Practice.* Palo Alto, CA, Health Markets Research, 1986.

Lerman D: *Home Care: Positioning the Hospital for the Future.* Chicago, American Hospital Publishing, Inc., 1990.

CHAPTER 36

Ambulatory Care

BARRY L. CARTER

INTRODUCTION

One of the most significant trends in health care has been the emphasis on shorter hospital stay and on outpatient care. This has led to hospital diversification into many areas including ambulatory care. Many conditions previously managed only in the institution are now handled on an outpatient basis. Broad-based support for innovative ambulatory care services was lacking until financial incentives forced major structural changes in the health care system.

In the past, unique ambulatory pharmacy services often received limited attention within institutional pharmacy practice. However, a persistent legion of ambulatory pharmacy practitioners believed that the model had major advantages for patient care and pharmacy practice. Ambulatory care is no longer on the horizon but has become the standard for health care delivery. This has greatly expanded the opportunities for ambulatory pharmacy practitioners. It will be the responsibility of organized pharmacy and academia to provide sufficient numbers of highly competent practitioners who can enter these settings and provide progressive clinical services.

The purposes of this chapter are to describe common ambulatory care settings in which pharmacy is involved, review the impact of ambulatory clinical pharmacy services, and outline standards of practice in these settings.

BACKGROUND

During most of this century, the trend in medicine has been toward greater specialization. In 1917, the first medical specialty board was organized (ophthalmology), and by 1948, there were 18 specialty boards.[1] During the 1950's, the vast majority of medical students entered specialty residencies and received training in tertiary-care centers. In the early 1960's, it became obvious that, if this trend continued, there would be a critical shortage of primary care physicians. During the mid-1960's, community pediatric, general internal medicine, and family practice programs were developed in academic centers.[2] These required different training sites, and some of the first were urban health centers that served indigent patients. However, this did not solve the problem of inadequate primary care for the majority of the population.

In 1966, two independent commissions recognized the potential crisis and the need for primary care training.[3] These were the "Citizens' Commission on Graduate Medical Education of the American Medical Association" (the Millis Commission) and the "Ad Hoc Committee on Education for Family Practice of the Council of Medical Education of the American Medical Association" (the Willard Committee).[4,5] In 1969, in part as a result of these findings, the American Board of Family Practice was developed and became the 20th medical specialty. For the next 15 years, specialty training in family practice, general internal medicine, and general pediatrics infused greater numbers of primary care physicians into private practice. However, even today, there is a critical lack of primary care providers and a maldistribution of those in practice. Small towns, rural areas, and indigent populations continue to have insufficient primary care. The problem of excessive numbers of specialists and lack of a solid primary care base is evident when medicine is compared to other professions (figure 36-1).[6]

One of the most significant events that restructured medical care occurred during the mid-1980's with attempts to control health care costs. These policies created major incentives for alternative health care delivery systems.[7] The emphasis on reduced hospital stay, outpatient procedures, and surgery resulted in a proliferation of ambulatory care centers, home health care services, and outpatient care. Another result was the growth of preferred provider organizations, health maintenance organizations, and primary-care networks.[7]

Hospital diversification has resulted in ambulatory centers within the hospital, adjacent to the hospital, or freestanding centers on the hospital grounds. Many hospitals have established satellites at distant locations within a city, which provide an automatic source of referrals to the hospital.[7]

The advancement of technology and training have also meant that many procedures are now performed in ambulatory settings. Outpatient surgery, sigmoidoscopy, endoscopy, exercise stress tests, and mammography are examples of procedures and tests that are becoming common in private physician offices.

DEFINITIONS AND PHILOSOPHY

"Ambulatory care" encompasses those health-related services that, by definition, are provided to patients who walk to seek their care. These services are provided to patients who are not confined to a bed in an institutional setting.[8] The term "ambulatory care" includes a wide range of service areas including outpatient pharmacies, emergency departments, primary care clinics, specialty clinics, ambulatory care centers, and family practice groups (table 36-1). This

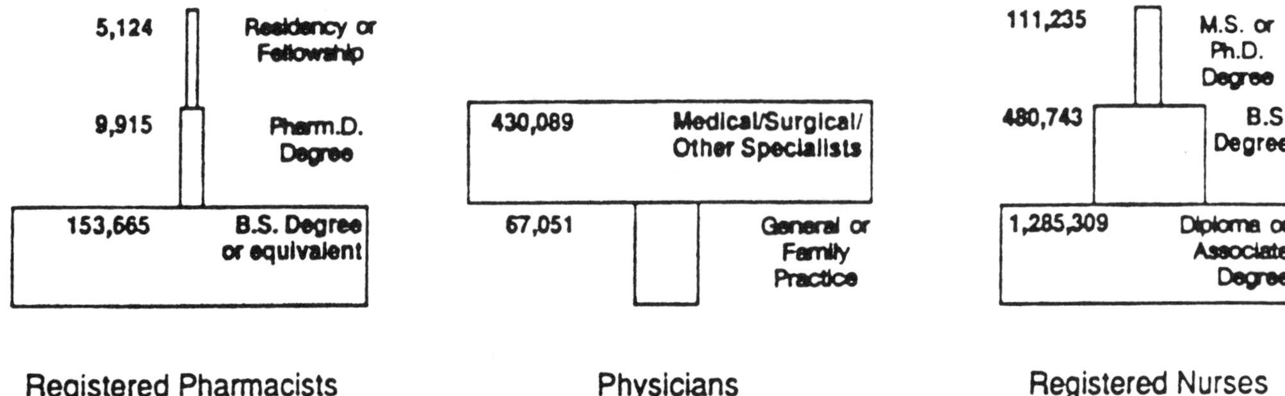

Figure 36-1. Educational differentiation of the pharmacy and nursing work forces and degree of specialization of the physician work force.

Reprinted with permission from Knapp KK, Letendre DE: Educational differentiation of the pharmacy workforce. *Am J Hosp Pharm* 46:2481, 1989.

chapter focuses on these ambulatory settings. Home health care, health maintenance organizations, residential homes, and some nursing home facilities are other examples of ambulatory care. These latter programs are covered elsewhere in this handbook.

Primary care is a subset of ambulatory care that has unique features and a specific philosophy. The three most common primary care specialties are general pediatrics, general internal medicine, and family practice. Rakel[3] provided a summary of the definitions for primary care derived from the American Board of Family Physicians and the Millis Commission, which states:

> Primary care is a form of delivery of medical care which encompasses the following functions:
> 1. It is "first-contact" care, serving as a point-of-entry for the patient into the health care system;
> 2. It includes continuity by virtue of caring for patients over a period of time, both in sickness and in health;
> 3. It is comprehensive care, drawing from all the traditional major disciplines for its functional content;
> 4. It serves a coordinative function for all the health care needs of the patient;
> 5. It assumes continuing responsibility for individual patient followup and community health problems; and
> 6. It is a highly personalized type of care.

Family practice is a specialty practice that is a subset of primary care:[3]

> The family physician provides continuing, comprehensive care in a personalized manner to patients of all ages and to their families, regardless of the presence of disease or the nature of the presenting complaint.... One of the essential functions of the family physician is the willingness to accept ongoing responsibility for managing a patient's medical care. Once a patient or a family has been accepted into the physician's practice, responsibility for care is both total and continuing.... The family physician's commitment to patients does not cease at the end of illness but is a continuing responsibility, regardless of the patient's state of health or the disease process.

Fry[9] stated, "We general practitioners... [have] the chance to observe and study changes in our patients and their disorders over many years, as though we were watching a continuous moving picture show. However, our hospital colleagues are not so fortunate; they have to peer at snapshots of patients and diseases as they present at the particular moment of referral."

"Primary care" by definition implies first contact into the medical system. Therefore, primary health practitioners must be prepared for patients who present with a wide variety of illnesses or multiple disease states. Many of these are conditions rarely managed by inpatient or tertiary care. In addition, problems with compliance and delayed adverse drug reactions must be identified and managed. Health practitioners who work entirely within inpatient or referral centers receive a skewed population that is not representative of overall health care problems. Rakel[3] addressed the issue of the breadth of knowledge required by the family physician, by quoting Fry:[9]

> Working in general practice broadens the mind and humbles the soul. It is very different from the sheltered world of hospital practice. It is as though we, in general practice, work in the natural habitat of the jungle, seeking and stalking our prey in its own environment, whereas our hospital colleagues have to function behind the bars of a zoo, dealing with patients and diseases in highly artificial situations.

Primary care physicians frequently practice either conceptually or physically with an interdisciplinary team. Primary care physicians frequently consult with social workers, dietitians, behavioral counselors, and clinical pharmacists. The primary care physician should be the leader of any interdisciplinary team. Patient care, teaching, and research activities should be provided by team members at a level and scope that correspond to their level of expertise. Interdisciplinary teams in ambulatory care function differently from their impatient counterparts, with one critical difference being communication between team members.

INTERPERSONAL COMMUNICATION

Good interpersonal skills are important in all areas of pharmacy practice. However, they are critical in ambulatory settings with interdisciplinary teams. In most ambulatory care clinics, there is no organized, structured team that visits the patient. Instead, a physician may be attending several patients at one time. Another team member may see selected patients only with the physician. In a group practice, there may be more than 20 patients in the clinic at one time. An individual patient may be in the office or clinic for only 30 to 60 minutes. Laboratory test results or serum drug levels may not return for 1 or 2 days after the patient's visit. These unique logistical characteristics can be very challenging to a clinical pharmacist. Because of these factors, excellent communication and followup are essential and must be provided by all team members.

Some patient care management roles will be delegated to the clinical pharmacist. This may include office visits or telephone followup to assess compliance or adverse reactions or adjust therapy. If the physician has delegated this authority, the clinical pharmacist must inform the physician about these patient interactions. Depending upon the severity or level of complexity, this may necessitate direct contact with the physician or simply documenting the information in the patient's medical record. Each member of the team must clearly understand his or her role definition within the team. This definition may change depending upon the setting or the philosophy of team members.

In ambulatory settings, a complex and personal relationship is established among the various health care members. Physicians who have trained in a primary care specialty understand their role as the team leader and coordinator of the patient's total health care. Generally, these physicians are very willing to accept recommendations from other health professionals. This delicate team relationship can easily be upset by someone who does not understand the practice philosophy or the role definitions within the team.

The successful clinical pharmacist must perform a balancing act with regard to interpersonal skills. This individual must not be passive or shy. Equally destructive is an individual who is aggressive, always right, and must "win" interactions. The latter characteristics have been observed in some pharmacy students and pharmacy clinicians who trained with inpatient specialty groups where aggressive personalities are more prevalent. Unless they are adaptable, these pharmacists may not be well suited for the ambulatory setting.

The effective ambulatory clinical pharmacist is knowledgeable and competent and must maintain a high level of communication with other team members.[10,11] The clinical pharmacist must have excellent writing skills in order to prepare consultations, newsletters, and memoranda. He or she must have the finesse to be assertive with recommendations to other team members while not being aggressive. There must be a team spirit that allows each to be willing to compromise when differences of opinion are expressed. These attributes do not come naturally, and in many cases must be developed in advanced ambulatory residencies or fellowships.

FUNCTIONS AND STANDARDS OF PRACTICE

The types of pharmaceutical services will differ from one setting to another. The new learning objectives for American Society of Hospital Pharmacists (ASHP)-accredited primary care residencies provide a good general description of the functions typically performed in ambulatory settings.[12] (See Appendix 36-A.)

This report went on to list 14 acute, 22 chronic, and 9 preventive care problems; it also discussed self-care, devices, emergency care, and family planning areas in which the ambulatory resident should have knowledge and skills. These should also be the goals and standards for ambulatory care clinical pharmacists.

Some ambulatory care clinical pharmacists serve very specialized settings, such as hypertension clinics or anticoagulation clinics. Others perform a great deal of primary care, patient assessment, and triage that is unique to some settings.

The level and complexity of clinical services will depend on the setting. In a program with comprehensive clinical services, the clinical pharmacist is integrated into the decision-making process with regard to drug therapy. This service must not be interrupted. In order to succeed in an ambulatory environment, the service must be continually provided.

Many ambulatory care pharmacists spend a considerable amount of time conducting research and publishing scholarly work. Most of these practitioners have responsibilities for teaching pharmacy students, residents and fellows, medical students, and medical residents.

AMBULATORY CARE SETTINGS

Many outpatient pharmacies provide only traditional pharmaceutical services. However, the focus of this chapter is the provision of comprehensive pharmacy services, which have been described in outpatient ambulatory pharmacy or group practices.[13-16] The importance of computer support and physical facilities in providing counseling and clinical services in busy outpatient pharmacies has been described.[17-19] These are discussed in other chapters of this handbook.

Primary Care Clinics

Clinical pharmacists practice in a wide variety of primary care clinics (table 36-1). A common model is the team of physicians and other health professionals in a general or specialty clinic.[20-23] In these settings, the clinical pharmacist functions as one of the interdisciplinary team members each time the clinic meets. In one study, the clinical pharmacist improved drug therapy documentation, improved patient compliance, decreased duplicate prescriptions, and prevented the risk of overdosage.[24] In a followup study, physicians referred patients to a clinical pharmacist and a nurse clinician.[25] Compared to a control group, study patients were more compliant (72 percent versus 20 percent) and blood pressure control was better (69 percent versus 29 percent). These were statistically significant, and the benefit remained after 4 years of followup of the active program. The cost savings resulting from reduced duplication of drugs, reduced office visits, and improved care greatly exceeded the cost to provide the service.

Table 36-1. Examples of ambulatory care settings and services

Outpatient Pharmacy Services
Community pharmacy
Hospital outpatient pharmacy
Emergency room
Private group practice
General Medicine Clinics (Primary Care)
Pharmacy clinic
Specialty Medicine Clinics
Hypertension
Anticoagulation
Diabetes
Pain
Rheumatology
Asthma or allergy
Pediatrics
General pediatrics
Asthma or allergy
Family Practice
Indian Health Service
Pharmacokinetic Monitoring Services
Home Health Care
Health Maintenance Organizations

A unique extension of these clinics is the pharmacy clinic.[26-30] Traditionally, these clinics developed as a method to provide refills to drop-in patients. However, many have expanded to pharmacist-managed assessment clinics in which a wide range of patients with multiple chronic diseases are seen. A medical director is available to consult with the pharmacists when needed. Patients are referred by physicians to the clinical pharmacists, who provide physical assessment, order laboratory tests, alter dosages, and change medications.

The value of these services was reported in a classic study by McKenney et al. in 1973.[31] The clinical pharmacist worked independently but maintained close communication with physicians in a model neighborhood comprehensive health program in Detroit. A group of hypertensive patients was divided into a control group and a study group. The study group received comprehensive education and monitoring when it received prescriptions. The pharmacist interacted frequently with the physicians in order to modify therapy caused by problems with compliance or adverse effects. Not only was compliance improved in the study group, but blood pressure control (as measured by the physicians) was better. When these services were discontinued, compliance and blood pressure control deteriorated.

One of the most successful pharmacist-managed ambulatory clinics has been the anticoagulation clinic.[32-38] Typically, physicians refer patients to the pharmacists, who obtain histories and laboratory results, make long-term dosage adjustments, and provide extensive patient education. The physicians maintain the responsibility for the overall care of the patient. A cost-benefit evaluation demonstrated that the pharmacist-managed clinic resulted in a marked cost avoidance by reducing complications and hospitalizations.[37] In 1985, the ASHP Research and Education Foundation established anticoagulation clinic traineeships. This program has allowed trainees to work in well-established anticoagulation clinics throughout the country.

Numerous studies have demonstrated the value of clinical pharmacists in the chronic management of hypertensive, diabetic, and anticoagulated patients.[14,20-22,35,36,38-42] These services have resulted in disease control that is at least as good as for conventionally managed patients. Clinical pharmacy services have also been well described in general pediatric clinics and pediatric allergy clinics.[43,44]

Family Practice

Clinical pharmacy services in family practice have been well established for nearly 20 years.[10,11,45-54] One of the earliest descriptions was of a program in the rural town of Mechanicsville, IA.[47,49] This model training site was developed by the Cedar Rapids Family Practice Residency and the University of Iowa College of Pharmacy. This model became one that many programs incorporated into private practice groups, especially in South Carolina.[45,50,51] The Area Health Education Centers in North Carolina and other States commonly incorporate a family physician-clinical pharmacist model into their programs.

Most clinical pharmacists in family practice work with one of the nearly 400 family practice residency training programs. Clinical pharmacy involvement with these programs continues to grow. In these settings, clinical pharmacists are less likely to serve as independent primary care providers. The majority of patients are seen by family practice residents in their educational training. The major functions of clinical pharmacists in these residency programs include patient service; education of residents, faculty, medical students, pharmacy students, and other health professionals; and research.[10,11] This does not mean, however, that clinical pharmacists cannot provide primary care in family practice residency programs. This author, and others, have developed practice programs with experienced faculty physicians who feel comfortable delegating responsibilities such as drug and dosage selection, long-term drug therapy management, and monitoring. Patients are seen by both the faculty physician and the clinical pharmacist. Diagnostic functions are performed by the physician. Drug and dosage selection, prescription writing, patient education, and plans for long-term monitoring are provided by the clinical pharmacist. Dosage adjustments, adverse reactions, and refills are managed by the pharmacist through either subsequent office visits or telephone followup.

Helling et al.[55] demonstrated that patient perceptions of their medical care were improved when they were seen by both a clinical pharmacist and a family physician. Brown and coworkers[56] used blinded physician/pharmacist peer review panels to assess the appropriateness of clinical pharmacist recommendations. In this study, 96 percent of the evaluations were implemented. The prescribing physicians rated 92 percent of the pharmacists' recommendations as moderately to very useful, and none were rated not at all useful. None of the recommendations were judged to be inappropriate by the review panel. Haxby and coworkers[57] evaluated pharmacist consultations with a physician questionnaire. In this study, 96 percent of recommendations were implemented, 97 percent of the consultations were rated very useful or mostly useful, and 77 percent of respondents felt that the consultation greatly improved or somewhat improved the clinical status of their patients.

Carter et al.[58] used a blinded physician/pharmacist review panel to compare the appropriateness of prescribing at four family practice model offices in the Iowa-affiliated network. Two of the offices had active clinical pharmacy services, and two had none. The peer-review panel evaluated overall prescribing (no pharmacist consultation) in the four offices. The appropriateness of prescriptions that were written following consultation with a clinical pharmacist was also measured at the two offices with these services. The blinded panel judged that significantly more prescriptions were "most appropriate" or "acceptable" in the offices with clinical pharmacists. In addition, the prescriptions that resulted from consultation with a clinical pharmacist were given the highest ratings for drug choice, dose, and benefit to the patient when compared to all other prescribing. These differences were statistically significant in spite of the consulted cases being judged significantly more difficult. Other studies have found that prescribing could be improved with educational intervention by a clinical pharmacist.[59,60] In addition, clinical pharmacy services in family practice have been shown to be cost effective.[61-63]

Pharmacokinetic monitoring services have been established in many ambulatory settings. However, the best-described program has been with the family practice group in Florida.[64-66] These authors have provided extensive information to establish a pharmacokinetic monitoring service in an ambulatory environment. In order to establish one of these services, the need for the service must be documented, the types of patients and volume of serum drug assays performed should be estimated, and then a proposal can be generated which describes the intended service. The unique feature of this type of service is that the pharmacist is directly inserted into the decision-making process each time a serum level is ordered. This provides a method to improve serum level determinations, offer physician education, and improve pharmacokinetic dosing.

The Indian Health Service

For many years, the Indian Health Service has been a leader in providing progressive primary care, clinical pharmacy services. Since 1972, pharmacists have been able to obtain didactic and clinical training, which enables them to become certified as pharmacist practitioners.[67] These pharmacists perform physical assessment and manage dozens of acute and chronic diseases using protocols.[68] In the pharmacist practitioner training program offered by the Indian Health Service, pharmacists are trained to provide primary care for most common medical conditions seen in primary care. However, they are not trained for major trauma, fractures, deliveries, or emergencies.[67] Protocols are initiated by the physician, which then allows the pharmacist to perform physical assessment, order diagnostic and laboratory tests and obtain x rays under these protocols.

The concept of the pharmacist as a primary care provider (e.g., physician's assistant) is more comprehensive in the Indian Health Service than in most ambulatory settings. This unique role has evolved as a result of the characteristics of this underserved population and is best suited for rural areas. It allows physicians to concentrate on the most complex patient management problems.

DEVELOPING AN AMBULATORY CARE PRACTICE

The most important aspect of developing an ambulatory practice is appropriate planning. The practice philosophy or team philosophy must be known and understood. This philosophy should be incorporated into the planning phase. For instance, is patient care the only mission of the practice? Is there any role for management of patients by a clinical pharmacist? Do medical residents or medical students have a major role, and how will this impact clinical pharmacy services? Is there a significant research program in progress or desired? The answers to these questions will determine the major thrust of any proposed clinical pharmacy service.

The administrator who plans to hire an ambulatory clinical pharmacist must ensure that the individual is competent and can effectively perform the standards of practice listed in Appendix 36-A. The pharmacist must have exceptional interpersonal skills and perform effectively in an interdisciplinary team. The administrator should strongly consider requiring advanced residency or fellowship training in primary care or family practice, as well as board certification as a pharmacotherapy specialist.

The types of potential pharmacy services can be obtained from references cited in this chapter and other ambulatory pharmacy literature. However, each setting or specialty practice will be unique. Some clinical pharmacy services or methods of providing the service will not be appropriate for all settings.

If personnel resources are limited, the scope of services may need to be limited when the service is initiated. For instance, a new practitioner in a group practice could not provide primary care services, a pharmacokinetic monitoring service, patient education, and physician education. However, some of these could be initiated. Once they are established, other services could be added.

One of the most important aspects of ambulatory care practice is the involvement of the clinical pharmacist in drug therapy decisions. This requires the pharmacist to be available and accessible when the patient is being seen. In large practices, it is not possible to interact during each prescribing event; therefore, a combination of methods for improving drug therapy may be necessary. These may include prospective chart review before patients present to the clinic, individual one-on-one supervision provided to physicians, and retrospective chart reviews to identify drug therapy problems that require correction. Koecheler and coworkers[69] identified six prognostic indicators that could be used to identify ambulatory patients with high risk of adverse outcomes. These included: (1) 5 or more medications in the drug regimen, (2) 12 or more medication doses per day, (3) medication regimen changed four or more times during the past 12 months, (4) more than three concurrent disease states present, (5) history of noncompliance, and (6) presence of drugs that require therapeutic drug monitoring. Clinical pharmacists in a very busy practice might focus their efforts on patients who meet these criteria and prospectively interact with their physicians to assist with decision making and plans for long-term management.

It is clear that successful ambulatory pharmacy services must be comprehensive and continual.[15] Some family practice, general medicine, or pediatric groups see patients 40 hours per week. If clinical pharmacy services are provided only 2 days per week or several hours each morning, their success and use will be limited. Clinical pharmacy services must be provided 80-90 percent of the time. This requires a strong commitment by the clinical pharmacist and the department that employs this person. In many circumstances, this level of service cannot be maintained (e.g., when the pharmacist is a faculty member). In this case, there must be methods to provide relief once the service is well established. This situation may necessitate having two pharmacists who share the clinical service responsibilities.

There should be ongoing evaluation of the pharmacy services. This may involve evaluations of physician satisfaction or use of the pharmacist, disease control, patient outcomes, or drug use reviews.

SUMMARY

The health care structure continues to shift to ambulatory care. This movement will provide additional opportunities for numerous types of ambulatory pharmacy services, including efficient outpatient pharmacies that provide prescriptions and comprehensive services to ambulatory patients.

In ambulatory care, the functions and clinical problems are so broad that general training is often insufficient. In the future, it will be necessary for ambulatory care pharmacists to complete advanced ambulatory residencies or fellowships. This is currently a requirement for many positions, and this trend will continue.

The vast majority of ambulatory practices described in this chapter were developed in Veterans Administration hospitals, ambulatory sites in tertiary medical centers, or residency training programs. However, comprehensive clinical pharmacy services are filtering into other ambulatory settings. It will be essential for pharmacist-physician practices to continue to develop in smaller hospitals and private practice. With the strong realignment of our health care system toward ambulatory care, there has never been a better opportunity for ambulatory clinical pharmacy practice.

REFERENCES

1. Langsley DG: Specialty training in clinical medicine. *Am J Hosp Pharm* 47:105-111, 1990.
2. Saward EW: The current role of the hospital in ambulatory care. *Bull NY Acad Med* 55:112-118, 1979.
3. Rakel RE (ed): *The Family Physician.* In *Textbook of Family Practice*, 4th Ed. Philadelphia, W.B. Saunders, 1990, pp 3-18.
4. Millis J: *The Graduate Education of Physicians.* Report of the Citizens, Commission on Graduate Medical Education. Chicago, American Medical Association, 1966.
5. Willard WR: *Meeting the Challenge of Family Practice.* Chicago, American Medical Association, 1966.
6. Knapp KK, Letendre DE: Educational differentiation of the pharmacy work force. *Am J Hosp Pharm* 46:2476-2482, 1989.
7. Black BL: Competitive alternatives to hospital impatient care. *Am J Hosp Pharm* 42:545-553, 1985.
8. Burns LA: Trends and initiatives in hospital ambulatory care. *Am J Hosp Pharm* 39:799-805, 1982.
9. Fry J: Common sense and uncommon sensibility. *J R Coll Gen Pract* 27:9-17, 1977.
10. Helling DK: Family practice pharmacy service: Part I. *Drug Intell Clin Pharm* 15:971-977, 1981.
11. Helling DK: Family practice pharmacy service: Part II. *Drug Intell Clin Pharm* 16:35-48, 1982.
12. Anon: ASHP supplemental standard and learning objectives for residency training in primary care pharmacy practice. *Am J Hosp Pharm* 47:1851-1854, 1990.
13. Baumgartner RP, Land MJ, Hauser LD: Rural health care: Opportunity for innovative pharmacy services. *Am J Hosp Pharm* 29:394-400, 1972.
14. Reinders TP, Rush DR, Baumgartner RP, et al: Pharmacist's role in management of hypertensive patients in an ambulatory care clinic. *Am J Hosp Pharm* 32:590-594, 1975.
15. Love DW, McWhinney BD: Ambulatory clinical practice programs. In McLeod DC, Miller WA (eds): *The Practice of Pharmacy*, Cincinnati, Harvey Whitney Books, 1981, pp 202-215.
16. Wallner JN, Still RP: Survey of outpatient pharmaceutical services in university hospitals. *Am J Hosp Pharm* 36:1193-1196, 1979.
17. Weissman AM, Solomon DK, Baumgartner RP, et al: Computer support of pharmaceutical services for ambulatory patients. *Am J Hosp Pharm* 33:1171-1174, 1976.
18. Miller RF, Herrick JD: Modernizing an ambulatory care pharmacy in a large multi-clinic institution. *Am J Hosp Pharm* 36:371-375, 1979.
19. Pierson JF, Hiner WO: Patient counseling in high-volume outpatient services. *Am J Hosp Pharm* 46:1990-1993, 1989.
20. Morton WA, Bridges ME: Pharmaceutical services in a medical screening clinic. *Am J Hosp Pharm* 35:574-578, 1978.
21. Stergachis A, Fors M, Wagner EH, et al: Effect of clinical pharmacists on drug prescribing in a primary-care clinic. *Am J Hosp Pharm* 44:525-529, 1987.
22. Tiggelar JM: Protocols for the treatment of essential hypertension and type II diabetes mellitus by pharmacists in ambulatory care clinics. *Drug Intell Clin Pharm* 21:521-529, 1987.
23. Schilling KW: Pharmacy program for monitoring diabetic patients. *Am J Hosp Pharm* 34:1242-1245, 1977.
24. Monson R, Bond CA, Schuna A: Role of the clinical pharmacist in improving drug therapy: Clinical pharmacists in outpatient therapy. *Arch Intern Med* 141:1441-1444, 1981.
25. Bond CA, Monson R: Sustained improvement in drug documentation, compliance, and disease control: A four-year analysis of an ambulatory care model. *Arch Intern Med* 144:1159-1162, 1984.
26. D'Achille KM, Swanson LN, Hill WT Jr: Pharmacist-managed patient assessment and medication refill clinic. *Am J Hosp Pharm* 35:66-70, 1978.
27. McKenney JM, Witherspoon JM, Pierpaoli PG: Initial experiences with a pharmacy clinic in a hospital-based group medical practice. *Am J Hosp Pharm* 38:1154-1158, 1981.
28. McKenney JM, Witherspoon JM: The impact of outpatient hospital pharmacists on patients receiving antihypertensive and anticoagulant therapy. *Hosp Pharm* 20:406-415, 1985.
29. Nelson LA, Cummings DM, Downs GE, et al: Financial impact of a pharmacist-managed medication refill clinic. *Military Med* 149:254-256, 1984.
30. Scrivens JJ Jr, Magalian P, Crazier GA: Cost-effective clinical pharmacy services in a Veterans Administration drop-in clinic. *Am J Hosp Pharm* 40:1952-1953, 1983.
31. McKenney JM, Slining JM, Henderson HR, et al: The effect of clinical pharmacy services on patients with essential hypertension. *Circulation* 48:1104-1111, 1973.
32. Reinders TP, Steinke WE: Pharmacist management of anticoagulant therapy in ambulant patients. *Am J Hosp Pharm* 36:645-648, 1979.
33. Davis FB, Sczupak CA: Outpatient oral anticoagulation: Guidelines for long-term management. *Postgrad Med* 66:100-109, 1979.
34. Nappi JM: Measuring the effectiveness of an anticoagulation clinic managed by a pharmacist. *Wisc Pharm* 6:164-168, 1980.
35. Cohen IA, Hutchison TA, Kirking DM, et al: Evaluation of a pharmacist-managed anticoagulation clinic. *J Clin Hosp Pharm* 10:167-175, 1985.
36. Garabedian-Ruffalo SM, Gray DR, Sax MJ, et al: Retrospective evaluation of a pharmacist-managed warfarin anticoagulation clinic. *Am J Hosp Pharm* 42:304-308, 1985.
37. Gray DR, Garabedian-Ruffalo SM, Chretien SD: Cost-justification of a clinical pharmacist-managed anticoagulation clinic. *Drug Intell Clin Pharm* 19:575-580, 1985.

38. Conte RR, Kehoe WA, Nielson N, et al: Nine-year experience with a pharmacist-managed anticoagulation clinic. *Am J Hosp Pharm* 43:2460-2464, 1986.
39. Sczupak CA, Conrad WF: Relationship between patient-oriented pharmaceutical services and therapeutic outcomes of ambulatory patients with diabetes mellitus. *Am J Hosp Pharm* 34:1238-1242, 1977.
40. Hawkins DW, Fiedler FP, Douglas HL, et al: Evaluation of a clinical pharmacist in caring for hypertensive and diabetic patients. *Am J Hosp Pharm* 36:1321-1325, 1979.
41. Morse GD, Douglas JB, Upton JH, et al: Effect of pharmacist intervention on control of resistant hypertension. *Amer J Hosp Pharm* 43:905-909, 1986.
42. Roberts RW, Stewart RB, Doering PL, et al: Contributions of a clinical pharmacist in a private group practice of physicians. *Drug Intell Clin Pharm* 12:210-213, 1978.
43. Levin RH: Clinical pharmacy practice in a pediatric clinic. *Drug Intell Clin Pharm* 6:171-176, 1972.
44. Ekwo E, Hendeles L, Weinberger M: Those who make decisions about management of children with asthma: Pharmacist-physician interaction. *Am J Hosp Pharm* 35:295-299, 1978.
45. Davis RE, Crigler WH, Martin H: Pharmacy and family practice: Concept, roles and fees. *Drug Intell Clin Pharm* 11:616-621, 1977.
46. Johnston TS, Heffron WA: Clinical pharmacy in family practice residency programs. *J Fam Prac* 13:91-94, 1981.
47. Juhl RP, Perry PJ, Norwood GJ, et al: The family practitioner-clinical pharmacist group practice: A model clinic. *Drug Intell Clin Pharm* 8:572-575, 1974.
48. Love DW, Hodge NA, Foley WA: The clinical pharmacist in a family practice residency program. *J Fam Pract* 10:67-72, 1980.
49. Perry PJ, Hurley SC: Activities of the clinical pharmacist practicing in the office of a family practitioner. *Drug Intell Clin Pharm* 9:129-133, 1975.
50. Robertson DL, Groh MJ, Papadopoulos DA: Family pharmacy and family medicine: A viable private practice alliance. *J Fam Prac* 11:273-277, 1980.
51. Robertson DL, Groh M: Activities of a clinical pharmacist in a private family practice. *Fam Prac Res J* 1:188-194, 1982.
52. Eichelberger BN: Family practice-clinical pharmacy opportunities in the community setting. *Am J Hosp Pharm* 37:740-742, 1980.
53. Maudlin RK: The clinical pharmacist and the family physician. *J Fam Prac* 3:667-668, 1976.
54. Moore TD: Pharmacist faculty member in a family medicine residency program. *Am J Hosp Pharm* 34:973-975, 1977.
55. Helling DK, Hepler CD, Jones ME: Effect of direct clinical pharmaceutical services on patients' perceptions of health care quality. *Am J Hosp Pharm* 36:325-329, 1979.
56. Brown DJ, Helling DK, Jones ME: Evaluation of clinical pharmacist consultations in a family practice office. *Am J Hosp Pharm* 36:912-915, 1979.
57. Haxby DG, Weart CW, Goodman BW Jr: Family practice physicians, perceptions of the usefulness of drug therapy recommendations from clinical pharmacists. *Am J Hosp Pharm* 45:824-827, 1988.
58. Carter BL, Helling DK, Jones ME, et al: Evaluation of family physician prescribing: Influence of the clinical pharmacist. *Drug Intell Clin Pharm* 18:817-821, 1984.
59. Gehlbach SH, Wilkinson WE, Hammond WE, et al: Improving drug prescribing in a primary care practice. *Med Care* 22:193-201, 1984.
60. Ives TJ, Frey JJ, Furr SJ, et al: Effect of an educational intervention on oral cephalosporin use in primary care. *Arch Intern Med* 147:44-47, 1987.
61. Chrischilles EA, Helling DK, Rowland CR: Clinical pharmacy services in family practice: Cost-benefit analysis I: Physician time and quality of care. *Drug Intell Clin Pharm* 18:333-341, 1984.
62. Chrischilles EA, Helling DK, Rowland CR: Clinical pharmacy services in family practice: Cost-benefit analysis II. Referrals, appointment compliance, and costs. *Drug Intell Clin Pharm* 18:436-441, 1984.
63. Nelson AA, Beno CE, Davis RE: Task and cost analysis of integrated clinical pharmacy services in private family practice centers. *J Fam Prac* 16:111-116, 1983.
64. Robinson JD: Pharmacokinetics service for ambulatory patients. *Am J Hosp Pharm* 38:1713-1716, 1981.
65. Robinson JD, Lopez LM, Stewaart WL: How to establish a pharmacokinetics consulting service for ambulatory patients. *Am J Hosp Pharm* 41:2048-2056, 1984.
66. Gums JG, Robinson JD: Pharmacokinetic monitoring in the community health-care setting. *Drug Intell Clin Pharm* 21:422-426, 1987.
67. Copeland GP, Apgar DA: The pharmacist practitioner training program. *Drug Intell Clin Pharm* 14:114-119, 1980.
68. Apgar DA: Clinical role in Indian Health Service. *Drug Intell Clin Pharm* 12:558-559, 1978.
69. Koecheler JA, Abramowitz PW, Daniels CE: Indicators for the selection of ambulatory patients who warrant pharmacist monitoring. *Am J Hosp Pharm* 46:729-732, 1989.

Appendix 36-A

FUNCTIONS PERFORMED IN AMBULATORY SETTINGS[12]

1. Conduct a patient interview and interpret the result of the interview.
2. List and explain the monitoring parameters and therapeutic endpoints for the safe and efficacious use of each drug used in a patient.
3. Prospectively monitor drug therapy for potential drug-drug, drug-laboratory test, drug-diet, drug-disease, and drug-condition interactions and recommend modifications in drug therapy, when appropriate, to minimize such interactions.
4. Use interviews, physical assessment skills, and interpretation of laboratory test results to monitor therapy for adverse and therapeutic effects.
5. Take a medication history, assess the patient's attitude toward compliance, and evaluate the influence of these factors on therapeutic response. Initiate strategies to correct noncompliant behavior.
6. Effectively counsel patients on drug use.
7. Serve on a health care team providing primary or consultative care.
8. Prospectively formulate individualized drug regimens based on the purpose of the medication(s), concurrent disease(s) and drug therapies, pharmacokinetic parameters of the drug(s), and the patient's clinical condition.
9. Competently devise individualized drug regimens and recommend adjustments based on therapeutic response.
10. Describe the clinical manifestations of potential toxicities associated with a patient's medication, assess the significance of the toxicity, and recommend an appropriate course of action.
11. Develop and conduct or assist in a collaborative clinical research project.
12. Evaluate drug studies in the literature in terms of research design, validity of results, and clinical applicability.
13. Communicate effectively with patients, physicians, nurses, other health professionals, and peers.
14. Manage a patient's drug therapy by:
    a. designing a drug therapy treatment plan, and advising prescribers on its implementation.
    b. using established therapeutic protocols, or
    c. independently prescribing or adjusting drug therapy in instances where supportive legislation exists.
15. Develop criteria for safe and effective drug use and coordinate drug use review and patient care audits.
16. Identify factors to measure the quality of care provided by the pharmacy service which could be used in the development of a departmental quality assurance program.
17. Explain the organization and operation of the outpatient pharmacy department. This could include physical accommodations, reference sources, computer applications, professional and supportive personnel, budgeting, relationships with other health care departments, assumed or designated responsibilities, and documentation of services.
18. Use personal computers to assist in the conduct of professional activities. These uses may include word processing, data base management, statistical analysis, graphics, and communication software.

CHAPTER 37

Pharmacy Service to Long-Term Care Patients

JAMES W. COOPER

Pharmacists must consult with patients and prescribers to prevent drug-related problems in long-term care or they will not have a place in health care delivery in the 21st century!

INTRODUCTION

The impact and cost savings of consultant pharmacist services in long-term care have been documented.[1,2] Problems of illicit nursing home practices, poor performance of health care professionals, and failure to detect and recognize problems in long-term care have been answered with expanded pharmacy involvement in the care of the chronically ill patient.

The purpose of this chapter is to present an overview of pharmacy services to long-term care patients, the scope of consultant activities, their legal and professional bases, and some as-yet unresolved problems in pharmacy care of the long-term care patient. A recent 2-year study has found that comprehensive drug regimen review of long-term care facility (LTCF) patients detects a significant drug-related problem (i.e., unwanted effect of drug therapy) every other month throughout their length of stay.[3]

The consultant pharmacist has been shown to decrease overall medication costs, adverse drug reactions and interactions, medication errors, hospitalization, and mortality rates of long-term care patients. In fact, when the consultant is no longer used, overall drug costs have been shown to increase markedly and subsequently decrease when consultant services are reinitiated.[4] The results of selected studies may be consulted for further substantiation of the vital role of pharmacists in long-term care.[5-8]

Consultant pharmacy is a blend of community and institutional practice. The three overlapping areas of professional functions are administrative, distributive, and clinical, and they are detailed in other publications.[10-17] The development of guidelines and standards for consultant pharmacy practice concerns three primary forces: regulatory, accreditation, and professional.

Federal regulations require consultant pharmacist activity in long-term care facilities (LTCF's) as a condition of participation[9,10] in Medicare reimbursement. In addition, there are Federal "indicators" for surveyor assessment of the performance of drug regimen review and overall pharmaceutical services.[11]

On a State level, at least one or more divisions of licensure, regulation, and/or reimbursement inspect each facility on at least an annual basis using Federal standards and regulations[10-12] as a basis for the facility's annual certification and reimbursement. Some LTCF's, especially those considered to be an extension of an acute care facility, seek other facility recognition by the Joint Commission on Accreditation of Healthcare Organizations (JCAHO).[12]

The Social Security Act also allows the States to work out a mechanism for payment of the consultant pharmacist separate from the fee paid to the provider pharmacist. Few States have elected to formalize this payment, and most have instructed facilities to pay for this service out of per diem rates. In addition, Federal regulations also allow States to work out a payment mechanism for compensation in unit dose systems, which to date only several States have elected. A common problem occurs when the provider is also the consultant, and the nursing home operator expects the consultant services free or at an unreasonable rate in exchange for the provider's prescription services. This has been considered illegal, and both the pharmacist and facility operator are subject to Federal penalties of fine and/or imprisonment.[13]

Federal and State surveyor expectations for consultant services, however, are being implemented on a gradual basis as the "state of the art" advances. Most pharmacists serving LTCF's are community pharmacists with little institutional practice training.

The main professional organizations for the consultant pharmacist are the American Society of Consultant Pharmacists (ASCP) and the American Society of Hospital Pharmacists (ASHP). In addition to the various standards and guidelines for administrative, distributive, and clinical services of ASHP intended primarily for the acute-care setting, ASCP has guidelines for consultant pharmacy services.[14] The American Pharmaceutical Association (APhA) has published a text on responsibilities for pharmaceutical services in the LTCF.[15] ASHP and ASCP have published supplemental standards and learning objectives for residency training in geriatric pharmacy practice.[16] APhA and the American Association of

Colleges of Pharmacy have published comprehensive standards for all areas of pharmacy practice.[17]

LONG-TERM CARE PATIENTS AND LEVELS OF CARE

The typical long-term care patient is more than 65 years of age and, as such, is termed "geriatric." More than three-fourths of persons found in long-term care are in this geriatric group. The most common diseases and conditions found in this group are arthritis, cardiovascular, and mental problems.[15]

In a paper that projects the use of medical care forward and backward from 1950 to 2050, institutional care is projected to consume a rapidly expanding share of the medical care budget in the next century, especially in the care of the aged nursing home patient, which is projected to increase to 12.8 per 1,000 population in 2050, greater than twice the 1975 rate of 5.4 per 1,000.[18] For the immediate future, nursing home expenditures are clearly one of the fastest accelerating categories of medical care expenditures, doubling between 1978 and 1985 ($15.8 to more than $32 billion) and are projected to double again before 1990 to about $76 billion, or about $1 of every $10 spent on health care in the United States.[19]

Within long-term care facilities there were, until October 1990, three levels of care. Skilled nursing facilities (SNF's) provide 24-hour nursing care and holistic personal needs and are intended to provide rehabilitative therapeutic goals for each patient. Intermediate care facilities (ICF's) provide more custodial than nursing care to those persons who can still provide some of their own personal needs. A subcategory of the ICF is that intended for the mentally retarded (ICF-MR) patient who is usually at the age range from childhood to early adulthood and needs some activities of daily living, nursing, and occupational and rehabilitative therapy.

As of October 1990, all LTCF's, whether SNF or ICF, are combined into one category known as "nursing facilities." This is a feature of the Omnibus Budget Reconciliation Act (OBRA).[a] Pertinent parts from the OBRA regulations for psychoactive drug use follow.

> The Omnibus Budget Reconciliation Act (OBRA) requires that long-term care facility patients be:
>
> 1. free from unnecessary drugs
> 2. free from chemical restraints
>
> Antipsychotic drugs must be used appropriately. Each patient must have a diagnosis or reason that indicates the use of an antipsychotic drug. These indications include:
>
> 1. Schizophrenia or schizo-affective disorders
> 2. Delusional disorders
> 3. Acute psychosis or mania with psychotic mood
> 4. Brief reactive psychosis
> 5. Atypical psychosis
> 6. Tourette's syndrome
> 7. Schizophreniform disorder
> 8. Huntington's chorea
> 9. Short-term symptomatic treatment of nausea/vomiting, hiccups, or itching
> 10. Dementia associated with psychotic or violent features that represent a danger to the patient or to others
>
> Antipsychotic drugs should not be used for the following reasons:
>
> 1. Restlessness, fidgeting, or wandering
> 2. Insomnia
> 3. Depression
> 4. Yelling, screaming, or crying out
> 5. Anxiety
> 6. Memory impairment
> 7. Uncooperativeness
>
> Reasons for the use of antipsychotic drugs must be documented on the physician's order sheet and in the patient care plan.
>
> Antipsychotic drugs must be used in the minimal dose necessary. This can be assured by:
>
> 1. Periodic tapering of the drug in an attempt to discontinue the drug if it is no longer necessary.
> 2. Using staff intervention to the utmost degree to control the patient's behavioral problem.
> 3. Monitoring and documenting the patient's target behavior to determine the actual effect of the antipsychotic drug on this behavior.
>
> The adverse effects of the antipsychotic drug should be closely watched for on a monthly basis. Movement disorders should be assessed every 6 months to annually using the Abnormal Involuntary Movement Scale (AIMS) or similar monitoring scale.

With the advent of prospective payment mechanisms for Medicare patients, those financing acute hospital care are looking to LTCF's and/or agencies such as home health and alternative health services as well as congregate housing, hospice, community physical and mental health centers, and personal care home options to lower the overall cost per patient case. For example, long-term hospital stays for extended courses of parenteral or enteral nutritional therapy or antimicrobial regimens may be a thing of the past with the same care available outside the institutional environment at a much lower case cost.

These additional lower and less costly levels of care can provide excellent opportunities for consultant pharmacist activity. Although the services of a pharmacist are now required only in LTCF's, there are no barriers to compensation of cost-effective consultant activity in a number of other areas, as discussed below.

Home Health Care and Other Agencies Serving Long-Term Care Clients

Studies[20,21] have indicated that a significant number of patients (one-quarter to one-third) have drug-related problems that may indicate the need for a legislated or regulatory mandate for the consultant pharmacist similar to that for the nursing home. Other agencies serving long-term care clients include area councils on aging, senior citizen centers, and community mental health centers.[22]

Alternative Health Services

This is an experimental program in some States where qualified individuals may take a candidate for ICF certification into their home for a fee that is much less than the usual

[a] *Fed Reg* 5 Feb 1992; 57(24):4516-33.

monthly nursing home cost. The individual agrees to supervise activities of daily living, food, laundry, and provide miimal medication supervision. It remains to be determined whether this will become a viable level of care, but the consultant and agencies providing referral and supervision of these patients should be aware of a potential consultation opportunity as well as the abuse potential of some "rest home" environments that sparked the scandals that rocked the nursing home industry in the 1960's, lest the cycle repeat itself.

Day Care

Adult day care centers are flourishing, usually as an extension of or associated with area senior citizen centers or councils on aging. Some States are promulgating specific regulations for their operation. Ideally, an adult day care center should be a licensed facility that provides an organized program of weekday, daytime therapeutic, social, and health activities aimed at rehabilitation to the self-care or personal level of family supervision, or as a further alternative to institutionalization. There appear to be a number of administrative, distributive, and clinical activities that can be efficiently and effectively provided by the consultant pharmacist.[23]

Congregate Housing

The high-rise apartment complex that offers a place to reside, a social system, and some administrative supervision of overall personal capability and security is a further opportunity for consultant pharmacist activity. One study has found that most drug-related problems in persons residing in this type of housing occur in those 75 years or older.[24] Improved compliance among a noncompliant geriatric congregate housing facility population has been shown with weekly consultant clinical pharmacist visits and special reminder packaging of medication.[25] It should be recalled that the key factor in drug-related hospital admissions, which are the reason for up to one-third of geriatric admissions, is noncompliance.[26]

Hospice

Holistic care of the terminally ill patient should involve the consultant pharmacist for medication monitoring and supervision, especially in the area of pain management.

Community and State Physical and Mental Health Centers

Most States have a public health emphasis in these areas that addresses the needs of the medically indigent patient. Without innovative consultant pharmacist activity, there is little doubt that excessive drug dosages, waste, pilferage, and drug-associated morbidity and mortality occur in this population.[27,28]

Personal or Self-Care

In this, the least expensive level of care, the opportunity for personal determination of care-associated expenses depends much more on the "individualistic" rather than "paternalistic" philosophy of health care, the educational level, and mental capability for learning proper self-care habits, as well as the consultant pharmacist's desire to teach patients or their families to take care of themselves. Numerous third-party payers are providing compensation for consultant educational activities with patients and families.[29] Although these services plus medication monitoring and supervision most logically arise from community pharmacy practice, there have been few studies documenting these expanded consultative roles.[29]

CONSULTANT FUNCTIONS

The administrative and distributive functions of the consultant pharmacist may be acquired by trial-and-error field experience. The clinical activity of the consultant pharmacist is the area in which most consultants acknowledge the greatest need for additional training.

Standards for baccalaureate and doctoral clinical education are set by the American Council on Pharmaceutical Education; for professional postdoctoral training, by ASHP; for residency training in long-term care (referred to as "geriatric residency"), by ASCP; and for fellowships, by the American College of Clinical Pharmacy. Post-doctoral training programs are usually administered through schools of pharmacy and pharmacy departments and private professional corporations and/or research groups.

The clinical activities of the consultant pharmacist can be viewed as a continuum of effort from the time the patient enters the LTCF, agencies, or pharmacy services through periodic evaluations and subsequent care.

Twelve areas of clinical responsibilities are listed below. Few consultants thus far have developed all areas to the point of minimal proficiency. This listing, therefore, represents a compilation of clinical activities now being performed that may be a goal for many and minimal proficiency for some consultants. They are:

1. Taking a complete drug history
2. Developing a problem list
3. Establishing and observing physical and laboratory parameters for the long-term care patient
4. Reviewing the patient-oriented medication regimen
5. Communicating clinically significant problems
6. Anticipating, preventing, and recognizing adverse drug reactions
7. Participating in patient care rounds and conferences
8. Taking part in pharmacotherapeutic, pharmacokinetic, and nutritional consultations
9. Monitoring medication regimen compliance by patient, family, prescriber nursing, and aide personnel
10. Educating patient, family, prescriber, and LTCF personnel
11. Providing objective drug information, retrieval, analysis and communications
12. Undertaking primary care and prescribing activities of the consultant pharmacist

A detailed review of all 12 areas is beyond the scope of this chapter and text. Drug regimen review is federally mandated.[11]

PATIENT-ORIENTED DRUG REGIMEN REVIEW

This function draws upon the first three activities and is based upon knowledge of the patient's previous drug use, verified problems, and parameters to be monitored on the individual patient's problems. The pharmacist reviews the patient's progress toward therapeutic endpoints to verify need for continued therapy or suggest changes that could improve patient response and/or prevent problems.

The review of the therapeutic regimen also involves assessment of the integrity of the distribution system (i.e., a checking for medication errors). The essential documents for patient-oriented drug review include the pharmacist dispensing records, records of drugs that have been administered to the patient (nurses' record and/or administration records), and the patient chart, especially orders, progress and nurses' notes, and laboratory sections. It is vital that detailed records of significant medication-associated incidents be maintained for physician, nurse, and/or pharmacist response; this may also be accomplished by keeping a nursing-pharmacy log on which all communicants sign off.[30]

Nevertheless, consultant pharmacists should keep records of all suspected problems to document their activities. On the other hand, they should not put in the chart any statement that they are unwilling to back in court testimony with qualified professional opinions or judgment. Adverse drug reactions should be listed in hierarchy form (suspected, potential, possible, probable) and appropriately noted in the patient's chart and monthly report of drug regimen review. Pharmacotherapeutic, pharmacokinetic, and nutritional consultations may arise from drug regimen activities. Nutritional problems are perhaps the most underaddressed and underreported problem in long-term care patients.[31]

Primary care by the consultant pharmacist in long-term care facilities is the most recent clinical activity of the consultant. The State of California allows consultant clinical pharmacists with doctoral-level training to provide primary care under physician supervision to SNF patients. The results of this practice innovation may provide a basis for further primary care functions for the consultant pharmacist.[32,33]

ADMINISTRATIVE ACTIVITIES

The consultant pharmacist in long-term care is, in many ways, like a hospital pharmacy director in that he or she must supervise all aspects of the comprehensive pharmaceutical services delivered to patients. Many of the chapters in this handbook document most of these activities. For the LTCF or agency, some differences may bear emphasis in the administrative area, including committee functions, in-service education, policy and procedure, and consultant reports.

Committee Functions

In examining the committee functions of the consultant pharmacist in LTCF's, one must consider, in particular, practical methods and expectations, committee purpose and responsibilities, along with an assessment of policy and procedure changes.

The three main committees with which the consultant should participate in LTCF's are the pharmaceutical services committee, infection control committee, and utilization review committee. Additional consultant functions that may take a committee format include in-service and patient and family education and patient care. Only the pharmaceutical services committee is discussed here. The pharmaceutical services committee was mandated until October 1, 1990, but is still important to quality long-term pharmacy care and should be a part of a Quality Assessment and Assurance Committee mandated by OBRA.

It should be noted that Federal surveyor standards employed by the various State field surveyors will look for documentation of the consultant's activities in each area, although the pharmaceutical services committee has been dropped from Federal requirements, as noted. In some cases, very specific endpoint guidelines have been developed. In each committee it is essential that:

1. All members understand the purpose and responsibilities of the committee.
2. Goals and objectives are realistic.
3. Adequate resource material is available, especially in patient data, literature references, and other input from consultant.
4. All must recognize resistance to change as human nature. Effective communications as to why change is needed may be helpful.
5. All must recognize that impasse may occur. This indicates the need for more documentation and discussion outside the formal meeting.
6. Even when new policies and procedures have been established, assessment of the implementation, effectiveness, and total system effects must be an ongoing responsibility of each committee member.
7. Agenda and activities must adequately document committee work.

The pharmaceutical services committee in the LTCF committee is analogous to the pharmacy and therapeutics committee in the hospital, and should consist of the provider and consultant pharmacist(s), administrator, one physician (ideally the medical director), and the director of nursing services. It has the responsibility for development and evaluation of written policies and procedures concerning drug therapy distribution, administration, accountability control, and use. The pharmaceutical services committée develops and annually updates the pharmacy policy and procedure manual. It further determines the level and types of medication services needed by the patient and how well the staff discharges these services.

Where possible, a formulary system should be developed to ensure availability of drugs determined by the medical staff to be the most effective and appropriate for therapy in the setting, secondary to costs. In addition, the pharmaceutical services committee has the overriding final responsibility for the optimal use of the medication modality of treatment in the facility. Some specific areas of concern would be minimizing medication or charting errors, anticipating and preventing adverse reaction and interaction, reducing irrational prescribing, and simplifying the drug administration procedure.

The pharmaceutical services committee must meet at least quarterly. The consultant's monthly reports and followup should be considered, and persistent communication difficulties remedied by committee (not consultant) letter to the individual prescriber. The consultant does not have to document change; only that attempt was made to communicate concerning problems. Some problem areas may involve multiple psychotherapeutic drugs, nightly hypnotic use, bowel care, vitamin and hematinic use, digoxin, and diuretic use without laboratory assessment of serum potassium and creatinine. Nursing followup should be noted, especially where serious medication errors have occurred.

In-Service Education

In-service education by the consultant pharmacist should be in the following three main areas:

1. A problem-oriented approach that addresses current problems with the drug distribution system, therapeutic effect, adverse drug reactions, inappropriate use of drugs, and the need for further assessment by observation and/or laboratory tests.
2. Review of specific patient therapeutic problems that could be avoided by better monitoring of drugs.
3. An ongoing review and testing on the practical pharmacology of the drugs most commonly used in the facility to ensure that staff members are familiar with the drugs that are being administered.

Patient and family education is important in avoiding drug-related problems. Unauthorized drugs, foods, and salt substitutes can create significant patient problems.

In self-care units or areas, studies show that 60 percent of uninstructed patients make errors in the use of their drugs. Patient education can reduce this to a 2-3 percent error rate via increased patient and family knowledge of therapy (what the drug is for, how to take it, what to expect, etc.).[33]

Policy and Procedure

The authority for the development of a policy and procedure manual comes from the pharmaceutical services committee of the facility. Although the pharmacist may provide a draft form of this manual, it is essential that all policies be workable for the nursing and medical staffs. In fact, rules proposed in 1980 as "conditions of participation" would have required this and have tacitly been enforced since this date.[10]

The pharmacy policy and procedure manual should cover all aspects of accurate drug use control and services, from acquisition of the drug through administration and observation of drug effects on the patient.

Pertinent policy and procedure points that should be considered in a comprehensive manual include:

1. Purpose of the manual
2. Policy and procedure authorization: Pharmaceutical services committee makeup
3. Pharmacist services agreement (provider and consultant)
4. Patient drug history and drugs brought into facility
5. Patient drug regimen review
6. Drug formulary and product selection
7. Drug ordering and delivery and distribution system
8. Emergency order provisions
9. Drug administration and documentation
10. Stop orders
11. Drug returns, discontinuation, and disposal
12. Discharge pass/leave of absence medications
13. Controlled substances
14. Bedside medications
15. Drug samples
16. Investigational drugs
17. Reports
18. Medication errors
19. Adverse drug reactions
20. Followup on problems

This should not be reviewed as an all-inclusive list of topics to be considered in a pharmacy policy and procedure manual. (See references at the end of this chapter for aid in the formulation of a complete policy and procedure manual.)[34,35]

The policy and procedure manual is a dynamic record of what will be done and how it will be done. Any dynamic system changes constantly, and the manual should be updated and revised at least on an annual basis by the pharmaceutical services committee.

Consultant Reports

Reports from consultants are used to document the need for their services as well as the performance of drug-related functions and responsibilities under contracts between institutions and/or agencies. For the purpose of this chapter, it is assumed that the provider and consultant may be the same person or two individuals.

Some facilities still encourage pharmacists to participate in a "paper consultant" activity. In the face of ever stronger Federal and State guidelines, this practice is certain to decline. More and more, "indicators" are being employed to determine facility and consultant compliance.

Federal regulations now specify that the report must be done at least on a quarterly basis. Monthly reports with a quarterly summary that might serve as a working agenda for the quarterly pharmaceutical services committee meeting are preferable, with consideration of administrative, distributive, and clinical (or patient-oriented) areas.

DRUG DISTRIBUTION SYSTEMS IN LONG-TERM CARE

The system by which drugs are ordered, filled, dispensed, administered, and recorded should be continually evaluated and revised to meet patient and facility needs as well as professional and regulatory standards. A drug distribution system is defined as the sum of activities that provide patient medications.

Staff members in LTCF's and agencies must be knowledgeable about the drug distribution system, or systems, used for their patients and residents. It is essential that the administrator, the director of nursing, and other members of the nursing staff accept the challenge to educate everyone who administers drugs and treatment under a nursing license.

At the same time, provider pharmacists—especially consultant pharmacists—need to cooperate in a plan that guarantees a thorough understanding of the drug distribution system. The ultimate goal is to ensure maximum efficiency and a minimum error rate, to cut down on waste in staff time and medications.

The policy and procedure manual, as written by the pharmaceutical services committee, should state what system is to be employed and how each distribution step is to be accomplished. This manual is a dynamic description of the system. Not only must it be understood by all, it also must be evaluated and changed to meet the needs of the facility as conditions dictate. This means that the pharmaceutical services committee should examine the policy and procedure manual at least annually to determine just how well the system is meeting the needs of safe drug distribution, the needs of the patient, and the needs of the facility.

PROBLEM AREAS IN DRUG DISTRIBUTION IN LONG-TERM CARE

The following problem areas may make it more difficult for the consultant to provide supervision of the distribution system:

1. Multiple drug providers
2. Incomplete or missing pharmacy dispensing records or failure to supply pharmacy dispensing records to the consultant
3. Incomplete or incorrect medication administration records and chart orders
4. Turnover of nursing personnel
5. Failure of all personnel to read, comprehend, and adhere to the pharmacy policy and procedure manual
6. Poor compliance with previous consultant recommendations
7. Failure to recognize that a problem exists

Unit dose or modified unit-dose distribution of drugs is essential to long-term care. "Unit dose" is strictly defined[36] as a 24-hour supply of unit-of-use packages of each medication recorded on a patient profile and medication administration record, and accounted for by nurse and pharmacist. In long-term care, a 3- to 7- and sometimes a 14-day supply of solid dosage forms only may be most feasible in current practice. Problems in unit dose systems may be noted.[37]

SUMMARY

This chapter has provided a brief overview of pharmacy services in long-term care. Please refer to the other chapters mentioned for additional information, as well as the citations and guidelines in the references.

REFERENCES

1. Cooper JW: Impact of the consultant pharmacist on health care: Past, present and future. *Consult Pharm* 3:342-345, 1988.
2. Cooper JW: Cost savings: The value of the pharmacist. *J Pharm Prac* 1(3):173-177, 1988.
3. Cooper JW: *Drug-Related Problems in Nursing Home Patients.* Binghamton, NY, Haworth Press, 1991.
4. Cooper JW: Effect of initiation, termination and reinitiation of consultant clinical pharmacist services in a geriatric long term care facility. *Med Care* 23:84-86, 1986.
5. Cheung A, Kayne R: An application of clinical pharmacy services in extended care facilities. *Calif Pharm* 23:22-25, 1975.
6. Thompson J, Floyd R: Cost-analysis of comprehensive consultant pharmacist services in the skilled nursing facility: A progress report. *Calif Pharm* 26:22-25, 1978.
7. Strandberg LR, Dawson GW, Mathieson D, et al: Effect of comprehensive pharmaceutical services on drug use in long term care facilities. *Am J Hosp Pharm* 37:92-94, 1980.
8. Kidder S: The potential cost-benefit of drug monitoring services in skilled nursing facilities. *Nat Assoc Ret Drug J* 19:21-22, 1978.
9. *Fed Reg* 93 p 228, 1974.
10. American Society of Consultant Pharmacists (ASCP) Special Bulletin, July 1980. HCFA 42 C.F.R. Parts 405, 442 and 483.
11. ASCP Special Bulletin, July 1982. Section 316 OFF Survey Procedures for Pharmaceutical Services in Long Term Care Facilities and Section 3161, Indicators for Surveyor Assessment of the Performance of Drug Regimen Reviews.
12. *Joint Commission on Accreditation of Health Care Organizations Manual 1992.* Chicago IL, Joint Commission on Accreditation of Health Care Organizations, 1992.
13. *Medical Assistance Manual.* Title XIX Part 6-160-30, US DHEW PHS, Washington, DC, 1965.
14. *Guidelines for Consultant Pharmacists Practicing in Long-Term Care Facilities.* Arlington, VA, American Society of Consultant Pharmacists, 1981.
15. Gerson CK (ed): *More than Dispensing.* Washington, DC, American Pharmaceutical Association, 1980.
16. Anon: ASHP supplemental standards and learning objectives for residency training on geriatric pharmacy practice. *Am J Hosp Pharm* 39:1972-1974, 1982.
17. Kalman SH, Schlegal JF: Standards of practice for the profession of pharmacy. *Am Pharm* NS19:21-35, 1979.
18. Russell LB: An aging population and the use of medical care. *Med Care* 19:633-643, 1981.
19. Kingston ER, Scheffler RM: Aging: Issues and economic trends for the 1980's. *Inquiry* 18:197-213, 1981.
20. Cooper JW, Griffin DL, Francisco GE, et al: Drug-related problems detected by consultant pharmacist participation in home health care. *Hosp Form* 20:643-650, 1985.
21. Solomon DK, Baumgartner RP, Weismann BR, et al: Pharmaceutical services to improve drug therapy for home health patients. *Am J Hosp Pharm* 35:535-537, 1978.
22. Jinks MA: Pharmacy-consulting service to agencies serving elderly clients. *Am J Hosp Pharm* 40:1542-1544, 1983.
23. Williams BR: The pharmacist in adult day care centers. *Today's Nursing Home* 5:19, 23-25, 1984.
24. Wade WE, Cobb HH, Cooper JW: Drug-related problems in a multiple site ambulatory geriatric population. *J Ger Drug Ther* 1(2):101-110, 1986.
25. Joyner JL, Hikmat FT, Catania PN: Evaluation of a medication-monitoring service for geriatric patients in a congregate housing facility. *Am J Hosp Pharm* 40:1509-1512, 1983.
26. Frisk PA, Cooper JW, Campbell NA: Community-hospital pharmacist detection of drug-related problems upon admission to small community hospitals. *Am J Hosp Pharm* 34:738-742, 1977.
27. Wade WE, Whaley JA, Cooper JW, et al: Pharmacist involvement in Georgia public health departments: Preliminary report of two pilot studies. *Ga Pharm J* 3:20-22, 1981.
28. Cooper JW, Doyal LE: Cost-effectiveness of the clinical pharmacist in community mental health center. *Med Interface* 2(11):44-48, 1989.
29. *ASHP Task Force Final Report on Payment for Pharmacy Services.* Bethesda, MD, American Society of Hospital Pharmacists, 1979.
30. Cooper JW: Monitoring drug therapy for the long-term care client. In Pagliano LA, Pagliano AM: *Pharmacologic Aspects of Aging.* St. Louis, MO, CV Mosby, 1983.
31. Cooper JW, Cobb HH: Nutritional changes in long-term care patients. *Nutr Supp Serv* 8(8):5-7, 1988.
32. Thompson JF, McGhan WF, Ruffalo JT, et al. Clinical pharmacists prescribing drug therapy in a skilled-nursing facility. *J Am Geriatr Soc* 32:154-159, 1984.
33. Cooper JW: Drug therapy in the elderly. Is it all it could be? *Am Pharm* NS18:25-26, 1978.
34. Caruthers KS: *Developing and Implementing a Pharmacy Policy and Procedure Manual for Skilled Nursing Facilities.* Sacramento, California Pharmaceutical Association, Academy of Long Term Care, 1977.
35. *ASCP Policy and Procedure Manual.* Arlington, VA, American Society of Consultant Pharmacists, 1981.
36. ASHP statement on unit dose drug distribution. *Am J Hosp Pharm* 46:806, 1989.
37. Davis N: A poor unit dose system versus a traditional system. *Hosp Form* 13:478, 1978.

CHAPTER 38

Decentralized Pharmacy Services

WILLIAM E. SMITH and DENNIS W. MACKEWICZ

Hospital pharmacy departments are responsible for the safe and effective use of drugs and drug products within the institution. Pharmacy personnel perform functions that relate to drug distribution and drug information in striving toward this objective. Decentralized pharmacy services have proven over the past 25 years to be an important action plan to achieve the "safe and effective use of drugs" for patients. Since the mid-1960's, hospital pharmacy services have evolved to meet these needs, frequently by decentralizing operations and staff in order to provide clinical services and a more efficient and less error-prone medication system. A decentralized pharmacy is an area located in the patient care parts of a hospital from which pharmacy personnel work and provide pharmacist clinical services and drug distribution services.

Hospital pharmacies historically have been centralized departments. A central area for drug storage is both a practical and a legal matter. As hospitals increased in size from 100-200-bed facilities to 400-500+ bed institutions, there has been a tendency to locate the central pharmacy away from inpatient care areas. Decentralized pharmacies have been an effective method for bringing pharmacy services closer to the patients and professional staffs.

The safe and effective use of drugs requires clinically competent pharmacists, systems, and services to deal with all patient care areas in cooperation with physicians and nurses. A decentralized service component maximizes pharmacists' communications and contributions to the professional staffs and the patient.

A completely decentralized pharmacy staff puts pharmacists and drugs close to the end users and facilitates the provision of necessary drugs and drug information in an effective manner. Although to some this may appear self-evident, the issue revolves around what the scope of pharmacy inpatient services should be. The rationale for providing "proactive" pharmaceutical services is discussed in this chapter in conjunction with the alternative centralized and decentralized approaches to providing these services.

PATIENT NEEDS

Drug use in the hospital setting has been studied and reported in the literature since the 1950's. These reports illustrate patient drug-related risks in the hospital setting with regard to the total "hospital medication system," which encompasses many steps beginning with a physician prescribing, a pharmacist dispensing, and a nurse administering each dose until the drug order is discontinued.

Medication Errors

Hospital medication systems have been reported to have an 8-20 percent medication error rate.[1-3] Medication errors are defined as the wrong patient, wrong drug, wrong dose, wrong route, and wrong time.

Drug Effects

Complications in patients resulting from drug use that have been reported include (1) adverse drug reactions, 5-30 percent of patients,[4] (2) prolonged hospitalization from adverse drug reactions,[5] (3) drug-modifying laboratory tests,[6] (4) drugs inducing blood dyscrasia,[7] (5) drugs affecting liver function tests,[8] and (6) drug interactions and teratology.[9]

Prescribing Errors

Medication prescribing errors by both private practitioners and house staff with regard to safe or effective dosage regimens, ambiguous and incomplete orders, inadequate laboratory test monitoring, and misinterpretation of the meaning of serum drug level results have been reported.[10,11]

From the patient's point of view, the hospital medication system that has the pharmacist dispensing from a central pharmacy location has frequently resulted in a high rate of errors, prolonged delays in receiving initial doses, significant drug complications, extended hospital stays, and increased expense. New drugs and drug delivery system technologies will be more complicated and more potent with high risks of toxicity. Hospital medication systems and the pharmacist's scope of clinical practice need to adapt to these advances in drug therapy if greater patient drug-related complications in the hospital setting are to be prevented.

The key question is, how can pharmacy services prevent and/or minimize patient drug related problems through the application of the pharmacist's clinical drug knowledge and the implementation of sound hospital medication systems?

NURSING NEEDS

The nurse plays a major role in the hospital medication system. Depending upon the scope of services provided by the pharmacy department, the nurse may order drugs from the pharmacy, prepare and reconstitute doses for administration, administer medications, record each drug administered, keep additional records for the controlled drugs received and administered, and maintain drug floorstock. Without adequate pharmacy support, the nurse would have to be knowledgeable about drug storage, dosage forms and strengths, the effects of each drug administered, and the safety of drugs intravenously administered. The nurse must also use an increasing number of drug administration devices with unique supplies, setups, and monitoring procedures. The nurse may also have to procure large and small intravenous (IV) solutions, add drugs using aseptic technique, and administer them in continuous, intermittent, or in some instances, patient-controlled devices. As a result, a great deal of nursing time is required for medication-related activities.

Each hospital must answer the following questions: Which drug-related activities should be performed by the nurse from quality of care, efficiency, and cost-effective points of view? Can the nurse, even with nurse specialization, maintain sufficient knowledge about all the drugs administered and apply the knowledge appropriately? Is the maintenance of sufficient knowledge realistic when at the same time the nurse must devote time to maintain nursing knowledge and skills required for quality patient care?

Generic drug names, therapeutic interchange of drug products, variable dosages depending upon the drug's salt form, more dangerous drugs such as oncology agents, are examples of continuing areas of confusion and potential errors. Adequate pharmacy support can assist the nurse with these potential drug areas of confusion. Registered nurse shortages, high staff turnover, and the ongoing use of registry nurses and part-time nursing employees make it very difficult to maintain a consistently experienced and a drug-knowledgeable nursing staff.

A centralized pharmacy service in hospitals frequently leads to many unanswered drug-related questions by a busy nurse. A decentralized pharmacy service more readily provides the drug-related activities and drug information support to the nurses when needed. A decentralized drug distribution system using a satellite pharmacy can improve the efficiency of the nurse compared with a centralized drug distribution system.[12]

PHYSICIAN NEEDS

The physician diagnoses the patient's medical problem and then prescribes a plan of therapy. The prescribing of drugs is frequently a critical aspect of inpatient care. Drug complications, identified previously, illustrate the physician's need for general and specific clinical drug information. Management of the patient's drug therapy by a pharmacist can reduce costly drug reactions and quicken the discharge of the patient from the hospital.

The usual sources of drug information to the physician include the medical service representative, *Physician Desk Reference*, journal articles, textbooks, drug data, and professional conferences. These sources are inadequate in meeting the physician's needs for drug information, particularly as it relates to complex patients with multiple health care problems and multiple drug regimens. Pharmacists who practice in patient care areas can provide clinical drug knowledge and experience to help physicians manage their patients' drug therapy.[13]

PHARMACIST NEEDS

Pharmacists' time in a centralized pharmacy system is likely to be dominated by dispensing duties and allow for minimal participation in providing drug information and clinical services to the hospital staffs. The professional relationships of the pharmacist with physicians, nurses, and patients are limited. A lesson to be learned from the past is the pharmacist's traditional practice in a central pharmacy, which provides a minimal scope of clinical services, does not adequately serve or meet patients', physicians', and nurses' drug-related needs.

In a decentralized environment, the pharmacist is able to relate directly to a patient's drug therapy needs as a result of easy access to the patient, nurse, physician, and medical record. Initial doses for a new order can be provided quickly. At the same time, drug information questions by the nurse can be answered quickly by the pharmacist. Pharmacists can develop expertise for particular patient care areas such as pediatrics, obstetrics and gynecology, medicine, and surgery when covering the same areas of the hospital over a sustained period of time. The pharmacist's inpatient therapeutic experience will include cases brought to the hospital by multiple physicians. Over time, the pharmacist can become an expert in understanding the significant patient variables for high-risk drug therapy. The pharmacist practicing in the patient care area needs to inform and communicate effectively with the nurse and physician. A rapport can be developed with the medical staff in which the pharmacist's input into drug therapy orders can be made before orders are written instead of just as a response to problems after the orders have been written. Many drug therapy needs can be addressed by the physician requesting the pharmacist to regulate a specific drug therapy following an approved protocol.

SERVICES AND EXPECTED PATIENT BENEFITS OF A DECENTRALIZED PHARMACY

Pharmacists practicing in hospitals have been active in developing new pharmaceutical services and systems directed toward reducing the problems associated with drug use. Such services and systems included unit dose drug distribution, patient medication profiles, drug information services, pharmacists practicing in patient care areas, and clinical pharmacokinetics. These services and systems have been associated with "clinical pharmacy" and provide significant benefits toward improved patient care while maintaining cost-effectiveness. The characteristics of a pharmacist's clinical practice in a decentralized pharmacy are described below. Expected patient benefits for each characteristic are also described.

Patient Care Rounds

Pharmacists accompany physicians making patient rounds, primarily teaching rounds. Participation occurs in providing drug information upon physician request or by the initiation of the pharmacist. The drug information provided to the physician frequently results in improvements in the patient's treatment plan.

Patient Interviews

Patient drug history information is obtained orally by the pharmacist to complete pharmacy records. Information may include prescription and over-the-counter drugs being taken, drug allergies, and attitudes about drugs as to which worked or did not work. Previous patient drug therapy problems, attitudes, and misconceptions as to what drugs worked or did not work are identified. Those drugs that do not work can then be avoided during hospitalization.

Patient Medication Therapy Monitoring

Patient charts are reviewed to determine if the patient is receiving safe and effective drug therapy. Drugs administered, pertinent laboratory tests, and the patient's diagnosis and medical condition are essential parts of the monitoring process. If changes in the drug therapy are desirable, the pharmacist discusses these with the physician. Potential and actual drug therapy problems are identified and communicated to the physician by the pharmacist. Safer and more effective drug therapy should result.

Physician Inquiry

Physician-initiated questions about patient drug therapy and general drug information questions are answered by the pharmacist. Safer and more effective drug therapy can result if questions are answered accurately and implemented in patient therapy.

Nurse Inquiry

Nurse-initiated questions about patient drug therapy, general drug information, and drug orders are answered by the pharmacist. More accurate drug administration and medication administration records, with greater drug knowledge by the nurse, result in safer drug administration for the patient.

Drug Information

The physician and pharmacist initiate drug information questions involving a patient's drug therapy problem requiring a search of the available literature for information in order to provide a response. The answers should result in safer and more effective drug therapy.

Cardiopulmonary Arrest Emergency Participation

The pharmacist is a member of the hospital's cardiopulmonary resuscitation team and participates by providing drug therapy assistance and the needed drugs. Pharmacist assistance with drug availability and drug therapy questions can facilitate resuscitation procedures.

Pharmacist-Regulated Drug Therapy Services

The pharmacist will develop and perform special drug therapy services as requested by the physician such as regulating anticoagulation, dosing of drugs in patients with compromised renal status, drugs affecting the blood and liver, aminoglycoside dosing, pain control, nutrition support, and aminophylline therapies. Safer, more patient-specific, and effective drug therapy should result.

Clinical Pharmacokinetics

The pharmacist schedules the appropriate time for drug levels to help ensure that test results are usable. Consultation services using the serum drug level and kinetic knowledge can be provided to modify the dose and/or dosing interval to prevent toxicity and ensure therapeutic efficacy. Unusable and unnecessary serum drug levels should also be eliminated.

Drug Usage Evaluation

Special drug case studies are conducted and educational programs provided to the medical, nursing, and pharmacy staffs by the pharmacist. Targeted incorrect and inappropriate drug prescribing of physicians should be corrected via educational programs. Costs and cost reductions of drug therapy can be defined and documented.

PHARMACIST PERFORMANCE CHARACTERISTICS

Pharmacists who practice in a decentralized pharmacy environment are able to greatly expand their professional knowledge and skills in the areas of patient service, teaching, and research because of the greater opportunities for clinical experience. To be successful in a decentralized pharmacy environment, pharmacists must have a commitment to high standards of patient care services. The decentralized pharmacy also provides ample opportunities for pharmacists interested in teaching and research. Working in the patient care environment requires clinical knowledge and skill, a commitment to lifelong learning, but also the important characteristics of initiative, self-accountability, and productivity. For the pharmacist to become a strong asset requires some specialization or concentration of time and energy into selected areas of clinical drug use.

DEPARTMENTAL ORGANIZATION AND OPERATIONS

What departmental organizational plan or structure is the most effective in providing services to meet patient, nurse, and physician drug-related needs? The first element is a drug distribution system that maximizes the use of nonpharmacists in the inpatient drug distribution system of the hospital. Many unit dose systems have been described in the literature. The benefits of unit dose distribution are more than just providing double-checks, reducing medication errors, and eliminating the drug waste seen in multiple dose systems. Unit dose systems also allow the pharmacist to delegate many of the nonprofessional drug distribution tasks to technicians and still maintain the necessary responsibility and supervision. A primary result from the use of technicians in conjunction with a unit dose system is pharmacist time for clinical services that otherwise may not have been available.

The patient drug profiles associated with a unit dose system also can provide a patient drug therapy record that can become the basis for the pharmacist's patient drug therapy monitoring system. Patient names, current drug therapies, and other information can be organized to easily review ongoing and new drug orders.

ADVANTAGES AND DISADVANTAGES OF A DECENTRALIZED PHARMACY SERVICE

Given a unit dose drug distribution system, use of pharmacy technicians, and patient drug therapy profiles, what are the advantages and disadvantages of centralized and decentralized pharmacy services? The following discussion deals first with this question and then examines alternative departmental organizational structures.

Pharmacy departments are usually referred to as either "centralized" or "decentralized." This depiction is an oversimplification, because most decentralized pharmacy departments are a mix of centralized and decentralized functions. Decentralized pharmacies frequently differ considerably in exactly what is decentralized and how. The way services are provided may also vary from shift to shift, from weekday to weekend. The following functions are all possibilities for either a centralized or a decentralized approach:

1. New order review by the pharmacist
2. First dose preparation
3. Unit dose preparation of ongoing orders
4. Unit dose checking by the pharmacist or trained technician
5. IV order review by the pharmacist
6. IV order preparation including admixtures and total parenteral nutrition
7. IV piggy back (PB) order reconstitution
8. IVPB order review by the pharmacist
9. IVPB order distribution to the patient
10. Prescription filling for discharged and special inpatients
11. Unit dose packaging
12. Pharmacokinetic consults by the pharmacist
13. Drug level ordering and/or scheduling by the pharmacist
14. Drug information questions directed to the pharmacist
15. Responses to drug information questions
16. Nonformulary drug request followup by the pharmacist
17. Pharmacist-patient interviewing as needed
18. Drug therapy regulation by the pharmacist
19. Drug therapy monitoring by the pharmacist
20. Adverse drug reaction monitoring by the pharmacist
21. Pharmacy charge processing

Several observations can be made about the activities listed above. First, some of these activities must be performed by the pharmacist; others can be performed by a technician or clerk. Second, some of these activities require the pharmacist to be outside the confines of the "pharmacy," whether it is located centrally or decentrally. Third, some of the nonpharmacist activities require immediate supervision; others require minimal pharmacist supervision.

An "ideal" configuration of a given pharmacy department must start first with a statement of the scope of pharmacist services. This statement should include what services are to be provided and when they will be available, i.e., 24 hours a day, day shift only, and so on. Then, how and where these services should be provided as efficiently and effectively as possible can be addressed.

Another issue to be considered is the relationship of any clinical service to the drug distribution system. In particular, the review of new drug orders usually is a part of the clinical pharmacist's responsibility prospectively, or it becomes a part of the clinical pharmacist's responsibilities to retrospectively review new drug orders from a clinical perspective beyond the "drug distribution pharmacist." The size of the institution may be a factor with regard to the use of pharmacy technicians as a whole, and this use may vary from day to day and shift to shift. The availability of space in decentralized areas or the lack of it for the centralized pharmacy may also dictate how the drug distribution systems are organized. The clinical services provided must then be woven into the basic configuration of the drug distribution systems.

There are many advantages to decentralization of pharmacy personnel responsible for providing drugs and drug information services to inpatients. These are listed below:

1. Drugs are immediately available for administration to the patient.
2. Drug control and accountability are greater.
3. Pharmacists communicate directly with physicians and nurses.
4. There is more space for the pharmacy as a whole and flexibility in reallocating or designing existing space in the central pharmacy.
5. Unique drug distribution systems are implemented to issue drugs to the nurse.
6. Pharmacist review of the chart or talk with the patient is efficient.
7. Drug information from the pharmacist is readily available to physicians and nurses.
8. Nursing time is reduced in drug distribution because more tasks are being performed by pharmacy personnel.
9. Pharmacist drug therapy specialization by patient care area is accomplished more effectively as a result of focused clinical experience.
10. Specialized pharmacist clinical services can be developed and efficiently provided, i.e., regulating a specific patient's drug therapy as ordered by the physician; heparin and oral anticoagulants, digoxin, aminophylline, aminoglycosides, nutrition support.
11. Pharmacists more readily perform clinical drug research and patient drug therapy quality assessment studies.

The disadvantages of decentralized inpatient pharmacy services are:

1. All clinical practice pharmacists must become proficient as supervisors to work effectively with technicians.
2. Pharmacists are usually responsible for both drug distribution and clinical services. Their time in non-drug-distribution activities is dependent upon the

availability and quality of pharmacy technicians and the technicians' ability to effectively organize their time to meet responsibilities.

3. Staffing flexibility is reduced when only one pharmacist with or without a technician is providing all inpatient pharmacy services for a specific patient care area when census levels are significantly above or below normal. Vacation and sick leave coverage must be carefully planned and provided for, including contingencies for personnel replacement when required.
4. Unrealistic expectations from nursing and physicians and excessive interruptions of the pharmacist and/or technician can reduce efficiency.
5. Drug inventory control within the department is more complex because of multiple pharmacy locations for the same drug, particularly infrequently prescribed drugs.
6. Communications within the pharmacy department are more difficult because the staff members practice in multiple physical locations.
7. More equipment is required, e.g., drug information references, refrigerators.
8. Patient acuity and resulting drug distribution workload may exceed the capacity of space and personnel in the small decentralized pharmacy units.
9. Use of technology to automate and mechanize the drug distribution system component of pharmacy services will require more hardware and software.

RELATIVE COSTS OF A CENTRALIZED AND DECENTRALIZED PHARMACY SERVICE

Cost is a very important part of the hospital's decision as to what form of pharmacy services will be supported. Costs can be divided into patient benefits, such as reduction in mortality, morbidity, and hospital patient days. Costs can also be divided into equipment, facilities, and personnel, with personnel costs being the most significant.

Equipment and Facilities

Equipment needs depend primarily upon the drug distribution systems employed. The equipment required for unit dose drug packaging and medication carts would not depend upon whether the pharmacy was centralized or decentralized. Intravenous admixtures and other sterile reconstitution and packaging done in decentralized areas of the hospital would involve the purchase of more biological safety cabinets.

Space in patient care areas is usually difficult to obtain, which has resulted in the development of several approaches to providing decentralized pharmacy services. Satellite pharmacies in hospitals were first described in 1960.[14] Hospitals that were originally built or remodeled with satellite pharmacies in mind generally have little trouble providing enough space to do the required drug distribution and clinical activities.

The size of a typical decentralized or satellite pharmacy would be 200-300 square feet to serve approximately 100 beds. Other variables that enter into planning and negotiating space are (1) the size of the hospital, (2) the physical layout of the hospital, (3) the number of patients per hospital floor, and (4) the number of nursing stations per hospital floor and per hospital. These are important, since all are determining factors for the number of required dose preparation and decentralized dispensing areas.

In the final analysis, the space for a decentralized pharmacy system may or may not be greater than the space of a centralized pharmacy. The cost difference is also affected if adequate space already exists in the nursing station area that can easily be converted into a satellite pharmacy. When space is not available for a satellite pharmacy, pharmacists have used a mobile cart system. Such systems generally use the decentralized clinical pharmacist to provide the immediate drug distribution needs of the patient, i.e., providing the initial doses. Ongoing drug needs may also be provided from the mobile cart or from a centralized drug distribution system.[15]

Computer systems can provide better communications within the hospital, such as patient tracking from the admitting department and laboratory results. Computer systems also allow transmittal of pharmacy orders from the patient care area to virtually any pharmacy location in the hospital building. The key issue concerning drug order entry into a computer system is whether the pharmacist ever sees the original physician order if the physician, nurse, or a clerk has entered the order directly into the computer. Unless the physician enters orders into a terminal directly, having nursing enter this information is error-prone and could forfeit the expertise provided by a pharmacist's interpretation of the order. Pharmacy computer systems can be used in both decentralized and centralized pharmacy operations for better communication within the department. For decentralized pharmacy operations, computer systems can offer more flexibility in staffing use and in splitting those functions that can be more effectively done centrally.

Personnel

The determination of personnel costs may rest only within the pharmacy department or may also include the impact of the pharmacy services on nursing time in the hospital medication system. It is suggested that comparative personnel costs for alternative systems and services be factored to a cost per patient day. In this way, personnel costs are reduced to a common factor for comparisons.

Several cost comparisons can be made as follows:

1. Centralized pharmacy service personnel costs per patient day
2. Decentralized pharmacy service personnel costs per patient day
3. Nursing personnel costs in medication-related activities prior to clinical pharmacy services (centralized and decentralized)
4. Nursing personnel costs in medication-related activities after clinical pharmacy services (centralized and decentralized)
5. Pharmacist and nonpharmacist personnel costs (centralized and decentralized)
6. Pharmacy personnel costs based on program elements, i.e., unit dose, IV admixtures, clinical services

All of these cost breakdowns will enable comparisons as to what the overall personnel cost results would be, depending upon the pharmacy service system configuration.

Ultimately, it is up to each hospital to determine from its own operational characteristics whether personnel costs will be greater or savings can be achieved from the implementation of a decentralized pharmacy service. The assumption that it will cost more because of increases in the pharmacy staff cannot be made until hospital-specific studies on personnel costs are completed.

FORCES THAT INTERFERE WITH DECENTRALIZED PHARMACY SERVICES

Many forces can interfere with providing decentralized drug distribution and clinical pharmacy services. They are described briefly below.

Attitudes and Behavior

Negative reaction by physicians may occur when pharmacists begin to expand beyond the drug distribution role and take a more active role in the patient care area. Some physicians may be outspoken against pharmacist involvement in clinical activities. Tactful communications are the key to gaining medical staff support when making recommendations on patients' drug therapy.

Oral communications to physicians are essential in lieu of written notes for the pharmacist to explain the rationale of a recommendation and to develop a positive relationship with the physician. Short, cryptic, written recommendations by pharmacists left in the patient's chart (not to be included in the final chart) for the physician to read when implementing pharmacist clinical services are not likely to attain the intended result. The relationship between physicians and the pharmacist may require an "evolution" over time within each medical specialty, gaining credibility one physician at a time.

Nursing managers may have reservations in supporting requests for "space" for decentralized pharmacies, which may be taking space away from "their" areas. Nursing managers may also envision the nurse to be primarily responsible for drug therapy knowledge and see the pharmacist's clinical activities of providing drug information to physicians and nurses as being costly and unnecessary.

Recognizing the dynamics and complexity of drug therapy in hospitals and the difficulty in maintaining knowledge current in drug therapy modalities is a key issue that must be clearly articulated by pharmacy management. Just as hospital pharmacy departments have prepared drug information newsletters for physicians, the nurse and administrator need to be made aware of new drug therapies and related issues aimed at their special "interests" with their specific communications from the pharmacy.

Implementing proactive pharmacy services and primary patient care such as pharmacist regulation of selected high-risk drug therapies via approved protocol may also be received with mixed reaction by physicians, nursing, and administration. Such pharmacist clinical services require periodic retrospective or prospective patient outcome audits to document a higher level of quality patient care than previously existed, as well as provide a means to evaluate and revise drug therapy protocols. Since such services require a physician order, the physicians ordering these services will view such services as being positive. Good communication with nursing is important in implementing such services. Certain procedures need to be defined, since the pharmacist will be writing chart orders affecting the nurse, and the pharmacist may want to adjust IV drug administration rates, which the nurse needs to know about.

Unless the administrator recognizes the patient care contribution the pharmacist can make in regulating selected drug therapy, an unsupportive attitude may result. A negative attitude could even result, since the time and effort by the pharmacist (paid from hospital revenues) to perform activities previously performed by the physician (not paid from hospital revenues) translate into more pharmacist staffing and higher payroll expenses. The hospital workplace is perhaps one of the most dynamic work settings in existence; the roles of the physician, nurse, pharmacist, and support staff continue to change in an attempt to use new technology and drugs to their best advantage. At one time, physicians personally added drugs to IV solutions for their patients and administered IV push drugs whenever required; this is now done primarily by hospital personnel. As long as quality patient care that is delivered efficiently and cost effectively are primary long-term goals of the institution, the pharmacist and pharmacy technician will continue to assume an increasing role in providing and improving patients' drug therapy in the foreseeable future.

Pharmacy Department

If pharmacy department facilities are lacking in space and equipment, adequate clinical services cannot be provided easily. Some pharmacy presence, including some space in the patient care area, is needed for the pharmacist to effectively provide nurses and physicians with a level of service that is impossible to provide from a distant central location. Decentralized order processing allows the pharmacists to maintain familiarity with "their patients" and makes it easier to resolve problem orders, clarify orders, and retrieve missing patient information. Pharmacists need to practice in the same patient care areas consistently to maintain patient care continuity and maintain a good working relationship with the physicians and nurses. A consistent practice area also allows for some specialization, so that pharmacists can focus on the high-risk drug therapies important for their patient care practice areas.

It can be expected that a pharmacist who is familiar with his or her patients can more easily and efficiently manage problem orders than can a pharmacist in a centralized location. A decentralized pharmacist is also in a position to expand his or her role in scheduling the times that medications are administered by working more closely with nursing to significantly improve the control of workflow into the pharmacy distribution area.

Dispensing first doses from a central location allows for greater control of inventory. Decentralized dispensing of first doses, on the other hand, may be accomplished with less delay because the order does not require delivery to and from the central pharmacy, and the amount of stock needed for this purpose can be kept to a minimum while avoiding uncontrolled floorstock.

Pharmacist Time for Information Functions

Hospital administration must support and approve a pharmacist staffing pattern to provide time for pharmacists' direct patient care functions. Without well-educated and interested pharmacists in clinical practice, these services cannot be provided.

Decentralized pharmacists must also be willing to work weekends and evenings in order to provide clinical services that can be counted on by the medical and nursing staffs. In fact, it is during these shifts that the nurse and physician may appreciate the expertise of a decentralized pharmacist the most in resolving problem orders and answering questions the nurse and physician would otherwise have to deal with themselves.

Legal Requirements

Present pharmacy State laws may limit the use of nonpharmacists, which can then minimize the amount of pharmacist time available for clinical functions. Federal laws continue to increase pharmacy time required for drug stock accountability records and paperwork, which can reduce the time for information and knowledge functions. Satellite pharmacies within the hospital are not usually defined legally as "pharmacies" by boards of pharmacy, thus avoiding the facility design requirements intended for licensed community pharmacies.

FUTURE CONSIDERATIONS

The new financial era for hospitals in the 1990's, driven by cost containment, diagnosis-related groups (DRG's), State rate-setting commissions, and price competition, may adversely affect the growth of clinical and decentralized pharmacy services. Pressures to reduce operational costs for providing care to inpatients is intense in U.S. hospitals. Creative thinking with realistic planning is needed by all hospital managers to provide the most cost-efficient and cost-effective care with a high level of quality. The scope of pharmacy services, like all other hospital services, will need to be redefined and defended with operational objectives, results, and patient care outcomes.

Decentralized pharmacy services will continue to be a cost-effective method for providing clinical pharmacy services in many hospitals. Hospitalized patients usually require a significant amount of drug therapy because of their increased acuity of care. Future drug therapy will increase in complexity. Hospital medication systems will need to be responsive in a manner to help keep patient stay to a minimum. Automation, mechanization, and continued use of pharmacy technicians will be necessary to cope with the volume of drug use in hospitals. New drugs and drug delivery systems will require pharmacists in clinical practice with greater drug knowledge and skills than currently are practiced.

REFERENCES

1. Hynniman CE, Conrad WF, Urch WA, et al: A comparison of medication errors under the University of Kentucky unit-dose system and traditional drug distribution systems in four hospitals. *Am J Hosp Pharm* 27:803, 1970.
2. Davis NM, Cohen MR: *Medication Errors: Causes and Prevention*. Philadelphia, Stickley, 1981.
3. Allan EL, Barker KN: Fundamentals of medication error research. *Am J Hosp Pharm* 47:555, 1990.
4. Ogilvie RI, Ruedy J: Adverse drug reactions during hospitalization. *Can Med Assoc J* 97:1450, 1967.
5. Barr DP: Hazards of modern diagnosis and therapy, the price we pay. *JAMA* 159:1452, 1955.
6. Young DS, Pestaner LC, Gibberman V: Effects of drugs on clinical laboratory tests. *Clin Chem* 21(5):1D-432D, 1975.
7. Swanson M, Cook R: *Drugs, Chemicals and Blood Dyscrasia*. Hamilton, IL, Drug Intelligence Publications, Inc., 1977.
8. Cluff LE: 5 Liver manifestations. *Major Prob Intern Med* 5:131-227, 1975.
9. Briggs G, Freeman RK, Yaffe SJ: *Drugs in Pregnancy and Lactation*, 3rd ed, Baltimore, MD, Williams & Wilkins, 1990.
10. Folli L, Poole RL, Benitz WE, et al: Medication error prevention by clinical pharmacists in two children's hospitals. *Pediatrics* 79(5):718, 1987
11. Lesar TS, Briceland LL, Delcoure K, et al: Medication prescribing errors in a teaching hospital. *JAMA* 263:2329, 1990.
12. Wadd WB, Blissenbach TJ: Medication-related nursing time in centralized and decentralized drug distribution. *Am J Hosp Pharm* 41:477, 1984.
13. Guglielmo BJ, Schweigert BR, Kishi DT, et al: Pharmacist-managed drug therapy in California hospitals. *Am J Hosp Pharm* 46:1366, 1989.
14. Carner DC: *New Concept in Hospital Pharmacies*. Indianapolis, IN, Tile and Till, 1960.
15. Lipman AG, Bair JN, Hibbard FJ, et al: Decentralization of pharmaceutical services without satellite pharmacies. *Am J Hosp Pharm* 36:1513, 1979.

CHAPTER 39

Hospital Pharmacy Equipment and Supplies

THOMAS R. BROWN and MARY MONK TUTOR

The opportunity to purchase new equipment and supplies for hospital pharmacy use is usually an exciting experience, especially when the purchase will improve profession capability. However, the procurement process can lead to anxiety and frustration when it becomes tedious and time consuming, and the results are unsatisfactory. In order to initiate a new patient care system, or plan, renovate, or remodel a facility or similar project, this procurement process plays an important role.

The procurement process for equipment and supplies requires an organized effort that will minimize the likelihood of problems and increase the potential for success. The process begins with a decision concerning what is purchased and then, more specifically, what features or characteristics are required to fulfill the need. Obviously, the type of item to be purchased dictates the degree of specifications required. The purchasing procedures in any institution may well define the procurement process at this point, but surveillance to expedite purchases may be required.

The more important components of the process of purchasing seem to involve the early considerations in the selection process and a number of considerations. Although many are self-evident, they are important and deserve reasonably exhaustive consideration.

EQUIPMENT CONSIDERATIONS

Before an item of equipment is purchased, a thorough investigation of motives, needs, and practical matters regarding the equipment is essential. A thought process that is not reasonably exhaustive may lead to a purchase that is disappointing at best. Consider the following items and questions in developing the logic for the purchase of equipment:

1. *Functionality.* Is the item what the department needs? Will it improve the service? Will it be a detriment to the service? What functions will it serve? Will the item perform the functions in a "hospital-specific" way?
2. *Personnel.* Does the pharmacy currently have personnel who can operate the equipment? If it involves a totally new environment, can current personnel adjust to a new way of working? Can the current facility manage the new equipment as well as personnel? Many other questions regarding personnel may be important locally.
3. *Cost.* Is the equipment worth the expense? Can the cost be recovered? Will the equipment generate new revenue? Is the expense unavoidable? Is the item comparatively reasonable in cost? Cost is a factor that must be weighed carefully, particularly relative to the quality of the item considered for purchase.
4. *Maintenance.* Is the item difficult to service, clean, repair, etc? Are repair facilities available? Are service agreements available, and, if so, what is the cost? Can the item be repaired in-house? Are maintenance manuals available (also repair manuals)? What about backup support if repair takes a long period of time? Are repair parts easy to obtain, and are they expensive? Is telephone assistance available for repair?
5. *Ease of use.* Are instruction manuals provided? Are they understandable? What about setup and demonstration after purchase? Are there special courses for users? Is there telephone assistance available for problems with use?
6. *Portability.* Will the equipment need to be moved? Can it be moved? Is the equipment flexible enough to meet changing needs or new facilities? Will alterations be needed if the equipment is moved?
7. *Lease versus purchase.* Is the equipment a short- or long-term need? What are the advantages of leasing? Is a service agreement included with leasing? Is it possible to lease now with a purchase option? There are many things to consider that may save money and headaches.
8. *Aesthetics.* Be sure to consider color, size, shape, placement, etc., in order to maintain or improve a pleasant workplace. Although often overlooked, it may be possible to obtain the needed equipment with all desired functions and aesthetics with little additional investment.
9. *Shared equipment.* Can a piece of equipment be shared with another department? Is it desirable to share the item?
10. *Reliability.* Is the manufacturer reputable? Are expendable supplies required that create a dependence on a single source in order to operate the equipment? Will supplies be reasonably available? Consider alternative sources.
11. *State-of-the-art.* Is this item last year's model? Will the next version (if foreseeable) make the current model obsolete? Can state-of-the-art be updated and maintained? Will the purchased model have to be replaced to keep up to date?

12. *Special requirements.* Does the equipment require special alterations to the building, or will it fit nicely into available space? What about requirements for water, electricity, light, etc.? Will it fit through the door? What about special temperature requirements? Many other factors must be considered.

These are but a few considerations that must be given careful, early attention in the decision to purchase an item. Many must be considered locally—do not overlook them.

SCOPE AND LIMITATIONS

The starting point for this compilation of suppliers of equipment and supplies was the second edition of the *Handbook of Institutional Pharmacy Practice.* Additionally, each issue of the *American Journal of Hospital Pharmacy* beginning with 1986 was reviewed to capture new companies and their products and/or new products from previously identified companies. The scope of the compilation is limited to those types of equipment and supplies the hospital pharmacist would need in planning a new facility, planning the expansion or remodeling of an existing one, or providing a new service within the institution. It was outside the scope of this compilation to include drug or drug-related products, equipment required for the large-scale manufacture of injections, tablets, capsules, liquids, etc., or to include commonly used articles that can be obtained locally by hospital pharmacists, such as common office equipment and supplies, carpets, etc. Added to the list of common equipment and supplies that was omitted in this compilation were administrative furnishings and filing equipment and supplies, which were also deemed to be reasonably available locally.

This compilation began with a list of approximately 800 companies with considerable diversity in products. The companies listed represent those that responded within a reasonable period of time (approximately 60 days) after a letter was mailed to a correct address. The first mailing revealed many incorrect (most were changes in address) addresses, and for those where a correct address could be obtained using resources that would be generally available to practitioners, a second letter was sent. In those cases, the 60-day clock began at that point. A number of companies failed to respond, and it is inappropriate to speculate the reasons for this failure; those companies are not included in the compilation.

To the extent possible, language provided by the manufacturers is used to describe the nature of the products. The section headings indicate the type of equipment and supplies. The "miscellaneous" section encompasses a wide variety of items that could not be placed in one of the other sections but deserved to be included in the compilation. Because of the dynamics of the industries that support pharmacy practice, particularly those dealing with equipment and supplies, it is impossible to guarantee that an individual supplier still offers specific equipment and/or supplies.

ENTERAL AND PARENTERAL INFUSION PUMPS

AVI Inc./3M
1120 Red Fox Rd.
St. Paul, MN 55112 — Small volume fusion systems; infusion pumps

BAXA Corporation
14-C Inverness Dr. East
Englewood, CO 80112 — Infusion pumps/enteral and parenteral

Baxter Healthcare Corporation
Pharmacy Division
1425 Lake Cook Rd.
Deerfield, IL 60015 — Infusion devices; volumetric pumps; pump sets; portable infusion pumps; syringe pumps

Controlled Flow Ltd.
12705 S. Kirkwood
Suite 220
Stafford, TX 77477 — IV flow regulators

Entech, Inc./Enteral Technology
Rte. 22 East
Lebanon, NJ 08833 — Enteral pumps/supplies

IMED Corporation
9775 Business Park Ave.
San Diego, CA 92131-1192 — Infusion pumps/controllers

IVAC Corporation
10300 Campus Point Dr.
San Diego, CA 92121-1579 — Syringe pumps/controllers/volumetric pumps; supplies

Ivy Medical Inc.
7411 Washington Ave. South
Minneapolis, MN 55435 — Infusion controller

MedFusion, Inc.
3450 River Green Crt.
Duluth, GA 30136 — Syringe infusion pumps/multiple infusion management system

O'Brien/KMI
320 Charles St.
Cambridge, MA 02141 — Enteral infusion pumps and sets

Parker Hannifin Corporation
17352 Von Karman Ave.
Irvine, CA 92714 — Ambulatory medication infuser; micropump

Pharmacia Deltec Inc.
1265 Grey Fox Rd.
St. Paul, MN 55112 — Ambulatory infusion pumps/implantable IV delivery systems/supplies

Razel Scientific Instruments, Inc.
100 Research Dr.
Stamford, CT 06906 — Syringe/drug pumps; supplies and equipment

COMPUTER SYSTEMS

AIMS/ACPI
485 Underhill Blvd.
Syosset, NY 11791 — Pharmacy management systems

Apothecary Software, Inc.
17810 S.W. Shasta Trail
Tualatin, OR 97062 — Specialized software for TPN/label printing/prepack/unit dose

Baxter Healthcare Corporation
Pharmacy Division
1425 Lake Cook Rd.
Deerfield, IL 60015 — Software/management system/kinetics system/nutritional assessment system

CPSI
501 Bishops Lane
Mobile, AL 36608 — Computer systems software

Cedar Systems, Ltd.
1520 N. Lincoln Ave.
Jerome, ID 83338 — Kinetic consultation software

ComCo Tec, Inc. 361 Frontage Rd. Burr Ridge, IL 60521	Computerized software pharmacy management system/drug distribution system
Compute-Rx, Inc. 4200 Park Place Ct. Glen Allen, VA 23060	Computer management system/computer software for impatient/outpatient services
Condor Corporation 2060 Oak Mountain Dr. P.O. Box 189 Pelham, AL 35124	Pharmacy software system
Continental Hlthcare Sys. 7300 West 110th St. Overland Park, KS 66210	Pharmakon 200 computer system
Datalogic Optic Elect. Bar Code Div. 301 Gregson Dr. Cary, NC 27511	Bar code reading systems
Datastat National Data Corp. (NDC) 1300 Picard Dr. Rockville, MD 20850	Pharmacy management system
Digimedics Corporation 280 Technology Cir. Scotts Valley, CA 95066	Complete inpatient/outpatient computer system
Enterprise Systems 2333 Waukegan Rd., Ste. E100 Bannockburn, IL 60015	Hardware/software for hospital materials management
First Coast Systems, Inc. 3035-3 Powers Ave. Jacksonville, FL 32207	Pharmacy management system/software
First DataBank The Hearst Corporation 111 Bayhill Dr. San Bruno, CA 94066	National drug data file; American drug interaction module; IV incompatibility module; prescription triage
Freedom Data Systems 47 Belknap Ave. P.O. Box 678 Newport, NH 03773	Software systems/supplies
Gamma Systems Services 401 Yelvington Ave., Ste. B Clearwater, FL 34615	Pharmacy software systems
Giles Scientific, Inc. 250 Mercher Sts. Ste. A301 New York, NY 10012	Computerized antibiotic susceptibility test system
HBO & Company 301 Perimeter Center North Atlanta, GA 30346	Clinipac and Clinstar pharmacy software system
Hann's ON Software 346 Kanan Rd., Ste. 201 Agoura, CA 91301	Computer software for pharmacy services
Health Care Consultants 627 Messapoag Ave. Sharon, MA 02067	Database management software
Inforite Corporation 1670 South Amphlett Blvd. Ste. 201 San Mateo, CA 94402	Portable data entry system/software
Management Systems Assoc. 100 E. Six Forks Rd. Raleigh, NC 27609	MasteRx pharmacy system
Medi-Span P.O. Box 68875 Indianapolis, IN 46268	Drug therapy screening systems; computerized drug product and clinical drug information
Medical Software Consortium P.O. Box 76069 St. Peters, MO 63376	Drug interaction/miscellaneous software
Medicom Professional Drug Systems 2388 Schuetz Rd. Ste. A-56 St. Louis, MO 63146	Medical information data bases
Micah Systems 340 Morgantown Rd. Reading, PA 19611	Pharmacy management system
Micromedex, Inc. 660 Bannock St. Denver, CO 80204-9989	Computerized clinical information systems
Milton Roy Analytical Products Div. 820 Linden Ave. Rochester, NY 14625	Software for use with spectrophotometers
Mumps Users' Group (MUG) 4321 Hartwick Rd., Ste. 510 College Park, MD 20740	Computer software
Orbis Systems, Inc. 4309-L Medical Center Dr. McHenry, IL 60050	Computer software for pharmacy and extended-care pharmacy
PRX Systems 5797 Central Ave. Boulder, CO 80301	Pharmacy management systems
Patient Medical Record 901 Tahoka Rd. Brownfield, TX 79316	Computerized medical record forms
Pharmacy Computer Svcs. 208 Northwest 6th, Ste. 2 Grants Pass, OR 97526	Hardware and software management system
Redwood Medical Computer P.O. Box 2286 Aptos, CA 95001	Pharmacy computer system
Renlar Systems, Inc. 2640 Palumbo Dr. Lexington, KY 40509	Complete computer hardware and software system
SDK Healthcare Inf. Sys. 1550 Soldiers Field Rd. Boston, MA 02135	Computerized pharmacy control system

STORAGE FACILITIES AND REFRIGERATORS

Akro-Mills Div. of Myers Ind. P.O. Box 989 Akron, OH 44309	Plastic bins/containers and hanging storage systems; emergency boxes
Bally Engineered Structure P.O. Box 98 Bally, PA 19503	Modular walk-in coolers/freezers; refrigeration supplies
Forma Scientific Mill Creek Rd. P.O. Box 649 Marietta, OH 45750	Refrigerator/freezers
Gem Refrigerator Co. 650 E. Erie Ave. Philadelphia, PA 19134	Pharmacy refrigerators & freezers
Hamilton Manufacturing Co. Two Rivers, WI 54241	Modular steel lab furniture
Health Care Logistics, Inc. 315 Town St., P.O. Box 25 Circleville, OH 43113-0025	Storage bins/racks
Kardex Systems, Inc. P.O. Box 171 Marietta, OH 45740	Movable shelf filing system
Kole Enterprises P.O. Box 020152 Miami, FL 33102-0152	General shelving/bins
Lab Line Instruments, Inc. Lab Line Plaza Melrose Park, IL 60160	Explosion-proof/flammable storage/refrigerators/ freezers
Lewis Systems 128 Hospital Dr. Watertown, WI 53094	Stack-n-nest containers/ shelving with plastic bins
Lyon Metal Product, Inc. P.O. Box 671 Aurora, IL 60507	Metal shelving/ lockers/cabinets/ benches/racks
MMI of Mississippi, Inc. 232 East Georgetown St. P.O. Box 488 Crystal Springs, MS 39059-0488	Modular storage units/shelf units/general casework/ systamodules for all pharmacy functions
Marvel Industries P.O. Box 997 Richmond, IN 47375	Biomedical/medical refrigerators
McKesson Corp. One Post St. San Francisco, CA 94104-5296	Storage facilities; control drug security cabinets; general purpose storage
Medi-Dose, Inc. 1671 Loretta Ave. Feasterville, PA 19047	Stackable trays/storage units
Medipak Customer Services P.O. Box 3248 Winchester, VA 22601	Plastic modular bins/storage racks; drawer organizers
Milcare A Herman Miller Company 8500 Byron Rd. Zeeland, MI 49464	Modular storage systems
NorLake Inc. P.O. Box 248 Hudson, WI 54016	Refrigerators/freezers/mini-room coolers
Omnimed, Inc. Pine Ave. P.O. Box 446 Maple Shade, NJ 08052-0446	Shelf bins/dividers; storage cabinets
Penco Products, Inc. Brower Ave. Oaks, PA 19456	Storage facilities/accessories
Precision Scientific Co. 3737 W. Cortlant St. Chicago, IL 60647	Safety refrigerators
Scott Company, Inc. 142 Flowers Rd. Terry, MS 39170	Refrigerators and freezers; flammable/explosion proof refrigerated storage
R.C. Smith 801 East 79th St. Minneapolis, MN 55420	Modular pharmacy storage facilities
Spacesaver Corporation 1450 Janesville Ave. Ft. Atkinson, WI 53538-9988	High density mobile storage systems
St. Charles Manufacturing 1611 E. Main St. St. Charles, IL 60174	General pharmacy casework
SystaModules Division of MISSCO Corp. P.O. Box 1059 Jackson, MS 39205	Modular pharmacy components and refrigeration; narcotic units
Waterloo Industries, Inc. P.O. Box 2095 Waterloo, IA 50704	Modumed center storage/narcotics storage

PHARMACY AND MEDICAL RECORD FORMS

Artromick International 4800 Hilton Corporate Dr. Columbus, OH 43243-4150	Visifile medication record system
Briggs Corp. P.O. Box 1698 Des Moines, IA 50306	Pharmacy and hospital forms
Health Care Logistics, Inc. 315 Town St., P.O. Box 25 Circleville, OH 43113-0025	Pharmacy forms
Kardex Systems, Inc. P.O. Box 171 Marietta, OH 45740	Patient record management system
Lionville Systems, Inc. Lionville, PA 19353	Nursing and pharmacy forms
Patient Medical Record 901 Tahoka Rd. Brownfield, TX 79316	Computerized medical record forms
Physician's Record Co. 3000 S. Ridgeland Ave. Berwyn, IL 60402	Pharmacy and narcotic record forms

Shamrock Scientific Spec. Systems, Inc.
34 Davis Dr.
Bellwood, IL 60104 — Pharmacy forms

Waterloo Industries, Inc.
P.O. Box 2095
Waterloo, IA 50704 — Medication carts/utility carts/emergency carts/plastic trays and accessories

EQUIPMENT AND SUPPLIES FOR MEDICATIONS AND MATERIAL HANDLING

Artromick International 4800 Hilton Corporate Dr. Columbus, OH 43243-4150	Medication carts/cassettes/control systems; cart locking/alarm system
Health Care Logistics, Inc. 315 Town St., P.O. Box 25 Circleville, OH 43313-0025	Utility carts
InterMetro Industries Corp. Advertising Dept. P.O. Box A Wilkes-Barre, PA 18705	Utility carts/shelving/crash carts/exchange carts/security carts/medication carts/storage bins/anesthesia carts
Kole Enterprises P.O. Box 020152 Miami, FL 33102-0152	Utility carts/bins/general accessories
Lakeside Manufacturing, Inc. 1977 S. Allis St. Milwaukee, WI 53207	Multipurpose carts, trucks, and accessories; medication carts; dollies
Lewis Systems 128 Hospital Dr. Watertown, WI 53094	Tote boxes/utility carts/work-in-process containers
Lionville Systems, Inc. Lionville, PA 19353	Medication carts; night cabinets; or drug management facilities; specialty carts
McKesson Corp. One Post St. San Francisco, CA 94104-5296	Med trays; night service cabinets
Medi-Crush Company 4801 West 4th St. Hattiesburg, MS 39402	Medication carts
Milcare A Herman Miller Company 8500 Byron Rd. Zeeland, MI 49464	Medication carts; dispensing units
Novak Company, Inc. P.O. Box 423 55 Old Field Point Rd. Greenwich, CT 06836	Pharmacy conveyor system
Omnimed, Inc. Pine Ave. P.O. Box 446 Maple Shade, NJ 08052-0446	Medication carts; narcotic cabinets; emergency drug box; all purpose carts
SystaModules Division of MISSCO Corp. P.O. Box 1059 Jackson, MS 39205	Multipurpose carts/tables/equipment

EQUIPMENT AND SUPPLIES FOR PACKAGING ORAL SOLIDS, ORAL LIQUIDS, INJECTABLES, AND MISCELLANEOUS PRODUCTS

Artromick International 4800 Hilton Corporate Dr. Columbus, OH 43243-4150	Packaging systems/labels/control drug packaging
Associated Bag Company 400 W. Boden St. Milwaukee, WI 53207	Zip lock bags/biohazard bags
Automated Prescription Sys. P.O. Box 868 Pineville, LA 71361-0868	Baker counting systems for oral solid medications
Baker Company, Inc. P.O. Drawer E Sanford, ME 04073	Laminar air-flow hoods/biological safety cabinets/supplies
BAXA Corporation 14-C Inverness Dr. East Englewood, CO 80112	Oral liquid syringe and ointment; filing equipment and supplies
Baxter Healthcare Corporation Pharmacy Division 1425 Lake Cook Rd. Deerfield, IL 60015	Needles; laminar air-flow hoods; ancillary supplies
Burron Medical Inc. Hospital Products Division 824 Twelfth Ave. Bethlehem, PA 18018	Liquid packaging equipment; filter needles and straws; vacuum transfer devices; oral syringe systems
B.W. Darrah, Inc. 115 S. 4th Ave. St. Charles, IL 60174	Reusable security control containers
Ertel Engineering Co. P.O. Box 3449 Kingston, NY 12401	Semi-automatic liquid fillers
Forma Scientific Mill Creek Rd. P.O. Box 649 Marietta, OH 45750	Laminar air-flow hoods/safety equipment
Germfree Equipment Mfg. Div. 7435 N.W. 41st St. Miami, FL 33166	Vertical and horizontal laminar flow hoods; fume hoods
Health Care Logistics, Inc. 315 Town St., P.O. Box 25 Circleville, OH 43113-0025	Oral solid and liquid packaging systems
Healthtek, Inc. 870 Gold Flat Rd. Nevada City, CA 95959	Flexible admixture containers/ambulatory infusion system/vial venting system
Kinematics and Controls Corp. 14 Burt Dr. Deer Park, NY 11795	Powder and liquid filler machines

LGS Health Products 14055 Cedar Rd. South Euclid, OH 44118	Pill splitter
Labconco Corp. 8811 Prospect Kansas City, MO 64132	Vertical laminar air-flow hoods/safety cabinets
Lionville Systems, Inc. Lionville, PA 19353	Unit dose packaging equipment/supplies
Lunaire Environmental, Inc. 4 Quality St., Box 3246 Williamsport, PA 11701	Laminar air-flow equipment/environmental rooms/incubators
MMI of Mississippi, Inc. 232 East Georgetown St. P.O. Box 488 Crystal Springs, MS 39059-0488	Laminar air-flow hoods/safety equipment/IV preparation modules
Markwell Medical Institute P.O. Box 085173 Racine, WI 53405	Button infuser for subcutaneous injections
Mayfield Printing Co. P.O. Box 469 Mayfield, KY 42006	Bags
Medi-Dose, Inc. 1671 Loretta Ave. Feasterville, PA 19047	Unit dose packaging and labeling system for solids, liquids, injections/light protection system/auto clavable bags/tote boxes and supplies
Medipak Customer Services P.O. Box 3248 Winchester, VA 22601	All types of containers for various dose forms; UV light containers; quick seal equipment
Milcare A Herman Miller Company 8500 Byron Rd. Zeeland, MI 49464	Unit dose packaging
National Instrument Co. 4119-27 Fordleigh Rd. Baltimore, MD 21215	Liquid filling machines, thermal impulse sealers
Pak Devices Inc. 4734 Spring Rd. Brooklyn Hgts, OH 44131-1098	Strip packaging equipment; label printing equipment
Pennsylvania Glass Prod. 430 N. Craig Pittsburgh, PA 15213	Glass droppers/dropper bottles/containers/ applicators
Pharmaceutical Innovators P.O. Box 308 West Union, IA 52175	Prepackaging equipment and supplies
Phenix Box and Label Co. P.O. Box 695 Olathe, KS 66061	Dispensing containers; bags; prescription tape
Popper and Sons, Inc. 300 Denton Ave. New Hyde Park, NY 11040	All types glass syringes; needles; pipettors
Production Equipment Inc. 17 Legion Place Box 236 Rochelle Park, NJ 07662	Prepackaging equipment for tablets and capsules
Prop'r Products, Ltd. 500 South Minnesota Ave. Sioux Falls, SD 57102	Liquid measuring/storage devices
Shamrock Scientific Spec. Systems Inc. 34 Davis Dr. Bellwood, IL 60104	Packaging machines; unit dose materials; medication containers; bags
Shaw-Clayton Plastics, Inc. 123 Carlos Dr. San Rafael, CA 94903	Hinged lid plastic containers
St. Charles Manufacturing 1611 E. Main St. St. Charles, IL 60174	Specialty hoods/fume hoods
SystaModules Division of MISSCO Corp. P.O. Box 1059 Jackson, MS 39205	IV preparation units with LAFH; general packaging and compounding units
Terumo Corp. P.O. Box 589 Elkton, MD 21921	Insulin syringes
U.S. Clinical Products 1900 Jay Ell Dr. P.O. Box 831667 Richardson, TX 75083-1667	IVA seals
Wrap Ade Machine Co., Inc. 189 Sargeant Ave. Clifton, NJ 07103	Strip packaging equipment/supplies

EQUIPMENT AND SUPPLIES FOR PRINTING AND LABELING

Briggs Corp. P.O. Box 1698 Des Moines, IA 50306	Labels and auxiliary labels/supplies
Health Care Logistics, Inc. 315 Town St., P.O. Box 25 Circleville, OH 43113-0025	Label/auxiliary labels/label management system
Mayfield Printing Co. P.O. Box 469 Mayfield, KY 42006	Computer labels; auxiliary labels; IV labels
Pharmex 207 Tuckie Rd. Willimantic, CT 06226	Labels/label systems; miscellaneous supplies
Phenix Box and Label Co. P.O. Box 695 Olathe, KS 66061	Computer labels; auxiliary labels
Shamrock Scientific Spec. Systems Inc. 34 Davis Dr. Bellwood, IL 60104	Labels and labeling equipment
Syntest Corporation 40 Locke Dr. Marlboro, MA 01752	Label printers
U.S. Clinical Products 1900 Jay Ell Dr. P.O. Box 831667 Richardson, TX 75083-1667	Pressure sensitive, preprinted labels

MISCELLANEOUS

A & D Engineering, Inc. 2165 W. Park Ct., Ste. M Stone Mountain, GA 30087	Analytical balances
Alsop Engineering Company P.O. Box 3449 Kingston, NY 12401	Stainless steel tanks, mixers, filters, and filtering apparatus
American Med Industries 505 Laurel Ave. Highland Park, IL 60035	EZ-swallow pill crusher
Apex Medical Corporation P.O. Box 1235 Sioux Falls, SD 57101	Medicating, dosing and administering aids
Artromick International 4800 Hilton Corporate Dr. Columbus, OH 43243-4150	Needle disposal system
Associated Bag Company 400 W. Boden St. Milwaukee, WI 53207	Disposable supplies
Baxter Healthcare Corporation Pharmacy Division 1425 Lake Cook Rd. Deerfield, IL 60015	IV filtration devices
Bernhard Industries, Inc. 300 71st St., S. 435 Miami Beach, FL 33141	Steam inhaler
Briggs Corp. P.O. Box 1698 Des Moines, IA 50306	File trays; narcotic cabinets; miscellaneous supplies
Brooklyn Thermometer Co. Dept. 853 Farmingdale, NY 11735	Environmental thermometers/ thermoregulators/ hygrometers/hydrometers/ recorders
Burron Medical Inc. Hospital Products Division 824 Twelfth Ave. Bethlehem, PA 18018	Specialty IV sets; flow control devices; miscellaneous IV supplies
CHEK-MED System 423 N. 21st St., Ste. 203 Camp Hill, PA 17011	Patient education system; identa-drug system
Contempra Furn Div. Fisher Scientific Corp. 922 Philadelphia St. Indiana, PA 15701	Complete lab furnishings/equipment
Controlled Environ Equip 3 Delta Dr. Westbrook, ME 04092	Contamination control MATS/wipers
Fisher Scientific Co. 1600 Parkway View Dr. Pittsburgh, PA 15205	Protective garments; lab equipment; chemicals; general lab supplies
Forma Scientific Mill Creek Rd. P.O. Box 649 Marietta, OH 45750	Environmental rooms/incubators; miscellaneous products
HEALTH-TEK, Inc. 870 Gold Flat Rd. Nevada City, CA 95959	IV filters; flexible admixture containers; ambulatory infusion system; infusion contamination tester
Health Care Logistics, Inc. 315 Town St., P.O. Box 25 Circleville, OH 43113-0025	Tablet crushers; suppository molds; security seals; miscellaneous supplies
Inforite Corporation 1670 S. Amphlett Blvd. Ste. 201 San Mateo, CA 94402	Portable data entry system
Inter Innovation LeFebure P.O. Box 2028 Cedar Rapids, IA 52406	Security systems and equipment; closed circuit TV; bullet resistive windows and supplies; safes and vaults
Kole Enterprises P.O. Box 020152 Miami, FL 33102-0152	Shipping equipment/supplies/ containers
Lab Line Instruments, Inc. Lab Line Plaza Melrose Park, IL 60160	Furnaces/heaters/mixers/ stirrers/incubators/general lab equipment
Lab Safety Supply Co. P.O. Box 1368 Janesville, WI 53547-1368	Safety equipment and supplies/personal protection storage and handling/hazard control
Lifescan Inc. 2443 Wyandotte St. Mountain View, CA 94043-2312	Blood glucose monitoring/management system
MMI of Mississippi, Inc. 232 East Georgetown St. P.O. Box 488 Crystal Springs, MS 39059-0488	Creative design services
Maddak Inc. Pequannock, NH 07440-1993	Home health care equipment and supplies
Mayfield Printing Co. P.O. Box 469 Mayfield, KY 42006	Prescription blanks; file folders; envelopes/ statements
Medi-Crush Company 4801 West 4th St. Hattiesburg, MS 39402	Medication crushing devices; plastic lockseals; tablet cutters; needle-syringe disposal; ambulatory med-minders; amber IV covers
Medi-Dose, Inc. 1671 Loretta Ave. Feasterville, PA 19047	Prescription supplies
Mettler Instrument Corp. Box 71 Hightstown, NJ 08520	Electronic balances and accessories
Milcare A Herman Miller Company 8500 Byron Rd. Zeeland, MI 49464	Administrative work environments; modular furnishings; computer furnishings
Millipore Corp. Bedford, MA 01730	Microbiology equipment supplies; filtration equipment/supplies; contamination anaylsis equipment

Milton Roy
Analytical Prod. Div.
820 Lindne Ave.
Rochester, NY 14625

Spectrophotometers/refractometers

R.C. Musson Rubber Co.
P.O. Box 7038
1320 E. Archwood
Akron, OH 44306

Floor mats/runners/carpet mats; anti-fatigue mats

Novak Company, Inc.
P.O. Box 423
55 Old Field Point Rd.
Greenwich, CT 06836

Rotary files/modular work stations/administrative furnishings

Nucleopore Corp.
7035 Commerce Cir.
Pleasanton, CA 94566

Laboratory equipment/supplies; filtration equipment/supplies

Omnimed, Inc.
Pine Ave.
P.O. Box 446
Maple Shade, NJ 08052-0446

Bags; safety control seals

Penco Products, Inc.
Brower Ave.
Oaks, PA 19456

Office storage products

Pharmacia Deltec Inc.
1265 Grey Fox Rd.
St. Paul, MN 55112

Infusion catheters and devices/patient aids

Pharmex
207 Tuckie Rd.
Willimantic, CT 06226

Patient information

Phenix Box and Label Co.
P.O. Box 695
Olathe, KS 66061

Anti-fatigue mats

Phonetics, Inc.
101 State Rd.
Media, PA 19063

Environmental monitoring system/security system

PlasTies
1500 East Chestnut Ave.
Santa Ana, CA 92701

Plastic products for packaging

Precision Scientific Co.
3737 W. Cortlant St.
Chicago, IL 66047

Incubators; water baths; vacuum pumps

Precision Systems, Inc.
16 Tech Cir.
Natick, MA 01760

Quality control equipment and supplies; osmometers

Pro-Tex International
P.O. Box 1038
5038 Salida Blvd.
Salida, CA 95368-0605

Protective disposable face shields

Pure Water, Inc.
P.O. Box 83226
Lincoln, NE 68501

Water purification systems; distilled water systems

Quest Medical Inc.
4103 Billy Mitchell
Dallas, TX 75244

IV delivery sets; filters

Shamrock Scientific Spec. Systems Inc.
34 Davis Dr.
Bellwood, IL 60104

Balances; miscellaneous equipment/supplies; filing system

R.C. Smith
801 East 79th St.
Minneapolis, MN 55420

Modular office furnishing/casework

Spectrex Co.
3580 Haven Ave.
Redwood City, CA 94063

Laser particle counter system for fluids

SystaModules
Division of MISSCO Corp.
P.O. Box 1059
Jackson, MS 39205

General office furniture

Teleautograph Corp.
8621 Bellanca Ave.
Los Angeles, CA 90047

Omnifax/business facsimile

Tennessee Mat Company
1400 Third Ave., South
Nashville, TN 37210-0186

All types of floor mats and matting/cushioned/runners/ anti-fatigue

U.S. Clinical Products
1900 Jay Ell Dr.
P.O. Box 831667
Richardson, TX 75083-1667

Chemo-protective gloves/garments/prep mats/bags; disposal system for needles

United Pacific Industries
P.O. Box 989
Everett, WA 98206

Latex and vinyl medical gloves

Valleylab
5920 Longbow Dr.
P.O. Box 9015
Boulder, CO 80301

Reusable TENS Electrodes

Vertex Industries, Inc.
23 Carol St.
P.O. Box 996
Clifton, NJ 07014-0996

Prescription balances

Waber Medical Specialties
Ste. 132
P.O. Box 2500
Honolulu, HI 96804

Vacuum tube cleaner for Baker counting machines

CHAPTER 40

Pharmacy Technicians

PAMELA A. PLOETZ and THOMAS W. WOLLER

The use of supportive personnel is well established in all aspects of pharmacy practice.[1] Pharmacy technicians have successfully assumed roles in institutional and community pharmacies, extended care facilities, home health care agencies, ambulatory clinic pharmacies, and mail order pharmacies. The increasingly widespread use of pharmacy technicians provides evidence that they are already an indispensable cog in the delivery of pharmaceutical care, and they will continue to assist the pharmacy profession in meeting society's needs.[2] The ability and willingness of pharmacy technicians to assume greater responsibility for the drug distribution process has enhanced many pharmacists' ability to expand clinical pharmacy services. This chapter explores the training, education, and role of the pharmacy technician in contemporary institutional pharmacy practice.

Pharmacy technicians are a subset of a broader group[1] called "supportive pharmacy personnel." The term "supportive personnel" refers collectively to all nonprofessional pharmacy personnel. The term "pharmacy technician" refers to someone who, under the supervision of a licensed pharmacist, assists with various technical activities of the pharmacy department that do not require the immediate judgment of a pharmacist.[1] Supportive personnel who are not considered pharmacy technicians include typists, clerks, delivery personnel, and secretaries. Pharmacy technicians are also differentiated from other supportive personnel by their increased level of education, training, and responsibility. Pharmacy technicians generally function within strict guidelines, policies, and procedures. Any deviation from same must be approved by a pharmacist. Other titles that have been used to refer to pharmacy technicians or other supportive personnel include "pharmacy technologist," "pharmacy aide," and "ancillary pharmacy personnel."

That pharmacy technicians exist as a necessary class of personnel is not doubted. The U.S. Armed Forces have been using pharmacy technical personnel since the 1940's. The profession has seen significant development over the last 10 years, evidence of which is the inception of the Association of Pharmacy Technicians (APT) in 1980. The APT has a current membership of more than 600 pharmacy technicians and is supported by a network of regional chapters throughout the United States. The American Society of Hospital Pharmacists (ASHP) has a technician member category, as do many State and local pharmacy organizations. Several States have also been active in recognizing the pharmacy technician through certification and registration programs. Five States now have some sort of registration system for pharmacy technicians. In addition, in 1981, the Michigan Pharmacists Association began an examination-based certification program that has seen more than 1,800 participants. In 1988, the Illinois Council of Hospital Pharmacists began a competency-based certification program that also has been successful. The Minnesota Society of Hospital Pharmacists conducted a demonstration project, completed in 1990, using pharmacy technicians to check unit dose cassettes, thereby freeing pharmacists to perform other patient care-related duties.

Overall, there has been strong organizational support for the development and nurturing of a technical class of personnel in pharmacy. In 1985, an ASHP invitational conference on directions for clinical practice in pharmacy, which was attended by educators, practitioners, and leaders in hospital pharmacy, identified the lack of appropriate technical personnel as a barrier to improving clinical pharmacy practice. Specific recommendations from that conference include standardization of pharmacy technician training programs, revision of unreasonable laws restricting technician use, and promotion of incentives for career-oriented pharmacy technicians.

In addition to organizational support, other factors contribute to the need for pharmacy technicians: economic, labor force management, and pharmacist role enhancement. Demand has increased for pharmacists in the clinical and patient care arenas. This, combined with a decline in the number of pharmacists available for employment, has created an environment that encourages appropriate use of technical personnel to perform some tasks traditionally performed by pharmacists. Pharmacists may then be freed to perform tasks for which they are uniquely trained. The economics of using pharmacy technicians rather than pharmacists to perform a certain task is quite simple. If a pharmacy technician can perform a task as accurately, safely, and efficiently as a pharmacist, it is in the best interest of pharmacy and society for the pharmacy technician to perform that task. However, optional use of pharmacists' and pharmacy technicians' time requires that any pharmacist time freed by a pharmacy technician be used in the patient care area to improve drug therapy. The net of these factors is that pharmacy technicians have a distinct role in institutional pharmacy practice, and that role is likely to expand in the coming years. The extent to which a pharmacy technician can assume responsibility for nontraditional tasks at a particular institution is largely dependent on institution-specific factors. For example, pharmacy technicians must be willing to accept the additional responsibility, and the pharmacists must be willing to delegate distributive tasks and assume a more clinically oriented role. Additionally, there must be a philosophical commitment on the part of department management staff to foster such role development.

POSITION DESCRIPTION FOR A PHARMACY TECHNICIAN

The position description for a pharmacy technician will define the functions and tasks for which the technician is responsible at a given institution. It should also define the level of authority of the technician and the title of his or her immediate supervisor. In most cases, functions performed by pharmacy technicians should be supervised by the licensed pharmacist working directly with the technician. The functions that a pharmacy technician performs in a hospital will vary greatly from institution to institution.

To a certain extent, regulatory processes play a role in defining the functions that can and cannot be performed by nonlicensed personnel. State law can dictate functions that can be performed only by pharmacists or those that can be delegated to technicians or other supportive personnel under the supervision of a registered pharmacist. Many State statutes have provisions that dictate a minimum ratio of pharmacists to technicians. The latter approach fails to take into account the ability for some departments to establish effective policies and procedures to safely delegate to technical personnel tasks that do not require such ratios. Defining certain functions that must be performed by a registered pharmacist allows each department to determine the other functions that will or will not be delegated to technicians after consideration of quality control mechanisms already in place.

The responsibility of a pharmacy technician can vary greatly within a hospital as well as from institution to institution. Within a department of pharmaceutical services in a hospital, a pharmacy technician may work in five or more distinct areas, each with its own unique duties for the technician. In a parenteral solution preparation area, the pharmacy technician prepares a wide variety of parenteral products, including antibiotics, large-volume parenteral solutions, cancer chemotherapy doses, and parenteral nutrition solutions. The technician is also typically responsible for labeling of the product, stocking of shelves, computer order entry, and possibly workflow coordination. The intravenous (IV) pharmacy technician is increasingly likely to encounter high-technology equipment and devices that assist in the preparation, distribution, and administration of medications. This trend is expected to continue as technology is better adapted to the drug distribution process.

In the unit dose area of a hospital pharmacy, the pharmacy technician profiles medication orders either manually or on a computer system, fills medication doses from physicians' orders or patient profiles, stocks shelves, and coordinates workflow. All patient-related work performed by a pharmacy technician must be done under the supervision of a registered pharmacist. Often the work will be double-checked by a pharmacist prior to distribution to the patient.

In the outpatient pharmacy of a hospital facility, the pharmacy technician may enter prescription orders into a computer system, fill medication orders for later verification by a pharmacist, interact with patients who are dropping off or retrieving their prescriptions, or otherwise assist the pharmacist with the daily duties.

Pharmacy technicians have also carved out less traditional roles in institutional pharmacy practice. For example, a pharmacy technician may be responsible for the record keeping and inventory of an investigational drug service. Pharmacy technicians have found positions in the management structure of pharmacy departments and have specialized in areas such as narcotic control, medication administration, computer programming, and purchasing. The common theme of these roles is that the pharmacy technician assists the pharmacist in a manner that allows the pharmacist to perform functions that only the pharmacist is trained to perform. For example, if a pharmacist working in an outpatient pharmacy is assisted by a pharmacy technician filling prescriptions, that pharmacist will have more time to spend counseling patients regarding appropriate drug therapy or reviewing patient profiles for drug interactions and therapeutic duplication. The appropriate delegation to pharmacy technicians of activities that were previously performed by pharmacists is one key to the expansion of clinical pharmacy services.

It is becoming increasingly common to see pharmacy technicians performing functions previously done only by a pharmacist. For example, intravenously administered chemotherapy doses used to be prepared by pharmacists, whereas today, in most hospitals, they are prepared by a pharmacy technician. The literature is replete with examples of nontraditional duties that a pharmacy technician has performed safely and accurately.[2-13]

Pharmacy technicians have developed roles in controlled substance distribution and record keeping, administration of medications, participation in an investigational drug service, and other unique areas of pharmacy practice. Future roles for pharmacy technicians will include more involvement in workflow management, high-technology drugs, and drug delivery devices and more extensive involvement in record keeping and documentation. Consideration of these principles may be helpful in looking for alternative roles for pharmacy technicians at a particular institution.

The position description of a pharmacy technician in an institution should contain a clear listing of the technician's daily responsibilities. It should be kept updated and be reviewed at least yearly for appropriateness. Appendix 40-A illustrates a sample of a pharmacy technician position description from the University of Minnesota Hospital and Clinic.

TRAINING AND EDUCATION OF PHARMACY TECHNICIANS

Although the ASHP has developed competency standards for technical personnel, the qualifications for becoming a pharmacy technician vary on a regional and even local basis. It is generally accepted that a pharmacy technician should have attained a high school diploma. The nature of work in a pharmacy often requires that a check of any prospective employee be completed to identify drug-related criminal convictions. This practice is a routine part of the employment screen in many hospitals. Beyond the diploma, minimum criteria are established based on the needs of a particular institution. Minimum qualifications should be based on the scope of responsibilities of the technician. Many hospitals have different levels or classes of technicians, depending on work assignment and predicated on the pharmacy technician level of training, with increasingly selective minimum criteria as responsibility increases. Many hospitals will require some level of training or equivalent experience to qualify for a particular position. Most multitier systems require a new pharmacy technician to begin at the lowest tier and move up as experience is gained and competence is demonstrated.

Pharmacy technicians entering the workforce for the first time may enter with some specific training or education. The ASHP has developed and conducts an accreditation program for pharmacy technician training programs. Many vocational and technical institutes offer pharmacy technician training programs that can be completed in 6-24 months. These programs combine didactic coursework with an experiential clerkship at a local hospital and require that the student meet predetermined objectives prior to attainment of the diploma. Some community colleges offer 2-year training programs designed to educate the pharmacy technician. The 2-year programs also combine didactic and experiential components and are generally more rigorous than the shorter programs.

Some people decide to become pharmacy technicians after attainment of a related baccalaureate degree, such as biology, at a college or university. Consequently, the newly hired pharmacy technician may or may not begin with education relating to pharmacy. Similarly, the new technician may or may not have experience in pharmacy or the medical field. As a result, most institutions have developed their own onsite training programs for newly hired pharmacy technicians. Many such programs have been described in the literature.[14-20] Most training of pharmacy technicians is done informally and on the job.

Even the best-educated, most experienced pharmacy technician will require some training at a new place of employment to learn policies and procedures unique to that institution and to become familiar with the duties and responsibilities for pharmacists and technicians at that hospital. The best training programs combine didactic, classroom-style training with an experiential component. There is a core of skills and knowledge that is considered to be essential for a pharmacy technician regardless of the practice site. The minimum required material includes review of policies and procedures, clarification of pharmacist and technician responsibilities, review of medical and technical terminology, aseptic technique, applicable laws, rules and regulations, and pharmaceutical calculations. Other topics should be included dependent on the responsibilities of the position. The experiential component may last 1 week to 6 months, again depending on the position. All training should be documented, and the documentation should be maintained in the employee's personnel file. Proper documentation increases the chances that crucial elements and details of training are not neglected, impresses the importance of the training on the trainee, and leaves no doubt as to what was included in the training session. A training checklist is a good documentation mechanism that can be signed by the pharmacy technician and trainer as objectives are met.

Once the initial training is completed, it is important to provide continuing education for pharmacy technicians. Examples of topics for pharmacy technician continuing education presentations include new drugs or types of drugs, new technology, safety issues, new techniques for preparation of medication, and ongoing research in the department or hospital.

The general lack of uniformity of training and education of pharmacy technicians can be attributed to the lack of national pharmacy organization-sponsored standards. Some direction in regard to technician training has been provided by the ASHP by offering publications on training guidelines and competency standards for supportive personnel.[21] ASHP also administers an accreditation program for pharmacy technician training programs that contains standards for training technicians.[22] This is the first step in attaining national uniformity in training and education for pharmacy technicians.

ROLE DEVELOPMENT AND JOB SATISFACTION

Few studies have been conducted to determine the level and character of job satisfaction among pharmacy technicians.[23-27] This topic will be of major concern over the next 10 years as technicians assume more nontraditional roles, resulting in an increased need to ensure job satisfaction. Several factors play a role in the job satisfaction of a pharmacy technician: compensation, perceived autonomy, job security, working conditions, recognition, and opportunity for advancement. These are concerns for pharmacists and pharmacy technicians alike. Attention to pharmacy technician job satisfaction will be necessary to ensure a motivated and qualified labor force.

Suggested methods to enhance the job satisfaction of pharmacy technicians include: providing continuing education, providing opportunities for advancement, keeping wages in line with other institutions, involving technicians in the decision-making process, providing opportunities for technicians to use creative abilities, and providing recognition for work well done.

Opportunities for job enrichment of pharmacy technicians will also come as a byproduct of pharmacists' greater clinical involvement. As the role of the pharmacist continues to evolve, so will the role of the pharmacy technician. The pharmacist is increasingly in demand to provide clinical, patient-oriented pharmacy services. In order to accommodate this goal, many tasks within the drug distribution system will be delegated to the pharmacy technician, with appropriate supervision by a registered pharmacist. This trend presents opportunities and challenges for pharmacy technicians. Job satisfaction in this scenario can be enhanced for technicians performing in roles with more autonomy and higher pay. Such a trend will also open the doors for professional advancement opportunities for the pharmacy technician.

FUTURE DIRECTIONS

Although pharmacy technicians are a recognized commodity in the workforce, there is a national lack of consensus on the role and qualifications of this group. The optimum use of pharmacy technicians in the near future will require that the profession of pharmacy come to consensus on many technician issues. In this spirit, ASHP, in 1987, appointed a task force on pharmacy technicians. The task force concluded, in part, that the pharmacist should expand the scope of pharmacy into more patient care-oriented activities and correspondingly delegate distributive activities to the pharmacy technician, with appropriate supervision.[28] In an effort to discuss this issue further, the ASHP Research and Education Foundation helped support the 1988 Invitational Conference on Technical Personnel in Pharmacy. The conference was attended by pharmacists, pharmacy technicians, and educators from all facets of pharmacy practice.

Among the consensus statements arrived at by this group was that "the needs and interests of pharmacy are subsumed by the broader needs of society."[29] Consensus statements were also developed on the topics of training, education, licensure, and supervision of pharmacy technicians. One of the conference conclusion statements describes well the future of pharmacy technicians: "The pharmacist must be willing to give up being a technician and more willing to embrace the roles and responsibilities of a health professional".[29]

REFERENCES

1. American Society of Hospital Pharmacists Task Force on Technical Personnel in Pharmacy: Toward a well-defined category of technical personnel in pharmacy. *Am J Hosp Pharm* 44:2560-2565, 1987.
2. Hogan GF: ASHP survey of use of pharmacy technicians-1985. *Am J Hosp Pharm* 42:2720-2721, 1985.
3. Directions for clinical practice in pharmacy. Proceedings of an invitational conference conducted by the ASHP Research and Education Foundation and the American Society of Hospital Pharmacists. *Am J Hosp Pharm* 42:1287-1342, 1985.
4. Woller TW, Kreling DH, Ploetz PA: Quantifying unused orders for as-needed medications. *Am J Hosp Pharm* 44:1347-1352, 1987.
5. Scala SM, Schneider PJ, Smith GL, Jr, et al: Activity analysis of pharmacy-directed drug administration technicians. *Am J Hosp Pharm* 43:1702-1706, 1986.
6. Woller TW, Roberts MJ, Ploetz PA: Recording schedule II drug use in a decentralized drug distribution system. *Am J Hosp Pharm* 44:349-353, 1987.
7. McGhan WF, Smith WE, Adams DW: A randomized trial comparing pharmacists and technicians as dispensers of prescriptions for ambulatory patients. *Med Care* 21:445-453, 1983.
8. Mahoney CD, Jeffery LP, Gallina JN: Pharmacy technician specialist: A career opportunity. *Am J Hosp Pharm* 36:1533-1536, 1979.
9. McLeod DC, Rhule D, Kitrenos JG, et al: Use of a pharmacy technologist to manage technicians' activities. *Am J Hosp Pharm* 35:1393-1394, 1978.
10. Phillips CS, Ryan MR, Roberts KB: Current and future delegation of pharmacy activities to technicians in Tennessee. *Am J Hosp Pharm* 45:577-583, 1988.
11. Becker MD, Johnson MH, Longe RL: Errors remaining in unit dose cassettes after checking by pharmacists versus pharmacy technicians. *Am J Hosp Pharm* 35:432-434, 1978.
12. Grogan JE, Hanna JA, Haight RA: A study of accuracy of pharmacy technicians working in a unit dose system. *Hosp Pharm* 13(Apr):194-199, 1978.
13. Woller TW, Ploetz PA: Expanding the role of the pharmacy technician. *Top Hosp Pharm Mgt* 9(1):35-49, 1989.
14. Idsvoog PB: Basic skills for hospital pharmacy technicians: Development of a programmed training manual. *Am J Hosp Pharm* 35:923-929, 1978.
15. Whisenant AD: Pharmacy technician training in the United States Army. *Am J Hosp Pharm* 41:2606-2614, 1984.
16. Fillmore AD, Schneider PJ, Bourret, JA, et al: Costs of training drug-administration technicians. *Am J Hosp Pharm* 43:1706-1709, 1986.
17. Phillips DJ, Smith JE: Six-month hospital based technician training program. *Am J Hosp Pharm* 41:2614-2618, 1984.
18. Smith TP, Adams RC, Brewer CD: Supportive personnel training program at a technical college. *Am J Hosp Pharm* 39:443-446, 1982.
19. Hanold LS, Leeds NH, Vogel DP: Implementation of a self-directed pharmacy technician training program. *Am J Hosp Pharm* 39:446-449, 1982.
20. Kaufman RL, Pistocco LF, Cotnoir GM: Development and implementation of a pharmacy technician training program. *Am J Hosp Pharm* 32:698-702. 1975.
21. American Society of Hospital Pharmacists: ASHP technical assistance bulletin on outcome competencies on training guidelines for institutional pharmacy technician training programs. *Am J Hosp Pharm* 39:317-320, 1982.
22. American Society of Hospital Pharmacists: ASHP regulations on accreditation of hospital pharmacy technician training programs. *Am J Hosp Pharm* 44:2741-2743, 1987.
23. Sanford ME, Fucchinetti NJ, Broadhead RS: Observational study of job satisfaction in hospital pharmacy technicians. *Am J Hosp Pharm* 41:2599-2606, 1984.
24. Noel MW, Hammel RJ, Bootman JL: Job satisfaction among hospital pharmacy personnel. *Am J Hosp Pharm* 39:600-606, 1982.
25. Mahoney CD, Gallina JN, Jeffery LP: A comprehensive program to increase job satisfaction among pharmacy technicians. *Hosp Pharm* 17:547-550, 1982.
26. Coburn MJ, Gagnon JP, Eckel JM: Job satisfaction among hospital pharmacy technicians in North Carolina. *Am J Hosp Pharm* 37:359-364, 1980.
27. Cortese LM, Greenberger DW, Schneider PJ, et al: Job characteristics and satisfaction of pharmacy technicians. *Am J Hosp Pharm* 44:2514-2518, 1987.
28. Final report of the ASHP Task Force on Technical Personnel in Pharmacy. *Am J Hosp Pharm* 46:1420-1429, 1989.
29. Technical personnel in pharmacy: Directions for the profession in society. Proceedings of an invitational conference conducted by the University of Maryland Center or Drugs and Public Policy and sponsored by the ASHP Research and Eduction Foundation, Oct 29-Nov 1 1988. *Am J Hosp Pharm* 46:491-557, 1989.

Appendix 40-A

POSITION DESCRIPTION OF A PHARMACY TECHNICIAN

DIVISION	01	General
CHAPTER	10	Department of Pharmaceutical Services
SECTION	15	Position Description
PART	05	Drug Distribution
SUBPART	30	Pharmacy Technician

Immediate Superior: Appropriate Section Supervisor or Pharmacist on duty during Supervisor's absence
Immediate Subordinate: None
Authority: Proceed within the expressed limits of established policies and procedures securing approval from the Supervisor or Pharmacist on duty for deviations from same.

Responsibilities

1. Be familiar with, understand, and comply with all policies and procedures affecting the scope of responsibility as compiled in the Department of Pharmaceutical Services Policy and Procedure Manual.
2. Respond to the Hospitals' Disaster Call at any time of day or night.
3. Work cooperatively with all Hospitals and Health Science Center employees and promote and maintain good interpersonal and interdepartmental relationships.
4. Maintain good relationships with the public in behalf of the Department of Pharmaceutical Services and the University of Minnesota Hospitals.
5. Advise Supervisor of malfunctioning equipment and unsafe equipment.
6. Make recommendation to the Supervisor as to how methods and procedures can be improved.
7. Observe and report to the Supervisor any unusual situations, occurrences, conditions, or complaints including those related to drugs, drug requests, drug usage, or security within the Pharmacy or the Hospitals.
8. Perform other related duties as assigned by authorized personnel or as may be required to meet emergency situations.
9. Keep work area in a clean and orderly manner.
10. Perform oral and/or written requests given by the Supervisor or other Pharmacists. Conflicting instructions should be resolved by the Supervisor or in his (or her) absence, the Administrative Pharmacy Officer.
11. Be accountable for the time period in which scheduled to work in dispensing area to the Supervisor or to the Pharmacist in charge. Notify the Supervisor or Pharmacist in charge when leaving the area assigned for breaks or meals.
12. Have all work checked by a Pharmacist.
13. When assigned to Inpatient area, perform duties according to Policy and Procedure on Inpatient Responsibility of Personnel (02-10-10-20). The ratio of technicians to pharmacists in this area shall not exceed 1 to 1.
14. When assigned to unit dose activities in the pharmacy satellites, perform duties according to Policy and Procedure on Technician Daily Procedures (02-20-10). The ratio of technicians to pharmacists in this area shall not exceed 3 to 1.
    a. Maintain adequate supplies of controlled substances on all nursing areas served by the satellite.
    b. Change unit dose medication cassettes.
    c. Periodically inventory the area and reorder additional supplies of drugs from Central Pharmacy as needed.
    d. Restock shelves in the dispensing areas upon receipt of stock replacement.
    e. Fill unit dose medication drawers.
    f. Prepare IV admixture solutions as required.
    g. Prepare extemporaneous package injectable and oral dosage forms.
    h. Fill new medication orders.
    i. Enter new medication orders into the computer.
    j. Type accurate and legible labels for IV admixtures, packaged doses, and pass/self meds.
15. When assigned to the Outpatient area, perform duties according to Policy and Procedure on Outpatient Responsibilities to Personnel (02-15-10).
16. When assigned to the IV Admixture Sterile Prep Packaging Service:
    a. Prepare IV Admixtures, Total Parenteral Nutrition Solutions (TPN), Antilymphocytic Globulin Solutions (ALG, ATG, IGG), skin test antigens, antibiotic piggybacks and syringes, and other sterile products as requested.
    b. Perform all clerical work associated with the IV Admixture Service such as calculations, computer processing, typing, coordinating, and workload statistics.
    c. Monitor credits returned, reissuing appropriate preparations and discarding expired ones.
    d. The ratio of technicians to pharmacists in this area shall not exceed 3 to 1.
17. When assigned as the Controlled Substance Courier, maintain adequate supplies of controlled substances on all nursing areas' maintained controlled substance floorstock.
18. Answer the telephone in assigned areas as per Departmental Policy and Procedures on Telephone Communications (01-45-05).

CHAPTER 41

Continuing Education

ROBERT J. HOLT

During the 20th century, entry-level pharmacy education has changed dramatically, expanding from a 2-year program to 5 and 6 years. In spite of its length and intensity, the professional program alone is insufficient training for the pharmacist to long remain a competent practitioner. Indeed, pharmacy educators often express the view that the new graduate is not ready to *be* a pharmacist at all; he or she is only ready to *become* a pharmacist. Proficiency and competence in a profession as complex and diverse as pharmacy can be developed and maintained only through a process of lifelong learning. Formal continuing education is one component of that process.

Continuing education programs for pharmacists are of relatively recent vintage, becoming widespread only in the last three decades. Begun as voluntary programs, early continuing education efforts were offered by pharmacy schools and professional associations to help practitioners keep up with the changes in practice. For the first time, in the mid-1960's, practitioners were required to participate in formal continuing education activities as a prerequisite for relicensure.[1] Today those pharmacists have been joined by the majority of their professional colleagues; as 1990 began, 42 boards of pharmacy in the United States required continuing education or were implementing such requirements, and 2 others had been granted the authority.[2] Thus, mandatory continuing education is a fact of life throughout most of the pharmacy profession.

FUNCTION OF CONTINUING EDUCATION

The essential function of continuing pharmaceutical education, however, is still the subject of much debate. Some practitioners consider it an employment or membership benefit, a "package" of lectures or manuals provided by the employer or association to meet the requirements of the board of pharmacy. A few view continuing education as an institutional training program, granting credit for the inservice education required to keep employees current on institutional practices. And some see it as credits to be applied toward some kind of certificate. All of these views focus on the participant's utility for the credit, not the educational content of the programming. Thus, they overlook the essential function of continuing education. As an educational entity, continuing education can be understood in terms of three basic models: the *update model*, the *competence model*, and the *performance model.*

The Update Model

Originally, continuing education programming was developed according to the update model, which maintains that continuing education "is intended to keep professionals up-to-date. It introduces new technology, new professional requirements, and updated information."[3] Underlying this approach is the assumption that pharmacy practitioners already possess the necessary skills for effective practice, that they have attained a satisfactory level of competence, and that provision of this new information will allow them to maintain that competence. If these assumptions are valid, the objective of continuing education programming is to convey new information as cost-effectively as possible. From this belief came the traditional continuing education seminar, bringing pharmacists together and presenting new information with minimal expenditure of time or money. The seminar approach is now firmly entrenched in the professional community; lectures are the standard against which other presentation methods are evaluated,[1,4] and participation in live programs is at least part of the continuing education requirement of several State boards of pharmacy.[2]

Many pharmacists, however, find it inconvenient to attend seminars because of time or distance, turning instead to alternative formats. Didactic continuing education can be accomplished through a variety of media. Correspondence courses and journal articles replace the spoken lecture with the printed monograph, again updating practitioners with new information. Courses on audiocassette tape perform the same function while maintaining the spoken word as the medium of communication. A recent review of programs listed by the American Council on Pharmaceutical Education (ACPE) revealed that monographs and audiotapes constituted the majority of programs offered to pharmacists, with audiotape being the most common medium.[5] Over the last decade, videotape has expanded continuing education opportunities by combining the lecture with visual reinforcement. Further, the last few years have witnessed the growth of computer-assisted instruction, using a written medium in an interactive format for reinforcement. The availability of update continuing education in a variety of media helps satisfy participants' individual preferences and improves access to continuing education for those who are unable to attend seminars.

By focusing on the dissemination of new information, however, such programming assumes that pharmacists will accurately select the information they need and that they possess the skills necessary to evaluate that information and skillfully apply it to practice. The update model, therefore, may or may not fulfill the actual continuing educational needs of professionals, offering some new technologies and information while overlooking others. Participants may rightly wonder, "Why this update and not that update?"[3] Further, some of their needs may go beyond the provision of new information.

The Competence Model

The competence model approaches continuing education as doing more than transmitting information; it introduces certain skills "the application of which leads to competence"[3] by the practitioner. Focusing on practitioner competence allows continuing education programming to revitalize existing knowledge with new applications and expand knowledge and skills by developing specialized expertise, thereby furthering specialization within the pharmacy profession. By incorporating skills in addition to information, the competence model includes more abstract disciplines such as logical thinking, personal and professional motivation, and improvement of self-image as a means of effecting better patient care. Continuing education providers who rely on the competence model view education as a lifelong endeavor: "Rather than just transmitting knowledge, we should attempt to teach how to identify and solve problems independently."[6]

Unlike update programming, the competence model of continuing education demands presentation media that go beyond the traditional lecture. Workshops, for example, bring pharmacists together for hands-on demonstrations and allow practice of new skills as they are learned. Workshops and other media that can teach skills, however, are usually quite labor intensive and thus more expensive than a traditional lecture. Some providers, therefore, use only a semblance of workshop medium and conclude with only a semblance of competence programming. Videotape presentations offer a less expensive alternative to the workshop and, if properly employed, videotape has the potential to demonstrate procedures and skills as a useful component of competence programming. Yet videotape courses often do little more than mimic a lecture format, transmitting information through nothing more than a recording of the lecturer and graphics in an update format. Workshops and videotapes, therefore, can effectively aid skills training or, like any other medium, offer nothing more than just another lecture.

Competence programming depends upon agreement about the competencies required of practitioners, an agreement that is not always present. The profession, however, can tacitly agree on certain technical skills, research techniques, analytical abilities, and other skills that are essential and others that may be valuable. By trying to teach those skills or competencies rather than simply providing information, a continuing education provider can implement competence programming, even if the final competencies are not fully accepted.

More important than the medium of presentation is the way in which the programming is evaluated. Programming developed according to the update model is most frequently evaluated using structure or process indicators, assessing who prepares materials, the mechanism by which the information is presented, and the level of knowledge included in the presentation. Some providers use questionnaires or written tests to assess changes in attitudes or the amount of information retained by participants, but such outcome evaluation is infrequent. Competence programming, however, demands an evaluation of educational outcomes, testing the knowledge and skills of participants both before and after the program to determine the effect on the competencies involved. Such programs are frequently evaluated through questionnaires or written tests, and an audit of the professional's performance, at least of specific skills, may even be performed to determine the effect of the educational experience.

The Performance Model

The third approach to continuing education, the performance model, goes one step further. Developed from job functions and practice performance, such programming relies on "carefully defined competency statements"[3] for the professional as he or she interacts with the entire health care environment. Performance programming incorporates the overall goals of a practice group, institution, or community in the educational planning process to gain a global perspective of the health system of which the professional is a part; from that understanding can evolve the individual practitioner's role and the means of fulfilling that role. Attempting to overcome the "hit or miss" nature of sporadic updating of information or the development or refinement of isolated skills, the performance model fuses the provision of information and skills into an understanding of the practice role within the entire environment. The objective is not merely to keep the professional informed, nor is it to keep him or her competent in certain areas. Instead, it is to educate members of the profession to fulfill their specific roles within the context of a health care community, with the ultimate goal being improved patient care. Practitioners must still master specific information and refine new skills, but they must also comprehend how the skills and knowledge interact with the rest of the system to improve patient care.

COMPONENTS OF EFFECTIVE PROGRAMMING

Cooperation

Programming developed according to the performance model, therefore, requires cooperation between professions to produce an integrated educational experience. Ideally, pharmacy schools, professional associations, and institutional employers should all work together, sharing their expertise and their understanding of practice to foster improvement in professional performance.[7] Admittedly, only those continuing education providers with a close working relationship with other health professions or institutions can readily produce such programming, but all providers can cooperate with their counterparts throughout the health care community to plan joint or complementary programs to the benefit of each.

Educational Principles

Yet more than cooperative planning is needed. To be effective, performance programming must be founded upon sound educational principles. A project conducted by the Illinois Council on Continuing Medical Education[8] analyzed eight studies of continuing education programs that produced changes in physician performance. It was found that five elements were common to all of the effective programs: (1) the target audience was specified and had (2) an identified learning need; (3) goals and objectives were clearly stated; (4) relevant learning methods with an emphasis on participation in a clinical setting were used; and (5) systematic evaluation was employed.

These programs, therefore, followed basic education methodology. The target audience specifically expressed a desire to learn. Participants all had identified a specific learning need, a gap between present and optimal performance. In each case, the study found that participants emphasized a patient need—performance behavior that was required for optimal patient care but which the physician was unable to provide. To be effective, therefore, programming seemingly should be directed toward those practitioners who recognize a specific educational need, not toward the general professional audience, and the needs that are addressed should be established cooperatively with practitioners, not solely by the continuing education provider.

Educational Goals

Once the needs are established, the educational goals should be made clear to everyone involved and strategies developed to fulfill those goals. If improved performance is the objective of continuing education, the educational experience should focus on performance, take place in a performance setting, and rely on the participation and performance of learners. Effective programming, therefore, will frequently take place in real or simulated practice settings and rely primarily on group discussions and practical procedures, learning methods requiring active student participation. The most common methods of delivering continuing education programming—all variations on the traditional lecture—do not follow the performance model, possibly a major shortcoming. Bringing pharmacists together for a seminar distinctly separates what is learned from where it is practiced. Even institutions that develop their own programming separate learning and practice; leaving the pharmacy, satellite, drug information center, nursing station, or other work area to attend an educational event in an "educational resource center" or conference room may detract from the practice performance aspect of the educational process. It is little wonder when pharmacists do not apply the learning to practice performance.

Systematic Evaluation

The final component of effective programming is systematic evaluation. Assessment methods should be determined as each learning experience is developed, basing the final evaluation on initial learning needs. To accurately evaluate learning, criteria must be developed in the early planning stages to assess whether the learning needs are satisfied and the educational goals are met. In performance programming, evaluation should focus on educational outcomes by auditing professional performance and its final outcome, patient care.

Continuing education is not an isolated activity; it is part of the entire process of lifelong learning. Cohesiveness, therefore, is an important factor in a provider's programming. The evaluation of one program is a basic factor in the planning of subsequent offerings. Further, educational programming may be sequential, relying on individual programs that build upon one another to form a unified curriculum. A provider, therefore, should assess educational outcomes not only for each offering, but after an entire series. Such a process was employed more than a decade ago in a major study funded by the National Science Foundation[9] of continuing education for engineers, and its use is expanding in pharmacy. Such sequential programming allows practitioners to develop more complex skills and integrate numerous performance objectives into an effective practice.

PROFESSIONAL REQUIREMENTS

Continuing education programming has become more sophisticated in the last decade, with many providers moving from the update model to competence or, on a limited basis, performance programming. The licensure requirements of the profession, however, have not always kept pace. Mandatory continuing education is the norm throughout the United States (table 41-1), yet most boards of pharmacy require a specific number of contact hours during the licensure period, not a specific level of performance or even much assurance of continuing education quality.

The simplest method of ensuring quality programming is accreditation of the provider, and most boards of pharmacy accept continuing education credits only from providers approved by the American Council on Pharmaceutical Education, the primary accrediting body in pharmacy education. The accreditation process, which results in "approved provider" status, is based on the ACPE Criteria for Quality, guidelines for evaluating the provider's planning structure, funding, and organization—structure and process indicators, not outcomes.

Not all practitioners, however, agree that continuing education should be mandatory. There is little doubt that "the responsibility to maintain professional excellence is inherent in the pharmacist's role."[10] The method of maintaining that excellence is the question.

Advocates of mandatory continuing education argue that pharmacy is a profession in transition. Only a few years ago, the pharmacist's primary function was distributive; today, professional competence includes at least the ability to evaluate drug information, monitor patient response to therapy, design drug therapy to improve the health of the individual, and communicate all of this information to others within and without the health care community. Further, many pharmacists practice in settings that demand specialized skills and knowledge, which cannot be fully developed during entry-level training. Thus, continuing education is essential to all pharmacists, and making it mandatory is the only way to ensure that all pharmacists obtain that which they need.

Those who advocate a voluntary approach counter that continuing pharmaceutical education must be individualized precisely because of these changes in the profession. General programs offered to fulfill the continuing education requirements imposed by boards of pharmacy do not meet the specialized needs of a profession in transition. It should be the self-imposed professional responsibility of each pharmacist to maintain competence, and the educational method and content should be the voluntary choice of the practitioner. Various approaches can be effective educational tools, including in-service training, informal education provided by colleagues, perusal of the professional and scientific litera-

Table 41-1. Continuing education requirements

Minimum participation in continuing education activities required by the board of pharmacy, listed as the number of contact hours required during each reporting period and the length of the period in years. Some jurisdictions have additional requirements.

Jurisdiction	Hours required	Reporting period	Jurisdiction	Hours required	Reporting period	Jurisdiction	Hours required	Reporting period	Jurisdiction	Hours required	Reporting period
Alabama	15	1	Illinois	30	2	Montana	15	1	Puerto Rico	35	3§
Alaska	15	1	Indiana	30	2	Nebraska	30	2	Rhode Island	15	1
Arizona	30	2	Iowa	30	2	Nevada	30	2	South Carolina	15	1
Arkansas	30	2	Kansas	15	1	New Hampshire	15	1	South Dakota	12	1
California	30	2	Kentucky	15	1	New Jersey	30	2	Tennessee	15	1
Colorado	–	–	Louisiana	15	1	New Mexico	15	1	Texas	12	1
Connecticut	15	1	Maine	15	1	New York	–	–	Utah	–	–
Delaware	30	2	Maryland	30	2	North Carolina	10	1	Vermont	30	2†
District of Columbia	–	–*	Massachusetts	30	2†	North Dakota	30	2	Virginia	–	–
Florida	30	2†	Michigan	30	2	Ohio	45	3	Washington	15	1
Georgia	30	2	Minnesota	30	2	Oklahoma	15	1	West Virginia	15	1
Hawaii	–	–	Mississippi	20	2	Oregon	15‡	1	Wisconsin	–	–
Idaho	15	1	Missouri	10	1	Pennsylvania	30	2	Wyoming	6	1

*Enabling legislation passed by the City Council; board of pharmacy published requirements of 15 hours for 1991 renewal period.
†Board of pharmacy requires at least 15 hours each year; participation in continuing education is reported biennially with license renewal.
‡An optional challenge examination is offered by the board of pharmacy in lieu of continuing education.
§A minimum of 10 hours is required in each year, but a cumulative total of at least 35 hours is required during the triennial recertification period.

Adapted with permission from National Association of Boards of Pharmacy, *NABP Survey of Pharmacy Law 1991-1992*, Chicago, IL, 1991.

ture, and personal research. Licensed health professionals such as pharmacists should have the personal initiative to continue their education and the ability to select the methods most appropriate to their needs.

Supporters of both sides in the debate are equally adamant, and neither seems able to sway the other. Despite these arguments, however, the future path is clear and mandatory continuing education is now the norm. Most professions, in fact, require at least some continuing education for relicensure: medicine, nursing, dentistry, many allied health professions, law, accounting, real estate, and several others are subject to mandatory continuing education in many States.

INSTITUTIONAL ROLE

In an environment imposing mandatory continuing education on its employees, the institutional employer has a threefold responsibility: (1) to ensure that employees remain or become proficient in their specific jobs, (2) to enable employees to maintain and improve the services within the institution, and (3) to ensure that employees remain or become proficient in the wider arena of their professions. The first two are frequently addressed through in-service training—educational efforts within an institution to address the needs, functions, and professional interactions occurring in the workplace. In-service training deals with the specific needs of the employer and trains the professional or other employee to complete specific tasks more effectively. Continuing education, however, addresses the institutional employer's third responsibility by providing the information, skills, and attitudes to fulfill the professional role in a number of settings.

The Joint Commission on Accreditation of Healthcare Organizations (JCAHO) affirms the institutional responsibility to maintain professional competence through continuing education. The quality assurance section of the JCAHO Standard on Pharmaceutical Services[11] states that the director of pharmacy services should be responsible for:

> Requiring and documenting the participation of pharmacy personnel in relevant education programs, including orientation of new employees, as well as in-service and outside continuing education programs.

Continuing education is necessary to quality pharmaceutical services, and the hospital has a distinct role in requiring participation.

The institution may fulfill this function by serving as its own continuing education provider. Indeed, many institutions are accredited by ACPE as providers, either individually or in conjunction with a larger group, offering continuing education in the work setting as a fringe benefit of employment. In such an arrangement, the hospital pharmacy is responsible for assessing the educational needs of its employees, planning and implementing programs to meet those needs, and monitoring employee performance to evaluate the effectiveness of the educational process. Such programs are usually offered during the workday and allow pharmacists, physicians, and other staff to share their expertise with colleagues through clinical case conferences, drug information conferences, open professional discussions, and journal reviews. Serving as its own provider, the institution incurs only a minimal financial obligation, an obvious benefit to the hospital; the employee pharmacist benefits by receiving free continuing education directed toward performance of his or her specific job. The education, however, is limited to the expertise available internally. More important, continuing education is a secondary function for the institution. With a limited commitment to continuing education, the provider may pursue the simplest path and focus only on the transmission of information rather than the development of professional skills, attitudes, and performance. The continuing education may not differ significantly from the in-service training that the institution also provides.

To overcome these limitations, the institution may delegate to outside agencies its obligation to provide continuing education, instead offering financial support, release time, or other incentives as an employee fringe benefit. Several approaches are available. Some institutions and groups contract for specific services, incorporating continuing education into the workplace while creating an objective distance with a contractual relationship. Such arrangements usually rely on both a continuing education committee within the institution and an independent provider from outside to develop and implement programming. The internal committee is an essential component in needs assessment and evaluation, and it serves as a liaison to monitor the quality of the programming from the provider and the effective participation of the institution.

Contractual relationships may be arranged to provide individual programs or long-term educational services; the latter may be more useful to the institution, since the provider then has the opportunity to ensure educational continuity and professional development, which are unavailable with single update programs. Depending on the provider's capabilities and the institution's needs, a contractual arrangement can significantly strengthen the pharmacist's continuing education experiences.

More commonly, however, the employer offers financial reimbursement or other compensation, allowing the employee to choose from among the programs available from pharmacy schools, professional associations, or commercial providers. Selection of appropriate, high-quality, continuing education is the responsibility of every pharmacist, but it can be particularly demanding when the institution provides little guidance.

ROLE OF THE PHARMACIST

As a continuing education participant, the pharmacist assumes a number of responsibilities. After all, any educational experience must be an active endeavor if it is to be truly effective; the passive participant cannot garner the full benefits available from the experience.

The pharmacist's first responsibility is assessing his or her professional abilities and performance requirements, often a difficult task. In its Statement on Continuing Education, the American Society of Hospital Pharmacists (ASHP)[12] suggests that the "institutional pharmacist should set for himself [or herself] personal educational objectives based on his [her] needs for performance improvement and his [her] career goals." All pharmacists recognize some of the gaps in their abilities, discrepancies between actual and desired performance; yet other gaps may go unnoticed. Further, even when pharmacists' career goals are clearly defined, they may not be fully aware of all the skills necessary to achieve these goals. Thus, practitioners "may often require assistance in identifying gaps ... [and] setting educational objectives and desired performance,"[12] as ASHP's statement further specifies. To help pharmacists identify their educational needs, a few continuing education providers are beginning to offer needs assessment, helping evaluate the areas in which practitioners are deficient and in which they are most skilled. Those deficiencies and skills can then be matched with career goals to identify the specific continuing education most needed. Yet few providers offer such services, and practitioners may be left to their own devices in determining their educational needs.

After determining his or her needs, however, the practitioner is still faced with the selection of providers and learning activities to meet those needs. By its "hit or miss" nature, update programming may satisfy an immediate need without providing the skills necessary for a changing practice, so emphasis should be placed on long-term educational approaches. As practice continues to change, more and more providers are offering new ways for the pharmacist to organize continuing education to develop long-term competencies.

During the last decade, many providers have moved toward such curricular programming; i.e., a sequence of continuing education programs, each of which builds upon the knowledge and skills of preceding offerings in the same way an academic degree curriculum is organized. Such sequences may be quite limited, consisting of only two or three programs on a single topic or in related areas. Some limited sequences seem to be designed for licensure requirements rather than educational content; they offer precisely the number of hours required for license renewal irrespective of the topic area. Others provide greater depth and include experiential components to develop skills and apply them to practice. As more programming becomes available in a curricular format, practitioners will be able to select programs that both fulfill their current professional needs and develop their potential for future practice.

Certificate programs are also based on the curricular model, but they are usually of greater magnitude. As defined in a 1989 joint conference of the American Association of Colleges of Pharmacy (AACP) and ACPE,[13] certificate programs are academically rigorous, contain both didactic and experiential components, and focus on new competencies rather than updating existing information. Certificate programs have been offered at least since 1984, when three were available from ACPE-approved providers,[5] but they became quite prominent and their number had expanded rapidly by the beginning of 1990. Because of the depth offered by certificate programs and the emphasis on practical competence, such programs may spur further specialization in pharmacy by offering the training necessary for specialized practice. Furthermore, the current emphasis on certificates has induced some boards of pharmacy to discuss curricular programming and certificate programs as the basis of mandatory continuing education.

Since curricular offerings, especially certificate programs, may provide academically rigorous postgraduate training, it may be argued that academic credit toward an advanced degree should be granted for their completion. Indeed, external degree programs are currently available, and the concept of using continuing education to earn the Doctor of Pharmacy or the Master of Science degree has received much attention in both the educational and professional literature.[5,14,15] One study found that many available home study continuing education courses were similar in content and depth to some advanced degree coursework,[5] indicating that a combination of didactic continuing education and on-campus training could feasibly attain the same goals as a traditional degree. Such a program, however, at least has the potential of making the degree a terminal goal, nullifying the concept of *lifelong* learning. Even if continuing education becomes widely applicable to advanced degrees, the essential function of continuing education will be unchanged.

The individual role of the pharmacist, therefore, is to identify educational needs and select the programs to satisfy them. Institutional pharmacists, however, often serve as providers, planning and implementing in-service and continuing education programs for their fellow professionals and other personnel. In this capacity, the pharmacist must also be familiar with mechanisms of assessing the educational needs of the department, educational methodology, and evaluation techniques. As an individual practitioner, the pharmacist is responsible for his or her own competence and performance; as a provider, the pharmacist must plan a sound educational curriculum which will maintain and improve the performance of the profession.

CONCLUSION

Continuing education can no longer be viewed as a necessary evil—a specified number of credits that must be obtained each year merely to renew a license. Pharmacists have an ethical obligation to remain current in the knowledge of the profession; maintain competence in the skills necessary for practice; improve their performance in relation to the entire health care environment; and help their colleagues, both pharmacists and others, obtain education of the same quality. Although it is not the only mechanism, continuing education is the most clearly defined, universally available medium to fulfill this obligation. And since employers benefit from the competence thus engendered, they have a collateral obligation to support continuing education, both financially and temporally. More than 20 years ago, Edmund Pellegrino[16] said, "After the degree is conferred, continuing education is society's only real guarantee of the optimal quality of health care." The obligation to the public and the profession is no less today.

REFERENCES

1. Nona DA, Kenny WR, Johnson DK: The effectiveness of continuing education as reflected in the literature of the health professions. *Am J Pharm Educ* 52:111-117, 1988.
2. National Association of Boards of Pharmacy, Chicago, IL: *NABP Survey of Pharmacy Law* 1991-1992.
3. Ansel HC: Some thoughts on continuing education and professional performance. *Am J Pharm Educ* 51:341, 1987.
4. Friesen AJ, Zinyk DE, Mah G: Mandatory continuing education in Alberta, Canada: The response to live programs and correspondence courses. *Am J Pharm Educ* 49:156-159, 1985.
5. Riley DA, Shannon MC, Nickel RO: Home study C.E. as possible components of pharmacy degrees. *Am J Pharm Educ* 49:154-156, 1985.
6. Nahata MC: The need to develop independent learners. *DICP* 21:543-544, 1987.
7. Phillips LE: Is mandatory continuing education working? *Mobius* 7(Jan):57-64, 1987.
8. Stein LS: The dilemma of CME: A third opinion. *AMA CME News* (July):2-11, 1980.
9. Morris AJ: The Return on Investment in Continuing Education of Engineers. Palo Alto, CA, Genesys Systems, 1978.
10. Jeffroy LP, Mahoney CD: Continuing education. In Brown TR, Smith MC (eds): *Handbook of Institutional Pharmacy Practice*, 2nd ed. Baltimore, MD, Williams & Wilkins, 1986, pp 597-600.
11. Joint Commission on Accreditation of Healthcare Organizations: *1990 Accreditation Manual for Hospitals*. Chicago, IL, Joint Commission on Accreditation of Healthcare Organizations, 1989.
12. American Society of Hospital Pharmacists: ASHP statement on continuing education. *Am J Hosp Pharm* 35:815-816, 1978.
13. AACP Board affirms certificate guidelines. *AACP News* (Dec):1, 1989.
14. APHA policy actions. *Am Pharm* NS22:369, 1982.
15. Karlitz K: How hospital pharmacists feel about their mandatory C.E. *Pharm Times* (Oct):110-112, 1987.
16. Pellegrino ED: Continuing education in the health professions. *Am J Pharm Educ* 33:712, 1969.

CHAPTER 42

Legal Aspects of Institutional Practice

VANCE L. ALEXANDER

With increasing frequency the institutional pharmacist is confronted with legal issues in his or her practice. For many years the use of drugs has been the target for strict control. Aspects contributing to the need for such control include the potential for abuse, misuse, and overuse, and the importance of establishing safe and efficacious uses. More recently, economic aspects have placed additional restrictions on drug control and distribution.

Often cited as one of the most regulated professions, hospital pharmacy also endures the heavy regulation placed on the hospital segment of the health care industry. The hospital pharmacist comes face to face with the legal aspects of practice in both straightforward and subtle ways. Control of scheduled drugs is decidedly the obligation of the hospital pharmacist. The statutes and regulations define the requirements that provide vast detail. However, subtle and emerging areas of law also control the practitioner. Antitrust implications of the drug distribution system and drug testing of employees are much less clear in their application. The institutional practitioner may encounter complex personnel management legal issues such as drug testing, Equal Employment Opportunity Commission terminations, and employment of impaired pharmacists. Almost any area of law could have a point of application for the hospital pharmacy practitioner.

It is not the intent of this chapter to provide the depth or breadth of the legal aspects of hospital pharmacy practice, but rather to alert the practitioner to some of the areas of concern. Hospital pharmacists should be intimately familiar with the State pharmacy practice act and other drug control laws and regulations such as the Comprehensive Drug Abuse and Control Act and the Poison Prevention Packaging Act. Such knowledge is essential. By being aware of the less obvious legal issues, the pharmacist can be sensitive to the need for assistance and direction from legal counsel.

SOURCES OF LAWS AND REGULATIONS AFFECTING THE PRACTITIONER

An understanding of the sources of laws and regulations is important in order that the institutional pharmacist may monitor and perhaps influence pertinent laws and regulations.

Legislatively Enacted Law

Law enacted by legislation is commonly called "acts" or "statutes." This source of law is the result of acts of elected officials through an elaborate system of lawmaking. Institutional pharmacists are familiar with the acts passed at the national and State levels. However, city and county ordinances also can affect practice. The law is generally codified and available to most public libraries. Examples of statutory law include the States' pharmacy practice acts and the recently passed Federal law, the Prescription Drug Marketing Act of 1987. Institutional pharmacists individually, or collectively through professional organizations, should closely monitor proposed legislation for its impact on practice.

Judicial Law

This form of law is made through the decisions of the local, State, and national courts. Courts reach thousands of decisions each day. Generally, only those cases that reach the appellate level are reported. Specialty publications report decisions from trial level courts and, to a limited extent, cases that were settled without a total trial.

Administrative Law

This is created by those agencies of the government charged with the responsibility to implement and enforce statutory law. As with legislatively and judicially created law, administrative law is made at all levels of government. Typically such law is called "regulations" or "rules" but also could include the decisions of administrative bodies.

Results from hearings or similar proceedings are a form of administrative law. As part of its adjudicatory power, an agency may use a hearing or like proceeding to hear violations of the agency rules, regulations, or statutes. State boards of pharmacy and the Drug Enforcement Administration (DEA) are examples of administrative agencies.

Certain procedures must be followed by the agencies in their rule-making function. Generally, there must be notice and an opportunity for comment on proposed rules or regulations. Similarly, such agencies must follow established procedures in their adjudication role. The practitioner should be aware that rules and regulations from other agencies and boards, such as the State department of health or the State department of medical licensure may have a direct impact on practice. Institutional practitioners also should establish some method to monitor proposed rules and regulations. These rules and regulations, once passed, have the effect of law until challenged and overturned.

Quasilegal Principles

Many quasilegal principles that affect the institutional practitioner are not actually laws but include standards and/or guidelines put forth by nongovernmental bodies. Such principles may be used for credentialing or attempts to standardize or upgrade a profession. Examples of these principles include the American Pharmaceutical Association's Standards of Practice for the Profession of Pharmacy and Code of Ethics and the Joint Commission on Accreditation of Healthcare Organizations' Standards. Each year the American Society of Hospital Pharmacists (ASHP) publishes *Practice Standards of ASHP,* containing more than 50 documents titled statements, guidelines, standards, technical assistance bulletins, and regulations. Although the courts have been reluctant to use these quasilegal documents as a measure of the standard of care, caution should be taken by organizations in publishing such principles.

DRUG USE CONTROL

Pharmacists' legal and societal mission is one of drug use control. This role continues to gain importance as more potent drugs become available. Abuse, both intentional and otherwise, of prescription and nonprescription drugs strengthens the need for the pharmacist in drug use control. Legislative acts have defined the legal responsibility of the pharmacist. The following sections provide an overview of the major legislative mandates of interest to institutional pharmacists.

Federal Food, Drug, and Cosmetic Act

For more than half a century, the legal basis for drug use control in this country has been the Federal Food Drug and Cosmetic Act. Passed in 1938, the act with its amendments provides the Federal Government with the authority to regulate drug products. The Food and Drug Administration (FDA) is charged with enforcement of the act. The law prohibits the introduction of foods, drugs, and devices—including diagnostic aids and cosmetics—that are misbranded or are adulterated. Through the adulteration provision, the Food and Drug Administration is able to regulate the purity and sanitation of drug products. The act provides for legend and over-the-counter drugs and the specific labeling required for each drug. Legend drugs may be dispensed only on the request of an authorized practitioner. States retain the responsibility of establishing who is an authorized practitioner in their jurisdictions. Drugs must have a demonstrated safety and effectiveness prior to introduction into the market. Labeling requirements allow only the promotion of approved indications for any prescription drug.

Investigational Drugs

Before a drug can be marketed, a new drug application must be approved by the FDA. Stringent and detailed regulations outline the procedures that must be followed to achieve approval. Before an unapproved drug can be tested in humans, the sponsor must file an investigational new drug form (IND) with the FDA. The same applies to an approved drug that is being investigated for use outside the approved labeling. The sponsor of the IND may be a drug company, a research facility, a physician, a pharmacy or pharmacist, or others. However, the investigators must be qualified by experience and training to conduct clinical research. Regulations provide that an institutional review board be established to monitor the use of investigational drugs and to ensure that the rights of patients are protected.

Hospitals and other health care institutions provide an excellent source of monitored patient care. Because of this, the institutional pharmacist often is involved with investigational drugs. Traditionally, the pharmacist is requested to control the supply and distribution of investigational drugs within the institution. Pharmacist involvement has both professional and financial implications. With increasing frequency, institutional pharmacists are becoming coinvestigators and primary investigators in clinical research protocols. In these situations, the pharmacist may be viewed as the expert on the clinical use of the drug. Additionally, the pharmacist may be considered the authority on the regulations of investigational drug documentation, use, and control. It is prudent for involved pharmacists to become thoroughly familiar with the sections of the Code of Federal Regulations devoted to the investigational drug process.

Unapproved Uses

As stated above, a drug manufacturer can only promote a drug for a use that is specified in its approved labeling. Questions often arise concerning the use of a drug by a physician that is clearly not within the approved labeling. The use may involve a dose, patient population, indication, or other matter contained in the approved labeling. The FDA has stated that such a use by itself does not violate the Food, Drug, and Cosmetic Act. However, where such use becomes *an investigational* use, it must then comply with the provisions of investigational new drug process.

As might be expected, the question may become, "What is an investigation?" The appearance of an investigation would include the collection of data on that use, employment of scientific process, blinding of a procedure or drug use, coding of drug products, and other indications. The use of drugs in an investigational manner without compliance with the regulations seriously jeopardizes the institution and the practitioners.

Comprehensive Drug Abuse Control and Prevention Act of 1970

Regardless of whose name may appear on the DEA controlled substances registration form, the leadership in most health care institutions looks to the pharmacist to ensure compliance with controlled substances regulations. The legislative basis for control of dangerous substances at the Federal level is the Comprehensive Drug Abuse Control and Prevention Act of 1970. Many State-controlled substances acts parallel this Federal legislation, often with only minor exceptions. Title 1 of this act deals with drug abuse, Title 3 addresses the import and export of controlled substances, and Title 2 covers other aspects of controlled substances regulation. This act is codified in United States

Code Title 21. Also, the regulations that enforce the act are found in the Code of Federal Regulations Title 21, primarily in Section 1300, et seq. The regulations appear to be designed with registrants other than institutional health care providers in mind and are in need of revision to accommodate realistic goals. Major areas of concern for the institutional practitioner include registration, record-keeping, and destruction of waste and unwanted controlled substances.

Registration

Registration is moderately direct. Initial registration is accomplished by completing a DEA form 224. The fee for registration is $60 for a 3-year period; however, Federal, State, and local agencies may have the fee waived with a proper certifying signature on the application. Manufacturers, wholesalers, distributors, pharmacies, and prescribers are required to register. It is important to note that separate registration is required for separate locations and separate activities.

Dispensing or administering, by a hospital or other similar institution, is not considered a separate activity in this context. The administering or dispensing of a narcotic drug for a narcotics-addicted patient is considered a separate activity under certain circumstances and would, therefore, require the institution to be registered as a narcotic treatment program. Security requirements for narcotic treatment programs are stringent. When a patient is admitted for a medical or surgical reason other than narcotics addiction, the use of the institution's methadone or other controlled substances for detoxification or maintenance would be appropriate.

A registration issue in which the institutional practitioner may become involved deals with physicians in training. The law mandates that prescribers be registered. A prerequisite to registration in the majority of jurisdictions is postgraduate internship or residency training. However, regulations permit physicians-in-training, as employees of the institution, to use the institution's registration. Such physicians-in-training must be assigned a suffix to the institution's registration number. Use of the institution's registration number requires compliance with the following:

1. The dispensing, administering, and prescribing are in the usual course of professional practice.
2. The physician is authorized or permitted to do so by the jurisdiction in which the physician is practicing.
3. The hospital or institution has verified that the physician is permitted to dispense, administer, and prescribe drugs within the jurisdiction.
4. The physician acts only within the scope of his or her employment in the hospital or institution.
5. The hospital or institution authorizes the intern, resident, or foreign physician to dispense and prescribe under its registration and assigns a specific internal code number for each physician so authorized.
6. A current list of internal codes and the corresponding individual practitioners is kept by the hospital or institution and is made available at all times to other registrants and law enforcement agencies upon request for the purpose of verifying the authority of the prescribing individual practitioner.

Record Keeping

Accountability is probably the most important aspect of the control of dangerous and addictive substances by the institutional practitioner. Records of inventory, receipt, and dispersal for drugs in all schedules are required. Although the controlled substances regulations make a distinction between prescriptions and medication orders, regulations for record keeping demand the same information. As practitioners are aware, the act and its attendant regulations categorize controlled substances into Schedules I through V. Regardless, no practical differences exist between schedules for record keeping for medication orders. It should be noted that although the inpatient medical record is considered the basic original record, pharmacists may find it prudent to employ a derivative record.

Destruction of Unwanted Controlled Substances

Because of the large volume of controlled substances required by institutions, unused, contaminated, or unwanted controlled substances can be burdensome for the institutional practitioner. Regulations describe the method for returning controlled substances to DEA and other agencies for destruction. Nonetheless, the institution may be allowed to dispose of controlled substances itself. The institution should petition the agent in charge for the DEA region. The request should delineate a complete description of the method for destruction, including how the destruction is witnessed.

Use of Tax-Free Alcohol

Hospitals have traditionally found it financially advantageous to use tax-free ethyl alcohol in laboratories, for sterilization and other nonbeverage purposes. The regulations for use of tax-free alcohol are found in Title 27 of the Code of Federal Regulations. By obtaining a permit from the Federal Bureau of Alcohol, Tobacco, and Firearms, hospitals, laboratories, and other designated entities can be exempted from the $12.50 per gallon tax. Tax-free alcohol may not be used for making food or beverages. Medicines made with tax-free alcohol may not be sold; however, institutions may make a separate charge for medicines compounded with tax-free alcohol and used on the premises.

In addition to Federal regulation of the sale and distribution of alcohol, States are also involved in the control of alcohol. Institutional pharmacists should carefully examine practices whereby patients are supplied with beer, wine, or other forms of alcohol. Local and State laws may require the institution to obtain a permit or license to dispense alcohol to its patients.

Poison Prevention Packaging Act

The intent of the Poison Prevention Packaging Act of 1970 is to reduce accidental poisoning of children. All indications show that the act has been successful toward that end. The act is aimed primarily at the packaging of "household substances" requiring child-resistant containers. However, the packaging requirements extend to both nonprescription and prescription drugs. Outpatient prescriptions must be dispensed in child-resistant containers, except for sublingual nitroglycerin tablets, sublingual and chewable 2.5-mg and 5-mg isosorbide dinitrate preparations, a limited number of memory-aid packaged drugs, and others. A complete list of the exceptions to the packaging requirements should be posted in outpatient dispensing areas. Further exception to the use of noncomplying containers is permitted on the request of the prescribing physician or the patient. Such orders should be made on an individual basis, since blanket orders by physicians are not valid. Although such a request for noncomplying containers is not required to be in writing, it is suggested that a form of acknowledgment by the patient be used. Of importance to institutional pharmacists is the exemption for drugs dispensed to inpatients in hospitals.

DRUG PRODUCT SELECTION AND ACQUISITION ISSUES

Antitrust

Because of the manner in which drugs are purchased by hospitals and other institutions, the courts have addressed the antitrust implications of these practices. For a variety of reasons, drug manufacturers have provided institutions with preferential pricing schedules. The core antitrust act prohibits price discrimination between different purchasers of goods of like quality and grade if the effect of such discrimination is likely to injure competition. By way of an amendment to the antitrust act, nonprofit institutions have an exemption when drugs purchased are for the institution's own use. Importantly, the court in its definition of own use has said:

1. Drugs purchased for use on the premises of a hospital are exempt under the act. Such use covers inpatients, outpatients, and emergency patients, etc.
2. Drugs purchased for take-home medications for inpatients, outpatients, and emergency room patients fall within the exemption. Drugs so dispensed must be for a "reasonable and limited time" and a continuation of or supplement to treatment administered at the hospital, which the patient still requires.
3. Drugs purchased for dispensing to hospital employees, students, and medical staff for their personal use or the use of their dependents are permissible. Dispensing to such persons for use by nondependents or for use in a physician's private practice is not exempt.
4. Drugs purchased for dispensing refills to former patients are far too removed from the hospital setting to fall within the exemption. Even if continued use of a drug is indicated, use beyond reasonable and limited quantities of initial take-home medication is not exempt from the act.
5. Walk-in prescriptions for persons with no present connection with the hospital cannot be filled with drugs purchased under the exemption. Occasional walk-in prescriptions, filled in emergency situations, although not necessarily permissible, would be considered of minor legal consequence. The court has further defined "own use" in relation to health maintenance organizations. Use of drugs purchased at special hospital prices may be dispensed to members of health maintenance organizations.

The practitioner should bear in mind that the courts have not prohibited the institution from providing pharmaceutical services and drugs to nonexempt patients. However, caution must be exercised to avoid the use of drugs purchased at preferential prices except for own use. The court has left options open to the institutional pharmacy as whether to maintain separate inventories in serving nonexempt patients or to use other means to comply with the use limitations.

Prescription Drug Marketing Act

This Federal legislation is aimed at curbing abuses in the legitimate chain of distribution of drugs. The regulations supporting this legislation have not been published, even though the effective date of the statute was July 22, 1988. The reader should note that the title is "Prescription Drug Marketing Act" and does not apply to over-the-counter medications. The basic provisions deal with reimportation, control of samples, sales restrictions, and registration of wholesale drug companies.

Reimportation

Reimportation is prohibited except by the manufacturer. Samples and coupons are restricted allowing drug sample distribution only by mail or common carrier or by manufacturer representatives. The law requires the submission of a written request for samples by the practitioner to include certain specified information. Records on the distribution of samples or coupons must be kept for 3 years. Proper storage of drug samples is established to ensure conditions that will maintain drug stability, integrity, and effectiveness, and freedom from contamination, deterioration, and adulteration. Annual inventories of drugs possessed by manufacturer and representatives must be maintained. Manufacturers must maintain a list of names and addresses of representatives who distribute samples and sites where samples are stored. The manufacturer also must provide notification of any drug convictions by its representatives and notification of drug losses.

Sales Restrictions

Sales restrictions for hospitals, health care entities, and certain charitable organizations were established. The law prohibits the sale, purchase, or trade of prescription drugs by a hospital or the sale, purchase, or trade of drugs donated or sold at reduced cost to charitable institutions except:

1. Pursuant to a valid prescription
2. To or from other hospitals or health care entities
3. To a nonprofit affiliate or other hospitals under common control
4. Members of the same purchasing group for own use
5. For emergency medical reasons

Registration of Wholesalers

The act requires the establishment of wholesale distribution controls. Wholesalers must be licensed by the State, using Federal guidelines. Although much confusion has ensued, the law requires controls on drug returns to wholesalers by hospitals and other health care entities. An interesting provision of the act allows for rewards up to one-half of criminal fines imposed to a limit of $125,000.

Contractual Considerations

Increased drug use, coupled with the increased cost of drug products, has placed enormous incentives for cost control on institutional pharmacy practitioners. Opportunities to reduce drug cost are sought. Whether through the bidding process or through the review of proposals presented by drug manufacturers or other vendors, the pharmacist will encounter situations involving contractual obligations. Because of the binding nature of contracts, pharmacists should exercise extreme caution in the purchasing process, including requesting and accepting proposals. For example, a standard "request for proposal" with terminology reviewed by legal counsel should be employed.

Drug Product Selection

With the repeal of the antisubstitution statutes, speculation arose that there would be a large increase in lawsuits involving drug product selection by pharmacists. The reported cases involving pharmacists' drug product selection have been extremely small. A malpractice carrier for pharmacists points out that there have been few published appellate court cases and that the number of claims is very small. It appears that the claims involve categories of drugs with known bioavailability problems, such as anticonvulsant drugs and thyroid drugs.

Institutional pharmacists can take steps to continue to maintain their low exposure on this issue. The institution should use a formulary system, involving an active pharmacy and therapeutics committee. The addition and deletion of drugs to the formulary by the pharmacy and therapeutics committee should be well documented, with the basis for the committee's actions clearly stated. With more products becoming available generically, criteria should be established and employed to determine which products are acceptable. Careful review of bioequivalence information from the FDA and other sources should be documented.

In its operation of the formulary system, the institution should ensure that prescribers consent to product selection procedures. Such consent can be current or general. Current consent allows the prescriber the option on each order to permit the use of the generic product. A general consent is a blanket consent, thus allowing the use of the formulary equivalent regardless of the name used by the prescriber unless otherwise indicated on a particular order. Although opposition has been expressed to the use of general consent, the author knows of no legal cases involving such consent.

LIABILITY

Liability for the practitioner can arise in several ways. Criminal liability can exist when there has been a violation of a statute. Depending on the severity and the penalties outlined by the statute, fines, imprisonment, and loss of property can result from criminal liability. Contractual liability arises as the result of a breach of an agreement. The agreement may have been implicit or explicit.

Product-Related Liability

Although historically, this category of liability has not been of great significance to institutional practitioners, the potential for such liability increases as institutional practitioners become involved in nondrug products. Breach of warranty theory may be employed in recovery attempts. Warranties may be express warranties, implied warranties of merchantability, or implied warranties of fitness for particular use. An express warranty is a written or oral statement about the product that is a fact, promise, or description of the product that becomes a part of the basis for the bargain. The implied warranties deal with products made in compliance with industry standards and being useful for the purposes for which they are sold. Drug administration devices and home health care products such as infusion pumps could increase warranty liability exposure.

Another theory involving products is strict liability in tort. This theory holds that a supplier should be liable if it places a product on the market that is in a defective condition unreasonably dangerous to the consumer. Under strict liability in tort, all components of the chain of distribution would be liable, regardless of the exercise of due care. Despite continuing attempts to use this legal theory, pharmacists have been held to be exempt. Liability also occurs as the result of the actions of others for whom responsibility exists to oversee and control.

Negligence

Often called "malpractice," professional negligence is perhaps the largest source of civil liability for the practitioner. Negligence exists when a practitioner—with an established duty to follow a standard of care—fails to attain that standard, resulting in injury to another individual. The institutional practitioner can better appreciate liability exposure with an overview of the elements of actionable negligence.

Duty

There must exist a duty to do a certain act or refrain from doing a certain act. The patient-pharmacist relationship creates certain duties. An individual also may assume a duty, for example, in the good Samaritan situation. Once that duty is created or assumed, the provider must act according to the standard of care. Questions about to whom the duty is owed also exist. It is reasonable to expect that a duty is owed to the patient, but a duty could also be owed to others. For example, in the provision of drug information to another health professional with a third-party patient injured, a duty to that third person may be asserted.

Standard of Care

Expert testimony will be used to establish what standard of care should be applied. Most often, "standard of care" is defined as that degree of care a reasonable and prudent pharmacist would use under similar circumstances. Local custom may not be the standard if it deviates from national standards.

Breach

A breach of duty is simply the failure to fulfill properly that duty and failure to achieve the standard. Failure to follow the law could be used to establish *negligence per se*.

Damages

For an actionable negligence claim to proceed, there must exist an allegation of damages. The damages to the patient may be physical, mental, and financial loss resulting therefrom. Other damages that can be considered include damage to a relationship such as husband-wife or parent-child relationship.

Causation

Even though damages have been sustained and a duty owed by the practitioner has been breached, it must be established that the particular breach caused that damage.

If all of those elements are present, as determined by the jury or the judge, the plaintiff collects absent any defenses. Damages also can include punitive damages if the conscience of the court is so offended by the defendant's behavior. An example of such behavior might be where a practitioner realized a mistake was made but failed to take timely corrective action.

Insurance

Because of the large increase in insurance cost, many large institutions are becoming self-insured. Many others provide malpractice insurance, covering their employees through insurance carriers. Practitioners should not assume that the institution provides insurance, but should investigate the existence and nature of coverage provided by the institution. If the institution does not provide malpractice insurance coverage, the pharmacist may obtain a policy at an inexpensive rate through the national pharmacy societies.

Whether coverage is provided by the practitioner or the institution, a careful reading of the policy should be undertaken to determine extent of coverage provided and the presence of defense or settlement clauses (is the practitioner's consent needed?). It should be determined if the policy contains exclusion to coverage, such as criminal or other acts. The practitioner should be aware of the conditions that must be met before coverage is provided, such as those related to notice, time periods, and attendance at hearings and trials.

CONCLUSION

In the practice of pharmacy in the institutional setting, the pharmacist must not only be thoroughly familiar with the long-established law, but must also remain alert to the new and the potential law. It is imperative for the practitioner to take an active role in maintaining knowledge of the legal aspects of the institutional setting.

ADDITIONAL READING

Brushwood DB: *Medical Malpractice: Pharmacy Law.* Colorado Springs, CO, Shepard's/McGraw-Hill, 1986.

DeMarco CT: *Pharmacy and the Law,* 2nd ed, Rockville, MD, Aspen Systems, 1984.

Fink JL III, Marquardt KW, Simonsmeier IM: *Pharmacy Law Digest.* Media, PA, Harwal Publishing, 1985.

Gibson JT: *Medication Law and Behavior.* New York, John Wiley & Sons, 1976.

Nielson JR: *Handbook of Federal Drug Law.* Philadelphia, PA, Lea & Febiger, 1986.

Strauss S (ed): *The Pharmacist and the Law.* Baltimore, MD, Williams & Wilkins, 1980.

Appendix 42-A

LEGAL ARTICLES IN THE AMERICAN JOURNAL OF HOSPITAL PHARMACY

Volume	Date	Page	Title
25	1968	528	Medication errors and legal implications of drug handling on the patient floor
26	1969	346	Taxability of income of hospital pharmacy residents in ASHP-accredited residency programs
26	1969	404	Legal responsibility of the hospital pharmacist for rational drug therapy
26	1969	537	Regulation on the sale of narcotics through hospitals and related institutions: Monkey on our backs?
27	1970	318	Federal legislation: An examination and prognosis
27	1970	684	Federal legislation: An examination and prognosis: Part II
27	1970	848	State union law: A look at the new Pennsylvania public employee relations act
27	1970	1011	Federal legislation: An examination and prognosis: Part III
28	1971	127	National health insurance: A look at what Congress is prescribing
28	1971	290	Comprehensive drug abuse prevention and control act of 1970
28	1971	707	State narcotic and drug abuse laws: A combination of ingredients
29	1972	168	Some legal considerations in the formation of a group practice
29	1972	774	Some legal considerations in the formation of a group practice: Part II
29	1972	970	The Florida "Institutional Pharmacy" Law
30	1973	168	The new methadone regulations
30	1973	723	PSROs and pharmacy
30	1973	1067	The legal basis for clinical pharmacy
31	1974	86	Some legal aspects of the hospital formulary system
31	1974	402	Health maintenance organization act of 1973
32	1975	212	Implications of certificate of need legislation for institutional pharmacy practice
32	1975	1159	Maximum allowable costs for medications in hospitals
33	1976	475	Current federal legislation
33	1976	572	Portland Retail Druggists Association v. Abbott Laboratories et al, part I
33	1976	648	Portland Retail Druggists Association v. Abbott Laboratories et al, part II
33	1976	814	Legal implications of preparing and dispensing drugs under conditions not in a product's official labeling
33	1976	937	The Federal Drug and Devices Act and the Drug Safety Amendments of 1976
33	1976	1049	Federal health planning, part I: Legislative background
33	1976	1211	Health planning, part II: The National Health Planning and Resources Development Act of 1974
33	1976	1308	Medical devices amendments of 1976
34	1977	90	Antisubstitution law changes and the hospital formulary system
34	1977	541	Effect of NLRB rulings and collective bargaining by hospital pharmacists
35	1978	81	Regulatory aspects of investigational new drugs
		729	Drug Regulation Reform Act
36	1979	85	Pharmacy inspections: Constitutional without a warrant?
36	1979	226	Patient package inserts and the pharmacist's responsibility
37	1980	537	Implications of the Lannett and Pharmadyne decisions
37	1980	1546	Legal standard of due care for pharmacists in institutional practice
37	1980	1656	Institutional pharmacist's guide to complying with PPI regulations
38	1981	218	Liability of the pharmacist as a therapeutic consultant
38	1981	222	Update on the Lannett and Pharmadyne decisions
38	1981	892	Role of JCAH standards in negligence suits
38	1981	1768	Legality of mandatory continuing professional education
38	1981	1949	Therapeutic substitution and the hospital formulary system
39	1982	1544	Pharmacists as a liability-reducing factor
40	1983	111	"Procompetition" and the continuing struggle to contain health care costs
40	1983	282	Legal implications of preparing and dispensing approved drugs for unlabeled indications
40	1983	439	Pharmacist liability for suicide by drug overdose
40	1983	739	Recent Supreme Court antitrust rulings in health care
41	1984	942	Medicare coverage of hospice care
41	1984	1115	Legal issues associated with the handling of cytotoxic drugs (special feature)
41	1984	2074	Legal aspects of termination of employment
42	1985	352	Legal aspects of outpatient drug transactions in nonprofit hospitals
42	1985	849	Repercussions of The Drug Price Competition and Patent Term Restoration Act of 1984
42	1985	1572	Robinson-Patman update: DeModena v. Kaiser Foundation Health Plan
43	1986	386	Legal implications of home health care by nonprofit hospitals
43	1986	1951	Legal implications of hospital resales of pharmaceuticals
45	1988	1115	Fee-for-service activities provided by drug information centers
45	1988	2118	The Prescription Drug Marketing Act of 1987
46	1989	1535	Drug Free Workplace Act
47	1990	1260	Complying with the National Childhood Vaccine Injury Act
47	1990	1804	Liability of dispensing to an inpatient an estrogenic drug without a patient package insert
47	1990	2082	The pharmacist as an expert witness
48	1991	114	Summary of 1990 Medicaid drug rebate legislation
48	1991	654	Requirements for certifiers of biological safety cabinets
48	1991	747	Criminal conviction for distribution of a drug not approved by FDA

CHAPTER 43

Pharmacist and Pharmaceutical Industry Relations

MICHAEL L. KLEINBERG and DAVID S. ADLER

In an editorial in the *American Journal of Hospital Pharmacy*, Zellmer[1] described the sometimes uneasy relationship between hospital pharmacists and pharmaceutical manufacturers:

> The purpose of contemporary pharmacy is the advancement of rational drug therapy. This purpose is incompatible with certain goals of the industry which include the promotion of drug product sales to generate profits and returns on investment. The patient-oriented roles to which pharmacy aspires (e.g., drug product selection, patient education and counseling, drug information services, management of drug therapy for chronic illnesses) require the pharmacist to be an independent practitioner. In order to establish and maintain credibility, the pharmacist must be free from any hint of alliance with the manufacturers and distributors of drug products.

The methods used by the pharmaceutical company to achieve its objectives are linked closely to the hospital. Most new drug entities are tested and evaluated in hospitalized or clinic patients, and the hospital pharmacist may be involved with a pharmaceutical manufacturer to develop and test a product. Mutual questions regarding drug stability, packaging, storage, and pharmacokinetics are answered in research protocols designed by a pharmaceutical company and the hospital pharmacist. Producing a product that will help the consumer and that can easily be controlled by the hospital will benefit both the pharmaceutical industry and the pharmacist.

DEFINING GOALS

In defining a relationship between the hospital pharmacist and the pharmaceutical industry, it is necessary to define the objectives or goals for each. A clear sense of the responsibilities of the pharmacist and the industry will facilitate an understanding of the interrelationships.

The hospital, for the most part, exists to perform one of four functions. These include patient care, education of physicians and other health professionals, laboratory and clinical research, and service to the community. An example of a hospital mission statement is shown in Appendix 43-A.

Defining the goals of the pharmaceutical industry is equally important. Those goals are: (1) to provide pharmaceutical products through research, (2) to promote pharmaceutical products in an ethical manner, and (3) to provide to the professional community information on pharmaceutical products.

In both examples, the goal of making a profit was not included. This, however, belongs in both statements. The hospital requires the production of revenue for growth and for upgrading of services and technology. The hospital is responsible to its owners, be it a private corporation or government owned. The pharmaceutical industry has a profit motive to continue its research activities and growth and is responsible to its shareholders.

By looking at the goals of both the hospital and the pharmaceutical industry, one can see how the relationship can be developed so that both groups may achieve their individual goals. Examples of this include development of drug distribution systems, innovative drug delivery systems, patient and professional educational services, and clinical and technical research activities. When both groups work together, both benefit. The hospital pharmacist is able to provide innovative distribution and clinical services, and the pharmaceutical industry is able to provide a product that can be used.

MEDICAL SERVICE REPRESENTATIVES

The medical service representative (MSR) or professional service representative is the liaison between the pharmaceutical industry and the hospital. The goals of the MSR are the same as those of his or her company, i.e., to obtain a marketable product and to sell that product. The MSR achieves these goals by interacting with various health professionals in the institution, including physicians, residents, interns, nurses, and pharmacists. The MSR may use many different approaches and resources to promote a product. Company literature, journal reprints, newsletters, and other promotional materials are often discussed with health care practitioners. The goals of the hospital and the pharmaceutical industry, however, should not be compromised by the inappropriate use or acceptance of gifts from drug companies by health care professionals. Promotional material should be educational in nature and should be useful to health care practitioners for the care and treatment of their patients.

The typical functions of an MSR are listed in table 43-1. Obtaining information on available drugs is important to the hospital pharmacist. This information should be concise and accurate. Such efficiency may be developed through the use of a form or format similar to the presentation of drug information as found in the American Hospital Formulary Service (AHFS) *Drug Information 1992.*

Table 43-1. Functions of a medical service representative

1. Provide current information on available drugs
   a. Dose
   b. Use (new use)
   c. Side effects
   d. Compatibility
   e. Pharmacology
   f. Pharmacokinetics
   g. New dosage forms
   h. Administration guidelines
   i. Reimbursement
2. Provide current information and possible solutions on company services or problems.
   a. Availability of continuing education programs
   b. Drug recalls
   c. Return goods
   d. Drug prices
   e. Back orders
   f. List on damaged drugs
   g. Assistance in order placement

Independent clinical studies should be part of the reference material used by the MSR. The MSR should be aware of any drug recall that the company initiates and should make arrangements to provide help in obtaining other supplies. In addition, during a hospital-wide disaster, the MSR should be available to provide help. Although functions of individual MSR's may differ, their main goal is to promote the products of their company. This promotion should be based on the cost-effectiveness of the product. In this way, the pharmacist and MSR will work together rather than in opposition.

Hospital MSR Standards

To maximize the usefulness of an MSR in the hospital, it is necessary to develop guidelines to control his or her activities. Without these guidelines, control over the type of information being disseminated, visits to restricted areas of the hospital, improper use of hospital personnel time, and inappropriate drug sampling may become problems. To control the MSR, specific guidelines or standards should be developed by the hospital through the department of pharmacy. These standards should be in writing and discussed with each MSR by the pharmacist. (See Appendixes 43-B, 43-C, 43-D, and 43-E for examples of guidelines and standards.) The pharmacist should keep a log of current MSR's with their telephone numbers and the date that the standards were discussed.

The standards should include the following information:

1. *Registration and orientation.* The hospital should identify those people who fall into the classification of an MSR. These people should be given appropriate orientation to hospital rules and regulations.
2. *Identification.* It is important for visitors to be identified when they are in the hospital. Proper identification should be displayed at all times.
3. *Authorized areas.* Various areas of the hospital may be off limits to the MSR. Such areas should be identified at orientation. The confidentiality of the patient and the patient's records must be maintained.
4. *New drug requests.* The mechanism to obtain a new product in the hospital should be outlined to the MSR. If the hospital has a formulary system, this should be explained to the MSR.
5. *Samples.* Drug samples left in various areas of the hospital may lead to inappropriate uses. Control of all drugs within the hospital is the responsibility of the pharmacy department.
6. *Exhibits.* Displays are one way to disseminate information to the hospital staff. Without proper control, displays may lead to confusion as to which drugs are presently available in the institution.

Improving Relationships

The MSR and the pharmacist should discuss problems and exchange ideas. An unusual increase or decrease in drug use may lead to out-of-stock items or to an excessive inventory. The pharmacist should be aware of any new use of a drug so that he or she may plan the inventory accordingly. In addition, if the pharmaceutical company is unable to supply its drug, the MSR should work with the pharmacist to maintain needed drugs. Medication errors continue to be a major problem in the hospital. Errors have occurred through poor naming of drugs, poor label design, and confusing or misleading packaging. The pharmaceutical industry should consult with the end users (pharmacists, physicians, and nurses) of their product before introducing new drugs or changing existing drugs. The pharmacist should continue to use the Drug Product Problem Reporting Program developed and coordinated by the United States Pharmacopeia.

Drugs that are no longer used or that are out of date are an added inventory expense for the hospital. The MSR should work with the pharmacist to obtain credit for the items. The pharmacist may want to itemize these drugs (see figure 43-1) or have the MSR perform this task. Pharmaceutical companies may want to change their product-dating procedures. If drugs were dated to expire only in January or July, the hospital pharmacist would be able to control returns and outdated items more effectively. An exchange of educational material would also benefit the pharmacist and the MSR.

The pharmaceutical company offers a great deal of educational material relating to its drugs and the diseases for which the drugs are effective. The pharmacist can use this information in promoting rational drug therapy to physicians and nurses. The pharmacist, according to several polls, is recognized by the public as a trusted health practitioner. That trust provides the pharmaceutical industry with a link to the public sector. The pharmaceutical industry should continue to provide pharmacists with a mechanism to educate members of the public on the drugs they are prescribed or select on their own. This continuous education will foster a more positive relationship among all segments of health care.

The pharmacist, in addition, may coordinate and participate in staff development programs. The MSR may increase his or her knowledge by attending these programs.

In recent years, pharmacists have increased their responsibility for drug product selection in institutional practice. The decisions for drug use in the institutional setting are

The Medical University Hospital

Return Goods Authorization

This hospital is hereby authorized to return the products listed below for credit, subject to the return policies of the company. Credit should be issued on a hospital purchase order. The credit memorandum should be sent to:

The Medical University Hospital
Accounting Department
26 Main Street
Anytown, USA

Return merchandise should be shipped to:

____
____
____
____

____
Company Name

____
Signature of Representative

Quantity	**Item description, size, N.D.C. number, etc.**

Figure 43-1.

usually made through the pharmacy and therapeutics committee, which is composed of physicians, pharmacists (including the director of pharmacy and the drug information service pharmacist), nurses, hospital administrators, and representatives from the laboratory. The MSR should establish good communication with the drug information service pharmacist.

To improve the relationship between the pharmaceutical industry and the hospital pharmacist, communication should be increased between the two. One strategy to improve this communication is to have a formal orientation program for the MSR. This orientation program may be used to discuss the standards for the MSR at the hospital and, in addition, to provide the MSR with information so that he or she becomes familiar with the various hospital systems. A thorough understanding of the purchasing system (bids, vendor registration, use of wholesalers), drug delivery system (unit dose, intravenous admixtures), and formulary system will aid the MSR in providing necessary services to the pharmacist.

Finally, communication between the pharmaceutical industry and the hospital pharmacist must be open and ongoing. The hospital pharmacist must communicate recognized needs to the industry, and the industry must strive to meet these needs. Scientific information regarding the physical nature (stability, compatibility, pH) and the clinical nature (pharmacokinetics) of a drug must be communicated to the pharmacist. Similarly, the pharmaceutical industry must efficiently communicate its needs to the hospital pharmacist.

REFERENCE

1. Zellmer WAP: Report on the study commission on pharmacy: Pharmacy and the pharmaceutical industry (editorial). *Am J Hosp Pharm* 33(Sept):893, 1976.

ADDITIONAL READING

Burkholder D: The role of the pharmaceutical detail man in a large teaching hospital. *Am J Hosp Pharm* 20:275-285, 1963.

Chren M, Landelfeld S, Murray T, et al: Doctors, drug companies, and gifts. *JAMA* 262:3448-3451, 1989.

Davis N, Cohen M: *Medication Errors: Causes and Prevention.* Philadelphia, George F. Stickley Co., 1983.

Hassan WE: Medical service representation-pharmacist relationship. In Hassan WE: *Hospital Pharmacy, 5th ed.* Philadelphia, Lea & Febiger, 1986, pp 213-224.

Industry peer review "opens" hospital. *Hospitals* 47(Jan):66-70, 1973.

Jeffrey LP: Communication between medical service representatives and physicians. *Am J Hosp Pharm* 15:584-585, 1958.

Katz S, Triboletti M: The pharmaceutical industry's obligation to clinical pharmacists. *Drug Intell Clin Pharm* 11:740-742, 1977.

Lipman AG: Therapeutic substitution (editorial). *Hosp Formul* 18(Sept):841, 1983.

Lipman AG, Mullen HF: Quality control of medical service representative activities in the hospital. *Am J Hosp Pharm* 31(Feb):167-170, 1974.

McEvoy GK (ed): *AHFS Drug Information 90.* Bethesda, MD, American Society of Hospital Pharmacists, 1990.

Phillips DJM, Smith JE: Hospital-based training for pharmaceutical manufacturer's representatives. *Am J Hosp Pharm* 40(Oct):1661-1663, 1983.

Santell JP, Birdwell SW, Scheckelhoff DJ, et al: Perception of the role of medical-service representatives in hospitals. *Am J Hosp Pharm* 47(Jun):1354-1359, 1990.

Stolar MH: The need to improve hospital investigational drug policies and procedures. *Hosp Formul* 18(Jan):79-82, 1983.

Turco S: What hospital pharmacists expect from a medical service representative (editorial). *Hosp Pharm* 9(4):126-128, 1974.

Zellmer WA: The euphoria factor (editorial). *Am J Hosp Pharm* 40(Jan):51, 1983.

Appendix 43-A

MISSION STATEMENT — University of California-San Diego (UCSD) Medical Center

University Medical Center is the only general acute-care institution in the area that serves as the primary teaching hospital for the School of Medicine at the University, and that is open to all members of the general population. As such, University Medical Center must simultaneously fulfill three principal missions:

- To deliver comprehensive, quality patient care that is responsive to the needs of the region as a whole and of the local community.
- To provide an environment appropriate for the education of physicians and allied health professionals.
- To provide an environment that supports and encourages clinical research.

In addition to these primary missions, the University Medical Center is committed to working closely with other hospitals, government agencies, health care organizations, and community groups to identify community health needs and problems and to contribute toward their resolution.

University Medical Center, in conjunction with the School of Medicine at the University, also will seek to provide selected services to patients from Mexico, Central and South America, and the Pacific Basin.

1. *Patient Care*

University Medical Center is committed to providing highly specialized services for the treatment of major illnesses in and injury to the population of the region as a whole, and primary and secondary services as required to meet local community needs and the educational and research objectives of the School of Medicine at the University. All patient care will be rendered in a personal and sensitive manner without regard to race, creed, or national origin. In discharging these responsibilities, University Medical Center will foster the growth and development of the clinically active faculty, other health professionals, and staff.

2. *Education*

University Medical Center, in concert with the School of Medicine at the University, is committed to educating physicians, nurses, and other health professionals to meet future health care needs. In order to produce professionals of competence and integrity with a broad view of health care and its roles in society, University Medical Center will maintain and develop a spectrum of primary, secondary, and tertiary services and will endeavor to attract a culturally and economically diverse patient population.

3. *Research*

Basic and clinical research are essential to continued advancement in the understanding and treatment of disease and to improvement in the health status of the population. Such research contributes substantially both to the general public well-being and to the educational and patient care missions of University Medical Center. University Medical Center is therefore committed to providing an environment conducive to clinical investigation.

4. *Community Responsibility*

University Medical Center recognizes the crucial importance of social, environmental, and economic factors in the health of the community. The Medical Center will take an active role in promoting, assisting, developing, and conducting programs leading to improvements in community health.

Appendix 43-B

PHARMACEUTICAL SALES REPRESENTATIVES COMMITTEE

General Information

This document has been developed by the Pharmaceutical Sales Representatives Committee to assist and guide all Pharmaceutical Sales Representatives who call upon the University of California Medical Center, San Diego.

A Pharmaceutical Sales Representative (PSR) is defined as the representative of a pharmaceutical company having products/services which are the responsibility of the Department of Pharmacy to evaluate or purchase.

Purposes and Functions

The Committee is a sub-committee of the Pharmacy and Therapeutics (P&T) Committee. The names of current members are available through the Director of Pharmacy.

The purposes and functions of the Committee are:

(1) Development, implementation, and enforcement of policies and procedures concerning the activities of the PSRs in the Hospital;

(2) Maintenance of effective communication between the Medical Center professional staff and PSRs;

(3) Efficient utilization of health care personnel time through implementation of the PSR guidelines;

(4) Provision of a forum for PSR peer review at the Medical Center.

Policies developed by the PSR Committee are forwarded to the Pharmacy and Therapeutics Committee. Upon approval, they are submitted to the Hospital Executive Committee. Policies are communicated to the Medical Center professional staff by means of DISCOURSE, the Drug Information Newsletter.

The Committee meets twice yearly, and as needed. Each meeting is scheduled three weeks before the next Pharmacy and Therapeutics Committee meeting. A nonmember PSR wishing to attend a meeting of the Committee should leave a note with the Department of Pharmacy Administrative Assistant. The Committee will then invite the representative.

The Committee will issue identifying badges. The badges will be maintained in the Department of Pharmacy office and will be worn by the representatives while in the Hospital. Badges will be picked up when coming to the Hospital and returned at the end of that visit.

Composition

The Pharmaceutical Sales Representative Committee is composed of three representatives from pharmaceutical companies and three members of the Department of Pharmacy, a physician-member of the Pharmacy and Therapeutics Committee, and the Director of Pharmacy.

Pharmaceutical Sales Representative members of the Committee are selected in accordance with the following criteria:

(1) Representatives who service the facility on a routine basis; and

(2) Representatives whose company's products involve several classes of drugs; and

(3) Representatives interested in serving on the Committee should submit their names to the Department of Pharmacy office by October 1st of each year. Recommendations will be requested from the Medical Service Society.

Terms of Office

A. Term of office will run from January to December.

B. Original committee members will hold office until December 1986; thereafter, one position will change each year and term office will run for three years.

C. If a vacancy should occur in mid-term, the Committee will be responsible for notifying other representatives of the vacancy. Representatives interested in filling this unexpired term will be requested to submit their names. A replacement will then be selected by the Committee.

Procedures for Newly Assigned PSRs

A. All newly assigned PSRs shall introduce themselves to the Administrative Assistant in the Pharmacy office and secure an appointment with the Pharmacist Purchasing Agent. If time permits, the Administrative Assistant will introduce the PSR to the Chief of Pharmacy.

B. During this initial meeting, the Pharmacy Administrative Assistant will provide the new PSR with:

(1) One copy of the PSR Guidelines; the PSR will sign for these guidelines.

(2) One copy of the PSR Guidelines for delivery to the PSR's District Manager.

(3) A list of names and telephone numbers of PSRs currently serving on the Committee.

(4) A brief orientation to the PSR Guidelines.

(5) A description of the Drug Information Service, Medical Center Purchasing Department, and Pharmacy Purchasing Section, and procedures for visiting these persons [in these areas].

C. Following the initial meeting, the PSR shall:

(1) Give the Administrative Assistant one business card bearing name, current address, and telephone number.

(2) Delete the previous PSR's card from the file maintained by the Pharmacy Administrative Assistant.

(3) Request the Pharmacy Administrative Assistant to order a name tag (a personal in-house authorization badge), payment to be made in advance. A temporary badge will be issued until the name badge is received ($5.00 check—Medical Service Society).

(4) Make an appointment with the Director of the Drug Information Service and the Director of Pharmacy to assure that appropriate information on the company's product is on file.

(5) Check for messages addressed to his/her predecessor.

(6) With the PSR Committee list provided, check to determine if a PSR on the Committee is at the Medical Center to be contacted for orientation. If a meeting cannot be arranged immediately, the

new PSR should contact a PSR on the Committee to arrange for orientation at a time convenient for both parties.

(7) Read the PSR guidelines thoroughly before attempting to contact Hospital Personnel and before the orientation by a PSR on the Committee.

(8) Check for PSR announcements.

Standard Procedures

A. All PSRs calling on the University of California Medical Center, San Diego, shall come to the Department of Pharmacy office prior to visiting other areas of the Hospital or Clinics. At each visit, a PSR shall secure an in-house authorization badge from the box on the PSR Bulletin Board. This badge is recognized by Security and will assist the PSR during visits within the Hospital. If the badge is lost, a $5.00 fee will be charged for replacement. A temporary badge may be obtained at the Pharmacy Office until a new badge is secured.

B. PSRs shall first inform the Director, Drug Information Service, and the Pharmacist Purchasing Agent of the therapeutic and supply-price aspects, respectively, of new or non-formulary drugs which they wish to discuss in the Hospital. No restrictions will be placed on discussions of such drugs in the Medical Center unless the Department of Pharmacy or the Pharmacy and Therapeutics Committee determines that the use is detrimental to patient care.

C. PSRs shall provide the Drug Information Service with monograph packets on new drugs released by their companies as soon as such information available. Information on changes pertaining to currently available drugs (i.e., indications, dosage, routes of administration, formulation, etc.) shall be provided to the Drug Information Service before discussion with Hospital personnel. A copy of any material to be distributed in the University of California Medical Center, San Diego, shall be left with the Drug Information Service.

D. Each PSR shall assure that a current address and telephone number are filed in the Pharmacy Office.

E. On each visit, PSRs shall check the PSR Bulletin Board for announcements and minutes of the PSR Committee meetings.

PSR Activities Within the Hospital

A. At any one time, only one representative per company shall visit a clinic or patient care area. Exceptions are permitted for a newly hired PSR who may be accompanied by the manager or a senior PSR during his/her training period, or with approval of the Director of Pharmacy.

B. Operating Suites and Delivery Suites: PSRs may only enter these suites by appointment.

C. Patient Care Areas: PSRs may only enter patient care areas on the invitation of a specific physician, nursing supervisor, or pharmacist. PSRs shall pass through such areas only when there is no convenient alternate route to their destination.

D. Respect for Individuals' Time: Physicians, pharmacists, nurses, and other professionals have manifold patient care responsibilities. Please respect their time and other commitments.

Sample Policy

A. Office Use: It is policy to discourage the use and storage of sample drugs in offices and clinics. The indiscriminate supply of samples can lead to misuse, and may encourage theft or diversion. However, a minimal number of sample drugs may be desirable in specific offices or clinics. The following rules apply:

(1) No samples will be left in any office or clinic without the expressed permission of the P&T Committee.

(2) Permission for specific samples may be requested only by faculty physicians.

(3) Faculty physicians may request permission to keep samples in their office or clinic by notifying the P&T Committee of their intent, naming specific samples to be stored, amounts needed, and storage conditions.

A written statement of the P&T Committee's decision will be sent to the physician.

B. Permission to keep specific samples can be given on an interim basis by the Chairman of the P&T Committee or Director of Pharmacy. This approval is valid only until the next scheduled P&T meeting.

C. No samples will be left in any hospital nursing unit, non-physician's office, or elsewhere on the premises, except as stated above.

D. Personal Use: Requests for sampling are discouraged. Physicians making such requests should be referred to the UCSD outpatient pharmacy. In special cases, drugs requested for a physician's own use shall be delivered directly to that physician. This policy also applies to nutritional products.

Rules for Enforcement of Guidelines for PSRs

A. A person or persons filing a complaint shall be interviewed by the PSR Committee or by the P&T Committee.

B. A PSR accused of an infraction shall be interviewed by the PSR Committee after the person filing the complaint has been interviewed.

C. The PSR Committee shall then decide if an infraction has occurred, determine the severity of the infraction, and make recommendations concerning any actions to be taken. Findings and recommendations must be forwarded to the full Committee for adjudication.

D. For minor infractions, an oral warning will be given, to be followed by a letter. For major or repeated infractions, greater penalties will be imposed, and a letter will be sent to the PSR's District Manager and/or to the home office.

E. Penalties will range from a written warning to exclusion of the individual from the hospital. (See C above.)

Appendix 43-C

UNIVERSITY OF CALIFORNIA, SAN DIEGO MEDICAL CENTER
225 West Dickinson Street
San Diego, CA 92103

Subject: Rules for Pharmaceutical Exhibits

1. Exhibits are held in the Cafeteria Small Dining Rooms, during the hours 7:00 am to 11:00 am on the first Wednesday of each month. These exhibits are open to the physicians, pharmacists, nurses, and other members of the hospital professional staff.
   a. All exhibits must be set up no later than 7:15 am on the exhibit date.
   b. No exhibit shall be dismantled and removed prior to 11:00 am.
2. Exhibitors may request exhibit space by submitting an application form along with a ten dollar ($10.00) registration fee. Checks should be made payable to the Medical Service Society. (See application procedures attached.) Exhibitors will check into the Pharmacy Administration office on the exhibit date and pick up a validated display permit and Vendor's Hospital Pass.
3. Exhibits will be kept to a reasonable size; a floor area not to exceed 4' by 5' is desired.
   a. Each exhibitor should be prepared to supply his/her own table, since a sufficient number may not be available.
   b. The exhibitors are responsible for returning the room to its original condition prior to the exhibit.
4. Only materials of an educational nature will be displayed and available.
   a. No drug samples, whether legend or non-legend, will be given out at displays.
   b. Representatives wishing to leave samples for a physician's personal use may leave the requested samples in the Pharmacy Department marked for the physician's attention. Representatives will not be permitted in other areas of the hospital for the express purpose of delivering samples.
5. Due to limited exhibit space, only one representative per exhibit space is permitted.
   a. Training and supervisory visitations are not exceptions to this rule.
   b. Exhibitors may not leave the display unattended.
6. Only those products approved by the Director, Department of Pharmacy, may be displayed. Normally, only Formulary Products will be approved for display.
7. UCSD Medical Center reserves the right to refuse displays to representatives who have previously violated "Regulations for Pharmaceutical Representatives" or these exhibit rules.
8. Exhibitors will keep a validated display permit in view during their exhibit.

Appendix 43-D

APPLICATION PROCEDURES FOR PHARMACEUTICAL EXHIBITS

Because a limited amount of exhibit space is available, it is not possible to accommodate all the pharmaceutical representatives who wish to exhibit each month. In order to assign exhibit space in as equitable a manner as possible, the following procedure for accepting applications for exhibits is in effect.

1. Each representative is assigned to one of three groups. Any representative whose company has displayed regularly at University Hospital since January 1979 was assigned to a group. Each group has 14 representatives assigned. Fifteen exhibit spaces are available.
2. The groups will be assigned to a specific month's exhibit on a three-month rotation. Participation of each company was reviewed in January 1982, and the groups adjusted accordingly.
3. The Alternate Group includes the pharmaceutical representatives who have not exhibited since January 1981, and all non-pharmaceutical representatives.
4. The representatives in groups I, II, and III have priority in submitting applications to exhibit in the specific month assigned.
   a. This priority must be exercised by the last Wednesday of the month preceding the assigned exhibit.
   b. Any exhibit space left vacant one week prior to the exhibit date is open to any representative in the Alternate Group, and any representative in the other two groups.
   c. Applications for vacant exhibit space may be made no sooner than the Wednesday morning preceding the exhibit date (i.e., one week prior to the exhibit).
   d. Applications for vacant exhibit space will be accepted in order of receipt.
5. If a representative does not use scheduled and verified exhibit space, no refund may be granted and the representative's exhibit privileges may be curtailed at the discretion of the Director of Pharmacy.
6. Responsibility for coordinating with other representatives, the room set-up, specific display locations, and refreshments is assigned to one representative, who is selected by exhibitors to represent the group. This representative is given the privilege of displaying each month.

Appendix 43-E

THE OHIO STATE UNIVERSITY HOSPITALS MEDICAL SERVICE REPRESENTATIVES GUIDELINES

I. General Information

These guidelines have been developed to assist and guide all Medical Service Representatives (MSR) who call upon The Ohio State University Hospitals. An MSR is defined as the representative of a pharmaceutical, chemical, or hospital supply company who enters The Ohio State University Hospitals to solicit the use of products/services which are the responsibility of the Department of Pharmacy to evaluate or purchase.

II. Procedures for Newly Assigned MSRs

A. All newly assigned MSRs shall introduce themselves to the department secretary and secure an appointment with the Assistant Director of Pharmacy in charge of purchasing.

B. During this initial meeting the Assistant Director will provide the new MSR with:
   1. A copy of the MSR Guidelines.
   2. An additional copy of the MSR Guidelines for delivery to the MSR's district manager.
   3. A description of the Drug Information Center, Pharmacy Purchasing, and University Purchasing.
   4. A brief orientation to the MSR Guidelines.

C. Following the initial meeting the MSR shall:
   1. Provide the secretary with three business cards bearing the name, address, and telephone number of inclusion to department files.
   2. Delete the previous MSR's information from the departmental file and update the file.
   3. Meet with the Drug Information Pharmacist to assure that appropriate information on the company's products is on file before calling upon other members of the hospital staff.
   4. Read the MSR Guideline thoroughly before attempting to contact any hospital personnel.

III. Standard Procedures

A. MSRs shall first inform the Drug Information Pharmacist and the Pharmacist Coordinator responsible for Drug Product Selection of the therapeutic and supply-price aspects of new or non-formulary drugs which they will discuss in the hospital. Please arrange interviews with these individuals at their convenience. No restrictions will be placed on discussion of such drugs unless the Department of Pharmacy determines that the use of the product is detrimental to patient care.

B. MSRs shall provide the Drug Information Center (DIC) with monograph packets on new drugs as soon as such information is released from the company. Similarly, information on current drugs (i.e., indications, dosage, routes of administration, formulations, etc.) shall be provided to the DIC before discussion with other hospital personnel.

C. Each MSR shall insure that the most current address and telephone number is on file in the Pharmacy office.

D. MSRs shall make an appointment through the Pharmacy secretary prior to visiting the Pharmacist Coordinator responsible for Drug Product Selection. The time for appointments is currently Tuesday, 1:00 pm - 4:00 pm. Pharmacy purchasing personnel will inventory and order all products needed by the department. MSRs shall confine all routine appointment requests to such matters as: price changes, credits, return authorization, bid notice, deliveries, and new product information (including new dosage forms, product revisions, etc.).

E. All MSRs shall notify Pharmacy purchasing personnel immediately of all product recalls, discontinuations and/or problems causing shipping delays as soon as such information is made known to them by the company.

F. MSRs shall assure that their company's catalog on file in the Department of Pharmacy is current, complete, and accurate regarding product availability. MSRs should come to the pharmacy receiving window in room 377, Doan Hall, ask for their company file, review and/or update the materials, and sign and date the file. This shall be done whenever necessary and at least once every six months. Files shall contain a current catalog listing all products and regular prices to wholesaler, sales and return policies, and a company profile.

G. MSRs shall be responsible for outdated or otherwise unusable drug products manufactured by their company before departure from the hospital following a visitation or promptly after notification via the memo file.
   1. If return authorization is required, MSRs shall sort, count, and list the products on the appropriate form.
   2. If authorization must come from the company, MSRs shall be responsible for obtaining such authorization.
   3. If no authorization is required, MSRs shall sort and list products on the Departmental Form.
   4. For non-returnable products, MSRs shall prepare a list and include prices and total value of the items to be discarded.

H. If the Department of Pharmacy has outdated products to return for credit, the MSR must complete authorization for their return before the appointment can begin.

IV. MSR Activities Within the Hospital

The MSR is a guest of the hospital and, as such, should provide his/her services in accordance with the accepted rules of conduct and in a manner which provides the greatest benefit to the hospital and its staff. MSRs are not permitted:

A. On any nursing or other patient care areas, Emergency Department, or Ambulatory Clinics except by invitation of a member of the medical staff, the Directors of Nursing or Pharmacy or their designee, or other hospital department heads.

B. To meet attending staff members, department heads, and designees except by appointment scheduled in advance.
C. To detail medical resident staff except by appointment.
D. To use the hospital paging system to arrange appointments.
E. To contact medical, nursing, or allied students except by invitation from a faculty member.
F. To prepare a formulary request form for an attending or resident physician's signature.
G. To call on members of the Pharmacy and Therapeutics Committee to review any pending formulary requests.
H. To attend medical and other educational conferences scheduled in the Hospitals and Medical School unless specifically invited by a member of the attending staff.

V. Drug Samples

A. Location of drug samples
1. Inpatient Areas — Drug samples shall not be stored in or dispensed from any inpatient area or the Emergency Department. No drug may be dispensed to any inpatient area unless it is dispensed by the Pharmacy Department.
2. Clinic Areas — Drug samples in the outpatient clinic areas shall be kept in a secure cabinet.

B. Drug samples permitted
1. Formulary Drugs — Formulary drugs will be permitted in the clinic areas. It is recommended that these samples be dispensed to:
   a. Those patients for which an initial starter dose is required; the amount dispensed should be sufficient to determine the effectiveness of the drug before a prescription is filled.
   b. Indigent patients who would not otherwise be able to have their prescription filled in a timely manner. The amount dispensed should be sufficient to allow them to make arrangements with a support agency such as Social Services.
2. Non-Formulary Drugs — Non-Formulary drugs will be permitted in the clinic areas if requested by the physician for a trial period only. If the product is found advantageous, a request for Formulary addition should be submitted.

C. Security
1. The designated nurse serving as the contact person for the Clinic area shall be responsible for managing inventories and returning outdated drugs to the MSR for disposal on or prior to the expiration date.
2. The MSR supplying the drugs will leave them with the contact person and will not be permitted in the drug room.
3. The MSR will be responsible for removing and destroying all outdated samples as needed (including recalled drug products).
4. No controlled drug samples shall be permitted.

VI. MSR Exhibits

A. Eligibility — Any pharmaceutical manufacturer producing or offering a therapeutically advantageous product or a specialty product shall be eligible to participate in pharmaceutical exhibits. A manufacturer having more than one division, each of which has separate products and a separate sales force, shall be entitled to exhibit each division's product as an independent company.
B. Exhibit Guidelines — MSRs participating in pharmaceutical exhibits within the Medical Center shall abide by the following guidelines. Failure to comply with these guidelines shall result in cancellation of any future exhibits by the MSR.
1. Each company presenting an exhibit shall be represented by a maximum of two MSRs.
2. No drugs shall be distributed at the exhibit. MSRs may take requests for drugs from physicians and shall deliver these to the physician at a later time.
3. Only stock drug packages shall be on display. Drugs of non-Formulary status on the University Hospitals' Formulary of Accepted Drugs which are displayed shall be accompanied by a sign noting that it is non-Formulary in the hospital.
4. Exhibits shall be open to Medical Center professionals only.
5. Individual invitations to hospital professional personnel to the exhibit are appropriate and shall be permitted if mailed or presented directly.
6. Exhibitors shall be responsible for cleaning up the exhibit area immediately after each exhibit.
7. No food is to be given out.
8. Physicians should be given the opportunity to walk by without interruptions.

VII. Violation of MSR Guidelines

Infractions reported to the Department of Pharmacy shall be directed to the attention of the Director of Pharmacy. A file of all infractions shall be maintained listing the implicated MSR, the company he/she represents, the nature of the infraction, investigation, and disciplinary action taken. These records shall be maintained for at least seven years.

The Director of Pharmacy may impose one or more of the following penalties on any MSR found to be in violation of these guidelines.

A. Oral and written warning to the MSR with notice of the decision sent to the individual or department filing the complaint.
B. Oral and written communication of the infraction to the MSR and to his/her district manager.
C. Loss of Pharmaceutical Exhibit privileges for one year.
D. Restriction to service calls upon the Department of Pharmacy and Purchasing for one month.
E. Restriction to the above departments for three months.
F. Restriction to the above departments for six months.
G. Restriction to the above departments for one year.
H. Letters from the Director of Pharmacy to the MSR, his/her district manager, and to the sales director of the company stating that the MSR is no longer permitted in the hospital.

Reprinted with permission from the Ohio State University Hospitals.

Backword

When the idea for a "handbook" in hospital pharmacy was first mentioned, it seemed straightforward enough! I had seen handbooks in other fields, notably marketing and management, and the logic was compelling. Simply recruit the leaders in each aspect of the field, and they write a definitive chapter, do a little editing (they're the experts, after all), and voilà!

Of course, things didn't work out *that* way, but they did work out. I believe the first two editions were real contributions to the literature of pharmacy practice. If that is true, of course, it is because of the leading practitioners who wrote the material.

It was my decision not to be involved in the third edition, and I am proud of the reason. Simply, it is that institutional pharmacy practice has grown so rapidly and become so sophisticated in the 15 years since I started with the *Handbook* idea that I no longer felt competent even to identify the leaders. But I'm happy to have *been* a part of that growth and to *be* a part of pharmacy's new age.

Mickey C. Smith

Index